MENDING BODIES, SAVING SOULS

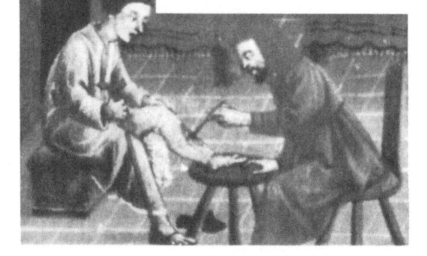

Guenter B. Risse, M.D., Ph.D.

Department of the History of Health Sciences
University of California, San Francisco

Mending Bodies, Saving Souls

A HISTORY OF HOSPITALS

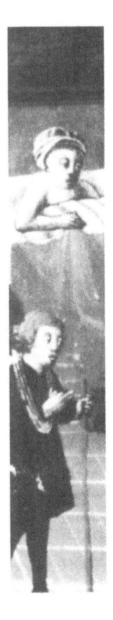

New York   Oxford
OXFORD UNIVERSITY PRESS
1999

Oxford University Press

Oxford New York
Athens Auckland Bangkok Bogotá Buenos Aires Calcutta
Cape Town Chennai Dar es Salaam Delhi Florence Hong Kong Istanbul
Karachi Kuala Lumpur Madrid Melbourne Mexico City Mumbai
Nairobi Paris São Paulo Singapore Taipei Tokyo Toronto Warsaw

and associated companies in
Berlin Ibadan

Copyright © 1999 by Oxford University Press, Inc.

Published by Oxford University Press, Inc.,
198 Madison Avenue, New York, New York, 10016

Library of Congress Cataloging-in-Publication Data
Risse, Guenter B., 1932–
Mending bodies, saving souls : a history of hospitals /
Guenter B. Risse.
p. cm. Includes bibliographical references and index.
ISBN 978-0-19-505523-8
1. Hospitals—History. 2. Hospital care—History.
I. Title.
[DNLM: 1. Hospitals—history. 2. History of Medicine.
3. Hospitals—history. 4. History of Medicine.
WX 11.1 R595m 1999] RA964.R57 1999
362.1'1'09—dc21 DNLM/DLC for Library of Congress 98-40966

9 8 7 6 5

Printed in the United States of America
on acid-free paper

To my wife, Sandy

CONTENTS

Preface, xiii

Introduction, 3

    Framework for a history of hospitals, 3
    Hospital narratives and case histories, 9

1. Pre-Christian Healing Places, 15

  Dreaming of Asclepius: Ancient Greek Temple Healing, 15

    A divine summons to Pergamon, 15
    Asclepius and his cult, 20
    Temple healing: Ideology and patronage, 24
    Staging temple rituals, 28
    Aristides' healing dreams, 33

  Collective Care of Soldiers and Slaves: Roman *Valetudinaria*, 38

    A young warrior becomes ill, 38
    Building a new professional army, 41
    Valetudinaria: Ideology and mission, 44
    Valetudinaria: Organization and staff, 47
    Soldiers and their care, 52

  Asclepieion and Valetudinarium: Confluence of the Sacred and Secular, 56

2. Christian Hospitality: Shelters and Infirmaries, 69

Early Christianity: A New Vision of the Sick, 69

    Edessa: famine, epidemics, and strangers, 69
    Christianity: Constructing a mission of healing, 73
    Christian welfare: Rise of the *xenodocheion*, 79
    "Slash and burn": Caring for the sick, 83

Healing at St. Gall: The Golden Age of Benedictine Monasticism, 87

    The abbot of St. Gall takes a fall, 87
    Benedict's monasteries: *Ora et labora*, 91
    Monastic caring spaces: Infirmary and hostel, 94
    Healing in monasteries: A community approach, 99

The Twilight of Western Monastic Supremacy, 106

3. Church and Laity: Partnership in Hospital Care, 117

The Pantocrator *Xenon* of Constantinople, 117

    Tales of a feverish poet, 117
    Post-Justinian Byzantium: Society, medicine, and *xenones*, 120
    Islam's *bimaristan* and Christianity's Pantocrator *xenon*, 125
    Theodoros Prodromos and life in the hospital, 130

"Our Patients, Our Lords": The Care of Pilgrims in Jerusalem, 134

    A pilgrimage to Jerusalem c 1172, 134
    Jerusalem and the Hospital of St. John: Mission and patronage, 138
    Feudal loyalty: Caring for "Our Lords the Sick," 143
    St. John's Hospital: Model for the world, 148

Hospital Agendas in Peril: Corruption and Early Medicalization, 153

4. Hospitals as Segregation and Confinement Tools: Leprosy and Plague, 167

Leper Houses, 167

A fateful second opinion, 167
Views of leprosy and the construction of stigma, 173
Locus of confinement: Anatomy of leper houses, 179
Institutional rituals, 184

Pesthouses or Lazarettos, 190

Trastevere: Rome's early plague spot, 190
Framing and fighting plague: Pestilence and public health, 195
Lazarettos: Makeshift isolation, cleansing, and treatment, 202
From Asclepius to San Bartolomeo: Purification rites, 208
Frameworks for early medicalization, 214

Welfare and Hospitals in Early Modern Europe, 216

5. Enlightenment: Medicalization of the Hospital, 231

Edinburgh, 1750–1800, 231

Wanted: A letter of recommendation, 231
Age of Enlightenment: Edinburgh and its infirmary, 236
Hospital patients and their management, 243
House of teaching: Clinical instruction and research, 251

Vienna, 1750–1800, 257

Seeking care: A tailor's fate, 257
Joseph II and Vienna's *Allgemeines Krankenhaus*, 259
Johann Peter Frank: Hospital director and Brunonian practitioner, 265
Clinicum practicum: The patient as teacher, 273

6. Human Bodies Revealed: Hospitals in Post Revolutionary Paris, 289

A former soldier seeks rest, 289
Ancien Régime: Paris and its hospitals, 293
Hospital reform: The fate of France's "curing machines," 300
Bedside and autopsy table: New approaches to disease, 309
Physical diagnosis: Laennec and the stethoscope, 314
Life at the Necker Hospital, 317
Parisian hospitals: Teaching and research, 325
The patient's body: Centerpiece of medical learning, 329

7. Modern Surgery in Hospitals: Development of Anesthesia and Antisepsis, 339

America: Warren and Anesthesia, 339

Living in a voluntary American hospital, 339
Philantropy in Boston: The Massachusetts General Hospital, 344
Management of pain: A professional goal, 349
First amputation under ether anesthesia, 1846, 354
The significance of ether anesthesia, 359

Scotland: Lister and Antisepsis, 361

From the Shetlands to Victorian Edinburgh, 361
Hospitalism and the "new" nursing, 366
Lister and the antiseptic system of surgery, 373
Infirmary life: An eyewitness account, 379
Providing aseptic surgery: A new role for hospitals, 385

8. The Limits of Medical Science: Hospitals in Fin-de-Siècle Europe and America, 399

Typhoid fever and Johns Hopkins Hospital, Baltimore, 1891, 399

A bartender with fever, 399
Hopkins and Billings: Genesis and gestation of a new hospital, 402
Osler, physicians, and nurses, 408
Life in the hospital: The healing power of water, 413
Science and religion: Partners in healing, 420

Cholera and Eppendorf General Hospital, Hamburg, 1892, 422

A frightful collapse, 422
Eppendorf General Hospital: Model for the world? 427
Cholera and hospital caregivers, 432
Back to water: Managing cholera at the Eppendorf Hospital, 439
Aftermath, 446

9. Main Street's Civic Pride: The American General Hospital as Professional Workshop, 463

An automobile accident in 1930, 463

"A public undertaking": American hospitals after 1900, 467
Madison, Wisconsin, and its general hospital, 475
Who pays? "Hospital-hotels" face the Depression, 482
A new national epidemic: Automobile accidents, 488
Efficiency versus humanity: Hospital life at MGH, 492
The road to financial health, 499

10. Hospitals at the Crossroads: Government, Society,
    and Catholicism in America, 1950–1975, 513

    A sudden heart attack, 513
    Serving the community: Buffalo and Mercy Hospital, 517
    Catholic hospitals: "The fairest flowers of missionary endeavor," 522
    Hospital life at Mercy Hospital, 1954, 525
    Another heart attack, 1974, 531
    The impact of Medicare, 535
    Catholic hospitals: Identity crisis and ethical guidelines, 540
    Wired for survival: Life in Mercy's CCU, 546
    "Moving forward under God," 553

11. Hospitals as Biomedical Showcases:
    Academic Health Centers and Organ Transplantation, 569

    Searching for a donor, 569
    From teaching hospitals to academic health centers, 576
    Quest for excellence: Moffitt Hospital and UCSF, 582
    Renal transplantation: Scientific, clinical, and professional contours, 587
    World class: Transplantation at UCSF, 594
    "Rebirth" at Moffitt Hospital, 599
    Making transplantation routine, 606

12. Caring for the Incurable:
    AIDS at San Francisco General Hospital, 619

    An early AIDS portrait: "Warren," 619
    San Francisco General Hospital: Tradition and evolution, 623
    Framing AIDS in the early 1980s: Lifestyle, cancer, or infection? 627
    Who "owns" AIDS in San Francisco? Planning Ward 5 B 633
    Gay pride: Patients' rights and responsibilities, 639
    The art of nursing: Life in Ward 5 B, 646

Managing death and dying, 652
The lessons of AIDS, 658

**Conclusion: Towards the Next Millennium:
The Future of Hospitals as Healing Spaces, 675**

Evolution of hospitals: A profile, 675
The new American spirituality, 679
Consumerism in medicine, 680
New managerial and financial imperatives, 681
Hospitals and the humanity of institutional care, 683

Index, 689

PREFACE

Books have varying gestation periods. Narrowly, mine can be reckoned as stretching for almost a decade, but in truth, it represents a much longer journey through the world of hospitals. During my childhood, I regularly accompanied my parents on their journey by train to a southern suburb of Buenos Aires for a visit with my mother's family. Shortly after leaving the main station, the tracks ran through Barracas, a working-class neighborhood dotted with storage depots and railroad yards.* Prominently located on a hill and exposed to the cleansing winds from the pampas stood a vast network of pavilions surrounded by trees and gardens. Several open squares were always filled with people, some milling around, others aimlessly wandering along the paved, diagonal pathways linking the various facilities. Housing only males, the Hospicio de las Mercedes was a nineteenth-century asylum, based on European models and built on ground previously selected by the Jesuits during colonial times for a convalescent home. Adjacent to it but separated by a tall wall was a similar hospice for women. All inmates wore the same type of uniform, a gray flannel suit or dress during winter, a lighter cotton outfit in summer. The institution, with its elaborate entrance gate on a street then called Vieytes, resembled the eighteenth-century French hospice or general hospital. It was a warehouse for the chronically ill, aged, disabled, and presumed lunatics, as well as vagrants and prostitutes collected from the streets. Needless to say, I became thoroughly fascinated by this city within a city and accosted my parents with more questions than they dared to answer.

Many years later, during my first year in medical school, I was confronted with an extreme shortage of cadavers for dissection. One of my teaching assistants casually suggested that I travel to the Mercedes Hospice and offer a bribe to the custodian at the institution's morgue for the purpose of dissecting one of the recent

*For details see Enrique H. Puccia, *Barracas en la Historia y en la Tradición*, Buenos Aires, Municipalidad, 1972, and Germinal Nogues, *Buenos Aires, Ciudad Secreta*, Buenos Aires, Ruy Díaz Sudamericana, 1996.

unclaimed corpses of a deceased inmate. Encouraged, I proceeded to the hospital that had intrigued me during my childhood. My ultimate destination, however, forced me to traverse the entire complex on foot, and I was soon overwhelmed and terrified by the sights and smells of this kaleidoscopic assembly of people, some gesticulating and talking to themselves, others asking me for handouts or running away at the sight of the white coat neatly folded over my arm. Needless to say, my dissection did not go well. In sharp contrast to the wrinkled wooden cadaver reeking of formalin at the Anatomy Department, my corpse at the morgue started bleeding heavily as soon as I made my first incision. The awesome experience of hospital life at the Hospicio de las Mercedes will remain with me forever.*

A year later, while studying human physiology, I came into contact with one of Bernardo Houssay's disciples, Miguel Covian. Fired from his academic post by the Fascist government of Juan Peron, Houssay, the 1947 Nobel-Prize winner in medicine, was carrying out research in a private mansion. After assisting Covian with his physiological experiments on rats concerning specific appetites, I attempted to duplicate this work with some of my schoolmates using guinea pigs, available at the Hospital Dr. Enrique Tornu, a municipal hospital devoted to the diagnosis and treatment of tuberculosis. In exchange for access to the plentiful laboratory animals, I performed menial clinical chores, including the physical examination of newly arrived patients. Divided into multiple 20-bed pavilions, the institution provided me with my first experiences of hospital life. It was winter time and frigid in the well-ventilated wards. The men wore colorful pullovers and scarves over their institutional pajamas, while the women in their nightgowns covered themselves with knitted morning jackets or *mañanitas*. Flushed cheeks made their haggard faces glow; the red lips were drawn into nervous smiles. Their sunken eyes glistened, an effect of the low-grade fever ravaging their bodies. They did not want to walk to the cold-water showers, preferring instead to complete the morning toilette by brushing their teeth and sprinkling themselves with cheap cologne to neutralize the smells emanating from their bodies. During rounds, most patients sat stiffly upright, their clothing loosened to allow the repeated and extensive auscultation of their chests. Given the shortage of nursing personnel, those who were ambulatory helped the bedridden, especially at the 10 AM lunchtime, when the first dish, a steaming but thin vegetable soup with a few potatoes, carrots, and noodles, was served from large pots placed on a food wagon together with "pancitos"—small, hard French breads. The soup was not popular, and all but a few spoonfuls used to soften the bread was left in the bowls in spite of the exhortations of the nurses who admonished the sick that the ward was not a restaurant.

This tightly knit community of patients, composed of young people, some with

---

*For a retrospective see R. Gonzalez Leandrini, "Sujeción y carencia. Cambio y continuismo en los hospitales de Buenos Aires (1870–1900)," *Asclepio* 42 (1990): 291–309. For details about the asylum, see Hugo Vezzetti, *La Locura en la Argentina*, Buenos Aires, Paidos, 1985.

advanced stages of the disease in their lungs, made a profound impression on me. Hospitalized for several months and subjected to a strict regimen of drugs until their sputum became free of bacilli, they usually remained cheerful and coopera- tive, socializing and helping each other to cope with the usual drudgeries of ward life. Before visiting hours, they tried to improve their appearance, with the women even putting on makeup and searching for clean clothes. Family members and friends circled the beds, distributing fruit, candy, cologne, and magazines. In Ar- gentina's pre-TV era, patients played cards and shared stories about their fami- lies, many of them living far away in the provinces. Many attended daily mass in a nearby chapel. A certain spiritual comfort, a relief from the fear of death—ever- present among them—pervaded the ward, revealing the importance of emotional support in a hospital setting. Not unexpectedly, the experience caused me to con- vert to a tuberculin-positive status and gave me a calcified lymph node in my lung.

Following a year of military service, medical school requirements prescribed a stint of emergency practice at another of Buenos Aires' archaic municipal hos- pitals. Through a schoolmate, I found a vacant position at the Hospital Guillermo Rawson, a decrepit pavilion-type hospital also located in Barracas behind the asy- lum.* As a newcomer, or *perro* (dog), the lowest extern on the staff, I dutifully spent 24-hour shifts every Saturday from February to April 1957. During each weekly rotation, I remained sleepless making frantic ambulance calls, embroiled in the chaos of injured crime victims, or interacting with hapless and dying, often resigned patients suffering from acute medical problems and their families bur- dened by abject poverty and despair.

In Rawson's *"sala de guardia"* or emergency room all of us worked without supervision—the chief resident and attending physicians were frequently unavail- able, socializing in their comfortable sleeping quarters—learning firsthand by trial and error from our unfortunate patients. Exposed to the trauma of pain and dis- ease, medical ignorance, and cultural shock, many of us on the Rawson shift joined in juvenile pranks during our brief intervals of idleness, a platoon of "men in white" desperately trying to exorcise the demons of a hospital practice from hell. Sumptuous meals, prepared by a special cook from food donated by grateful pa- tients, contrasted with the meager fare provided to patients. Attended by hospi- tal officials, physicians, priests, and special guests, such banquets turned into ex- tended soirees, with junior medical students and young women of dubious repute providing the entertainment. Only later did I discover that these surreal experi- ences now etched in my brain were almost carbon copies of events that took place in similar Parisian *salles de garde* a century earlier.†

---

*M. Gandini, "Hospital municipal Guillermo Rawson, 1868–24 de mayo 1968. Reseña historica," *Prensa Med Argentina* 55 (1968): 1913–25.

†For details from a nearby hospital see Maximo Deysine, *Sala de Guardia: Memorias de Hospital,* Buenos Aires, Ed. Galena, 1987.

This veritable nightmare was followed by calmer service in a small, private institution as I worked the night shift from July 1957 to January 1958 attached to the surgical service of the Hospital Aleman—the German Hospital. Reserved for members of the German community living in the metropolis, this aging pavilion-type institution in the affluent district of Palermo had been founded in 1867, but new facilities were being readied. The patient population was middle class and friendly, reassured by the presence of a German-speaking staff of caregivers who shared their ethnic values. Moreover, in sharp contrast with the Rawson Hospital, this institution possessed the most modern diagnostic equipment and a competent clinical laboratory to ensure state-of-the-art medical care. Here I not only experienced a pronounced shift in the social status of the patients but also confronted a radical change in institutional discipline. From the medical director down, a quasi-military authoritarianism borrowed from imperial German models still prevailed, tinged with latent sympathy for the Third Reich. Needless to say, I did not last very long and was fired for taking an unauthorized leave.

I spent the rest of my practical year in the medical service of another municipal hospital in Buenos Aires, the Hospital Dr. Juan Fernandez, a modern medium-sized facility also in Palermo, under the direction of professor Juan J. Beretervide, my thesis advisor. In all, my exposure to a combination of traditional French clinical and German scientific laboratory-based medicine proved invaluable for my future medical and historical activities.* Finally, following my 1958 graduation from the University of Buenos Aires School of Medicine, I won a competition for a residency at the famous Hospital Militar Central in Buenos Aires, a large high-rise building and flagship of the powerful military establishment in Argentina, where as a civilian I was thankfully exempted from many army regulations. My short service—I had accepted a position in the US—was uneventful and fruitful, but it provided me with a new appreciation of the importance that military authorities accorded to health care in the lives of a soldier and his family.

My first American hospital experience came in late 1958 after I started a rotating internship at Mercy Hospital, a Catholic community institution in Buffalo, New York. Many of my own experiences at Mercy are reflected in the first part of Chapter 10. In 1994 I returned to carry out archival research and conduct interviews with patients and staff. Some of the sisters, nurses, and attending physicians I had known in the years 1958–59 were still around, eager to reminisce about the good old days. In the belief that total immersion would be good for my study, I spent a full week living again in the old section of the institution, ensconced in the "bishop's room." Sleeping on a standard hospital bed, I was once again lulled to sleep by the hum of multiple compressors placed in a former atrium and on

---

*The influence of the French Medical School on Argentine medicine is explained in R. Carillo, "Influencia de la Facultad de Medicina de Paris sobre la de Buenos Aires," *Quipu* 3 (1986): 79–89, and by the same author in *Teoria del Hospital*, Buenos Aires, Eudeba, 1974.

the nearby rooftops and awakened during early mass by the sounds of a choir singing in the chapel. Hearing my name paged over the loudspeaker system brought back bittersweet memories.

In 1960, my fledgling medical career as a general internist brought me next to the Henry Ford Hospital in Detroit, a prominent private teaching hospital, with its new 17-story outpatient facility completed in 1955. Under the able leadership of Robin Buerki, the institution had joined other group practice clinics and hospitals such as the Lahey, Ochsner, Cleveland, and Mayo hospitals to form a consortium involved in the planning of international conferences and other educational activities.* Ford Hospital had already recognized the importance of shifting care from the hospital to clinics, thus anticipating current efforts to train students and house staff in ambulatory settings. One of my three-month assignments was to work in an outpatient clinic devoted to individuals suffering from psychosomatic ailments, one of the fountains for popular holistic models of illness. Another two-week rotation in medicine was devoted entirely to making housecalls on patients currently in treatment but unable to come to the clinic. I will always remember with relish the challenge of getting around the city and enjoying the hospitality of those I visited.

After a brief interlude in Argentina, my hospital experience came to include another middle-sized Catholic institution, Mount Carmel in Columbus, Ohio, where I spent 1962–63 as assistant chief resident in medicine. This experience signaled my transition to history—my special love since early school days—and I used my free time to investigate options for reentering academia and obtaining another doctoral degree to become a clinician-historian. Still, I continued to have contacts with medicine and its institutions, first at Billings Hospital of the University of Chicago, and then the University Hospital of the University of Minnesota in Minneapolis. After 1971, my academic appointment at the University of Wisconsin also brought me into contact with Madison General Hospital, a medium-sized, city-supported private institution, where I participated in a number of educational programs. Because of that hospital's active institutional history program, archival materials, and an ongoing program of interviews with former staff members, I also decided to feature this hospital in this book.

Finally, this study was prompted by my current residence in California, especially in the Bay Area, which exposed me to one of the largest and most competitive health care markets in the country and perhaps in the world. My arrival more than a decade ago coincided with the first drastic actions of the federal government in shifting from generous reimbursement schemes to prospective payment plans for San Francisco's hospitalized Medicare patients. As will be pointed out, this development had a significant impact on all academic medical centers, in-

*Details are provided in Patricia Scollard Painter, *Henry Ford Hospital, The First 75 Years*, Detroit, Henry Ford Hosp Assoc., 1997.

cluding Moffitt Hospital at the University of California, San Francisco (UCSF), my academic home, periodically ranked among America's best. My early exposure to the mixed blessings of managed care through the popularity of the Kaiser Permanente system was another factor in the conception of this project. In 1997, Kaiser of Northern California ranked as the top integrated health care system in the nation, followed in sixth place by another giant corporate San Francisco provider, Catholic Health Care West. In my present academic position, I personally interviewed most of the protagonists of my last stories. Visiting the wards, making rounds, and observing hospital life were invaluable experiences informing this book. Perhaps the most moving event of all was the time I spent in the AIDS ward at San Francisco General Hospital, an institution affiliated with UCSF and consistently ranked as the best hospital in the nation for the care of this disease since the opening of this unit.* A recent visit to the city's former almshouse, now devoted to rehabilitation and hospice care, brought back images of earlier ward experiences during my medical school years. Thus, my hospital collection spans more than half a century. It includes public and private institutions, academic and community hospitals, and religious and military establishments.

Like all historical accounts, this one is necessarily personal and incomplete. To fully understand hospital life and the plight of the patients, I have included much detail about diagnoses, caregiving efforts and treatments. Since the Enlightenment, hospitals have become the main engines in the production of medical knowledge, sites for the display of cutting-edge diagnostic procedures and therapeutic interventions. Hospital history is closely linked to the history of medicine and the stories that follow are imbedded within some of the more salient moments of our medical past. After walking along miles of corridors, enduring countless bland cafeteria meals, and spending long hours in the wards with anxious patients, I wanted to search for the historical roots of my multiple experiences and share my impressions with the reader. In doing so, I am very conscious of the numerous gaps remaining in this story. Given my medical training, the focus in modern times remains on general institutions, leaving aside special hospitals devoted to particular diseases or organ systems. Another important omission is asylums, already the focus of excellent studies. The selection of a Catholic hospital also reflects my own religious affiliation, suggesting the need for further studies of other religiously sponsored establishments. A more detailed examination of hospital architecture and its importance in shaping institutional life will be presented in a separate volume.

For twentieth-century developments, the tilt toward hospitals in the United States was a function of my ability to secure the necessary clinical documentation

---

*These yearly surveys are conducted and published by *U.S. News and World Report* in a July issue of this magazine and on the Internet. Top honors in 1997 went to Johns Hopkins Hospital in Baltimore, followed by the Mayo Clinic and Boston's Massachusetts General Hospital.

in my capacity as an academic or staff physician. As quintessential voyeurs, historians attempt to organize the past and attempt to give it meaning within the context of contemporary developments and perceived problems. Ultimately, perhaps, our interpretations say more about ourselves, our personal values, our interests, and our world views than about those we attempt to portray. As we age, we all become primary sources for historical information. Except for one aborted admission for a dubious diagnosis of appendicitis, I have been on the staff side of hospital life, but I am fully aware that such virginity will not last.

The scope of this project required the counsel and assistance of numerous scholars, librarians, archivists, research assistants, as well as the cooperation of hospital patients, physicians, and administrators whose stories I followed and documented. The debts I have incurred cannot possibly be repaid. Among those who provided manuscripts and unpublished material or helped translate excerpts were Randall Albury, David Barnes, Fritz Dross, Jackie Duffin, Alfons Labisch, Howard Markel, Rebecca Ranson, Deirdre O'Reilly, Barbara Schürman, Victoria Sweet, Claudia Stein, Karen Veit, Dora Weiner, and Donald Zukin. Rosemary Stevens carefully read the second half of my manuscript and provided me with useful criticism and more importantly, much needed encouragement. I am also grateful for the comments and suggestions of Nancy L. Ascher, Robert Bartz, Ronald Batt, William Bynum, Luke Demaitre, Marilyn E. Flood, Caroline Hannaway, John Henderson, Robert Jütte, Christopher Lawrence, John Malfa, Francis Moore, Vivian Nutton, Paul Potter, Earl Thayer, Morris Vogel, Daniel L. Weiss, Ursula Weisser, Juliane C. Wilmanns and the reviewers of my manuscript. At UCSF, special thanks go to research assistants Leif Brown, Halle Lewis, Rebecca Ratcliffe, Andrea Richardson, Matt Wray, and Patricia Zimmermann, as well as our graduate students Caroline Acker and Colin Talley. Further research was conducted by Cynthia Ronzio (Baltimore), Jennifer Munger (Madison), and Jean Richardson (Buffalo).

All historians depend on a cadre of dedicated and resourceful archivists and librarians to uncover and provide the documentation critical for the success of a book. I would like especially to acknowledge Nancy Zinn and Robin Chandler from our own institution, together with John Parascandola, Phillip Teigen, Steven Greenberg and the entire staff at the National Library of Medicine. Richard J. Wolfe and Tom Horrocks at the Countway Library, Nancy McCall at the Allan M. Chesney Archives at Johns Hopkins and all their collaborators were quite helpful. My appreciation also extends to Henry Behrnd and Sue Baranowski, of Meriter Hospital, Madison, Wisconsin, together with Lilli Sentz at SUNY Buffalo and Linda Karch at the Health Sciences Library of Mercy Hospital of Buffalo for providing access to important documentation. Special thanks to Diane Jones, head nurse of San Francico General Hospital's AIDS ward, and Juliet Melzer, transplant surgeon at UCSF's Moffit Hospital, who allowed me to witness the drama of the wards. In addition, I am beholden to Michael Barfoot and Lisa McDonald at the Archives of Edinburgh University, Julia Sheppard at the Contemporary Medical Archives Centre of the Wellcome Institute for the History of Medicine in London, and Karl Holubar of the Institut für Geschichte der Medizin at Vienna University. Finally, the staff of our History of Health Sciences Department deserves special appreciation, especially JoAnn Lopez for her dedication to this project. Last but not least, I would like to thank the various hospital staff members and patients, as well as their friends and relatives, who were willing to be interviewed. Without their participation, this book would never have been written.

San Francisco   G.B.R.
August, 1998

MENDING BODIES, SAVING SOULS

INTRODUCTION

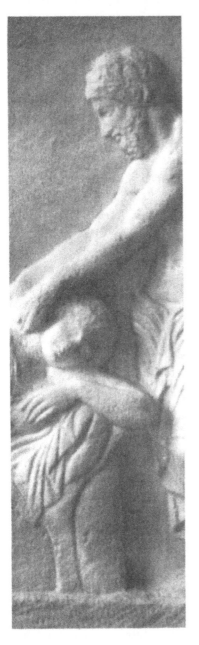

A hospital is only a building until you hear the slate hooves of dreams galloping upon its roof. You listen then and know that here is no mere pile of stone and precisely cut timber but an inner space full of pain and relief. Such a place invites mankind to heroism.

Richard Selzer
Taking the World in for Repairs, 1987[1]

Framework for a history of hospitals

For a century, hospitals have been among society's most valued institutions. Yet dramatic changes in today's medical practice are forcing a shift from hospitals to ambulatory settings and home care. Mergers and closings are now commonplace. Most of us were born in hospitals and return on the average about seven times before dying there. Hospitals are extolled for providing the means of lifesaving procedures and miraculous recoveries while simultaneously being criticized for their high costs, impersonality, and in-house infections. A current consumer guide even warns prospective patients that "the words *hospital* and *hospitality* come from the same root. And with that their relationship ends. Hospital patients don't find much hospitality nowadays. Tolerance is more like it. And confusion. And neglect. And unbelievable expense."[2] How did this happen?

To assess with greater clarity the nature of the hospital in the Western world and its place in medicine and society, we must examine its origins and evolution. Above all, we must probe the social and cultural currents that have set the hospital on its trajectory to our time. Such forces include the changing definitions of health and illness, shifts in the ecology of disease, the role of religion, and the fluctuating sense of responsibility for welfare and health care that societies in the West have had. Moreover, the more recent history of hospitals is inextricably linked to developments in the modern science and the practice of medicine; they also function as sites for professional training and clinical research. In sum, hospital history is cultural, social, and medical history.[3]

To depict the evolution of the hospital in broad strokes is to present a lifeless universe. The generic hospital is an abstraction. In reality, there are only particular hospitals, each with its unique name, patrons and mission, buildings, staff, and patients. The nature of a hospital's organizational "culture" is a reflection of its size, purpose, and mission.[4] Religious affiliation and the socioeconomic status of the patients play equally important roles. Location often determines the nature of an institution's population. Its operation depends on a hierarchically arranged workforce featuring managers and professionals at the top, supported by groups of less skilled workers. Thus, hospitals acquire their own identities, reinforced by architectural features and interior furnishings. Each composite personality, moreover, rests in great measure on traditions and staff behavior. "A hospital may be likened to a hive. What gives it character is not its queen but its workers and producers," wrote Harvey Cushing in 1930, referring to the Massachusetts General Hospital.[5] For its part the in-patient's "journey" is divided into a succession of rituals designed to provide meaning, structure, and continuity while demanding personal attention and participation. The sight of nurses, doctors, patients, and volunteers circulating through corridors and lobbies, the crackling sounds emanating from the public paging system, and even the smells wafting from wards and kitchens combine to shape a hospital's distinctive ambiance and character, which have a powerful impact on newcomers and visitors alike.[6]

A complete historical reconstruction of hospitals from charitable guest houses to biomedical showcases presents a formidable challenge.[7] How can one reduce the enormous variability displayed by hospitals at any historical moment and geographic locale to a common denominator when in fact each establishment is the distinctive and proud product of a prominent patron or a defined community?[8] The sheer volume and diversity of information suggested the chronological presentation of a few representative examples. I therefore decided to portray the key developments as a series of distinct episodes, like snapshots in a photo album or scenes in a play. This sequential presentation features a particular hospital in each time and place. Most examples represent poignant moments in hospital history that illustrate critical shifts in institutional frontiers. To tell each story, six basic aspects of hospital life are examined in depth: mission, patronage, organization, staff, patients, and ritualized caring activities.

A hospital's ideology, vision, and policies are the result of both converging and conflicting values and goals that change according to perceived social and health needs, political contexts, and economic fluctuations. From a religious point of view, hospitals have always been instruments of hope and pious benevolence. Based on ancient ancestors, the Christian *hospitalitas* has shaped the hospital's charitable mission, specifically Matthew's six works of mercy depicted in the New Testament. Social control and other rationales for welfare have also inspired hospital services over the ages, helping communities cope with the catastrophic displacements caused by famines, wars, and epidemics. Moreover, the early Christian institutions became an important source of political power for Church leaders, secular rulers, and, later, the local authorities of modern states. As recipients of gifts, endowments, and capital, many hospitals were involved with local and regional economies. With the permanent addition of physicians and surgeons to their caregiving staffs during the Renaissance, many institutions evolved into sites for the development of professional agendas, notably clinical training and research. By the eighteenth century, hospitals were tangible and symbolic expressions of the Enlightenment's commitment to rationality and progress. In our own medicalized society, hospitals are linked to the high value and utility we accord scientific and technologically assisted care. At the same time, new efforts to create "patient centeredness" seek to modify current science and technology-centered management operations and hospital environments to ensure the delivery of a more humane care.[9]

Because of their importance and status in a given community, hospitals have always been in the public eye. Fluctuations in image and reputation shaped admissions and generated public support. From charitable pledges and vows of religious devotion in the first millennium A.D. to humanitarian dedication since the Enlightenment, hospitals have actively portrayed themselves as houses of God and science. Hospital buildings were promoted as architectural landmarks, their monumental exteriors as expressions of religious piety and sources of civic pride. Like cathedrals, awe-inspiring interiors sought to calm the weary and the sick. Beginning in the eighteenth century, however, institutional crowding and cross-infections produced high institutional death rates, creating a long-lived negative image in which hospitals were categorized as "gateways to death." Such dreaded and pervasive epidemics of "hospitalism" precluded middle-class acceptance of hospital care until an optimum degree of institutional organization and cleanliness could be ensured. At the beginning of the twentieth century, gleaming high-rise buildings and home-like interiors proclaimed a vision of asepsis, professionalism, and comfort, illustrated in brochures and annual reports. In America, hospitals needed favorable images in the increasingly competitive medical marketplace of the century. In more recent times, the media have focused almost obsessively on the drama of hospital life, particularly in emergency and operating rooms, stressing the saving of individual patients' lives, the heroics of caregivers, and the availability of state of the art of medical technology.

The issue of patronage and sponsorship of hospitals is also critical for understanding their particular mission. Ownership and the social meaning of being a benefactor gradually moved from ecclesiastical leaders, emperors, kings, and wealthy individuals to state governments and private corporations, lay confraternities, municipal authorities, and academic institutions. What began as a personal display of faith and charity by Church members was transformed by rulers into a pageant of wealth and influence. Later, local sponsors demanded social control or physical rehabilitation, building monuments to civic or ethnic pride, scientific progress, and academic excellence. For many, hospitals still embody the human gift relation, a moral commitment to giving and receiving removed from the purely commercial realm and its cold, bottom-line mentality.[10]

Over time, each hospital functions as a unique environment, shaped by its geographic location, architectural design, size, internal organization, and financial base. Past notions of disease-causing miasma or vapor suggested that hospitals be erected on high ground, downwind, and away from population centers. Southern exposure was sought for the presence of cleansing sunlight, and proximity to streams was important for water supply and sewage disposal. In modern times, vertical or horizontal complexes are linked by a maze of corridors, tunnels, and bridges. A hospital's internal spatial organization has traditionally been shaped by its function. From simple dormitories adjacent to churches, hospitals redefined and successively fragmented their interior into wards, private rooms, nursing stations, operating and examining facilities, laboratory and radiology areas, intensive care and neonatal units.

From their inception, hospitals were organized according to official sets of rules first borrowed from monastic models of discipline and later adapted to lay schemes designed to ensure the social control of inmates. Since finances and fiscal accountability were critical aspects of hospital operations, institutions were supplied with a hierarchical system of management that followed monastic standards before being replaced by household practices during the Enlightenment and by business yardsticks in our own century. Historically, the mix of hospital income obtained from personal gifts and endowments, municipal taxes, private subscriptions, and, later, direct patient payments or health insurance reimbursements determined the viability of an institution, as well as the scope and quality of the services rendered. Patronage over the disbursement of such revenues was a perennial source of power struggles between hospital sponsors and administrators. Since the Middle Ages, financial irregularities have often resulted from lack of supervision and personal greed. The issue of accountability was closely linked to a particular hospital's mission and the patron's control over endowments. Further bureaucratization and mercantilist agendas since the Enlightenment generated a host of other issues, including attempts to maintain institutional autonomy and improve efficiency.

Hospital governance and staffing implemented the mission and intentions of the sponsors. In the early stages of their evolution in Byzantium, Christian hospitals demanded great sacrifices from those who committed themselves to aiding the sick. Hospital service was a form of penance. Vocation and total devotion were rewarded within the Christian framework of good works. Until the late Middle Ages, religious personnel remained in leadership positions, staging ceremonies and participating in caregiving. A subsequent division of labor required administrators, aided by accountants and attorneys, to sift through the hospital's financial and legal affairs. Spiritual care remained in the hands of priests, while physical nurturing became mostly the responsibility of religious and lay women because of the perceived domestic roots of these tasks. A medical presence in hospitals occurred only gradually, from consultants to salaried staff members during the Renaissance. Providing diagnostic, surgical, and therapeutic tasks, medical professionals in the late eighteenth and nineteenth centuries took over administrative functions regarding the selection and discharge of patients. They also created training programs and set up clinical experiments. More recently, in the twentieth century, hospitals have dramatically expanded their administrative staffs in the face of institutional complexity, hiring the ancillary personnel needed to perform the multiplicity of managerial and technologically assisted caregiving tasks.

Hospitals were usually launched in response to perceived needs in their surrounding populations. From the beginnings of hospitals in Byzantium, the selection of patients was prompted by the presence of local disasters such as famines, wars, and epidemics, reflecting a shifting ecology of disease. Social class, age, and economic status were also determining factors, as exemplified by the admission of the poor, homeless, and aged. Often, from the Middle Ages on, urbanization, as well as segregation of stigmatized groups such as lepers and plague victims, played a role. Within a more medicalized context, the issue of physical recovery began to loom larger after the Renaissance, based on more optimistic notions of health and illness. Subsequent medical triage systems in the nineteenth century sought to accept and divide new patients according to contemporary disease classifications. The growing tendency in this century to allow people with acute rather than chronic conditions into an institution rested on medical, social, and economic factors such as the improved management of medical and surgical emergencies, the availability of health care insurance, and the desire to return the sick to productive lives. Finally, the makeup of hospital populations was closely linked to patients' expectations and their willingness to accept authority, whether religious or medical. In recent decades, the concept of entitlement regarding health care, insurance status, and new judgments about the outcomes of medical intervention have further influenced patient composition.

From their beginnings in Byzantine Christendom, hospitals organized care through a series of activities and routines capable of accomplishing their institutional mission and fulfilling their sponsors' intentions. These rites tended to be executed by the establishment's staff, and their range reflects both institutional goals and the nature of the problems exhibited by those allowed to enter. From our vantage point, a hospital's activities throughout history can be broadly divided into religious ceremonies, hospitality and custodial care, and medicosurgical interventions. Medieval religious admission rituals included penance and the Eucharist, followed by purification ceremonies—the washing of feet and issuance of new clothing. Meals were preceded by fasting and followed by prayers, and other chores such as the laying on of hands were similarly routinized. Daily mass, anointing, and vigils for the dying were carefully choreographed. To this day, making beds, and the bathing and grooming of patients, are still part of nursing routines, performed in rotating shifts.

During the Enlightenment, a program of visiting hours for family and friends became another rite. By this time the medical profession had its own rituals, including daily visits, teaching rounds, reports, and entries in ward journals. Prescriptions of food and medicines were dictated and entered on boards attached to individual beds. Daily pulse and respiration readings were followed by later nineteenth-century temperature measurements. This information was collected and displayed in individual patient charts together with other diagnostic procedures and the caregivers' progress notes. Among medical professionals, surgeons were the most dramatic, their operations carried out since the eighteenth century in amphitheaters with large audiences in attendance. Thanks to the emergence of the clinical laboratory, the almost daily phlebotomies and other bodily samples for multiple biochemical tests have added another diagnostic ritual. Two critical factors shaping hospital work in the late twentieth century are the state of medical knowledge and technology and the shifting quality of the patient–nurse and patient–physician relationships. The former has given rise to additional rituals, including new technical methods of body imaging, while patients now face teams of busy caregivers, a barrier to forging healing relationships. Hospitals have been and continue to be dramatic stages populated by a diversified staff that performs a series of rites encoded with numerous meanings.

Indeed, for those who enter its space, the experience of the hospital includes a series of formal initiations and routine activities. These functions, created over time, were meant to establish institutional order and convey a number of religious, humanitarian, and medical meanings to patients anguished by disability and pain. Hope was expressed that the ordeal would end in healing. Segregation of the sick from the healthy was among the earliest aims of hospitals. This separation allayed the fear of contamination gripping the healthy but compounded the isolation of the sick. This segregation was, and continues to be, accomplished through the use of rituals and costumes that symbolized the transition to patienthood. To this day, admission ceremonies tend to confirm and sanction the perceived sick role. In early Christian times, the sick entered a religious realm that required purity of body and soul, accomplished by prayers, confession, and communion, as well as washings and a change of clothing. In modern times, secular "induction" measures include the application of wrist bands for identification purposes and the surrender of private clothes. Like prison inmates in their distinctive garb, hospital gowns are designed to provide easy access to the body by caregivers, thus spotlighting the gulf between patients and the rest of the hospital microcosm. In their capacity as guardians, nurses, physicians, and assistants sometimes wear their own distinctive uniforms according to seniority and rank, a practice now increasingly abandoned and thus contributing to patient disorientation.[11]

Hospital narratives and case histories

Personal narratives are currently quite popular in historical discourse. They provide an alternative mode of viewing the world and expressing elementary human emotions and concerns distinct from official documents and texts. In medicine, the patient was traditionally a valuable source of information about illness in everyday life, only to be silenced by the technology-assisted physical and chemical probes of our century. In addition to framing the evolution of hospitals, this book illuminates the human dimensions of hospitalization. One of its central organizing themes is depicting the world of hospitals and asking: how therapeutic was the hospital environment in the past? Each institutional journey examines social and professional issues and presents details of patient management. Here personal narratives are central in understanding the patient experience. Whether expressing themselves orally or in writing, sick individuals in the past as well as the present have been quite capable of articulating their experiences, presenting them as dramatic stories of suffering and redemption. Some traced their own illnesses, placed them in historical perspective, and used language and discourse shaped by the social and cultural contexts in which they experienced these illnesses. In more recent times, other historical narratives were embedded in medical jargon, sharply critical of medicine. In a world increasingly distrustful of experts and professionals, recent patient narratives constitute a complementary source of empirical knowledge.[12] However crafted, the stories provide valuable insights into the universe of meanings and emotions surrounding patienthood. For those sufferers who talk or write about their experiences, their sharing often has a healing quality that contributes to the recovery of others.[13] Yet, despite the richness and importance of such narratives, a patient-centered ethnography of hospital life is still in its infancy.[14]

As depicted by contemporary narratives, going to a hospital resembles a journey to a foreign, exotic land, an often too common pilgrimage in which patients cross into a world of strange rites, miraculous interventions, and frequent death. For those who tell or write their stories, this approach allows them to attach a social value to the events surrounding their hospitalization, making the experiences transitory and capable of being endured with courage and patience. From admission to discharge, the unknown and often hostile environment must be negotiated from a position of weakness and disadvantage. The conception of the hospital as a house of crises and rituals is therefore useful not only for interpreting the choreography of institutional routines but also for understanding the experience of hospitalization for patients. Like many other life journeys, hospital stays can induce profound personal mutations, including changes in lifestyle and spiritual growth.[15]

The words of the sick help us to connect to the past and reconstruct the context of their sufferings. I am particularly indebted to the writings of Oliver Sacks, especially his autobiographical narrative *A Leg to Stand On*, published in 1984 (the date of my two last case studies). Sacks' status as a wounded healer who recognizes himself in a patient and his sensitivity to the dehumanizing aspects of modern hospitalization resonate powerfully with other patients' accounts I obtained during a series of interviews. Another work, Arthur W. Frank's *At the Will of the Body*, also relates a personal account of a struggle with a heart attack and cancer.[16] A medical sociologist by training, Frank combines emotion with analysis as he sifts through his illness experiences. While functional recovery has largely replaced spiritual concerns, the once key issues of sinful causality, need for penance, and some form of redemption still echo powerfully through the wards and corridors of the modern hospital. In our quest to attend to bodily ills, we may be neglecting the spiritual dimensions of sickness and recovery. Hospital history is human history; the personal drama of experiencing suffering reflects basic aspects of human nature filtered through contingent cultural, social, and medical frames.

To provide thematic coherence, my parade of historical hospitals is rooted in the experiences of several patients. On the assumption that we all share a fundamental humanity across time and space, the spotlight is on their lives and institutional journeys. The idea came to me while perusing Michael Crichton's early work *Five Patients: The Hospital Explained*, a selection of individual clinical stories based on his experiences as a medical student in 1969 at the Massachusetts General Hospital.[17] Crichton used this approach to illuminate some of the profound changes affecting American medicine in the 1960s. Hospitals are never neutral spaces. They constitute a keen weathervane detecting shifts in both medical and social currents. I wish to stress the fragmentary and uneven quality of these sources. Most members of our society suffer in private; they may reveal some of their somatic complaints but repress their feelings. Often, hospitalization is an experience worth forgetting, instead of being revisited in word or on paper. To supplement personal accounts, I have obtained additional data from surviving clinical records in collections of older medical journals and institutional archives.[18] Extensive personal interviews with some patients, their relatives, and caregivers flesh out the more recent stories. Since this information was confidential, it was often modified to respect the patient's privacy. The final chapter featuring Warren J., the patient suffering from AIDS, is an exception. His family and friends very much wanted his story told as a contribution to our historical understanding of this disease.[19]

Few firsthand accounts from earlier historical periods survive, and some of the case studies had to be built around them. The story of Aelius Aristides, the second-century Roman orator, is well known but was never presented within the institutional framework of a Greek healing temple. Aristides' chronicle was written as a quest for health advice, and his sojourn at the Asclepieion in Pergamon proved personally empowering: he not only learned to handle his physical disabilities but also gained a greater appreciation of himself and the meaning of life. In the following section, the letters from a Roman soldier to his father anchor a brief view of imperial military life and the possible uses of a unique institution: the *valetudinarium*. In turn, the dramatic accounts of famine and epidemic disease in fifth-century Edessa create a concrete backdrop for the emergence of the Christian shelter in Byzantium, the ancestor of all subsequent charitable institutions in the Western world dealing with the poor and sick.

The brief tale of a tenth-century *infirmarius* at the famous monastery of St. Gall allows a glimpse into the anatomy and life of a Benedictine infirmary and the treatment of its injured abbot. Another personal account was sketched by the twelfth-century poet Theodoros Prodromos in Constantinople. His illness was eventually managed at the new Pantocrator Hospital in that city. Prodromos' humiliating and painful treatments document the early medical presence in the evolution of Christian shelters devoted to the sick. A few decades later, the death of a pilgrim in the Holy Land was chronicled together with the most famous medieval institution for sick pilgrims: the Hospital of St. John in Jerusalem. For the subsequent centuries, most sick people and their sufferings remain poorly documented. Reports such as a fifteenth-century request for the examination of a leper and the census of a makeshift lazaretto in seventeenth-century Rome for plague victims furnished the necessary scaffolding for two separate stories of social stigma and institutional separation.

By the eighteenth century, the further medicalization of hospitals provides the historian with collections of complete clinical cases, preserved and even published for research and teaching purposes. However, the patients themselves were now silent, their suffering increasingly categorized within competing disease categories and expressed in professional terms. A pair of near-contemporary fever patients, one in Edinburgh and the other in Vienna, symbolize the new hospital medicine as practiced and taught in two of Europe's most famous institutions. I deliberately juxtaposed these stories as examples of two opposing medical systems of the time, represented by two well-known Scottish physicians, William Cullen and John Brown.

Of similar pedigree is the story of a French veteran who came to a small Parisian hospital in 1818 just before R. T. Laennec, its resident physician, published his new auscultatory findings. Laennec presumably dictated the case to one of his interns, but the account allows for an in-depth look at the dramatic shifts in knowledge and power associated with the new mapping of the human body. Three decades later, a young Irish domestic hospitalized at the Massachusetts General Hospital became the first person subjected to ether anesthesia for a major surgery, the amputation of her leg. For surgery to flourish, however, hospitals needed to cleanse their premises to avoid the dreaded institutional contagion. Margaret Mathewson's personal account of her hospital experiences with Lister and the Nightingale nurses at the old Royal Infirmary of Edinburgh during the 1870s is a unique document, since most poor people at the time remained illiterate. This story mirrors many of the more recent narratives in which illness, although a painful hardship, became a vehicle for spiritual growth and redemption.

In the early 1890s, the new science of medicine was challenged by the onslaught of two widespread infectious diseases: typhoid fever and cholera. With the help of published clinical records, we can observe the battle against those diseases at two of the most prominent and most modern hospitals in the world: Johns Hopkins Hospital in Baltimore and the Eppendorf General Hospital in Hamburg. In both instances, the promises of science for the treatment of these scourges remained unfulfilled. More effective was the surgical management of an accident case in 1930. The patient received treatment in a typical general hospital supported by the city of Madison, Wisconsin, in the American Midwest. The story, unfolding during the Depression, was captured through clinical notes, administrative records, oral histories, and personal interviews. A similar combination of patient narratives, clinical records, and interviews with relatives and caregivers forms the basis for two comparative portraits of patients who suffered heart attacks in 1954 and 1974. Both men were hospitalized at Mercy Hospital, a Catholic institution located in Buffalo, New York. The 20-year interval between these admissions revealed the growing importance of noninfectious diseases. It also allowed a glimpse of the profound changes in hospital organization, management, and medical treatment.

Ten years later, two urban San Francisco institutions, Moffitt Hospital and San Francisco General Hospital, displayed the stark contrasts between an academic tertiary-care institution performing kidney transplants and a municipal establishment taking care of indigent, uninsured residents. Here again, extensive interviews with patients, relatives, and caregivers were supplemented with medical and administrative records to flesh out the individual institutional trajectories. The patients' impressions, emotions, and clinical progress represent a near-contemporary record of hospital politics, finances, and institutional life in two of America's most famous establishments. Moreover, these last chapters illuminate the significant changes in the healing relationship between patients, their nurses and physicians, and the birth of the much-heralded San Francisco model of caring for AIDS, now employed throughout the world.

NOTES

1. Richard Selzer, *Taking the World in for Repairs*, London, Penguin Bks, 1987, p. 238.

2. Charles Inlander and Ed Weiner, *Take This Book to the Hospital with You, A Consumer Guide to Surviving Your Hospital Stay*, rev. ed., New York, Pantheon, 1991, p. 3.

3. For a brief synopsis see L. Granshaw, "The hospital," in *Companion Encyclopedia of the History of Medicine*, ed. W. F. Bynum and R. Porter, London, Routledge, 1993, vol. 2, pp. 1180–1203. See also *The Hospital in History*, ed. L. Granshaw and R. Porter, London, Routledge, 1989, and *History of Hospitals*, ed. Y. Kawakita et al., Tokyo, Ishiyaku EuroAmerica, 1989.

4. M. Gerteis and M. J. Roberts, "Culture, leadership, and service in the patient-centered hospital," in *Through the Patient's Eyes*, ed. M. Gerteis et al., San Francisco, Jossey-Bass, 1993, pp. 227–59.

5. Harvey Cushing, *The Personality of a Hospital*, Boston, White & Home Co., 1930, pp. 8–9. See also J. G. Houghton, "Determinants of the culture and personality of institutions," in *Integrity in Health Care Institutions: Humane Environments for Teaching, Inquiry, and Healing*, ed. R. E. Bulger and S. J. Reiser, Iowa City, Univ. of Iowa Press, 1990, pp. 141–47.

6. D. S. Kornfeld, "The hospital environment: Its impact on the patient," *Adv Psychosom Med* 8 (1972): 252–70.

7. The classic article on this subject remains H. E. Sigerist, "An outline of the development of the hospital," *Bull Hist Med* 4 (1936): 573–81.

8. For the United States, a recent valuable collection is D. E. Long and J. Golden, eds., *The American General Hospital: Communities and Social Contexts*, Ithaca, Cornell Univ. Press, 1989. The nation's premier resource on hospital history is the Center for Hospital and Healthcare Administration History in Chicago.

9. M. Gerteis and M. J. Roberts "Introduction," *Through the Patient's Eyes*, pp. 1–15.

10. "A considerable part of our morality and our lives themselves are still permeated with this same atmosphere of the gift, where obligations and liberty intermingle. Fortunately everything is still not wholly categorized in terms of buying and selling. . . . We posess more than a tradesman morality." Marcel Mauss, *The Gift*, trans. W. D. Halls, New York, Norton, 1990, p. 65.

11. The isue of "situational propriety" and social order is discussed by Erving Goffman in *Behavior in Public Places*, New York, Free Press, 1963. The author stresses that individuals modify their behavior according to the social spaces they occupy.

12. G. Williams and J. Popay, "Lay knowledge and the privilege of experience," in *Challenging Medicine*, ed. J. Gabe et al., London, Routledge, 1994, pp. 118–39.

13. For a collection of patient autobiographies see Jens Lachmund and Gunnar Stollberg, *Patientenwelten; Krankheit und Medizin vom späten 18. bis zum frühen 20. Jahrhundert im Spiegel von Autobiographien*, Opladen, Leske & Budrich, 1995.

14. For a review of the pertinent literature during the past decades see R. Zussman, "Life in the hospital: A review," *Milbank Q* 71 (1993): 167–85. One recent example is Sydney Lewis, *Hospital: An Oral History of Cook County Hospital*, New York, New Press, 1994.

15. A valuable source is Anne Hunsaker Hawkins, *Reconstructing Illness, Studies in Pathography*, West Lafayette, Ind., Purdue Univ. Press, 1993.

16. Arthur W. Frank, *At the Will of the Body*, Boston, Houghton Mifflin Co., 1991. His discussion on hospitalization and medicine as rites of passage is found on pp. 131–32.

17. Michael Crichton, *Five Patients: The Hospital Explained*, New York, A. A. Knopf, 1970.

18. A special issue of *Literature and Medicine* edited by J. T. Banks and A. H. Hawkins is devoted to "The Art of the Case History." See especially the introduction by the editors: *Lit Med* 11 (Spring 1992): vii–xi, and K. M. Hunter's article "Remaking the case," 163–79.

19. Another recent account of terminal AIDS is Amy Hoffman, *Hospital Time*, Durham, Duke Univ. Press, 1997.

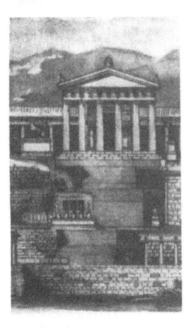

1

PRE-CHRISTIAN
HEALING PLACES

DREAMING OF ASCLEPIUS: ANCIENT GREEK TEMPLE HEALING

> Neither belonging to a chorus nor sailing together nor having the same teacher is as great a thing as the boon and profit of being a fellow pilgrim to the temple of Asclepius and being initiated into the first of the holy rites by the fairest and most perfect torch-bearer and leader of the mysteries.
>
> Aelius Aristides (ca. 117–180 AD)[1]

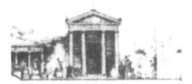

A divine summons to Pergamon

During the early summer in about the year 145 AD, Aelius Aristides, a famous and wealthy orator from Mysia, in Asia Minor, dreamed that the Greek healing god Asclepius had invited him to visit the Asclepieion at Pergamon for a cure. Temporarily living in Smyrna, one of the most important urban centers in the region, Aristides, by his own admission, was not well. After buying a house in the city, he had for the past six months shuttled to nearby warm springs seeking relief. Months earlier, as the unspecified symptoms of his illness intensified, Aristides had visited a local temple dedicated to the Egyptian goddess Isis, offering "at her command" two geese. There, in another dream, the gods Sarapis and Asclepius appeared before him, "marvelous in beauty and magnitude."[2]

Aristides had already been contacted by Asclepius the previous winter, an event that forever changed his life. In a dream, Asclepius simply ordered Aristides to henceforth walk barefoot as much as possible, presumably to help toughen up his ailing body. "Great is Asclepius!, the order is accomplished!" confided Aristides to his diary.[3] As the season proceeded, he received a second divine command ordering him to travel to the nearby warm springs but to bathe in an adjacent river. Aristides accomplished this feat bravely on a windy, rainy, cold afternoon, seemingly without further harm, since he later indicated in his notes that "this was the first miracle" performed by Asclepius.[4]

In a sense, Asclepius' initial advice to Aristides imitated the recommendations of classic athletic coaches bent on hardening their trainees' bodies. It marked the beginning of a steady stream of visions and dreams, both within and outside temple precincts, through which the healing god guided the Roman intellectual's subsequent life. Among the divine commands was a request to record the dreams and eventually make them public for the benefit of the sacred cult. In the work *Hieroi Logoi* ("an account of the apparition of the god who makes a revelation"), Aristides reveals that "I made a copy of my dreams, dictating them, whenever I was unable to write myself."[5] This story recalls Aristides' 20-year odyssey, during which he repeatedly visited the Asclepian shrines.[6]

Aristides was possibly born in October 117 AD into a wealthy land-owning family in Mysia, northeast of Pergamon. In accordance with his social status, he received a liberal education in Smyrna, followed by studies in rhetoric under Herodes Atticus in Athens. Back in Pergamon, Aristides came to enjoy the social and political advantages of Roman citizenship in an age of relative peace under the rule of emperor Antoninus Pius (138–161), Hadrian's successor. Here, the cult of Asclepius was experiencing a belated renaissance, and some of the god's shrines were being rebuilt and honored by the Antonine rulers. Hoping to propitiate the powerful god, senators and members of the equestrian order had placed new inscriptions and buildings within the temple's precincts. Closely associated with Zeus, Athena, and Dionysus, Asclepius appeared to eclipse some of the traditional Olympian deities by the second century AD.[7]

Aristides recalled falling ill in Egypt while traveling on the Nile near Elephantine a few years earlier. Concerned, he had turned to the healing god Sarapis, attending the god's spring festival. Sarapis, closely associated with his female counterpart, the goddess Isis, was a Hellenized blend of the ancient Egyptian deities Osiris and Apis. Both Sarapis and Isis were venerated throughout the Roman empire and featured among their attributes the power to heal.[8] Prognostication and diagnoses through dreams had been practiced since pharaonic times, and the increasingly individualized relationships sought with deities during Aristides' time made such dreams an excellent medium for personal contact. Both Roman tolerance for foreign religions and the progressive syncretism exemplified in the

Sarapis-Asclepius association promoted the expansion and popularization of such cults throughout the empire, particularly among the educated classes. Ancient oracles enjoyed fresh popularity, and fortune tellers successfully plied their trade. Although there is no explicit mention, Aristides could also have learned at Elephantine about the pre-Hellenic worship of Imhotep, the legendary Egyptian architect, whose rise from a venerated public official and patron of scribes to sage and healer had resulted in a popular cult that included incubation—the practice of sleeping in temples or sacred places for oracular purposes—votive inscriptions, and yearly festivals with striking parallels to the cult of Asclepius.

In spite of his visits to the Egyptian shrines, Aristides returned home still suffering from symptoms suggestive of a respiratory ailment. Back in Smyrna, he now faced a widespread problem described by Galen during the Antonine era: how to find a competent physician. It was difficult in cities to distinguish among the resident *medici*, whose educational backgrounds and reputations defied assessment. Practitioners who seemed to spend most of their time socializing with the rich were worthless, in Galen's opinion. His solution to this dilemma was that prospective patients be self-reliant and skeptical, learn a great deal about medicine themselves, and aggressively question would-be healers about their knowledge and skills. Unfortunately, this approach demanded a considerable amount of time and energy, something that the aristocratic classes, including Aristides, seemed unwilling to divert from their quests for pleasure, travel, and unhealthy lifestyles.[9] To Galen's chagrin, medical charlatans continued to prosper.[10]

We know little about Aristides' career and health until about a year later, when, again during the winter, he decided to travel by land to Rome to further his budding career. "I set out for Rome in the middle of winter, though I was already sick at home from the rain and a cold," he writes, adding that "I paid no heed to my present ailments but trusted to the training of my body and to my general good luck." As he hurried his travel party along and staying at inns where "more rain came in through their roofs than from the sky," Aristides' symptoms only grew worse, now including nagging toothaches. "I was very worried about my teeth falling out," he tells us, "so that I held up my hands to catch them. I was absolutely prevented from taking nourishment, except only milk. Then I first noted the shortness of breath in my chest and I was attacked by strong fevers and other indescribable things."[11]

While Aristides' voyage to the capital seemed less than propitious, conditions in the Roman empire under Antoninus Pius were said to have been orderly and stable. The massive military apparatus established by Trajan and Hadrian was still fully operational, the existing fortifications consolidated.[12] Tolerance for multiculturalism and justice prevailed. Antoninus' *pax Romana* gave ailing cities, especially in Greece and Asia, a welcome economic boost, while military recruits from provincial communities were allowed to become citizens as they joined the legions.

In a speech the following spring at the Athenaeum in Rome, Aristides extolled the current political stability and its favorable effects on educated people in the empire like himself.[13]

Once in Rome, where he had arrived in early spring, Aristides bitterly complained that "my intestines swelled, I trembled with cold, shivering ran through all my body, and my breath was impeded." Upon requesting medical aid, he was subjected to the routine practices of purging and wet cupping: "the doctors produced purges, and I was purged for two days by drinking squirting cucumber, until finally there was a bloody discharge." The approach represented the therapeutic rationale of Greek healing craftsmen and their descendants. Unfortunately, matters failed to improve "and fevers attacked me, and now everything was despaired of, and there was not any hope even of my survival." In the end, "the doctors made a [superficial] incision, beginning from my chest all the way down to the bladder. And when the cupping instruments were applied, my breathing was completely stopped, and a pain, numbing and impossible to bear, passed through me and everything was smeared with blood, and I was excessively purged."[14]

To understand these treatments, one must be aware of the theoretical principles that guided ancient Graeco-Roman therapeutics. Classical humoralism was based on a set of notions about human functioning derived from domestic and folk views of bodily behavior in health and disease. Within such a framework, the body was said to be composed of four inextricably mixed elements and humors endowed with particular qualities. In addition, persons were believed to possess an individual humoral blend that defined their bodily constitution. Nature was destiny since this combination not only dictated individual bodily form, but also determined mental status and susceptibility to particular disorders. Classical disease concepts were largely predicated on bodily behavior in processes of internal poisoning and external wound development, interpreted as humoral stagnation and putrefaction. When introduced into the organism, all substances capable of altering the healthy balance could be considered poisons. They were either inhaled, ingested, or acquired through direct contact.

To counter such effects, nature possessed healing powers. Indeed, the ancients described the presence of a natural healing force within the human body, activated as soon as the healthy balance became threatened by a poison or another noxious influence.[15] Natural healing could occur through a process of selective humoral *pepsis*, or cooking, with the body driving out all excess or corrupted humors during critical moments of the disease process. Such an expulsion was accomplished through the body's natural exits (by "derivation," or withdrawal), including vomiting and diarrhea, bleeding, sneezing and coughing, sweating and voiding urine, as well as through menstrual and vaginal flows. At other times, nature tried to rid the body of dangerous substances by creating alternative exits, often through the surface of the skin, presumably to avoid excessive humoral ac-

cumulations near vital organs. All natural depleting efforts followed particular evo-
lutionary paths toward slow and gradual "lysis" and recovery, punctuated by so-
called crises, sudden and dramatic humoral discharges.

Aristides was well aware that humoral disturbances were the result of complex interactions between the body's individual constitution, diet, environment,
lifestyle, and behavior.[16] Human organisms possessed a natural tendency toward
balance among their various components through the production of new humors
and the elimination of wastes. Constant renewal was achieved through food and
drink. The body acted as a veritable cooking vessel capable of boiling and blending the ingested ingredients to build new solid and fluid parts.[17] Air and climate,
food and drink, sleep and exercise, and mental activity were all considered essential for life and the preservation of physical and spiritual harmony. Health management or regimen prominently featured diet to achieve and sustain the humoral
adjustment.[18] Frequently, the body sought to return to a healthy state by selectively discharging some excess humors, especially if they were still in a "raw" or
"uncooked" stage.

Therapeutic interventions such as those employed by classical practitioners
and described by Aristides sought to imitate natural healing efforts. Physicians
feared that if the body's natural efforts seemed to fall short or if their timing was
off, sickness could become established permanently through a deposit of noxious
substances, leading to chronic conditions and death. Practitioners, therefore, were
encouraged to imitate the natural healing actions without causing additional bodily harm, a therapeutic injunction frequently violated, as in Aristides' case. Treatment consisted in the medicinally assisted expulsion of all poisons through the
usual excretory organs by the employment of emetics, purgatives, cathartics, enemas, expectorants, diuretics, and bloodletting. Agents capable of accomplishing
more than one or two of these expulsive functions were considered *panaceas*, or
cure-alls. Healers similarly searched for specific antidotes (*theriacs*), with their
emetic and purgative qualities, to neutralize bodily poisons.[19] These compounds
were created by combining viper flesh or scorpions with other ingredients. Indeed, the selection of medicines was frequently guided by notions of signs and
sympathy whereby plants, animals, and minerals were believed to disclose their
healing qualities through physical clues linked to disease manifestations.

At other times, ancient practitioners chose alternative routes for such an expulsion. If the natural exit of the noxious humors was felt to be impeded, insufficient, or dangerous, adherents of Hippocrates and Galen also followed nature
by creating artificial diversions or revulsions. This meant that particular areas of
the skin were designated as substitute exits for the expulsion of poisons and uncooked humors. To accomplish their goals, healers massaged, irritated, scarified,
and burned the skin, then employed cups or leeches, blisters, and running sores
to extract the offending poisons from the vicinity of vital internal organs. The ex-

pectation was that, once herded into discrete but far less dangerous blisters, pustules, and abscesses near the surface of the skin, poisonous humors became visible to the practitioner, who could promptly drain them.[20]

In sum, classical therapeutics was based on a coherent humoral framework of bodily functioning in health and disease. This theory was quite simple and easily understandable to both healers and their patients. Holistic in approach, it lent itself to individualized adjustments, mostly executed within the sick person's home environment with the employment of domestic resources and the help of family networks. Respectful of natural developments, such ancient treatments expected to imitate or follow the spontaneous evolution of self-limited disease processes. In doing so, humoral therapy frequently claimed success, thus confirming the healers' clinical knowledge, judgment, and skill.

Languishing in Rome, Aristides decided to return home in early fall. While traveling by sea, however, his suffering increased. By the time he reached Miletus around October, Aristides admitted that "I was unable to stand, and my ears had become quite deaf, and there was nothing which did not trouble me." Later, he recalled that "when I was brought from Italy, I had contracted by ill luck many varied ailments from constant sickness and the stormy weather."[21] Once Aristides landed in Smyrna a month later, he wrote that "the hardest and most difficult thing of all was that my breathing was constricted. With much effort and disbelief, scarcely would I breathe forcibly and rarely, and a constant constriction of my throat followed and I had fits of shivering." Moreover, he added that "my palatal region was in very bad condition, and the rest as well."

Now, at Aristides' request, "doctors and gymnastic trainers assembled. The doctors were wholly at a loss not only as to how to help, but even to recognize what the whole thing was. Neither could they help nor recognize the variety of my disease." Finally, he reported that "they agree on, that I be brought to the warm springs, since I was not even able to bear the climate in the city."[22] Still feeling sick by early summer, Aristides set out from Smyrna for the shrine of his favorite healing god, accompanied by his foster father Zosimus.

Asclepius and his cult

In the surviving literary sources, Asclepius is first mentioned in Homer's *Iliad*, depicted as an ordinary mortal and father of two healers, Machaon and Podaleiros, who had joined the Greek coalition against Troy.[23] Alternatively, Asclepius was also considered to be a pre-Homeric chthonic (under the earth) or subterranean spirit from Thessaly, hidden in caves with lizards and snakes. Given this aspect of his nature, he was associated with fresh well water bursting in the form of springs from the depths of the earth or damp dew placed on plants and flowers. By about 700 BC, Hesiod stressed Asclepius' heroic background and provided him with a family, a wife called Epione and several daughters, among them Hygieia, who was often portrayed as Asclepius' healing partner and companion. As a hero, Asclepius and his entire family were responsible for prosperity and health.[24]

Another mythical origin was proposed by the poet Pindar in his third *Pythian Ode*, composed during the early fifth century BC. Here Asclepius is depicted as the son of Apollo, the god of health, and a mortal woman, Coronis, daughter of King Phlegyas of Trikka in northern Greece. Eventually, according to Pindar, he became an excellent healing craftsman. "All who came to him sick with festering sores, or with limbs wounded by shiny bronze or far-hurled stones, or with bodies that were wasting from the scorching summer or chilly winter, he loosened and delivered from their assorted aches and pains, attending some with soothing spells, making others drink comforting potions, or wrapping their limbs all round in bandages, or setting them back on their feet through surgery."[25] However, when in his zeal, greed, and arrogance he restored a dead person, Hippolytos, to life, he was struck by a thunderbolt of the angry Zeus, who condemned him for violating the universal order of nature. Pindar's story implies the existence of divine rules that impose limits on human ambitions, as well as on the healing art.[26] The myth of Asclepius as a hero—a man of superhuman strength, courage, and ability—and a skillful healer seems linked to Thessaly and Trikka, in particular, and contrasts with a later formulation in Epidaurus. Other myths portray the paradoxical nature of Asclepius: "he was the sickness and the remedy . . . himself afflicted, and because he was a divine patient, he also knew the way to heal."[27] In this sense, Asclepius could also be viewed as a wounded healer—he was even said to have died and been resuscitated—someone who had suffered but could also heal. Because of his background and his tragic experiences, he possessed the qualities to understand those who came to him in search of help.

The cult of Asclepius possibly originated in Thessaly, gradually spreading south until the god, now an Epidaurian, began to be worshipped there alongside Apollo Maleatos but without a temple of his own.[28] By the fifth century BC, however, Asclepius had become the main focus of the Epidauran temple complex, prompting the construction of a new temple to him circa 430 BC. At this point, fear of disease may have become rampant throughout ancient Greece, especially after the plague that devastated Athens. This temple construction is said to have occurred during a time of rapid urbanization, civil strife, and tension between rich and poor in the nearby city of Argos. In fact, Epidaurus was actually attacked by an Athenian force while the epidemic was raging back home. In any event, located six miles from the town of Epidaurus in a broad valley, the Asclepian precinct quickly became the proud home of a pan-Hellenic healing cult.[29] This expansion coincided with the rise of secular Hippocratic healing and, in Athens, with the first appearance of public physicians. Even the island of Cos, presumably the home of Hippocrates, had a functioning Asclepieion from about 420 BC on, located on a hill slope above the newly refounded capital city.[30]

At Athens, the healing god had been conveyed by ship from Epidaurus to the port of Piraeus in the late 420s BC, representing a radical shift in religious outlook for a community in which magical healing had been restricted to local shrines devoted to several heroes. Asclepius' apparent success led 12 months later to the establishment of a second shrine dedicated to him on the slopes of the Acropolis. This was perhaps a tribute to the enterprising Epidauran priesthood vigorously promoting their local deity as a national god in an attempt to reap greater benefits for their own temple complex. Another export reached Pergamon, Aristides' destination, where around 370 BC another shrine was founded outside the city by a certain Archias, believed to have been healed at Epidaurus. Asclepius was similarly carried to Rome around the year 293 BC, supposedly following an epidemic outbreak. Legend had it that the deity's voyage from Epidaurus came in the form of a sacred snake that allegedly left the ship at Tiber Island and slithered into a temple erected there for the Roman god Faunus, a local version of Apollo.[31] Shaped as a sun ship pointing downstream, this small island was said to possess a sacred well and an obelisk. In Rome, the god was henceforth worshiped under the Latin name Esculapius. During imperial times, the island reputedly featured an impressive temple complex with hostels, baths, theaters, and gymnasiums staffed by many attendants designed to accommodate the crowds at festival times. Given the god's growing reputation as a healer, Romans were said to have abandoned sick slaves on the island, ostensibly for Asclepius to cure them.[32]

From the remaining evidence, it appears that shrines dedicated to the god, called *Asclepieia*, were mostly erected in valleys at favorable wooded locations near hot or cold springs but also near caves outside of towns. While water had obvious symbolic cleansing qualities in ancient Greece, the existing springs also possessed oracular powers since good spirits were said to live in the mountains and groves of cypress or olive trees surrounding them. The sacred land or *hieron* was always marked off by an enclosure called a *temenos*, separating it from profane space by stones or a wall surrounding the whole complex. At Epidaurus, a special path or "sacred way" linked the town with the temple. A roofed gate or *propylon*, with ramps at either end, provided access and opportunities for prayer. Water basins must have allowed visitors to purify themselves symbolically before stepping into a sacred area. Most enclosures had a temple, image, and altar, but others simply consisted of a grove, spring, or cave in the countryside. At some places, there were also a number of peripheral shrines devoted to other deities. Sacred dogs—a dog was said to have protected Asclepius as an abandoned toddler—and snakes were said to roam and slither freely on the grounds.

In some locations, caves were the original places of worship, eventually replaced by regular temples. Buildings usually faced east, aligned with the entrance to the compound. Most were raised above the ground by a base three steps high; a peristyle surrounded the whole building. According to religious tradition, a temple's large door was turned toward the rising sun and often remained the only source of light for the interior. Many temples, including the one located at Epidaurus, had a porch leading to the inner room. This chamber or *cella* featured a statue of the god facing the entrance. Cult images in ancient Greece were normally made of wood, but ivory or marble figures were also used. Perceived color changes of these images could be interpreted as important omens. Asclepius was usually depicted as a middle-aged, bearded man wearing an ankle-length tunic slung across the left shoulder, barefoot or clad in sandals. Gazing up, his expression was grave but serene, his body often leaning on a snake-entwined staff or walking stick used by Greek travelers or diviners. The sacred serpent, a harmless and widely distributed species, reflected the god's mystical link with the earth, although numerous symbolic interpretations connected this animal with qualities of wisdom, shrewdness, divination and prophecy, rejuvenation, rebirth, or restoration.[33] At Epidaurus, the statue of Asclepius, perhaps made of ivory and gold, depicted the god sitting on a seat grasping his staff, his other hand above the head of the serpent, with the figure of a dog lying by his side. Finally, the room also displayed a number of tables or *trapezai*, used to collect and exhibit food offered to the gods.

Another prominent feature was the altar, located in the open air, opposite the temple entrance and often in front of a temple door. This was the usual locus of sacrifice and death, next to a burning fire and with a perforated offering table that allowed sacrificed blood or donated wine to seep into the ground. In ancient Greece, a temple's reputation, especially in this instance the efficacy of its divinity's healing powers, was based not only on its antiquity but also on the nature and quality of its votive offerings. A number of *stelae* or plaques scattered around the temple area commemorated miraculous cures.

The other key building was the *abaton*, reserved for those visitors who wished to remain and sleep on the premises. Often this feature could simply be a long, narrow building with an open portico supported by columns and oriented toward the south. In some temples, this arcade was not available and supplicants simply lay on the ground, either in the open air close to the temple or in the temple itself. At Epidaurus, the *abaton* was apparently located near a sacred well, adjoining a bath house to the east. As various temples began to stage more elaborate and extended festivals in later centuries, separate guest lodgings located inside or outside the sacred enclosure were erected. Some of them were temporary structures also employed by priests. During Aristides' lifetime, Antoninus Pius erected a permanent building at Epidaurus that allowed women in childbirth and the dying to be housed beyond the sacred precinct. The huge hostel is said to have contained about 180 rooms in its four courts. Epidaurus also is said to have featured a stadium and gymnasium, as well as a banqueting hall for special use during festivals. At Pergamon, a separate open-air auditorium or theater built into the hillside provided seating space for thousands of spectators.[34]

Also at Epidaurus, the Asclepieion had a circular peristyle structure called a *tholos*, a beautiful building with a conical roof and subterranean passages. This prominent feature of the temple complex had six concentric platforms for spectators and at the bottom a central pit, perhaps the source of a sacred spring where visitors bathed. Pausanias reported the presence of testimonial plaques describing divine cures. The ritual purpose of the tholos remains obscure, but it could have been another locus for ritual purification and sacrifice, even perhaps a mock grave or cenotaph for Asclepius himself, celebrated as a chthonic hero.[35]

At first, the baths were merely an adjunct to the temple, reserved for the preliminary purification. Over time, however, they underwent a significant process of expansion and elaboration, with the construction of several pools and artificially heated rooms creating a sauna-type setting. At Epidaurus, facilities for communal hot and cold bathing became available to all visitors. This transformation into spas during the Roman empire went along with the celebration of multiple festivals and athletic events. By the time of Augustus' reign, more than 300 temples dedicated to Asclepius existed throughout the Roman empire, impressive testimony to the god's popularity in the Mediterranean world and beyond.[36]

Temple healing: Ideology and patronage

From the ninth century BC on, Greek civilization became a "temple culture," establishing places of cultural identity and prestige in which citizens could interact with the divine. As dwellings of gods and goddesses with various attributes, temples became spaces organized around a set of religious principles and beliefs. As in other contemporary cultures, religion was inextricably linked to everyday life in ancient Greece.[37] Eschewing a central orthodoxy, numerous ubiquitous gods protected all human activities and provided for particular needs, including health. All important transactions, both public and private, needed religious sanction and propitiation. This also meant harnessing divine power and creating an orderly system of communication with the divine to ensure a measure of social and emotional stability. Temples can be seen as social systems facilitating communion as well as bestowing meaning upon human events, including suffering, illness, and death.

Although intimately connected with the Greek polis structure, temples celebrated the supernatural. Access to the divine world occurred through oracles, prophecy, and divination, thus creating a reassuring channel of communication frequently sought in times of personal and communal difficulties, especially during crises.[38] Religious activities were usually organized by groups, either a family, residential district, professional organization, or the city itself, with full participation reserved for its citizens.[39] Individual cults competed for status and resources. Most temples were built on polis land by a decree and under the supervision of the city-state, although private initiatives (as in the case of the Asclepieion in

Athens) were also possible.[40] Different poleis worshipped the same gods but structured their cults according to local myths, traditions, and practices. At any rate, private worshippers provided most of the support for the cults. Later, powerful patrons such as Alexander the Great made some donations to Epidaurus. Thus, temples became distinctive and prestigious religious centers, symbols of city political and economic power. This association linked them to the fortunes of their patrons and to ancient Greece in general, extending well into the Hellenistic period and the time of Roman conquest.[41]

Ancient Greeks made clear distinctions between the divine and human realms. Numerous communications with the divine were carried out through the performance of religious rituals. As in other cultures, Greek religion constituted a key social ordering principle concerned with basic existential needs.[42] By the fifth century BC, it is said that Greece witnessed a gradual decline in the traditional civic religions with their community-oriented rites and festivals. In response to rising individualism, particular citizens began searching for cults offering spiritual comfort for their own anxieties. This apparent shift led to the growing popularity of divinities whose attributes could be crafted in such a way that these gods could better respond to personal feelings and needs. Among the gods, then, a particular worship of Asclepius could have provided challenges to the traditional polis-centered religion. Other gods of the Greek pantheon, notably Apollo, had been endowed with certain healing powers, but these abilities were now concentrated on one particular deity. Visiting Asclepius, therefore, seemed to open up the exciting prospect of a face-to-face encounter with a god within the sacred enclosure of his own temple.[43]

The Asclepieion at Epidaurus became a pan-Hellenic and eventually an international institution of worship, the destination of countless visitors, who enriched the city's reputation as well as its coffers. Since Asclepius was not perceived as a politically oriented deity, his wide appeal was probably never in question.[44] He was frequently worshipped for preserving the health of an individual supplicant, his family, and even an entire community or city. In the fourth century BC, the town sent out representatives or ambassadors to central and northern Greece, Macedonia, Thrace, Sicily, and Italy for the purpose of promoting the cult and collecting funds to improve the sanctuary. Whether these actions were solely expressions of religious devotion or also deliberate planning by a self-interested Epidauran priesthood remains unknown. Temples were not self-sufficient institutions; they were expensive to run and depended on the donations of worshippers.

As life expectancy dropped in the fourth century BC and as growing inequality in income increased the morbidity and mortality of the poorer sectors of the Greek population, awareness of health matters must have increased. Perhaps for the first time, sickness and its cure were now identified as legitimate and self-contained areas of a divine and professional domain. In an effort to expand their healing options, which ranged from divine intercessions by Apollo, opinions of healer seers, magicians, surgeons, athletic trainers, and herbalists, the ancient Greeks may also have targeted human disabilities as the proper concern of a former healer turned hero and now a major deity: Asclepius. Thus, Asclepian healing could have become an important option for ordinary sufferers in antiquity.[45] The simultaneous rise of the cult of Asclepius and the Hippocratic craftsmen may thus be seen as products of new attitudes toward both suffering and recovery from illness. Whether the cult of Asclepius preceded the new concerns or was simply the result of such changes in attitude is difficult to establish.[46]

Possible linkages between new Greek health concerns, demographic shifts, warfare, and changes in the contemporary ecology of disease are not too farfetched. Between the ninth and fifth centuries BC, the country's topography and infrequent land communications had probably kept the various regions fairly isolated from one another, thus preventing the rapid transmission of epidemic disease. However, population growth and gradual urbanization not only increased the complexity of ancient Greek society but also created ideal conditions for additional disease burdens, injury, and death. Given the nature of the terrain, agricultural expansion remained limited, and with the lack of adequate distribution networks, recurrent food shortages occurred because of lower yields both in Greece and in other areas of the Mediterranean. Greater population density and its corollary increase in contagious diseases, both respiratory and gastrointestinal, must have adversely impacted the urban centers. At this time, the emergence of tertian and quartan malaria in low-lying coastal areas may also have begun as the transmitting African mosquito vectors (anopheles) became established.[47] From the available evidence, the average life expectancy of Greeks between 650 and 150 BC was about 38 years.

By the fifth century BC, hints of an increased burden of disease in Periclean Athens and beyond are numerous. Here, population growth outstripping the countryside's agricultural resources may have been especially significant. A decline in life expectancy in the densely populated areas of Attica was a distinct possibility, due perhaps to a combination of war, famine, and disease. An obvious example was the dramatic epidemic in Athens in the 420s BC immortalized by Thucydides. This episode generated panic among the local population, which tried very hard to appease Apollo, who was blamed for having sent the scourge.[48] At the port of Piraeus, an early epidemic beachhead, the incidence of infection could also have been high. In response, the Greeks worshipped their established gods, including Athena and Hygieia at the Acropolis, but whether the arrival of Asclepius in both locations coincided with these epidemic outbreaks is unclear. During the next century, however, increased civil strife and earlier changes in labor manpower (including slavery) allegedly caused significant social dislocations, unemployment, and homelessness. While numerous epidemics swept over the peninsula, an extensive network of small sanctuaries dedicated to Asclepius and his healing family emerged throughout Attica.[49]

Not surprisingly, given his status as a powerful healer, Asclepius—according to Plato—became the patron hero of wandering, healing craftsmen—also identified as Hippocratic physicians based on the fame of one of them, Hippocrates of Cos, who practiced their art. The term *Asclepiads*, or fictive "sons or servants of Asclepius"—already common after 500 BC—must have lent prestige and identity to such lay practitioners (*iatroi*) and should not be interpreted as a priest-physician designation.[50] There were no overt signs of competition between the practices of the new "Hippocratics" and the healing taking place in an Asclepieion. Although their authority as healers was a function of personal knowledge and skill, their formal linkage to a divine power could have only expanded their appeal among the pious living in ancient Greece's polytheistic society. Indeed, in Athens, the *iatroi* regularly came together to worship and made sacrifices to Asclepius.[51] Diseases were considered divine insofar as they were caused by nature, including the weather and earthly exhalations, a proposition accepted by philosophers and lay healers alike. Hippocratic writers did not renounce this concept either. Among their rational tenets, it was widely accepted that because the medical art dealt with changes of a divine nature, it was similarly a gift of the gods. Even plant remedies were characterized as "the hands of the gods" and thus were seen as elements acting within a divine system of nature.[52]

Like other contemporary deities, Asclepius gave meaning to suffering and made efforts to rid supplicants of their anguish. As in Aristides' case, simple prayer to the gods was certainly considered a valid recourse and perhaps a less costly substitute for a temple visit. The prospect of a pilgrimage to an Asclepian shrine and establishment of a relationship with the god, however, provided an even stronger impetus for achieving a cure.[53] The adventures of travel and arrival in the sacred precinct heightened hope. Fueling the visitors' expectations were the temple's inscriptions and testimonials. Sacrifices, ceremonies, and at last incubation contributed to anticipation and self-reflection. Contact with the divine, and the god's commands or recommendations for restoring function and well-being, provided additional healing power. Finally, personal narratives of successful outcomes were important sources for achieving trust and faith in the power of the healing god. In ancient Greece, divine dreams and their interpretations were considered legitimate forms of acquiring knowledge, both for Hippocratics and for devotees of Asclepius.[54] Human medicine was limited, and its practitioners were conscious of their potential for iatrogenicity as they tried to relieve suffering. There was a widespread expectation shared by the healing craftsmen and the public at large that incurable patients should seek help from the gods for their illnesses. In fact, an early prognosis became an important action in establishing a reputation.

This issue prompts a consideration of the healing hierarchy in ancient Greece, a topic of great obscurity. As in other cultures, Greek domestic ideology stressed family care as a labor of love, presumably including responses to illness. Such informal activities were almost always carried out by the women living in a household, who provided emotional support and nursing care, perhaps supplemented by consultations with friends and neighbors. Additional counsel could have been sought from itinerant diviners, herbalists or "root cutters," midwives, gymnastic trainers, and Hippocratic healing craftsmen. There is even evidence of patient visits to physicians' homes or *iatreia* for further advice. These *iatreia* resembled other Greek homes in featuring a number of guest rooms. Some appear to have been outfitted for consultations or even surgical procedures. It is conceivable that at times the established healing craftsmen may have followed the practice of normal Greek hospitality, temporarily assigning rooms to their guest-patients while continuing to administer certain treatments or monitoring convalescence.

Staging temple rituals

In Greek temples, the reigning god—in this case Asclepius—was master of the house or *temenos*. Local political organizations and their elected officials, however, were usually in charge of the temple's administration, funds, and buildings. Sacred enclosures provided refuge and even asylum from persecution. The principal elements of a Greek cult were prayer, sacrifice, and setting up votives.[55] A wide cross section of the Greek citizenry came to the Asclepieion, including children accompanied by their parents. In surviving testimonial plaques, women predominate slightly over men. A traditional taboo prohibited birth and death—regarded as impure—from taking place on the premises. Reasons for a temple visit ranged from petitioning to prevent illness and giving thanks for continued good health to, most frequently, seeking a cure for disease or disability. A brief examination of the surviving testimonials reveals that visitors suffered from a great variety of illnesses, from trivial headaches and worms to crippling injuries, paralyses, infertility, and even blindness.[56] Greek temples were open to the public only during regularly scheduled sacrifices and special annual festivals. At that time, everyone was allowed to "come to" and "turn to" the gods. The supplicants, some after extensive travel, entered through the gates and usually said a prayer at the *propylon*.

Once in the compound, newcomers went through a series of preliminary preparations designed to ensure their *katharoes*, or moral and physical purity, before approaching the divine. An Epidauran inscription quoted by the writer Porphyry suggested that "pure must be he who enters the fragrant temple; purity means to think nothing but holy thoughts."[57] Rules and ceremonies varied somewhat both in time and in place. Those who entered the precinct were provided access to the temple's sacred well, where ceremonial ablution or bathing was accompanied by purification rituals that included the use of brimstone and laurel.[58] This was sometimes followed by a change of dress to a white garment that symbolically identified the wearer as qualified to participate in religious ceremonies. During festivals, visitors were provided with special clothes for public processions. The worshippers usually proceeded to the sacred locus of the temple early in the morning and faced the rising sun. Many forms of worship took place outdoors at altars in front of the temple. Prayers were integral parts of the liturgy, usually structured and divided into three parts, including an invocation of the god, offer of a gift by the person making the prayer, and finally the request itself. In certain instances, the statue of the god could also be touched.

Sacrifice was central in all Greek religious cults. It usually took the form of animal killings followed by an ensuing ritual meal. At the Asclepieion, purified visitors usually made preliminary sacrifices or offerings to the god in the form of honey or cheese cakes, loaves of bread, roasted meats, and fruits laid upon the table before the god's image in the temple. Animals to be sacrificed were sometimes led to the god's image before ritual slaughter. Some of their parts were burned on the sacred fire, and the remaining meat was placed on tables to be consumed later within the sanctuary or perhaps served in adjoining banquet halls.[59] Sacrifices of cocks or roosters (identified with dawn) were traditional. For a person who woke up feeling cured in the morning after having dreamed of Asclepius, this was a relatively inexpensive and appropriate gift.[60]

Some of the ceremonies took place in the temple itself, which was opened each morning to let the visitors in. "Now the day is breaking and more people are crowding in, . . . for the door is now open and the curtain has gone up," wrote the poet Herondas at the Asclepieion of Cos.[61] The curtain he referred to was part of the elaborate daily ritual performed by the priests to awaken the statues, pull the veils hiding their faces, and feed them. Each night, the gods were then veiled again and put to sleep. At Pergamon, the destination point of Aelius Aristides, regular services were held among the priests in the morning and evening before the temple was opened to worshippers and incubants. The priesthood (a chief priest and several assistants) was primarily recruited from among members of wealthy families, often linked to the local civil administration. Physicians were seldom found among the priests. Additional grounds-keeping duties were performed by young boys hired to light and maintain the altar fires and bear incense.

Barefoot supplicants entered the temple wearing white robes without rings or belts. Here they said their vows, combining petition and thanksgiving. Special hymns were sung in praise of the divinity by the visitors and sometimes by a temple choir. Visitors knelt before the god's statue; others read the marble tablets mostly located outdoors and inscribed with testimonials of previous divine cures. Displaying permanent gifts or *anathemata* from grateful visitors was a very old practice in ancient Greece. These exhibits were intended to impress the visitors further and strengthen their faith in the healing abilities of Asclepius. At Epidaurus, accounts of miraculous cures from earlier centuries survived as testimonials to divine power. Recorded in the third person and inscribed on stelae of stone or *iamata*, these personal experiences were written in prose or poetry and simply provided the names of the cured individuals, their places of birth, and the popular diagnoses or descriptions of the afflicted body parts, as well as Asclepius' successful healing procedures.[62]

Perhaps the goal of a temple visit was to forge a state of Aristotelian "catharsis" whereby rituals containing melodies and dances could ameliorate the anxiety and depression of the afflicted.[63] Individual visitors formulated their healing requests and promised some act of gratitude or gift in return. Some cures may have occurred in the sanctuary itself without recourse to incubation. Most petitioners, however, patiently waited until the evening to be summoned by priests to the *abaton*. At most temples dedicated to Asclepius, guests such as Aristides walked at twilight to this "sacred dormitory," where priests assigned each of them a pallet, sometimes stone divans called *klinai* covered with animal skins. Following another prayer by the supplicants, the priests demanded silence, put out the lamps, and departed. A mixture of physical exhaustion from the voyage and the ceremony must have conflicted with the heightened state of mental excitement and anticipation generated by the dramatic temple rituals.

Divination is one of the oldest practices of humankind. Like other cultures before them, the ancient Greeks placed great importance on the value of prophecies and oracles. Traditionally, Greeks had sought advice and solace by sleeping in a place considered sacred because of its association with chthonic powers and heroes. Messages received during sleep or drowsiness were said to have true prognostic value and were treated the same way as other cognitive processes in reaching decisions and charting one's future plans.[64] From Hippocrates to Galen, ancient physicians also accepted the legitimacy of dreams for their diagnostic and prognostic efforts. In fact, Galen even admitted that a vision of Asclepius was responsible not only for many diagnoses, but also for his choice of a medical career.[65] However, not all dreams were deemed equally important. Those reflecting routine thoughts and actions had no value, while others were considered to have been merely caused by food and drink and the resulting humoral imbalances. The real prognostications of the soul were linked to god-sent dreams such as those experienced in an Asclepieion.

For Artemidorus of Daldis, a near-contemporary of Aelius Aristides and Galen, for example, "dream prescriptions of the gods are on the whole simple and without riddles. Indeed, whenever the gods prescribe salves, poultices, foods or drinks, they employ the same names that we are in the custom of using."[66] In fact, divine prescriptions were always linked to prevailing medical theories and practices. The stuff of healing dreams reflected familiar ancient healing wisdom, including dietary advice, surgical interventions, and the administration of certain drugs. Physical measures such as bathing and bloodletting seemed to be common. Indeed, many of the recorded cures were traditional Greek folk practices also employed by Hippocratic craftsmen. Dreams functioned either as cures themselves or as agents for these cures. Riddles or puns were often an essential part of dreams in need of interpretation before a cure could take place. Thus, many of Asclepius' cryptic messages often required the assistance of the temple priests. Some assistants apparently expanded on the divine prescriptions, adding further items to the proposed curative regimen.[67]

In the temple's *abaton*, the anxiously awaited event was this face-to-face encounter in dreamland with an approachable, kindly deity. Dressed in his robe and holding a staff, or accompanied by a snake or dog, Asclepius would make personal visits. Since both animals were alternate forms of the god's epiphany, dogs and snakes played important healing roles. Petitioners often reported being touched by the tongues of snakes and dogs instead of seeing the god personally. In Aristophanes' comedy *Plutus*, one man had his sight restored by two snakes, which appeared from the depths of the temple and licked his eyes.

In most respects, however, the god was expected to behave like any other contemporary healing craftsman, only operating more decisively and competently. First, he would ask questions, then give guidance or advice, and end with a reassuring prognosis. As always, all such epiphanies were shaped by the dreamer's own expectations, and the authoritative answers could themselves be therapeutic, diminishing the incubant's anxiety and uncertainty. The dream became the central vehicle of communication between the divine and human realms. Some individuals dreamed that they were physically touched or even operated on. Many cures were instant and wondrous. At times, the recommended remedies needed to be initiated or continued after departure from the temple. According to Galen, Asclepius not infrequently also asked supplicants to compose odes, comic skits, or songs. These were designed to correct the *ametria* or imbalance of their emotions.

Miracles were expected, but whether Asclepius always came through is unknown.[68] All mystery cults promised their initiated a form of rebirth, a new life, or a way to overcome suffering and death.[69] Asclepius' precincts were destinations for the worried, anxious, and sickly. Temple rituals stressed the importance of faith and emotion in healing. Every vision was a mystery, shaped by the supplicant's expectations and framed by previous sickness experiences and familiarity with healing strategies. Sufferers remained the most important partners in this temple curing. For each visitor, the key was to find the meaning of one's own anguish and to discover one's future fate through divine contact.[70] Admitted skeptics and doubters were sometimes punished by the god, who demanded unconditional trust. The available, albeit fragmentary, evidence suggests that temple healing displayed great similarity with prevailing domestic and medical routines. In Aristophanes' *Plutus*, Asclepius was to be garbed as a physician and portrayed with mortar, pestle, and a box while preparing a plaster with hot spices and vinegar to be applied to the eyes of one of the supplicants. In fact, Asclepius' ability to function as a contemporary healing craftsman of unusual power and ability distinguished him from other gods and their miraculous cures.[71]

As time went on, recorded dreams, explanations of Asclepius' epiphanies, and the range of his advice appeared to become more comprehensive and detailed. Many fourth-century BC inscriptions at Epidaurus seemed miraculous advertisements. The lame, blind, and deaf gratefully and unquestionably placed themselves in the hands of this all-powerful god. During Hellenistic times, Asclepius appears to have been increasingly asked for specific medical and surgical advice. Perhaps this occurred because more informed and perhaps more assertive supplicants such as Aristides considered a temple visit as a sort of second medical opinion. Asclepius responded by widening the range of his recommendations, further articulated and recorded by an expanding priesthood. Perhaps such a redefinition of boundaries between the divine and human worlds followed efforts to place pagan gods into specialized categories and expose their oracles to competition with other types of explanations.[72] By the time Aristides consulted the god, Asclepius had become for some the supreme and most trusted advisor. He was frequently consulted about matters of personal behavior and vocation, diet, and physical fitness, including bathing, as well as strictly medical treatments.[73]

One illustrative example of this broader role played by Asclepius is recorded in an inscription left at Epidaurus by another Roman visitor, Julius Apellas of Idrias, who apparently suffered from indigestion and went to visit the god at the temple. In this particular case, Asclepius ordered the man to rinse his sore throat with cold water and use anise oil for headaches. Moreover, he was to drink lemonade and protect his head for two days since it was raining. For a beverage, Asclepius ordered milk with honey to create a laxative effect while also prescribing a vegetarian diet consisting of bread, cheese, parsley, and lettuce. In addition, Apellas was told by Asclepius to walk barefoot around the temple's upper colonnade, exercise vigorously (including on a swing), use hot water baths enriched with wine, and, for a drachma, get body rubs of mustard and salt from an attendant. This prescribed treatment apparently went on for days, inside and outside the sanctuary, and was to be combined with sacrifices by the patient to Asclepius, his wife, and the Eleusian gods.[74]

Following the divine consultation or cure, supplicants who had not done so previously were encouraged to offer a sacrifice or make a number of dedications, a donation sometimes suggested by the god himself during the healing dream. In Aelius Aristides' times, but perhaps much earlier, the priesthood switched from gift items to cash, imposed directly on supplicants at the sanctuary. Other, more affluent and grateful visitors gave cocks and pigs, coins and jewelry, ceremonial vases and clothing. Those with even more resources commissioned or purchased statuettes, plaques, and so-called votive offerings, often prominently displayed together with the plaques. In time, many of the donated objects made of precious metals were melted and recast into elaborate cult furnishings or sold by the priests to obtain further endowment funds for the maintenance of the sanctuary.

Usually inscribed with the name of the donor, most *ex-voto* figurines were separate body parts. Eyes, ears, hands, legs, feet, and genitalia were particularly popular, suggesting that perhaps they were the presumed loci of a disability cured by Asclepius. These objects, however, made of terra-cotta, ivory, bronze, gold, or silver, rarely depicted evidence of disease. They could well have represented the normal human shape expected by the supplicant after divine intervention. Older pieces could be buried. All donated items had to be carefully inventoried and stored in treasuries, thus keeping a number of assistants and accountants busy. Many of the gifts seemed to have been available for purchase in a wide range of quality and quantity at stalls surrounding the shrine.[75]

In addition to the regular sacrifices and ceremonies, temples also organized major yearly festivals—called the *Asclepieia*—for large groups of people at important temple sites in the ancient world. These celebrations were apparently great public occasions focusing on the central performance of a sacrifice at an open-air altar in full view of the participating crowds. At Athens, a statue of Asclepius was carried from the center of the city to the temple at the acropolis. At Epidaurus, celebrations seem to have been scheduled for nine days in late April after the conclusion of the festival of Poseidon at the Isthmus of Corinth. The visitors assembled in town and, together with local residents, marched in solemn procession to the sanctuary carrying their sacrificial animals.

Following some purification ceremonies, hymns were sung, and the priests usually sacrificed a bull to Asclepius. The crowds then attended theatrical performances, musical contests, and athletic games. They temporarily occupied lodging houses located outside the sacred gates. At Pergamon, the religious calendar was marked by three great annual festivals during which poetic contests and nightly vigils took place in honor of the god. Visitors also listened to laudatory speeches extolling the god's many virtues. These expansions of religious ritual during Hellenistic times and later in imperial Rome may have demanded staff increases to service an ever broader range of functions. One example was the appointment of Galen as surgeon of gladiators performing at the Asclepieion of Pergamon, a position he held early in his medical career. Others identified there at the time of Aelius Aristides were two wardens, a herald, door keeper, custodian of keys, and bath attendant, as well as a chorus responsible for singing the ritual hymns.

Aristides' healing dreams

When Aelius Aristides and his foster father, Zosimus, journeyed to the Asclepieion of Pergamon, this temple had apparently regained some of its former splendor and popularity. Two centuries earlier, Pergamon had been the capital of the Attalid empire, a city endowed with a magnificent acropolis and library. However, subsequent political and cultural developments had led to the city's stagnation, a development bound to affect the cult of Asclepius. Under the Flavian emperors, however, the healing god supposedly began to stage a gradual comeback as the "Pergamene god," and there are suggestions that his sanctuary was significantly refurbished and expanded thanks to a number of donations by Roman noblemen during Hadrian's rule. By this time, gods and goddesses perceived to be sympathetic to the needs of individuals, whether Greek or Egyptian, were increasing in public favor. This apparent popularity possibly cut across social classes and may have prompted the programs of temple repair and expansion.

As in Epidaurus, the enclosure was linked with the nearby city along a sacred way, and access to the complex was possible only through a grandiose marble *propylon* flanked on one side by a library containing a statue of the deified Emperor Hadrian. The principal buildings were arranged along the east side of a large rectangular plaza closed on the other three sides by colonnades. A small theater was joined to the outside of the northern colonnade, with a suite of flushing latrines to the south. The central temple, recently completed by a friend of Aristides, the consul Rufinus, was dedicated to Asclepius. It was an impressive circular building, probably with a domed cupola—similar to the Pantheon in Rome—with connections to the sacred well sought for ritual bathing. Instead of using a separate *abaton*, incubants apparently slept in alcoves located in the shrine itself, which had quadrangular and semicircular niches around a statue of the god. In addition to some stelae depicting healing testimonials, the Pergamene temple featured dedicatory inscriptions by members of the provincial Roman elite who were keen to have their names in close proximity to the powerful divinity. At the western end of the central court stood a theater that could accommodate a few thousand spectators. Three separate wells served the entire enclosure. Temple visitors generally must have stayed in accommodations available nearby in the city.[76]

As at other shrines, regular temple services in Pergamon were held twice a day, in the morning and evening, at which time the sacred lamps were lit. As darkness enveloped the compound, both Aristides and Zosimus were conducted into the temple for their expected epiphany. After the warden extinguished the lights, the supplicants were left alone. On the first night, Asclepius appeared only to Zosimus, speaking through a family friend, the consul Salvius, not an uncommon event. Advised through a proxy, Aristides reported that the god "gave me medicines, of which the first was, as I remember, the sap of balsam. I had to use it while bathing and going from the warm water to the cold. Next there was soap mixed both with raisins and other things." The Hippocratics had already stressed the important role that pure drinking water and baths played in health,[77] and the Roman bathing practices had been woven into the rational therapeutics recommended by Galen and other medical authors.[78]

After this first encounter with the deity through Zosimus' dream, Aristides decided to continue bathing in the nearby river. Because of his status and family connections, and the fact that he owned no property in the city of Pergamon, Aristides was invited to remain within the temple complex, living in the house of one of the wardens, aptly named Julius Asclepiacus. His symptoms, however, apparently remained unchanged: "I had catarrhs and difficulty with my palate, and everything was full of frost and fire, and my stomach trouble was at its peak," he confided, describing the suffering that forced him to remain indoors throughout the summer.[79] Faced with this turn of events, Aristides sought further advice. A new dream startled him: "First he [Asclepius] commanded that I have blood drawn from my elbow," possibly up to 60 pints.[80] Whatever the actual amount, this divine instruction seemed to astonish even the veteran temple wardens, who admitted that they had never witnessed a recommendation for such an extensive series of phlebotomies.[81]

While Aristides proceeded to comply with Asclepius' bloodletting orders, probably with the aid of a physician, the next divine command insisted that part of the blood should be drawn from the forehead, an order also given to another incubant, a Roman senator. Coupled with the bloodletting, Asclepius told Aristides to take a bath in the Caicus River, located at some distance from the sacred precinct. This prescription was successful. Aristides commented afterward that "the comfort and relaxation which ensued was very easy for a god to understand but not at all easy for a man to conceive of or write about."[82]

An affluent landowner, Aristides apparently stayed at the Asclepieion of Pergamon for the next two years, calling this period of his life a "time of inactivity" during which he persevered in his allegiance to Asclepius and trained his willpower so as to comply with all divine commands. Perhaps the Asclepieion at Pergamon provided respite from the presumed stresses of everyday life to a select population composed of a coterie of politicians, philosophers, poets, and aristocrats. In a more relaxed, spa-like atmosphere, the baths, theatrical performances, concerts, and athletic games may have provided needed distraction.[83] After six months of care that also included poultices and drug prescriptions popular at the time, Aristides complained that "my body was remarkably weak so that for a long time I did not at all leave the room where I lay."[84] In spite of his prostration, the god continued to test the orator's stamina, ordering him to bathe three times in the river flowing through the city. To the consternation of new friends who insisted on accompanying him, Aristides set out on a stormy, rainy day, reaching the flooded river banks with his party. Tossed around in the churning water and battered by debris, he searched for calmer waters behind some rocks. As he emerged from the current, he felt warm and much improved: "much steam rose up, and I was red all over."[85] Commenting later on another bath ordered by Asclepius in the sea at Elea, the port of Pergamon, Aristides admitted that "I know that such things have been prescribed for many people. But first of all, in itself, the action of the god is rather wonderful, since he often and frequently revealed his power and providence."[86]

Throughout the ordeal, the orator's compliance with divine advice demonstrates the key role played by water as a religious symbol and a traditional therapeutic tool. His dreams provided successive suggestions for purifying baths in rivers, wells, and the ocean, as well as abstinence from warm baths and unreasonable exercise in summer.[87] Other divine recommendations transmitted through dreams were dietary and medicinal, thus imitating the traditional restorative regimen prescribed by contemporary practitioners associated with nearby thermal baths, including those in Smyrna.[88] The advice ranged from enemas, vomiting, and purging to bloodletting and dietary restrictions. Mental stimulation could be obtained through attendance at games and theatrical functions at the temple complex.

Before arriving at the Asclepieion, Aristides had evidently given up the study of rhetoric because of his physical discomfort and mental depression. After residing for a few months at the temple, however, he received another divine summons to return to his work and promptly complied by giving a number of speeches at the temple's theater.[89] Moreover, at that time, "Asclepius the Savior also commanded us to spend time on songs and lyric verse and to relax and maintain a chorus of boys. There would be no end of saying how many other things we also enjoyed from this advice, for high spirits and self-sufficiency. But the children sang my songs, and whenever I happened to choke, if my throat were suddenly constricted, or my stomach became disordered, or whenever I had some other troublesome attack, the doctor Theodotus, being in attendance and remembering my dreams, would order the boys to sing some of my lyric verse. And while they were singing, there arose unnoticed a feeling of comfort, and sometimes everything which pained me went completely away."[90]

Soon Aristides took his choral group to public performances staged in honor of Asclepius within the sacred precinct. These occurred especially during the great festivals, scheduled for January, March, and especially August, when games, poetic contests, and nightly vigils kept the temple crowds entertained. However, Aristides' stay at the Asclepieion consisted of periods of relative well-being and high spirits marred by periods of physical infirmity and despondency. As another winter season returned, he described once more his many sufferings. For days and nights "the flow from my head and the turmoil in my chest continued," and his breath "caught in my throat and seared." Bedeviled by headaches, he could not keep any food down and finally despaired: "my expectation of death was always so great that I did not even have the courage to call my servant." Confined to bed, unable to rise, and wrapped in woolen blankets, Aristides spent days in a closed room: "day was equal to night and the nights were sleepless instead of the days."[91]

In his diary, Aristides portrayed himself as Odysseus, a pilgrim on a journey of self-discovery, learning to deal with his physical frailties under the divine tutelage of the most powerful of gods, Asclepius. His personal relationship with the deity had grown strong, and he now followed unconditionally the advice provided by his savior in dreams, even if the recommendations were questioned by Aristides' own medical consultants. For him there was clearly no real choice between listening to physicians or to his god. One of his contemporaries, the famous physician Galen, had observed similar instances of this strong healer–patient bonding and compliance while working at the temple: "Even among ourselves in Pergamon we see that those who are being treated by the god obey him when on many occasions he bids them not to drink at all for fifteen days, while they obey none of the physicians who give this prescription. For it has great influence on the patient's doing all which is prescribed if he has been firmly persuaded that a remarkable benefit to himself will ensue."[92] Despite his periodic sufferings and anguish, Aristides remained devoted to Asclepius and the miraculous prescriptions. Following an exhaustive regimen of baths, diet, and exercise, he tried to increase his bodily strength while regaining his confidence as a poet and public speaker. In a telling passage of the *Sacred Tales*, he observed that whenever the god prescribed a regimen, it "brought to my body and to my spirit salvation, strength, comfort, ease, high spirits, and every good thing."[93]

If Aristides had initially sought out Asclepius for unbiased medical advice in the midst of conflicting and discredited medical recommendations, subsequent events suggest that the extended stay in Pergamon's healing temple facilitated the development of a close personal relationship between them. Unlike the more commonly known one- or two-night stay in an *abaton*, believed to be characteristic of the cult in ancient Greece and in Hellenistic times, our visitor remained in the sacred precinct for years, not only pursuing physical health but also acquiring insight and meaning concerning his life as an orator and a human being. If Aristides was indeed a true representative of people belonging to the contemporary Roman ruling classes, the mystical experiences so vividly portrayed in the *Sacred Tales* demonstrate Asclepius' ascendancy to a position of supreme divinity, endowed with personal attributes and powers not unlike those of another, gradually competing god: Jesus Christ.

Of course, it remains to be seen whether Aristides' temple experiences were the exception or the rule. Individuals with far less threatening symptoms and anxious to settle simple lifestyle questions—should I walk barefoot or not?—now sought extensive and repeated advice while enjoying their stay in the temple complex. Indeed, Aristides appears to have moved effortlessly in a restricted circle of distinguished provincial Greeks and Romans, all passionate followers of the healing god, people who endowed the temples and immortalized their charitable proclivities on marble columns. Attending to the daily whims of these "pilgrims" was a small army of servants and retainers. Aristides also regularly consulted a physician, Theodotus, presumably living in the nearby city of Pergamon. This professional was used not only as another sounding board for dream interpretations, but also as an executor of the divine medical prescriptions.

After leaving Pergamon, Aristides seems to have traveled extensively through a number of Greek and Asia Minor cities and to Rome, presumably achieving the literary prominence that had eluded him earlier. Because of frequent chest colds during the next few years, he returned for short periods to the Pergamon sanctuary for further divine counsel. About a decade later, Aristides is said to have even paid a visit to the famous Asclepieion at Epidaurus. Most of his symptoms were respiratory until about the 160s AD, when he contracted an ailment then sweeping across the Roman empire from the east that may even have caused Galen's precipitate departure from Rome. Aristides' recovery, however, was followed by intestinal troubles. He eventually died on his estate in Asia Minor around 188 AD at age 63, allegedly of "consumption."[94]

Almost 80 years later, Asclepius' magnificent temple complex at Pergamon was destroyed by a powerful earthquake and never rebuilt. Indeed, with the rise of Christianity, the Greek god of healing became a direct competitor to Christ. Christians sought to discredit Asclepius by portraying him as evil.[95] Given their local character, financial insecurity, and discredited priesthood, Asclepian and other pagan temples became targets of the new religion. The cult was finally prohibited after 391 AD as Christianity became the official religion of the Roman empire and its temples were systematically destroyed. Their ruins in places such as Epidaurus and other sites gave way to Christian churches.

COLLECTIVE CARE OF SOLDIERS AND SLAVES: ROMAN VALETUDINARIA

The health of the army may be preserved by situation, water-supply, season, medicine, and exercise. It is the constant duty of senior officers, commanding officers, and generals to seek diligently that sick soldiers should be brought back to health by suitable food and cured by the skills of the doctors.

Flavius Vegetius (fl. 385 AD)[96]

A young warrior becomes ill

Several decades before Aelius Aristides' first visit to the Asclepieion of Pergamon, an enlisted marine fell ill on the warship *Neptune*. Part of the *Classis Augusta Alexandrina* or Alexandrian fleet, this vessel was temporarily anchored in the port of Alexandria with orders to sail for Syria. Indeed, Claudius Terentianus' illness may well have occurred in the summer of the year 115 AD, toward the end of Emperor Trajan's reign (96 BC–116 AD). Severe riots had broken out in Egypt under the governorship of Rutilius Lupus while the emperor was involved in his Parthian campaign. Trajan was completing his sweep of Mesopotamia, having conquered Nisibis and entered into an alliance with Abgar, prince of Osrhoene. At a time when the emperor needed every legionary to consolidate his Eastern provinces, Jewish revolts in Judea, Cyprus, and Cyrene perhaps lay at the root of the orders Terentianus received to proceed to Syria.[97]

Since the time of Augustus, the Roman emperors had assigned considerable value to the presence of an organized fleet in the eastern Mediterranean. After all, the *Mare Nostrum* was truly Rome's internal lake and an avenue for imperial expansion. Plied by a great variety of ships, it was the main route for commerce and communication with Asia Minor, Palestine, Egypt, and northern Africa, as well as Britain and northern Europe. Protecting these routes that linked the empire with Asia and India called for the establishment of several naval bases, including those at Misenum and Ravenna. The unfortunate side effect of such travel must have been to facilitate the transmission of human infections from one port to another, contributing to the spread of epidemics.[98]

Since Terentianus, like the bulk of the contemporary Roman armed forces, was illiterate, he hired a scribe who wrote in Latin to communicate his sudden illness to his father, Tiberianus. The old man seems also to have been a Roman official, perhaps still active in nearby Palestine. Somewhat apologetically, Terentianus discussed his ill-fated enlistment, which must have been quite recent. Although he had initially aspired to become a legionary, his application had been rejected by army recruiters based on an unsatisfactory report written by a certain Marcellus. Everybody at the time knew that, among the imperial armed forces, the Roman navy was an inferior service. Insisting that he in no way hated Marcellus for what he had done, Terentianus made it clear, however, that his enlistment in the Roman navy was hardly his first choice but merely—for his father's sake—an option to settle down, as he put it, "lest I seem to you to wander like a fugitive."[99]

While a military career loomed as an increasingly attractive option for idle young men from the provinces, the public at large continued to view imperial soldiers with a mixture of admiration and trepidation. The soldiers' growing professionalism generated a series of laudatory commentaries from the emperor, linking military readiness to the stability of the empire, a return to reason, and respect for human values. On the other hand, many civilians still influenced by the preimperial images of violence, rape, and looting, continued to portray soldiers as dangerous barbarians, prisoners of their desires, and a threat to public welfare.[100]

In a second letter to his father, written somewhat later, Terentianus complained that as he lay sick on board the ship, someone had stolen his assigned mattress and pillow. Angry and somewhat depressed, he demanded the assistance of his *pater familias* or household head in securing a transfer from the Roman navy to an army cohort. As he explained, "nothing will be accomplished without money and letters of recommendation will have no value unless a man helps himself."[101] We do not know the origins of our warrior's family, but evidence like this suggests that he may very well have belonged to the new middling classes joining the provincial bureaucracy and army under Trajan's rule. In Terentianus' time, the social level of the recruits was definitely higher than that of Republican army draftees a century earlier. Opportunities for upward mobility existed throughout the empire, in part due to a more sophisticated economy and relative peace. Elites living in many imperial cities had achieved public positions. A new cosmopolitanism once more mixed Greek and Latin cultural traits.

Rookies or *tirones* such as Terentianus who were just beginning their military careers were appalled by their spartan pay and multiple deductions. Moreover, navy infantrymen were among those at the bottom of the pay scale, but this fact failed to deter the recruits from overspending to retain the trappings of their previous social position. Besides reporting on his bad health, Terentianus' correspondence and that of other soldiers reveals their multiple requests to relatives for money and care packages containing supplementary food, clothing, and other amenities. In exchange, some of these enlisted men offered to send their generous kin exotic local trinkets, food, and spices.

In time, Terentianus' plea for a transfer apparently was effective, since he soon reported to Tiberianus that he had recovered his health and was now a legionary, transferred from his ship to a military camp outside the city of Alexandria. Perhaps money had undone what Marcellus' unfavorable letter of recommendation had accomplished earlier. In any event, he was now off the boat, out of the navy, and looking forward to better pay and higher status. Unfortunately, his troubles had only begun. Soon thereafter, he informed his father that a riot had broken out in the city and he was again ill, worried, and helpless: "my illness is at this moment no laughing matter, and it is even necessary that I be fed by someone else as you will hear when you come to the city"[102]

Terentianus' transfer coincided with the consolidation and organization of the Roman imperial army under Trajan. It now boasted close to 500,000 men, including some 180,000 legionaries forming 30 legions, with many enlisted provincials from places other than the Italian and Spanish peninsulas. Unlike earlier times, Roman armies were now stationed along permanently fixed and clearly delineated frontiers that divided the empire from its barbarian neighbors. Big frontier towns, fortified camps, and lines of fortifications commanded the emperor's concern. Popular with his troops, Trajan had paid particular attention to military organization, insisting on strict order and discipline. As under the Flavians, the Praetorian cohorts remained 10 in number, but alongside them appeared a special body of legionaries—Roman citizens—the *equites singulares Augusti*. Perhaps Terentianus was one of them.

Between the years 106 and 112 AD, shortly before our legionary's illness, Trajan had rounded off the frontier in the East, creating a new province of Arabia with its capital in Petra. By 115, a successful invasion of Armenia and upper Mesopotamia had ended with the capture of the Parthian capital.[103] Trajan, meanwhile, dealt with a revolt of Jews in a number of areas, including Mesopotamia and the island of Cyprus, finally losing control of his new Parthian province before dying suddenly of a stroke in the year 117. In a final letter, Terentianus disclosed the reason for his inability to depart for Syria: a "violent an attack of fish-poisoning made me ill, and I was unable for five days to write you anything, not to speak of going up to you."[104] Indeed, still debilitated from his latest illness, Terentianus was also slightly wounded as he helped put down a local disturbance, but his subsequent experiences in Alexandria or elsewhere were not recorded. We do not even know whether he was treated at the barracks by military physicians. Had Terentianus, however, been stationed at the empire's northern frontier, he could have been brought to a special military institution created to care for sick and wounded Roman soldiers: the *valetudinarium*.[105]

Building a new professional army

A number of historical circumstances had favored creation of the *valetudinarium*, a space designed for valetudinarians, or individuals deficient in *valetudo* or health. Before the time of Emperor Augustus (27 BC–14 AD), medical services for Roman soldiers were mostly ad hoc, temporary, and highly dependent on the individual generals in charge of the legions. The Republican army had been composed of conscripted citizens, whose high-risk activities could be handsomely rewarded by valuable booty. Military campaigns were short, and citizen armies promptly disbanded. However, even before the empire was created, a reputation for caring for warriors became an important attribute for effective military leadership. During their brief military careers, opportunity, uncertainty, and self-preservation must have been the lot of these conscripts. Most Roman soldiers were keenly aware of the health risks involved in their service, perhaps fearing illness more than battle injuries. If soldiers were disabled, their superiors arranged for transportation, medical care, and convalescence behind enemy lines. Those who were wounded could be treated on the field or in their tents, or, if in friendly territory, lodged in private houses or returned to their families for convalescence. This was still the case during the civil wars of Julius Caesar.

Under Caesar, the army had already become a highly efficient and professional body without, however, providing comprehensive medical services. In an effort to give encouragement and boost morale, Germanicus, for example, accompanied by his wife, Agrippina, made rounds visiting his troops at the base camp on the Rhine in 15 AD, making sure that dressings were provided to all the wounded. At times, the emperor or his subordinates paid for the so-called home care of injured soldiers forced to remain far from their families.

During Augustus' reign, dramatic changes occurred as the emperor established a new volunteer and professional army of about 400,000 men.[106] The imperial goal was to transform the military into a cohesive and permanent fighting force capable of defending the vast Roman frontiers that now extended from the Atlantic to the west, the Rhine and the Danube to the north, the Black Sea, Asia Minor, and Palestine to the east, and Egypt and North Africa to the south. At this point, the population of the Roman Empire was estimated at about 50–60 million people, with high birth and death rates and an average life expectancy at birth of 25 years.[107]

To ensure high levels of recruitment, the imperial authorities went to great lengths to make military life seem attractive. Traditional stereotypes of crude, violent, pillaging Roman warriors had to be erased. A new image of organization and discipline was projected. Downplaying the previous harshness and brutality of military life, the new army was portrayed as a civilizing influence and a protector of communities. Regular (albeit low) salaries, enrollment bonuses, and the opportunity to learn a trade were important incentives. Not only was military pay, the *stipendium*, standardized, but the period of service became fixed at a maximum of 20 years. In addition, soldiers were to receive medical care, a generous retirement grant, and free burial.

Not surprisingly, these benefits provided new recruits with a career security virtually unknown in contemporary civilian Roman life. Yet Roman soldiers like Terentianus were forbidden to marry, nor could they acquire land in the areas where they were garrisoned. Deductions for rations and an obligatory savings plan diminished the actual cash payments, making them lower than those of artisans and workers, although soldiers received periodic gratuities and imperial gifts. Previous specified bounties for veterans—sometimes in the form of land allotments—were partly abandoned in favor of cash awards, which were much more meaningful and eagerly welcomed by former urban soldiers. To enjoy the fruits of their retirement, members of the armed forces usually remained in the service as long as possible.

During the first century AD, the construction of a professional identity for imperial soldiers succeeded. Lofty rhetoric proclaimed that the military forces secured freedom for all citizens of the empire. Dedicated service to their supreme commander-in-chief—the soul of the world—was believed to be based on special personal qualities and skills that separated soldiers from the *paganus* or civilian.[108] In the end, the Roman army constituted an extraordinary mix of ethnic, national, and social groups unprecedented in civilian life. On average, professional soldiers were better educated and capable of accepting their role as defenders of the empire and its values. As always, issues of masculine identity, valor, sacrifice, and adventure must have combined with the more prosaic ones of companionship and financial security.

The development of a northern Roman frontier or *limes* beyond the Alps also occurred during the reign of Augustus as part of a gradual process of territorial consolidation. Initially, together with the Gaul region, Julius Caesar had brought the area near the Rhine under Roman control in 55–53 BC. However, the rivers Rhine and Danube were not true borders in terms of military defense. Although Rome's global concept of power and territory was based on natural boundaries, both rivers were perceived not as effective barriers but as important routes of access, transportation, and commerce.[109] For Rome, the *limes* were perceived to be zones of economic marginality, studded with small communities incapable of sustaining thousands of troops. This was especially a burden in the Danubian provinces. Since local markets were limited, food supplies had to be shipped to these outposts, leading to the development of social and commercial ties with populations beyond the frontier itself.

Thus, the Romans established legionary forts on great European rivers primarily for commercial and supply purposes, not for defense. This influx of provisions included cattle, horse, sheep, and iron imports from northern Germany. Within a few decades, an economically prosperous corridor developed on either side of this frontier led by a new native elite.[110] Following the imperial campaigns against the Germans across the Rhine and Danube rivers by Germanicus, the permanent stationing of legions on the frontier began under Emperor Tiberius (14–37 AD). In subsequent years, the original bases on the left bank of the Rhine were rebuilt and extended. The cold Central European winters demanded the establishment of semipermanent camps, forts, and depots at intervals along the northern borders of the empire. Preventive measures were taken to avoid unhealthy sites for this construction. Tiberius was praised for providing soldiers with food, baths, and even physicians.

Based on architectural designs proposed nearly half a century earlier by Vitruvius, the Romans went on to build a number of permanent fortresses—*castra stativa*—in Germany, Eastern Europe, and Scotland for the protection of their western and northern frontiers. This development continued unabated throughout the next century.[111]

By the time Claudius Terentianus was able to join the army, Rome had built numerous forts throughout the northern border of its empire and had established civilian towns in these regions populated by a mixture of Romans and local dwellers. Most of the forts in this network along the Danube River—Vindobona, Carnuntum, Brigetio in Upper Pannonia. Novae, Durostorum and Troesmis in Lower Moesia—were endowed with their own *valetudinarium*.[112] Thus, Rome, at the beginning of the second century AD, was busy building an extensive communications network and promoting commerce from the Lower Rhine to the Danube and the Black Sea. In the process, the old Greek coastal cities were revived and urban life, Greek in character, even developed inland as far as Moesia in central Europe. In the year 107, Thrace was also raised to the status of a Roman province, and for the first time, the empire under Trajan was composed of clearly marked, well-organized provinces. Therefore, the establishment of military *valetudinaria* can be seen as the product of a new imperial military policy creating a paid professional army and permanently stationing its multinational legions at Rome's frontiers beyond the Alps after a century-long process of conquest and colonization. Moreover, the new institutions benefited from the empire's prosperity, which gave rise to important programs of public works.

Valetudinaria: Ideology and mission

In classical antiquity, social welfare was never directly linked to any religious cult. In ancient Greece, philanthropy consisted of a series of services to other citizens but lacked specific identification with the poor. Given the prevailing ideology of equality concerning political rights and social status, members of a Greek polis evidently made no distinctions between rich and poor. In fact, Greek and Roman ideals envisioned altruism as a series of civic activities benefiting the entire community. This attitude reflected social, economic, and political conditions prevailing in Greece during the classical period of the fifth and fourth centuries BC, when most members of the population were still landowners. In theory, the state was viewed as a community of self-governing citizens providing gifts to each other and their commonwealth. No rewards in a presumed afterlife were linked to such displays of largesse.

Basic forms of Greek welfare were based on two principles: reciprocity and desire for social recognition. All activities of a benevolent character were based on models of exchange. To function properly, respect and good works needed to be mutual. There was the presumption that, given life's uncertainties, benefactors could quickly become receivers of aid. A record of good deeds ensured such mutual aid, often expressed as love of mankind or *philanthropia*, and variously applied to parents, old people, friends, guests, and fellow citizens. The desire for social acceptance also pervaded antiquity as individuals strove for status and recognition. Dispensing gifts was viewed as an expression of superior status and helped fashion a successful social life. As a result of such views, hospitality remained mostly a private affair, dispensed to family and friends.[113]

Within these ideological boundaries, there was initially no public duty toward the sick in ancient Greece. Illness remained a private concern. As noted earlier, the cult of Asclepius was merely another valuable diagnostic and therapeutic alternative. Care provided by medical craftsmen was one option for individuals who wanted to transcend domestic healing routines. Normally, ancient Greek craftsmen advised individuals with health problems at the marketplace or went to the patients' homes. If the craftsman was established well enough to forego an itinerant career, diagnoses and treatments could also be provided at his home, the *iatreium*. Some practitioners received appointments and became salaried in a community, available to treat all members of a polis free of charge.[114]

This nonreligious and egalitarian view of welfare contrasted sharply with atti-

tudes popular in ancient Egypt. There, since early dynastic times, welfare had traditionally been a social ethic and a government policy embedded in religious values. The land belonged to the pharaohs, and the population had neither rights
nor powers, but were obliged to provide services to the state under rules imposed
by a priestly bureaucracy. Under those circumstances, Egyptians accepted sharp
distinctions between rich and poor and formulated a series of ethical principles
designed to safeguard and aid the latter. Gods and rulers were enjoined to be especially protective of the poor, shielding them from excessive exploitation. The
same can be said about the charitable Egyptian focus on widows, orphans, the elderly, the homeless, and wandering strangers. Temples, in turn, provided hospitality, food, and asylum. Moreover, good works were not only important for one's
social standing but essential for a favorable final reckoning following death, a centerpiece of Egyptian religious beliefs. Eventually, the ancient Egyptian formula
of providing food for the hungry, water for the thirsty, clothing for the naked,
and remedies for the sick, blind, and crippled became a central theme in Judeo-
Christian welfare and the core of Christian good works to be evaluated at the last
judgment.[115]

Ancient Israel, in turn, adopted most Egyptian welfare views, with the additional belief that the poor were a special, religiously sanctioned group or God's
chosen people. Since the social and economic conditions in Palestine were quite
similar to those of Egypt, the masses also needed to be protected from the rich.
Thus, provision of assistance and hospitality was also a religiously sanctioned act,
and those who begged were expected to receive alms and other forms of aid. As
everywhere else, temples were considered to be places of political and economic
asylum where people could escape from their hostile masters. During religious festivals, selected poor individuals, strangers, widows, and orphans were similarly
provided with alms, food, and gifts.

In imperial Rome, social welfare schemes initially followed the Greek egalitarian model and thus failed to distinguish between rich and poor people for purposes of providing aid. As in Greece, the philanthropic drive focused on family
and friends. Sympathy for strangers was considered irrational, a character flaw
bound to result in unjustified aid.[116] Pagan social ethics imposed all welfare duties on the *pater familias* and restricted all aid to his extended family. The concept of *xenones* or guest rooms in private houses was apparently expanded to include buildings specially designated for guests or temporary residences for foreign
officials. Relations among individuals were still conceived in equal terms, although
economic conditions in the empire gradually created a large mass of dispossessed
urban poor who still retained their civil and political rights. In sickness, strong
emphasis continued to be placed on self-help and household medicines.

Changes in the attitude of the wealthy toward the poor were prompted in part
by Stoic philosophy in imperial Rome, as represented by Seneca and Marcus Au-
relius. According to Plutarch, aristocratic virtue, generosity, and piety could be

synonymous. Among gifts to be distributed to needy Romans were the *alimenta*, funds designated to support children of poor citizens who were now considered special wards of the emperor. More influential on shifts in the character of welfare were the changes in socioeconomic conditions experienced in the empire's western provinces, which possibly led to the adoption of more oriental forms of political and economic organization. For his part, Trajan displayed public generosity by perfecting the service of *frumentationes*, a permanent distribution of free grain to those among the urban proletariat entitled to it. In tandem with the ruler, the aristocracy also perceived new responsibilities toward the poor, but civic benefaction remained sporadic and not always specifically aimed at the poor.[117] At the same time, however, Stoic and other systems of pagan philosophy remained indifferent to physical suffering and pain, and seemed incapable of explaining the apparent randomness of disease and death, all part of nature's laws.

Rome's failure to fully develop a concern for the welfare of the poor was, in part, a result of its status as a slave society. In the process of building an empire, slavery had been closely linked to military expansion and colonization. Thousands of slaves were sent from the conquered provinces to Italy; before the end of the last century BC, slaves comprised well over 30% of the peninsula's total population. As in ancient Greece, slavery became an essential component of a Roman economy based on food production in individual households. Groups of Roman slaves on large agricultural estates produced larger surpluses than free subsistence farmers, thus increasing the productivity of labor without additional costs. Agricultural slaves typically worked on large estates in chain gangs and lived in primitive dormitories under the authority of a slave overseer or steward. In time, slaves began to occupy a wide spectrum of social positions, from powerful urban administrators in the emperor's household to vulnerable members of rural slave gangs employed as agricultural workers on large estates in southern Italy and Sicily. In between, many artisans and domestic servants were also slaves. The same was also true of architects, singers, and actors. Even Roman physicians of all persuasions trained some of their slaves as healers. On average, an upper-class Roman employed dozens of enslaved servants. Given the presence of such an underclass of powerless, exploitable individuals in virtually all walks of life, Romans degraded manual labor through its association with slavery and neglected to recognize the plight of the free poor.[118]

Slavery was exceedingly cruel. In the second century BC the Roman senator Cato recommended that worn-out slaves be sold or disposed of. Many masters simply abandoned sick slaves in public squares to fend for themselves, only to reclaim them if they recovered their health and strength. Whether slavery became somewhat humanized through the influence of Stoic philosophy remains unclear. Slaves were often portrayed as household enemies, untrustworthy, cunning, always running away and seeking asylum at shrines and sanctuaries, where they simply changed hands and became captives of the deity. Certain slave owners certainly expressed affection for individual slaves such as nursemaids, secretaries, managers, and healers, but this may have been part of a myth-making effort that sought to protect masters from acknowledging the misery they caused. Defenseless and totally helpless, slaves remained on the margins of Roman society, legally impotent and socially dead.

With the end of compulsory military service in imperial Rome, landowners began to have their lands worked by free tenants, precipitating a decline in agricultural slave labor from the first century AD on. This development should also be considered against the background of a steadily declining population. As revealed by Columella in his work *De Re Rustica* (60–65 AD), rapid turnover of workers was gradually replaced by a more conservative approach that sought to protect and extend the productivity of existing slaves and cattle. Henceforth agricultural slaves were seldom freed. Changing conditions demanded a new approach: instead of freely disposing of their dysfunctional slaves, landowners sought to treat and rehabilitate them in special shelters or *valetudinaria*, while sick farm animals were similarly rounded up and subjected to veterinary care.

Perhaps the selection of soldiers and slaves as recipients of medical care was related to their shortage and rising economic value.[119] The loyalty of foreign soldiers and slaves, and their physical performance, hung in the balance. Moreover, aid was perhaps offered because both groups were engaged in work that forced them to be away from the family networks traditionally responsible for assistance. Soldiers and slaves thus became attached to their military camps and masters' farms. Care in a *valetudinarium* was part of the bargain struck between the emperor and military rookies such as Terentianus or between the landowner and his slaves. This bargain included shelter, food, entertainment, and medical attention. In the end, the *valetudinaria* failed to spread to the rest of the civilian population. By contrast, civilians, rich and poor, continued to rely on their traditional family system of domestic and folk healing, balneotherapy, advice from private or public physicians, and temple healing.

Valetudinaria: Organization and staff

Our best evidence about the civil *valetudinaria* comes from the large imperial households, where efforts were seemingly made to preserve the health of their slaves. Tacitus and Seneca talked about the existence of special sick rooms presumably for the treatment of slaves. These private hostels may have belonged to a few wealthy landowners and were located in the countryside during the first century AD. In *De Re Rustica*, Columella mentioned that among the responsibilities of an estate administrator or *vilicus* was the care of exhausted or injured slaves dispatched to the *valetudinarium* for a few days. These establishments seem to have been mostly small shelters or dormitories erected by owners for the rest and rehabilitation of their most valuable slaves. Thus, like its later military counter-part, the civil *valetudinarium* probably focused on the welfare of a special group of individuals considered important for the political economy of the early empire. As Columella declared, "Attention of this kind is a source of kindly feeling and also obedience. Moreover, those who have recovered their health, after careful at-tention has been given them when they were ill, are eager to give more faithful service than before."[120]

In its basic form, the institution was possibly designed to take care of depen-dent workers who could be considered extended members of a landowner's *fa-milia*. This function can be seen as an expansion of traditional caring responsi-bility placed in the hands of the *pater familias*. We can assume that the civil *valitudinarium*, under the supervision of the owner's wife, was staffed by other slaves professing some medical knowledge, trained perhaps by their masters or briefly apprenticed to other physicians. In their efforts to make slaves productive, many landowners trained them in basic medical matters and even sent them out to treat other sick people for gain, a practice that Trajan attempted to restrict in 108 AD. Oddly, we know of no civil *valetudinarium* after 80 AD.

According to the remaining evidence, military *valetudinaria* were located only on the northern imperial frontier at the rivers Rhine and Danube. Roman forts in that region conformed to a rectangular plan with streets laid out on a grid. Al-though military tactics and strategy largely dictated the general location of forts and fortresses, hygienic criteria were also important. As Flavius Vegetius later de-clared, "as far as situation is concerned, do not keep the troops in an unhealthy region in the vicinity of marshes that bring diseases, on arid plains or hills lack-ing trees to provide shade.... Do not allow the army to use water that is un-wholesome or marshy, as drinking bad water, just like poison, causes illness for men."[121] Thus, the Romans normally erected their towns on well-drained ground, often on a hillside, adjacent to a river. Fresh water was mostly obtained from wells dug within the fort itself. These permanent complexes were obviously intended to mitigate adverse climatic conditions and make up for the lack of other local in-frastructures, including suitable boarding houses and roads.[122]

Before the advent of such fortresses, especially on the northern frontier, tem-porary tents probably served as field hospitals. Now, however, previously scat-tered collection points and sites of emergency care could be concentrated and fun-neled into a separate structure located inside the fort's perimeter, either near the outer wall away from the center of the town, or near the *praetorium*, on the *via principalis*. This placement could possibly have been made in deference to the *valetudinarium*'s inmates, who thus pursued their recovery in a quieter part of the fortress. In some instances, a further buffer was provided in the form of a line of storerooms located along the street frontage. Carefully constructed, these perma-nent buildings devoted to the sick and wounded were of brick and stone. Most surviving examples have been found in Germany, Britain, and Hungary.[123]

The design of a Roman *valetudinarium* reflected its perceived function of bringing together and housing a considerable number of individuals in need of care. The design was probably inspired by the popular Persian peristyle plan extensively employed since Hellenistic times in urban Mediterranean architecture. The building was shaped in the form of a hollow rectangle with four wings surrounding a central courtyard or garden. This inward focus provided relative closure to the street for privacy and rest. In some cases, the entrance to the building led to a large receiving room, the *atrium*, with rooms or cubicles arranged around the peristyle, with its adjacent latrines and courtyard. The number of rooms appears to have had a standard relationship to the number of legionaries stationed in a given fort. One cubicle was provided for every 60 enlisted men, an estimate that would have allowed at any time the accommodation of 5–10% of a unit's personnel in the hospital.[124] The inside courtyard furnished light and fresh air, as well as protection from rain and wind.

The ruins of the oldest *valetudinarium* were discovered in the fort of Aliso, near Haltern, Westphalia, presumably built as early as 9 AD during the reign of Emperor Augustus. Within the fort's walls, the Romans utilized the typical rectangular design, with rooms symmetrically arranged on both sides of a middle corridor. The architectural plans of a similar institution from the first century AD at Vindonissa, or Windisch, in Switzerland disclose two large halls, one at the entrance, the other in the courtyard, employed perhaps for meeting and dining functions. A number of small rooms behind the portico were presumably reserved for administration and nursing staffs. Two passageways from the central corridor allowed access to the central courtyard. The patients' rooms were arranged on both sides of this central corridor, circling around the building, and could be entered only from a small vestibule or chamber located between every two rooms.

This design, common to all extant *valetudinaria*, may have been formulated to reduce noise and prevent the intrusion of dust, common in all well-traveled corridors. The arrangement also created an additional barrier to contagion when some of the inmates required isolation. The vestibule had doors on all four sides leading to two-patient rooms, a common corridor, and a small storage space in the back, perhaps reserved for supplies. Apparently, each of the 60 rooms was large enough to accommodate about three individual beds. This arrangement must have allowed for adequate ventilation and plenty of light.[125] Spatial fragmentation also facilitated monitoring and social control, two important aspects of army and hospital life. Inmates could be kept under close observation by staff members or sentries posted in the vestibules.

During the reign of Claudius, a similar establishment was erected around 50 AD at Novaesium (Neuss) on the Rhine near Cologne. Of interest is the fact that nearly 100 medical and pharmaceutical instruments were found in one of its rooms—perhaps reserved for surgical treatments. A presumed operating room was furnished with a number of fireplaces, not only for warmth and ventilation but perhaps also for heating cautery irons.[126] At Vetera, near Xanten, a camp and supply depot on the lower Rhine built of stone in Nero's time (54–68 AD) could hold two legions. Here the *valetudinarium* was also located inside the fortified walls, adjacent to the main road and near the gate. Seventy small wards were arranged in pairs on either side of the central corridor with a capacity of four beds each. Other rooms have been tentatively identified as physicians' quarters, a dispensary, a mortuary, and isolation wards. In addition, there was a suite of baths with attached latrines.[127]

The Roman fortress at Novae, on the Danube, seat of the Legio I Italica, also possessed its own *valetudinarium*, one of at least seven such establishments on the shores of the river west of the town. Built on orders of Trajan, they featured a number of refinements such as roof tiles and windows. At Novae, a three-room complex identical to that at Novaesium opened into the central corridor. Walls were coated with several layers of plaster, and the average rooms had windows to provide more light and space for four to six cots. When excavated, the floors displayed several layers of yellow gravel, perhaps periodically spread for hygienic reasons. There were also traces of protective mats. Some rooms presumably had central heating, although portable stoves would have been needed throughout the building during winter.[128] Baths, admission areas, and operating rooms can also be surmised from the ruins, together with a shrine or cult room dedicated to Asclepius and Hygieia, deities mentioned in some inscriptions. This linkage between sacred and lay healing was not unusual. At Carnuntum, in Britain, a bust of Asclepius was found among the ruins of that *valetudinarium*, and at Chester, in or near the legionary building, were two altars evidently dedicated to Asclepius and Hygieia.[129]

By the 70s AD, staff arrangements within a military *valetudinarium* followed a standardized pattern. Like other buildings in the fort, the institution was under the control of the camp prefect or *praefectus castrorum*. His deputy, usually a former chief centurion, was the *optio valetudinarii* in charge of the hospital's administration, concerned with the physical upkeep of the establishment as well as the feeding and care of the sick. He requisitioned special food and medical supplies and supervised the team of physicians and assistants. Larger institutions could boast the presence of a *librarius* who looked after accounts, wrote orders, and composed reports. Another individual, the *optio convalescentium*, was put in charge of convalescent warriors, a post available in both the Roman army and navy.[130] With regard to nursing functions, most legionaries possessed basic wound-healing skills, and in emergencies could aid each other on the battlefield. However, the *valetudinarium* also possessed so-called *capsarii* or dressers (the *capsa* was a round box containing bandages and dressings) who had already received some institutional training from a senior staff physician or *medicus*. Like all posts in the military medical service, nursing positions were open to promotion, including advance to *medicus*. Other auxiliary medical personnel included the *seplasiarius*, a man responsible for supplying ointments for wound healing.[131]

Although the Romans never had an official and separate medical corps, by 150 AD approximately 500–800 physicians and surgeons had found employment in the armed forces. Their numbers and experience varied considerably according to the size and prestige of the military unit and its geographic location. On average, each legion of 6,400 men featured a total of 20 physicians, while auxiliary troops had 5. All medical personnel possessed normal military ranking, with the highest, *medicus sesquiplicarius*, available only in a legion. The auxiliary cavalry or *alae* boasted a medicus *duplicarius*, and infantry battalions or cohorts had their *medicus ordinarius*, usually in charge of the dressers. In both pretorial fleets, most doctors were listed as *medici duplicarii*. All physicians and surgeons took an oath and were bound by military law. After 20–25 years of service, they usually retired and returned to civilian medical practice. Instead of joining the armed forces, some *medici* actually remained civilians and for an honorarium worked occasionally as consultants.[132]

Following the reforms of Augustus, many early recruits who became *medici* were ambitious Greeks entering the army after acquiring some hands-on medical experience in the civilian sector. For the first century, over 90% of the entering physicians came from the Hellenized East. As immigrants, their status was usually quite low in Roman society, and they competed in the medical marketplace with other freedmen, slaves, and traveling drug sellers. Touting their higher educational background, these new arrivals needed to overcome the widespread Roman prejudice against Greeks, and many of them joined the army as the best available option to make a decent living.[133]

The reasons Greek physicians aspired to a military career were based on the significant differences in social position they held in the two halves of the empire. In the East, large cities such as Alexandria and Smyrna were prosperous urban centers. Many physicians there were members of the local provincial aristocracy who routinely associated with senators and magistrates (as the example of Theodotus and his patient Aristides at Pergamon attests). In the former Hellenistic commonwealth, medicine was an established and admired profession, intimately involved in public affairs. In the West, by contrast, 80% of the available physicians lacked full civil rights during the first century AD. No physicians were members of the senate or the magistracy, and only a few played small roles in the associations of freedmen. As immigrants, they could not own land in a society primarily based on agricultural wealth. Since in the West there were fewer large cities where physicians could earn a living entirely from medical practice, many of the Greek practitioners were forced into an itinerant status.

In the Roman empire, civic physicians and specialists needed official recognition from a town council to enjoy immunity from local taxation, but after the financial restrictions imposed by Emperor Antoninus Pius around 150 AD, tax immunity was reserved for a handful of physicians, depending on the size of a town. The choice of those so-called immunes was left to lay town councils concerned with a candidate's morals and abilities. Only constant good performance guaranteed the continuation of immunity. In contrast, the army provided this legal recognition to all of its members, and *medici* and other medical specialists received exemptions and protections similar to those of the civil immunes. Training of *medici* in the empire mostly involved continued apprenticeship. Most Roman physicians at this time were general practitioners variously versed in dietetics, drugs, and surgery. The Roman army offered considerable opportunities for young physicians who had already practiced in various civilian settings, but others got their entire training while enlisted. Among the praetorian troops, no distinctions between physicians and surgeons are known.[134]

Among the functions of the military medical corps was not only the care of soldiers wounded in battle but also the prevention, control, and treatment of infectious diseases, a major source of casualties. Military physicians focused on diet, exercise, and hygiene. In the forts, the *medici* certainly needed to pay attention to the provision of fresh water and to ensure proper waste disposal. During campaigns on the frontier, wounded soldiers were usually treated first on the battlefield by medical assistants or *capsarii*. This first aid could be followed up in a *valetudinarium* if such an establishment was available in the nearby fort. Further treatment, including possibly surgery, was usually performed by the unit's own *medicus* and dresser.

Soldiers and their care

For soldiers such as Claudius Terentianus, health and fitness were essential conditions for enrolling in Trajan's army. There was a plethora of candidates, and recruiters were in a position to select individuals of higher social standing. The average age of a soldier was 18–23 years. After an initial examination, the recruits were sent for a four-month training course.[135] As Claudius found out, transfers were part of a Roman soldier's life. One well-established principle in the new professionalized army was that promotions always involved a change of unit. Recruits eager to climb the ladder tried to be transferred more frequently, although very few actually managed it. The price could have been a greater burden of disease, particularly for those recruited from rural areas as they came in contact with each other and were bivouacked near dense urban populations, a problem that perhaps affected Terentianus' health in Alexandria. The reason was their lack of immunity to many common diseases, especially if they came from distant provinces with different disease ecologies.[136]

In the Roman army, soldiers fell prey to acute infectious diseases, especially fevers, more often than battle-induced trauma. Combat was sporadic, but living in crowded frontier conditions carried greater risks. Moreover, exposure to new diseases from contacts with barbarians living across the imperial boundaries must have been another threat. Injuries from accidents caused by routine construction, maintenance chores, and frequent military drills may have added to the burden. In Britain, for example, the First Cohort of Tungrians under Hadrian (ca. 121 AD) listed 296 men, including 1 centurion. Of these, 31 (over 10%) were listed as unfit because of illness, and another 15 (about 5%) were said to be actively suffering from diseases. Six were classified as wounded (2%), and 10 more were said to be suffering from inflammation of the eyes (over 3%), a staggering total of over 20% casualties of disease in this sample.[137]

By contrast, little is known about the health of slaves. In his *proemium* to the work *De Medicina*, Celsus (25 BC–25 AD) dismissively remarked that medical practice in civil *valetudinaria* was purely empirical instead of being based on reasoning. Comparing its activities to veterinary practice and foreign healing practices, Celsus believed that it was geared to the lowest common denominator instead of paying "full attention to individuals."[138] At least 80% of the working Roman population was primarily engaged in agriculture. Indeed, human labor constituted the chief engine of the Roman economy. As a consequence of the often ruthless exploitation of such workers, slaves must have frequently suffered from malnutrition, physical exhaustion, and disease.

Whether stationed at the northern frontier or, like Terentianus, near the city of Alexandria, the Roman army with its network of military camps and *valetudinaria* became a key factor in the delivery of an increasingly standardized Greco-Roman medicine based on the tenets of classical humoralism. Troop mobility and contact with frontier populations probably also allowed the military *medici* to learn new information from local healers while disseminating their own professional knowledge and techniques.[139] As always, no real boundaries existed between human and animal medicine.[140]

Traditionally, battlefield injuries had an aura of legitimacy and heroism, while periodical sickness, as Terentianus tells us in his letters, was less glamorous, even somewhat embarrassing, a nuisance for otherwise young, healthy men at the top of their physical form. Officers and soldiers routinely tended to ignore the impact of disease on army readiness, trusting in the physical conditioning and capacity for recovery of the troops.[141] Medical attention in a *valetudinarium* probably flowed naturally from the personal professional bond that each warrior felt with his disabled comrade. Contemporary classical medical texts stressed the importance of nursing and of letting nature take its course. The basic theoretical underpinnings for all healing strategies were still based on the balance of bodily humors and their qualities.[142]

Roman medicine outside or inside a *valetudinarium* tended to stress practical problem solving. An expanding number of drugs had already been compiled by Dioscorides (ca. 40–90 AD), apparently also a military physician, in his *Materia Medica*.[143] Surgery, in turn, while necessary, was always perceived as dangerous. The main emphasis was on restoring health through rest, diet, exercise, and a few drugs. The basic military diet was essentially vegetarian, including beans, peas, lentils, and cabbage. Corn and cheese were basic staples. Soldiers were often stereotyped as gluttons, trying to supplement their martial rations with condiments and local delicacies. Legionaries received unleavened army bread—*panis militaris*—and on the frontier the most popular salted meats were beef, mutton, and pork. Other meals were prepared with chicken, duck, and goose, as well as fish and oysters. Figs were said to promote wound discharge. In addition to vinegar and water drinks, medicinal wine was popular as a restorative, although plain rainwater was employed for convalescents. Contrary to peasant prejudices against baths as luxury practices that would soften not only the skin but a warrior's discipline, dietary prescriptions were often supplemented by the use of warm and cold baths.

Since no narrative from a Roman legionary dispatched to a *valetudinarium* has been found to date, Terentianus' correspondence with his father remains the only narrow window into the sufferings of an imperial soldier. We may infer that his so-called fish poisoning most likely resulted in a stomach disorder. According to Celsus, the "commonest and worst complaint" in such cases was gastric paralysis, associated with vomiting and even pain, in which the stomach was unable to retain food, thus compromising nutrition and leading to weight loss and wasting. In such cases, the army *medicus* attending Terentianus would have prescribed the use of cold drinks, including water to elicit further vomiting and thus cleanse the stomach. Others gave cupfuls of dry wine seasoned with resin until the vomiting ceased. Since an astringent action aimed at restoring the natural contractions of the stomach was most desirable, other drinks would have included radish and mint juices, as well as sweet and sour pomegranates. Similar external strategies called for the placement of a cloth or sponge soaked in vinegar or a refrigerant plaster over the stomach. If further action was required, the attending physician could also apply some heated copper cups to the upper abdomen. Warm baths were deemed harmful, but cold water could be poured over the body. To recover bodily tone, patients such as Terentianus were allowed to swim in cold spring or river water, a recommendation reminiscent of Asclepius' orders to Aristides at Pergamon.[144]

Surgery at the time of Celsus was a legitimate and respectable branch of medicine, although mostly a last resort, given the rudimentary level of anatomical knowledge and the frequency of postoperative infections. Elective surgery included trephination for the removal of damaged cranial bones using bronze-crown trephines. Lithotomy excised bladder stones. Battle wounds presented military surgeons with few alternatives to surgical intervention. Speed was always crucial, especially in limb amputations. Given the contemporary weapons technology, most frequent battle injuries were flesh wounds from cutting weapons such as swords, lances, and daggers, and from projectiles such as arrows, spears, sling bullets, and artillery bolts. Gangrene remained one of the scourges of early surgery, often leading to amputation and death. Soldiers who sustained serious internal injuries generally had a poor chance of survival even if cared for in a *valetudinarium*.[145]

In Roman military medicine, the key wound-healing strategies were to first arrest bleeding, then prevent inflammation, and finally promote closure and restoration. We should assume that Terentianus had merely sustained a superficial flesh wound, the most common and safest, according to our medical authority, Celsus. Everybody knew that young adults healed more readily, especially if they were strong, well nourished, and otherwise healthy. Wounds were allowed to bleed freely for the removal of impurities and matter that could help produce an inflammation and transform the retained humors into pus. If not enough blood flowed from the wound, supplementary bloodletting from an elbow vein was recommended. If the flow was excessive, another maneuver was to apply some cups to a part of the skin distant to the wound in an effort to divert the circulation. Finally, the gap in the skin was filled with dry lint, pressed down by hand with a sponge dampened in cold water, vinegar, or wine. For even better results, the lint to be applied to the wound could also be soaked in vinegar.[146]

After Terentianus' bleeding had been arrested, the *capsari*, or more likely the *medici*, may have applied iron rust and verdigris to keep the wound dry. Similar procedures would have taken place in a *valetudinarium*. Pain was a manifestation of nature's healing powers, but decoctions of opium poppy and henbane were administered if it was intense.[147] Butter with rose oil and honey kept the skin soft. Linen bandages pressed the margins of the wound together, and the patient was given light food. By the third day, the bandages were uncovered for the first time, dead tissue and pus were washed away with cold water, and a similar dressing was reapplied. Retractors or small sharp hooks held the wound edges apart.

Most Roman surgical instruments were made of copper and its alloys, especially bronze and brass, cast or forged.[148] Routinely, the extent of the inflammation was checked again on the fifth day, and if the wound appeared to be white or red, thin and soft, this was considered to be a favorable sign.[149] Until the lesion had completely closed, the surgeon probably employed warm water to keep Terentianus' wound clean. Pitch and turpentine were other choices to accomplish this most important goal. Another option was the use of iron-made cautery instruments, the fiery but versatile "bloodless knife" applied to stop bleeding wounds, remove abscesses, promote discharge from skin lesions, or stop the spread of gangrene. Such painful procedures were believed to foster a soldier's endurance for physical suffering while speeding up healing.

In the end, Claudius Terentianus recovered from both his episode of fish poisoning and his wounds. After a prudent period of convalescence, he was pronounced fit to return to his unit. In his last letter, he thanked his father, Tiberianus, for having visited him during his ordeal. But not all credit for the recovery went to the military physicians who presumably attended him. Like Aristides, Terentianus was a pious man, indicating that he continued to pray daily for both his father's and his own health "in the presence of our lord Sarapis and the gods who share his temple."[150]

ASCLEPIEION AND VALETUDINARIUM: CONFLUENCE OF THE SACRED AND SECULAR

Should the Greek Asclepieia, as well as Roman military and slave *valetudinaria*, be considered forerunners of hospitals?[151] Pain and suffering are perennial human experiences, often difficult to articulate. In classical times, expectations of recovery and cure were limited, in part because of scanty medical knowledge and the ethical posture of contemporary healers, whose preoccupation with personal reputation and income dictated extreme caution. Often these individuals were reluctant to assume responsibility for cases presumed to be life-threatening. Although, in the view of Greeks and Romans, illness could be caused by the gods and its cure lay in their hands, most individuals apparently shied away from general and impersonal explanations and looked for unique causal chains that embraced aspects of their own lives and personal fate.

Healing deities such as Asclepius and Sarapis and their temples were expressions of ecological, demographic, and cultural characteristics unique to the classical world. They functioned as centers of medical advice and prognosis, even specific treatment. Individuals seeking counsel came for brief visits, primarily for incubation and dream interpretations designed to ameliorate suffering and seek cures for many conditions deemed serious or hopeless. At the temple, the emphasis was on divination and prognosis, coupled with supernatural therapy. Except for the prescribed rituals, supplicants remained in nearby cities and shelters outside the sacred precinct. No explicit mentions of regular food distributions—except perhaps for banquets during festivals—or actual nursing of the sick were recorded, but these activities may have taken place in nearby hostels.[152]

In a broad sense, the Asclepieia may have fulfilled the criteria of establishments created for healing purposes. These temples provided carefully controlled spaces conducive to healing. Imposing buildings, statuary and offerings, bathing facilities, staff, and religious ceremonies all contributed to the physical and spiritual recovery of the visitors. By coming to an Asclepieion, health seekers entered into an association with the god not unlike that of a client seeking a commodity.[153] In fact, within the religious pluralism present in imperial Rome, Aelius Aristides frequently shuttled from one cult to another, shopping for a divinity that could aid his recovery. In spite of his pronouncements, these visits did not imply a strong commitment to any one religious cult. Aristides' visits described the sacred precinct as a safe harbor providing worshippers with serenity and repose.[154] His example at Pergamon demonstrated that at least during the early Roman Empire, medical and dietetic advice based on contemporary insights into health and disease could also be provided within a religious framework. A century later, during the turmoil created by successive epidemics and social dislocation, there are hints that some Asclepieia near cities of the Eastern Roman Empire even became shelters for the sick and displaced. In doing so, these temples merely extended their original mission of protection and assistance.

Roman soldiers who had joined the volunteer imperial army of Augustus and his successors had similar expectations when they were injured or became sick, like Terentianus, far away from their traditional sources of care. First aid from comrades and dressers on the battlefield was essential, but for those stationed at Rome's northern frontiers beyond the Alps, more was at stake. Like the Asclepieia, the *valetudinaria* provided the facilities, trained staff, and rituals that contributed to both spiritual and physical healing. Dispatched to the *valetudinarium* following a triage process, the sick and injured legionaries may have felt reassured. Their confinement in a quiet, limited area shared with two or three other comrades was restful and therapeutic.[155] The prospect of an extensive period of recovery and rehabilitation under the care of physicians in a *valetudinarium* was a morale builder. Nursing and medical routines focused on the evolution of wounds, the management of broken limbs, and the care of other acute illnesses. Soldiers lingered only as long as their medical caregivers considered prudent before a return to active military duty was indicated. Chronically disabled individuals were probably discharged from the army and sent home to be cared for by their families. Recovery based on the self-limited nature of many ailments helped to buttress the belief in the efficacy of the all-powerful gods and their inspired healing craftsmen. In the final analysis, the very existence of healing spaces within the protective walls of a frontier fort communicated to soldiers the message that the emperor and his army cared for them as individuals, that they were valuable assets to the Roman state. Following Augustus, Roman emperors were frequently portrayed as a powerful healers in their own right—even linked to Asclepius and Sarapis—whose magic could endow the *valetudinarium* with therapeutic qualities.[156]

Every healing act is a mystery. The organization of rituals in places such as the Asclepieia was in consonance with traditional temple routines guiding the interaction of the sacred and the profane. Access to the sanctuary was linked to notions of Greek piety and purity, with strict regimentation of dress and conduct. Ambulatory suppliants followed prescribed bathing and prayer formulas. A priestly caste of attendants furnished a rigid set of daily scheduled observances. Visitors listened to inspirational speeches—Christians would have called them sermons—and sang hymns in honor of the healing god. After the various ceremonies, many of the visitors lingered at nearby hostels. Similar objectives could be achieved in the military and perhaps slave *valetudinarium*. Feeding, bathing, wound dressing, or drug-prescribing routines, and perhaps even prayers, followed. Language, symbols, music, and costume all worked together to establish and enforce social cohesion among the ill. In both venues, faith and emotion must have been critical factors facilitating recovery.

At the temple, visitors could find the meaning of their suffering and their lives' destinies directly through communion with Asclepius. Cut off from their usual surroundings and temporarily bound within a divine enclosure, they looked forward to the expected epiphany and personal advice from the god. Temple cures represented an emotionally charged encounter with the powers of life and death, as the deity personally visited each supplicant and provided advice or performed cures. This healing relationship had the potential to satisfy individual needs, including restoration of confidence and self-esteem. In the Roman *valetudinarium*, such a religious dimension was apparently also retained, since there is some evidence of shrines or stelae devoted to healing gods. In a *valetudinarium* inscription from Augustan times, the medicus of the fifth cohort of praetorians in Rome, Sextus Titius Alexander, made an offering "in honor of Asclepius and the good health of his fellow soldiers."[157]

Finally, temple visitors and *valetudinarium* inmates had a common goal: they all wanted to be healed. Although each sufferer had a personal disability or plight, the assembled sick would have interacted and shared their stories and feelings. Physical proximity provided opportunities for intimate communication. Prescribed rituals of bathing, praying, singing, sleeping, and attending theatrical functions and sport spectacles encouraged socialization. Baths and drug prescriptions could have extended the range of therapeutic options. At the temples, construction of a relaxing spa atmosphere became a catalyst for the formation of social groups, often divided by class and gender. What provided such places with distinctive healing potential was the fact that both temple supplicants and soldiers were temporarily placed in distinct physical environments and social situations. Together with staffs of priests and attendants, the imposing buildings were therapeutic shelters promising safety and protection. Often, this search for mutual acceptance, the trading of illness narratives and remedies, should have diminished the anxieties surrounding suffering and disability, thus proving therapeutic. In the end, the Greek healing temples and Roman military hospitals of antiquity undoubtedly structured and possibly ameliorated human suffering. They provided spiritual and sometimes physical relief and thus fulfilled their expected therapeutic roles. The motto "Enter a good man, leave a better one," inscribed on the Asclepieion at Lambaesis in Africa, eloquently spoke to patients in antiquity, keenly aware of the limitations of the healing art but always hopeful of the power of gods and the skill of surgeons to relieve suffering and promote recovery.[158]

NOTES

1. Ludwig and Emma J. Edelstein, *Asclepius, A Collection and Interpretation of the Testimonies*, Baltimore, Johns Hopkins Univ. Press, 1945, vol. I, *Testimonies*, p. 203. The chronology of Aristides' life events is somewhat contested by at least a decade. For details about Aristides' career and contemporaries see G. W. Bowersock, *Greek Sophists in the Roman Empire*, Oxford, Clarendon Press, 1969, and more recently Graham Anderson, *Sage, Saint, and Sophist: Holy Men and their Associates in the Early Roman Empire*, London, Routledge, 1994.

2. Charles A. Behr, editor and translator, *Aelius Aristides and the Sacred Tales*, Amsterdam, A. M. Hakkert, 1968, p. 251. All subsequent quotations are based on this English translation. More recently, Aristides' text can also be found in Aelius Aristides, *The Complete Works*, trans. C. A. Behr, 2 vols., Leiden, Brill, 1981–86.

3. Behr, *Aristides*, p. 224.

4. Ibid., p. 233.

5. Ibid., p. 223. A literary analysis of Aristides' work is L. T. Pearcy, "Theme, dream, and narrative: Reading the Sacred Tales of Aelius Aristides," *Trans Am Philol Assoc* 118 (1988): 377–391.

6. Aristides' illness narratives shed light on the management of life problems by a wealthy contemporary within the context of Roman cultural values. I am adopting the approach outlined by Arthur Kleinman. See his *The Illness Narratives: Suffering, Healing, and the Human Condition*, New York, Basic Books, 1988, especially the preface. I am well aware of Vivian Nutton's recent admission that, unlike their more modern counterparts, historians of ancient medicine "can rarely be sure of even the most basic of facts" (personal communication).

7. For details see H. Idris Bell, *Cults and Creeds in Graeco-Roman Egypt*, Liverpool, University Press, 1957, and more recently Reginald E. Witt, *Isis in the Graeco-Roman World*, Ithaca, NY, Cornell Univ. Press, 1971.

8. T. T. Tinh, "Sarapis and Isis," in *Jewish and Christian Self-Definition*, ed. B. F. Meyer and E. P. Sanders, London, SCM Press, 1982, vol. 3, *Self-Definition in the Graeco-Roman World*, pp. 101–17. Aristides mentions the Egyptian god Asclepius-Imouthes (Imhotep) in one of his writings. See Edelstein and Edelstein, *Asclepius*, vol. I, *Testimonies*, p. 167. On Imhotep see G. B. Risse, "Imhotep and medicine: a reevaluation," *West J Med* 144 (1986): 622–24.

9. Galen, *On Examinations by which the Best Physicians are Recognized*, Arabic version trans. into English by A. Z. Iskandar, Berlin, Akademie Verlag, 1988. See also V. Nutton, "The patient's choice: a new treatise by Galen," *Class Q* 40 (1990): 236–57.

10. Vivian Nutton, "Healers in the medical marketplace: Towards a social history of Greco-Roman medicine," in *Medicine and Society: Historical Essays*, ed. A. Wear, Cambridge, Cambridge Univ. Press, 1992, pp. 15–58, and more recently, by the same author, "Medicine in the Greek world, 800–50 BC" in Nutton et al., *The Western Medical Tradition, 800 BC to AD 1800*, Cambridge, Cambridge Univ. Press, 1995, pp. 11–38.

11. Behr, *Aristides*, pp. 235–36.

12. Albino Garzetti, *From Tiberius to the Antonines, A History of the Roman Empire AD 14–192*, trans. J. R. Foster, London, Methuen & Co., 1974, pp. 441–71.

13. James H. Oliver, *The Ruling Power: A Study of the Roman Empire in the Second Century After Christ through the Roman Oration of Aelius Aristides*, Philadelphia, American Philosophical Society, 1953, p. 902. Oliver suggests April 23, 143 AD as the date of this speech.

14. Behr, *Aristides*, p. 236.

15. Max Neuburger, *The Doctrine of the Healing Power of Nature throughout the Course of Time*, trans. L. J. Boyd, New York, Homeopathic Medical College, 1926. For a comparative discussion see G. E. R. Lloyd, "Epistemological arguments in early Greek medicine in comparative perspective," in *Knowledge and the Scholarly Medical Traditions*, ed. D. Bates, Cambridge, Cambridge Univ. Press, 1995, pp. 25–39.

16. The classical roots of what Islamic authors called "non-naturals" are explained by L. J. Rather, "The six things 'non-natural,' " *Clio Med* 3 (1968): 337–47, and L. Garcia Ballester, "On the origin of the 'six non-natural things' in Galen," *Sudhoffs Arch* 32 (1993): 105–15.

17. V. Nutton, "Humoralism," in *Companion Encyclopedia of the History of Medicine*, ed. W. F. Bynum and R. Porter, London, Routledge, 1993, pp. 281–91. For a recent summary, see I. W. Müller, *Humoralmedizin: physiologische, pathologische und therapeutische Grundlagen der galenischen Heilkunst*, Heidelberg, K. F. Haug, 1993.

18. I. M. Lonie, "A structural pattern in Greek dietetics and the early history of Greek medicine," *Med Hist* 21 (1977): 235–60, and G. E. R. Lloyd, "The transformations of ancient medicine," *Bull Hist Med* 66 (1992): 114–32.

19. For details, see Gilbert Watson, *Theriac and Mithridatium: A Study in Therapeutics*, London, Wellcome Historical Medical Library, 1966.

20. William Brockbank, "Cupping and leeching" and "Counterirritation," in *Ancient Therapeutic Arts*, Springfield, IL, C. C. Thomas, 1954, pp. 67–102 and 105–34.

21. Behr, *Aristides*, p. 236.

22. Ibid., pp. 237–39.

23. The issue of Asclepius' Homeric identity is discussed in Edelstein and Edelstein, *Asclepius*, vol. II, *Interpretation*, pp. 1–22. Others have proposed that his origins should be sought in Anatolia or farther to the east, since the name could be derived from the Hittite words *assul* ("well-being") and *piya* ("to give"), thus meaning "health giver." O. Szeemeny, "The origins of the Greek lexicon Ex Oriente Lux," *J Hellenic Stud* 94 (1974): 154.

24. According to Jennifer Larson, the family context, often depicted on votive reliefs, reinforced populist values and supplied further opportunities to worship other family. Hygieia, for example, was very popular at numerous temples but not at Epidaurus. See her *Greek Heroine Cults*, Madison, Univ. of Wisconsin Press, 1995, pp. 58–77.

25. Pindar, *Third Pythian Ode*, trans. J. Sandys, Loeb Classical Library, London, Heinemann, 1915, lines 47–53, as quoted in Robert Garland, *Introducing New Gods: The Politics of Athenian Religion*, Ithaca, NY, Cornell Univ. Press, 1992, p. 117.

26. A story elaborated by Pausanias (fl. ca. 175 AD) explained that Phlegyas, father of Coronis, accompanied his pregnant daughter to Epidaurus, where she gave birth to her child by Apollo. The newborn Asclepius was then abandoned in the mountains, where goats fed him under the protection of a dog. A shepherd eventually found the divine orphan, whose healing powers quickly became known to all.

27. Howard C. Kee, *Miracle in the Early Christian World*, New Haven, Yale Univ. Press, 1983, pp. 78–104.

28. Other authors also argue on archeological grounds that a "new" Asclepius was constructed in Epidaurus, his attributes consonant with those of his previous adversary, Zeus.

See C. Benedum, "Asklepiosmythos und archäologischer Befund," *Medizinhist J* 22 (1987): 48–61.

29. For details see Richard Caton, *The Temples and Ritual of Asklepius at Epidaurus and Athens*, Liverpool, University Press, 1900, and R. A. Tomlinson, *Greek Sanctuaries*, New York, St. Martin's Press, 1976.

30. For Cos see Susan M. Sherwin-White, *Ancient Cos: An Historical Study from the Dorian Settlement to the Imperial Period*, Göttingen, Vanderhoeck & Ruprecht, 1978, and Elizabeth M. Craik, *The Dorian Aegean*, London, Routledge & Kegan Paul, 1980.

31. A translation of the pertinent text by Livius describing the event can be found in Edelstein and Edelstein, *Asclepius*, vol. I, *Testimonies*, pp. 431–51.

32. See C. Triebel-Schubert, "Die Rolle der Heilkulte in der römischen Republik: Eine Einführung zu ihrer politischen Funktion," *Medizinhist J* 19 (1984): 303–11.

33. Garland, *New Gods*, pp. 116–35. See also F. Rosenthal, "'Life is short, the art is long': Arabic commentaries on the first Hippocratic aphorism," *Bull Hist Med* 40 (1996): 226–45.

34. Alison Burford, *The Greek Temple Builders at Epidaurus*, Liverpool, Liverpool University Press, 1969.

35. R. A. Tomlinson, *Epidaurus*, Austin, Univ. of Texas Press, 1983.

36. C. Kerenyi, *Asklepios-Archetypical Image of the Physician's Existence*, trans. R. Mankheim, New York, Pantheon Books, 1956.

37. For background information see W. Burkert, *Greek Religion*, trans. J. Raffan, Cambridge, Harvard Univ. Press, 1985.

38. C. Sourvinon-Inwood, "What is polis religion?" in *The Greek City from Homer to Alexander*, ed. O. Murray and S. Price, Oxford, Clarendon Press, 1990, p. 303.

39. Sourvinon-Inwood, "Polis religion," pp. 295–322.

40. An excellent case study is Sarah B. Aleshire, *The Athenian Asklepieion: The People, Their Dedications, and Their Inventories*, Amsterdam, J. C. Gieben, 1989.

41. W. Burkert, "The meaning and function of the temple in classical Greece," in *Temple in Society*, ed. M. V. Fox, Winona Lake, IN, Eisenbrauns, 1988, pp. 27–47.

42. For an anthropological understanding, consult the work of Clifford Geertz, especially his "Religion as a cultural system," in *The Interpretation of Cultures*, New York, 1973, pp. 87–125.

43. See the important article by L. Edelstein, "Greek medicine in its relation to religion and magic," *Bull Hist Med* 5 (1937): 201–46. A good summary of the cult is provided by Ralph Jackson, *Doctors and Diseases in the Roman Empire*, Norman, Univ. of Oklahoma Press, 1988, pp. 138–69. See also Hector Avalos, *Illness and Health Care in the Ancient Near East: The Role of the Temple in Greece, Mesopotamia, and Israel*, Atlanta, Scholars Press, 1995.

44. See L. B. Zadman and P. S. Pantel, *Religion in the Ancient Greek City*, trans. P. Cartledge, Cambridge, Cambridge Univ. Press, 1992.

45. Similar conclusions were expressed by the Edelsteins. See "Social and political implications of divine healing" in *Asclepius*, vol. II, *Interpretation*, pp. 173–80.

46. Edelstein and Edelstein, *Asclepius*, vol. II, *Interpretation*, p. 123. Readers should realize that there is presently only fragmentary evidence for these conjectures, but raising them is nevertheless useful for probing reasons for the cult's growing popularity.

47. For an overview see Robert Salares, *The Ecology of the Ancient World*, Ithaca, NY, Cornell Univ. Press, 1991, pp. 225–93. Also valuable is Mirko D. Grmek, *Diseases in the Ancient World*, trans. M. Muellner and L. Muellner, Baltimore, Johns Hopkins Univ. Press, 1989.

48. There is an extensive literature on the "plague" of Athens, generated in part by

medical professionals anxious to diagnose the disease responsible for the epidemic. See, for example, D. M. Morens and R. J. Littman, "Epidemiology of the plague of Athens," *Trans Am Philol Assoc* 122 (1992): 271–304, and J. Longrigg, "Epidemics, ideas, and classical Athenian society," in *Epidemics and Ideas: Essays on the Historical Perception of Pestilence*, ed. T. Ranger and P. Slack, Cambridge, Cambridge Univ. Press, 1992, pp. 21–44.

49. On the possible linkage of epidemic disease and temple worship see J. Mikalson, "Religion and the plague of Athens," in *Studies Presented to Sterling Dow*, ed. A. L. Boegehold et al., Durham, Duke Univ. Press, 1984, pp. 217–35.

50. Edelstein and Edelstein, *Asclepius*, vol. II, *Interpretation*, pp. 53–64. See also L. Edelstein, "The Hippocratic physician," in *Ancient Medicine*, ed. O. and C. L. Temkin, Baltimore, Johns Hopkins Univ. Press, 1967, pp. 87–110.

51. V. Nutton, "The medical meeting place," *Clio Med* 27 (1995): 3–25.

52. H. von Staden, "Incurability and hopelessness: the Hippocratic Corpus," in *La Maladie et Les Maladies dans la Collection Hippocratique*, ed. P. Potter, G. Maloney, and J. Desautels, Quebec, Ed. du Sphinx, 1990, pp. 75–112. Contrary to earlier historians' assumptions, recent scholarship shows that this religious basis remained a strong stimulus for further medical studies and clinical observations. See Robert Bartz, "Hippocratic Practice: Context and Ethos; Lessons for contemporary Patient–Physician Relations," M.A. thesis, Univ. of California, San Francisco, 1997.

53. Edelstein and Edelstein acknowledged the importance of the visitors' confidence in Asclepius and their expectations as potent factors in temple cures. See *Asclepius*, vol. II, *Interpretation*, pp. 162–63. For an examination of the tacit beliefs about illness see R. Gordon, "The healing events in Graeco-Roman folk-medicine," *Clio Med* 27 (1995): 363–76.

54. G. E. R. Lloyd, *Magic, Reason, and Experience: Studies in the Origin and Development of Greek Science*, Cambridge, Cambridge Univ. Press, 1979, especially pp. 10–58.

55. S. Guettel Cole, "Greek cults," in *Civilization of the Ancient Mediterranean. Greece and Rome*, ed. M. Grant and R. Kitzinger, New York, C. Scribner's Sons, 1988, vol. 1, pp. 887–908.

56. Lloyd, *Magic, Reason, and Experience*, p. 46.

57. Edelstein and Edelstein, *Asclepius*, vol. I, *Testimonies*, p. 164. A still useful source is Alice Walton, *The Cult of Asklepios*, reprint, New York, Johnson Reprint Co., 1965.

58. Robert Parker, *Miasma, Pollution and Purification in Early Greek Religion*, Oxford, Clarendon Press, 1983, pp. 207–34.

59. See articles in M. Detienne and J. P. Vernant, eds., *The Cuisine of Sacrifice Among the Greeks*, trans. P. Wissing, Chicago, Univ. of Chicago Press, 1989.

60. A vivid prayer recorded by Herondas at Cos reveals the spirit of this sacrifice: "Come graciously and receive this cock, the herald of our walls at home whom I offer to you as a slight addition to your meal. . . . Put up our little tablet to the right of Hygeia." See J. R. Oliver, "The sacrificing women in the temple of Asklepios," *Bull Hist Med* 2 (1934): 507.

61. Ibid., p. 509.

62. Edelstein and Edelstein, *Asclepius*, vol. I, *Testimonies*, pp. 294–309.

63. Walter Burkert, *Ancient Mystery Cults*, Cambridge, Harvard Univ. Press, 1987, p. 113.

64. J. Pollard, "Divination and oracles: Greece," in Grant and Kitzinger, *Civilization*, vol. 1, pp. 941–49.

65. Galen's theories are presented in S. M. Oberhelman, "The diagnostic dream in ancient medical theory and practice," *Bull Hist Med* 61 (1987): 47–60.

66. Quoted in S. M. Oberhelman, "The interpretation of prescriptive dreams in ancient Greek medicine," *J Hist Med* 36 (1981): 418. See also F. Kudlien, "Galen's religious be-

liefs," in *Galen: Problems and Prospects*, ed. V. Nutton, London, Wellcome Institute, 1981, pp. 117–30.

67. Lloyd, *Magic, Reason and Experience*, pp. 40–46.

68. Edelstein and Edelstein cite one instance where a Roman patient "did all that devotees are wont to do but he obtained nothing that contributed to health" (Cassius, Historia Romana) in *Asclepius*, vol. I, *Testimonies*, pp. 198–99. For a general treatment of this subject see E. R. Dodds, *The Greeks and the Irrational*, Berkeley, Univ. of California Press, 1960.

69. Burkert, *Ancient Mystery Cults*, p. 112.

70. Edelstein and Edelstein, *Asclepius*, vol. II, *Interpretation*, pp. 163–73. For a psychoanalytic view consult C. A. Meier, "The dream in ancient Greece and its use in temple cures (incubation)," in *The Dream and Human Societies*, ed. R. Callois and G. E. Grunebaum, Berkeley, Univ. of California Press, 1966, pp. 303–19.

71. Edelstein and Edelstein, *Asclepius*, vol. II, *Interpretation*, p. 101.

72. See E. Kearns, "Order, interaction, authority: Ways of looking at Greek religion," in *The Greek World*, ed. A. Powell, London, Routledge, 1995, pp. 511–29, especially p. 519.

73. Edelstein and Edelstein, *Asclepius*, vol. II, *Interpretation*, p. 104. However, the case of Aristides may have been somewhat unique.

74. For a translation of the inscription see Edelstein and Edelstein, *Asclepius*, vol. I, *Testimonies*, p. 248. See also R. Herzog, *Die Wunderheilungen von Epidauros*, Leipzig, Dieterich'sche Verlagsbuchhandlung, 1931, as quoted by Kee, *Miracle in the Early Christian World*, pp. 88–89.

75. See W. H. D. Rouse, *Greek Votive Offerings*, Cambridge, Cambridge Univ. Press, 1902.

76. For details see O. Deubner, *Das Asklepieion von Pergamon*, Berlin, Verlag für Kunstwissenschaft, 1938.

77. See, for example, "Airs, waters, and places," in *Hippocratic Writings*, ed. G. E. R. Lloyd and trans. J. Chadwick and W. N. Mann, New York, Penguin Books, 1978, pp. 153–58.

78. For an overview of contemporary therapeutic modalities see V. Nutton, "Therapeutic methods and Methodist therapeutics in the Roman Empire," in *The History of Therapy*, ed. Y. Kawakita et al., Tokyo, Ishiyaku Euro-America, 1990, pp. 1–35. See also Galen, *On Hygiene, A Translation of Galen's Hygiene (De sanitate tuenda)*, by Robert Montraville Green, Springfield, IL, C. C. Thomas, 1951.

79. Behr, *Aristides*, p. 232.

80. Ibid., p. 232. According to Vivian Nutton (personal communication), the amount is questionable since the text is not at all clear on this point.

81. For a discussion of bloodletting in antiquity see Peter Brain, *Galen on Bloodletting*, Cambridge, Cambridge Univ. Press, 1986, and S. Kuriyama, "Interpreting the history of bloodletting," *J Hist Med* 50 (1995): 11–46.

82. Behr, *Aristides*, pp. 232–33. Nutton mentions an account of the popularity of cold baths by a certain Antonius Musa, based on a similar treatment of emperor Augustus, as well as a later account by Pliny about successful cold water treatments. See V. Nutton, "From medical certainty to medical amulets: Three aspects of ancient therapeutics," *Clio Med* 22 (1991): 17.

83. Based on the experience of Aristides, it is tempting to speculate that this was indeed the case. There is, however, no solid evidence to answer these questions, and the issue of a shifting role for the temples of Asclepius must remain a hypothesis until further evidence becomes available.

84. Behr, *Aristides*, p. 233.

85. Ibid., p. 234.

86. Ibid., pp. 234–35.

87. V. Boudon, "Le rôle de l'eau dans les prescriptions médicales d' Asclepios, chez Galien et Aelius Aristide," *Bull Corresp Hellenique* suppl. XXVIII (1994): 157–68.

88. W. Heinz, "Antike Balneologie in späthellenistischer und römischer Zeit; zur medizinischen Wirkung römischer Bäder," in *Rise and Decline of the Roman World*, ed. W. Haase and H. Temporini, Berlin, de Gruyter, 1996, Part II: Principale, vol. 37.3, pp. 2411–32, and J. Benedum, "Der Badearzt Asklepiades und seine bithynische Heimat," *Gesnerus* 35 (1978): 20–43. See also E. Craik, "Diet, diaita, and dietetics," in *The Greek World*, ed. Powell, pp. 387–402. For earlier Hellenistic practices see W. D. Smith, "Erasistratus' dietetic medicine," *Bull Hist Med* 56 (1982): 398–409.

89. Behr, *Aristides*, p. 255.

90. Ibid., pp. 261–62.

91. Ibid., p. 235.

92. Edelstein and Edelstein, *Asclepius*, vol. I, *Testimonies*, p. 202. For a discussion of Galen's relationship to Asclepius see Kudlien, "Galen's religious belief," pp. 117–30

93. Behr, *Aristides*, p. 238.

94. See B. Meinecke, "Consumption (tuberculosis) in classical antiquity," *Ann Med Hist* 9 (1927): 379–402, and W. D. Sharpe, " Lung disease and the Graeco-Roman physician," *Annu Rev Respir Dis* 86 (1962): 178–92.

95. During his brief reign, emperor Julian the Apostate (331–63), Constantine II's successor, elevated Asclepius to the status of a supreme sun god, patron of divination and a direct competitor of Christ as a healer of both body and soul, a blasphemy in the eyes of pious Christians. See G. W. Bowersock, *Julian the Apostate*, Cambridge, Harvard Univ. Press, 1978, and especially Polymnia Athanassiadi, *Julian: An Intellectual Biography*, London, Routledge, 1992, p. 167.

96. Flavius Vegetius, *Epitome rei militaris*, as quoted by R. W. Davies, "The Roman military medical service," in *Service in the Roman Army*, ed. D. Breeze and V. A. Maxfield, Edinburgh Univ. Press, pp. 209–10.

97. See Garzetti, *From Tiberius to the Antonines,* pp. 308–73.

98. Following the hypotheses of William McNeill, the naval traffic could have fostered a single expanded disease pool for all coastal cities, including forts at the frontier on the great rivers Rhine and Danube built by Trajan during his early reign. See his *Plagues and Peoples*, Garden City, NY, Anchor Books, 1976, pp. 77–147. For details on the Roman Navy, see C. G. Starr, *The Roman Imperial Navy,* Cambridge, W. Heffer, 1960.

99. H. C. Youtie and J. G. Winter, eds., *Papyri and Ostraca from Karanis*, 2nd series, Ann Arbor, Univ. of Michigan Press, 1951, letter 467, p. 31.

100. A most useful treatment of the cultural identity of imperial Roman soldiers is J. M. Carrie, "The soldier," in *The Romans*, ed. A. Giardina and trans. L. G. Cochrane, Chicago, Univ. of Chicago Press, 1989, pp. 100–37.

101. Youtie and Winter, *Papyri and Ostraca*, letter 477, p. 62

102. Ibid.

103. Ibid., letter 478, p. 66.

104. Ibid.

105. For an overview see V. Nutton, "Roman medicine, 250 BC to AD 200," in *The Western Medical Tradition,* pp. 39–70.

106. More information can be found in J. B. Campbell, *The Emperor and the Roman Army*, Oxford, Clarendon Press, 1984.

107. For details see L. J. F. Keppie, *The Making of the Roman Army*, London, B. T.

Batsford, 1984, and Brian Campbell, *The Roman Army, 31 BC–AD 337, A Sourcebook*, London, Routledge, 1994.

108. Carrie, "The soldier," p. 103.

109. V.A. Maxfield, "The frontiers: Mainland Europe," in *The Roman World*, ed. J. Wachter, London, Routledge & K. Paul, 1987, pp. 139–97.

110. See C. R. Whittaker, *Frontiers of the Roman Empire: A Social and Economic History*, Baltimore, Johns Hopkins Univ. Press, 1994, especially chapters 1 and 2.

111. Garzetti, *From Tiberius to the Antonines*, pp. 334–37.

112. H. Schönberger, "The Roman frontier in Germany: An archeological survey," *J Roman Stud* 59 (1969): 144–97.

113. For more information see A. R. Hands, *Charities and Social Aid in Greece and Rome*, Ithaca, Cornell Univ. Press, 1968.

114. L. Cohn-Haft, "The public physicians of ancient Greece," *Smith College Stud Hist* 42 (1956): 1–91.

115. Details can be found in Hendrik Bolkestein, *Wohltätigkeit und Armenpflege im vorchristlichen Altertum*, Utrecht, A. Oosthoek, 1939.

116. See E. A. Judge, "The quest for mercy in late antiquity," in *God Who Is Rich in Mercy: Essays Presented to D. B. Knox*, ed. P. T. O'Brien and D. G. Peterson, Sydney, Macquarie Univ. Press, 1986, pp. 107–21. See also Rodney Stark, *The Rise of Christianity*, Princeton, NJ, Princeton Univ. Press, 1996, pp. 209–15.

117. Garzetti, *From Tiberius to the Antonines,* pp. 348–49.

118. T. E. J. Wiedemann, "Slavery," in *Civilization of the Ancient Mediterranean, Greece and Rome*, ed. M. Grant and R. Kitzinger, New York, C. Scribner's Sons, 1988, vol. 2, pp. 575–88. For more details see K. R. Bradley, *Slaves and Masters in the Roman Empire, A Study in Social Control*, New York, Oxford Univ. Press, 1987.

119. See Arthur E. R. Boak, *Manpower Shortage and the Fall of the Roman Empire in the West*, Ann Arbor, Univ. of Michigan Press, 1955.

120. Lucius J. M. Columella, *On Agriculture (De Re Rustica)*, trans. H. Boyd Ash, Loeb Classical Library, Cambridge, Harvard Univ. Press, 1960, vol. III, p. 183.

121. Vegetius, in Davies, "Roman military medical service," p. 210. For more information see C. D. Gordon, "Vegetius and his proposed reforms of the army," in *Polis and Imperium: Studies in Honor of Edward Togo Salmon*, ed. J. A. S. Evans, Toronto, Hakkert, 1974, pp. 35–58. Vegetius wrote his *Epitome rei militaris* in the years 384–395 AD, but most of the issues he dealt with were already important centuries earlier.

122. H. von Petrikovits, "Die Innenbauten römischer Legionslager während der Prinzipatszeit," *Abhand Rhein Westfalen Akad Wiss* 56 (1975): 118–24.

123. A. Johnson, *Roman Forts of the First and Second Centuries AD in Britain and the German Provinces*, London, A. & C. Black, 1983. See also L. Murray Threipland, "The Hall Carleon, 1964: Excavations on the site of the legionary hospital," *Archeol Cambrensis* 118 (1969): 86–123.

124. The literature on this subject is quite limited. Among the older works is W. Haberling, "Die Militärlazarette im alten Rom," *Militärärztliche Ztschr* 38 (1909): 441–47, and Theodor Meyer-Steineg, *Krankenanstalten im griechisch-römischen Altertum*, Jena, G. Fischer, 1912.

125. D. Jetter, *Geschichte des Hospitals*, Wiesbaden, F. Steiner Verlag, 1966, pp. 1–7.

126. Rembert Waterman, *Ärztliche Instrumente aus Novaesium*, Cologne, H. Druck KG, 1970. For an update of this research see R. Jackson, "Roman doctors and their instruments: Recent research into ancient practice," *J Roman Archeol* 3 (1990): 5–27.

127. R. Schultze, "Die römischen Legionslazarette in Vetera und anderen Legionslagern," *Bonner Jahrbücher* 139 (1934): 54–63.

128. L. Press, "Valetudinarium at Novae and other Danubian hospitals," *Archeologia* 39 (1988): 69–89.

129. See Lynn F. Pitts and J. K. St. Joseph, *Inchtuthil: The Roman Legionary Fortress Excavations, 1952–65*, with contributions by T. Cowie et al., London, Society for the Promotion of Roman Studies, 1985.

130. J. C. Wilmanns, "Zur Rangordnung der römischen Militärärzte während der mittleren Kaiserzeit," *Ztscht Papyrologie Epigraphik* 69 (1987): 177–89.

131. K. D. Fischer, "Zur Entwicklung des ärztlichen Standes im römischen Kaiserreich," *Medizinhist J* 14 (1979): 165–75. See also V. Nutton, "Roman medicine: Tradition, confrontation, assimilation," in *Rise and Decline of the Roman World*, part II, vol. 37.1, pp 49–78.

132. R. W. Davies, "The medici of the Roman armed forces," *Epigraphische Studien* 8 (1969): 83–99, and by the same author "Some more military medici," *Epigraphische Studien* 9 (1972): 1–11. See also Juliane C. Wilmanns, *Der Sanitätsdienst im Römischen Reich*, Hildesheim, Olms Weidmann, 1995.

133. H. A. Callies, "Zur Stellung der Medici im römischen Heer," *Medizinhist J* 4 (1964): 18–27. See also V. Nutton, "Archiatri and the medical profession in antiquity," *Papers British Schools Rome* 45 (1977): 260–70. For another opinion see E. Kuenzl, "Die medizinische Versorgung der römischen Armee zur Zeit des Kaisers Augustus und die Reaktion der Römer auf die Situation bei den Kelten und Germanen," *Bodenaltertümer Westfalens* 26 (1989): 185–202. A brief summary appeared in *Soc Ancient Med Newsletter* 20 (1993): 85–86.

134. Jackson, *Doctors and Diseases*, pp. 112–37. See also this author's article "Roman medicine: The practitioners and their practices," in *Rise and Decline of the Roman World*, part II, vol 37.1, pp 79–101.

135. J. C. Wilmanns, "Tauglichkeitskriterien für den römischen Militärdienst," in *Bewertung der Gesundheit-Beurteilung militärischer Tauglichkeit*, ed. E. Grunwald, Bonn, Beta Verlag, 1989, pp. 31–50. See also G. R. Watson, "Conscription and voluntary enlistment in the Roman army," *Proc African Class Assoc* 16 (1982): 46–50.

136. These hypotheses are based on modern understandings regarding the epidemiology of infectious diseases and the shifts in immunity of the populations being affected by these illnesses.

137. A. K. Bowman and J. D. Thomas, "A military strength report from Vindolanda," *J Roman Stud* 81 (1991): 62–73.

138. Celsus, *De Medicina*, trans. W. G. Spencer, Loeb Classical Library, Cambridge, Harvard Univ. Press, 1960, vol. I, p. 35, and R. J. Hankinson, "The growth of medical empiricism," in *Knowledge and the Scholarly Medical Traditions*, ed. D. Bates, Cambridge, Cambridge Univ. Press, 1995, pp. 60–83.

139. Kuenzl, "Die medizinische Versorgung," pp. 186–89.

140. V. Nutton, "Medicine and the Roman army: A further reconsideration," *Med Hist* 12 (1968): 260–70.

141. J. C. Wilmanns, "Der Arzt in der römischen Armee der frühen und hohen Kaiserzeit," *Clio Med* 27 (1995): 171–87.

142. G. E. R. Lloyd, "The hot and the cold, the dry and the wet in Greek philosophy," *J Hellenic Stud* 84 (1964): 92–106.

143. See John M. Riddle, *Dioscorides on Pharmacy and Medicine*, Austin, Univ. of Texas Press, 1985.

144. Celsus, *De Medicina*, vol. I, pp. 401–05.

145. R. Watermann, "Aus dem Alltag des Truppenarztes," *Deutsches Ärzteblatt* 62 (1965): 24–29.

146. Celsus, *De Medicina*, vol. II, pp. 71–72 and 77–81.

147. J. Scarborough, "The opium poppy in Hellenistic and Roman medicine," in *Drugs and Narcotics in History*, ed. R. Porter and M. Teich, Cambridge, Cambridge Univ. Press, 1995, pp. 4–23.

148. For a sample see Lawrence J. Bliquez, *Roman Surgical Instruments and Minor Objects in the University of Mississippi*, Göteborg, P. Astroms, 1988.

149. An excellent description is provided by Guido Majno, *The Healing Hand: Man and Wound in the Ancient World*, Cambridge, Harvard Univ. Press, 1975, pp. 360–74. See also Jackson, *Doctors and Diseases*, pp. 112–37.

150. Youtie and Winter, *Papyri and Ostraca*, letter 478, p. 66. Whether Terentianus actually went to a nearby temple in Alexandria remains unknown. Among the Egyptian gods possibly sharing Sarapis' temple were Isis and even Asclepius.

151. This problem has been frequently discussed. See, for example, G. Harig, "Zum Problem 'Krankenhaus' in der Antike," *Klio* 53 (1971): 179–95. For a comparative overview see U. Lindgren, "Frühformen abendländischer Hospitäler im Lichte einiger Bedingungen ihrer Entstehung," *Hist Hospitalium* 12 (1978): 32–61.

152. Edelstein and Edelstein, *Asclepius*, vol. II, *Interpretation*, p. 176.

153. The issue of the "client cult" has been described by Rodney Stark and others. See Stark, *The Rise of Christianity*, pp. 205–08. For more details see Thomas Robbins, *Cults, Converts, and Charisma: The Sociology of New Religious Movements*, Beverly Hills, Sage, 1988.

154. See Edelstein and Edelstein: *Asclepius*, vol. I, *Testimonies*, p. 203, and vol. II, *Interpretation*, p. 112.

155. A comparative analysis of such care is also contained in G. Harig and J. Kollesch, "Arzt, Kranker, und Krankenpflege in der griechisch-römischen Antike und im byzantinischen Mittelalter," *Helikon* 13/14 (1973–74): 256–92.

156. See G. Ziethen, "Heilung und römischer Kaiserkult," *Sudhoffs Arch* 78 (1994): 171–91.

157. Inscription CIL 6.20, cited in Campbell, *The Roman Army*, p. 104.

158. Inscription on the Asclepeion in Lambaesis, Africa, quoted in Edelstein and Edelstein, *Asclepius*, vol. I, *Testimonies*, p. 164.

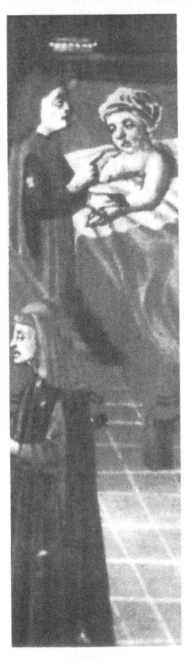

2

CHRISTIAN HOSPITALITY

Shelters and Infirmaries

EARLY CHRISTIANITY: A NEW VISION OF THE SICK

Then the king will say to those on his right hand: come, blessed of my Father, take possession of the kingdom prepared for you from the foundation of the world, for I was hungry and you gave me to eat; I was thirsty and you gave me to drink; I was a stranger and you took me in; naked and you covered me; sick and you visited me.

St. Matthew, The Last Judgment, 25: 34–36[1]

Edessa: Famine, epidemics, and strangers

Late in the year 499, the "Blessed City" of Edessa in southeastern Anatolia, with an estimated population of about 10,000, experienced a great crisis. Frequent wars in the surrounding countryside four years earlier had already destroyed entire villages and ruined the fields. This situation was blamed for an epidemic of boils and swellings during which many inhabitants apparently went blind. By the fall of the year 499, agricultural failures in the surrounding rural areas multiplied due to swarms of locusts devouring the remaining crops. As a result, a multitude of country refugees began streaming into the city.[2] Wrote Joshua the Stylite in his chronicle (composed in 507 in Syriac): "And the sick who were in the villages, as well as the old men and boys and women and infants, and those who were tortured by hunger, being unable to walk far and go to distant places, entered into the cities to get a livelihood from begging, and thus many villages and hamlets were left destitute of inhabitants . . . the pestilence came upon them in the places to which they went and even overtook those who entered Edessa."[3]

Now an important Christian enclave and seat of a bishopric, the ancient city of Edessa near the Syrian desert had become part of the Roman Empire perhaps at about the time that the legionary Claudius Terentianus was languishing in Alexandria. Located on the caravan route to Persia and India, this urban center had also been strongly influenced by Jewish settlers and their traditions, but Christianity had grown dramatically during the first centuries, rapidly gaining its first recruits from among the urban upper and middle classes of Greco-Roman society.[4] This development was greatly aided by a steady decline in living conditions and population in what had been quite prosperous regions under the Antonine emperors.

After the year 200 and even earlier, the Mediterranean region had been periodically afflicted by prolonged, severe draught, triggering repeated famines, and epidemics.[5] Sickness became a source of constant anxiety in the ancient Near East. Perhaps as a result of frequent commercial contacts with the Far East over the Silk Road, two separate disease pools, East and West, came together, with grave consequences for the entire region.[6] Even before the Antonine plague of 165–180, a considerable number of Roman urban centers had probably achieved a sufficient population density to sustain imported contagious diseases. Perennial sanitary problems contributed to the spread of infectious diseases and higher mortality.[7] Ailments resembling smallpox, measles, and plague repeatedly decimated populations and paralyzed political and social life.[8] Fueled by the famines, civil unrest, and extensive migrations from rural areas to urban centers, both endemic and epidemic diseases decisively contributed to the progressive demographic and economic decay of the people living in the Byzantine Empire.[9]

As economic conditions worsened in an environment of political infighting, population decline, and commercial downturn, citizens lost interest in civic affairs and their apathy contributed to a breakdown of municipal government in Byzantium. Greater dependence on imperial support spurred the creation of a vast central bureaucracy operating from the capital. Yet geographic conditions in Asia Minor and Greece, characterized by small, isolated valleys surrounded by mountains and few broad plains or navigable rivers, hampered political centralization efforts. Throughout subsequent centuries, the Byzantine Empire basically remained a federation of cities, each responsible for the political and economic welfare of its surrounding territory.

During Emperor Constantine's reign (313–337), the Diocletian persecutions of Christians were quickly reversed and an official policy of toleration was instituted. A new imperial capital city away from Rome became necessary to govern the Eastern lands. This prompted the establishment of Constantinople in 330, with its strategic access to commercial routes. Constantine also promoted doctrinal and disciplinary unity within the Christian Church, still raked by a number of disputes. Since 321, the Church had been authorized by Constantine to receive legacies and tax exemptions, as well as private assistance for construction projects. In 346, the emperor declared Christianity the empire's official religion, a move that triggered long-standing conflicts between church and state.[10]

A few decades earlier, Edessa had come firmly into the orbit of Byzantium after Constantine's successor, Julian, concluded a treaty with Persia that identified and consolidated their respective frontiers. The event also contributed to a growing antipathy between Christians and Hellenized Jews, with the latter becoming pawns in a struggle spearheaded by the pagan emperor against the growing power of Christianity. In urban centers such as Edessa, even without the influx of strangers, the breakdown of social organization was also due to recurrent epidemics and a drastic decline in population.[11] In fact, Edessa's population at around the year 100 had been estimated at about 80,000, but at the time of Joshua's experiences toward the end of the fifth century, it had dwindled to a mere 10,000.[12]

Informed in 499 of the impending catastrophe, Eusebius, Edessa's bishop, set out to visit the emperor personally in Constantinople. His goal was at least to request a remission of taxes, an indication of the power now placed in the hands of local bishops, who had taken over roles originally reserved for the local aristocracy before Edessa became a heavily Christian enclave. Apparently anticipating Eusebius' needs, the region's governor, Demosthenes, had already obtained emergency funds voluntarily donated by the landowners and had the treasure delivered to the emperor for distribution. To avoid sending the bishop away empty-handed, the emperor gave him money to pay for food and other supplies. After Eusebius returned to Edessa, Demosthenes himself went to Constantinople for more supplies, leaving Eusebius in charge of the stricken city.

In the meantime, the hungry refugees wandering about Edessa's streets were "picking up the stalks and leaves of vegetables all filthy with mud, and eating them."[13] Eusebius responded by ordering the release of grain from public stores and placing more bread for sale in the market. According to Joshua, famine and pestilence were now seriously threatening the city. The newcomers "were sleeping in the porticoes and streets, and wailing by night and day from the pangs of hunger, and their bodies wasted away." Indeed, the "the whole city was full of them and they began to die in the porticoes and in the streets."[14]

Bishops such as Eusebius were aware that the simple provision of food, water, shelter, and nursing allowed some of the sick to recover instead of dying miserably in the streets, thus reducing mortality and strengthening civic morale. During the fourth century, the Church had acquired not only significant political power, but also resources to care for its poor. Leading converted provincial aristocrats promoted a new urban constitution centered on the Christian bishop and his clergy.[15] Like other cities in the Eastern Roman Empire, Edessa adopted the social tenets of the new Christian welfare. According to the historian Sozomenos, the local ecclesiastical authorities had already sponsored in 373 a shelter or guest house—a *xenodocheion* or *xenon*—for the needy in response to a severe famine. The establishment was placed under the leadership of a hermit, Ephraim the Syrian, who had come out of seclusion. These foundations mirrored developments elsewhere in the empire, inspired, in part, by the original availability of Jewish hostels for pilgrims throughout Palestine. Since ancient times, Edessa's fame had been linked to the presence of several springs with alleged healing qualities, including one, the well of Job south of the city, functioning until Emperor Antoninus Pius' time but now surrounded by shrines dedicated to the saints Cosmas and Damian, who were buried there.

Not only was Edessa at the crossroads of commerce, but by the fifth century it was quickly becoming an important destination for scholars and countless visitors who considered it a place of healing. The availability of Greek manuscripts, the presumed presence of the apostle St. Thomas' body, and sacred relics from a number of martyrs attracted pilgrims from Mesopotamia, Persia, Syria, and Asia Minor. Further attractions were the presumed existence of correspondence between Jesus and the former king, Abgar, as well as a portrait of the Savior.[16] Moreover, Edessa was the locus of an extensive translation project that sought to render Greek documents, including theological and medical treatises, into Syriac. Most of those participating in this enterprise, however, were followers of Nestorius, an abbot of Antioch, who had been declared heretical at the third ecumenical council of Ephesus in 431. During the last decade of the century, the Nestorians had been forced to leave Edessa for Persia.

By this time, Edessa's shrines dedicated to Christian martyrs were known for their healing power. Performing miracles, saints or "holy men" such as the twins Cosmas and Damian protected the fields and helped the infirm. Their bones were often believed to be resting places of the Holy Spirit, and dust from their graves was a valuable relic to ward off or cure sickness. Later, Rabbula, another bishop of the city between 411 and 435, founded around 420 another institution nearby specifically devoted to the sick and dying poor, a so-called *nosokomeion* or sick house, with separate facilities for men and women. Here attendants and even physicians were actively engaged in caring functions. Nearby, another hostel, created around 450, sheltered several lepers.[17]

In November 499, Joshua observed that the pestilence had become worse, and a month later, when frost and ice affected the homeless, "the sleep of death came upon them during their natural sleep."[18] The spectacle of crying children and infants in every street hovering over the bodies of their dead mothers was said to be heartbreaking. "Dead bodies were lying exposed in every street, and the citizens were not able to bury them," Joshua recalled.[19] At this point, two priests from Edessa's main house of worship "established an infirmary among the buildings attached to the Great Church of Edessa. Those who were very ill used to go in and lie down there; and many bodies were found in the infirmary which they buried."[20] As the combination of foul weather, famine, and disease took its toll, Edessa's summer and winter bathhouses, with their extensive colonnades, were also pressed into service. "The governor blocked up the gates of the colonnades attached to the winter bath and laid down in it straw and mats, and they used to sleep there, but it was not sufficient for them."[21]

Under these dramatic circumstances, the city council or *curia*, composed of well-known city personalities or *curiales*, delegated all authority to a smaller emergency committee endowed with executive power. This group was consulted by the governor, and a decision was made to set up several more shelters. According to Joshua, "when the leaders of the city saw this, they too established hostels, and many went in and found shelter in them. The Greek soldiers too set up places in which the sick slept, and charged themselves with their expenses."[22] In spite of these measures, mortality remained high. The community expressed its solidarity by attending many of the funerals. Of those placed in the shelters and nursed, many still "died by a painful and melancholy death," although surrounded by those devoted to their care.[23]

Christianity: Constructing a mission of healing

Christianity, which was well established in cities of the Eastern Roman Empire by the time of the disaster at Edessa in 499, was well suited to a population beset by famine, disease, and social disorder.[24] Capable as it was of providing not only an ideology of salvation, but also charity and material assistance to the homeless and poor, it satisfied the longing for relief, hope, and community experienced by the ethnically diverse and uprooted people of the eastern cities, including Greek natives, Roman conquerors, Hellenized Jewish immigrants, and traders from the Far East. Joining this religion ensured membership in a dedicated network of believers whose family values protected orphans and widows and whose nursing services were eagerly sought during earthquakes, fires, and epidemics. Christianity thus became the basis for a new social solidarity eminently suited to the periodic chaos afflicting the urban dwellers.[25]

The result was the institutionalization of philanthropy and the creation of establishments to shelter and feed the poor, care for the sick, assist widows and the aged, and raise orphans. Building on the pagan concept of *agape* or love of God, Christians created a new vision of charity by equating their sufferings to the vicissitudes of Christ's brief sojourn on earth.[26] The mutual love between God and humans was distinct to Christian dogma and energized all actions aimed at assisting others. Instead of the reciprocal hospitality that had prevailed in ancient Greece and the family-oriented obligations of the Romans, Christianity adopted ancient Egyptian and Jewish models of social welfare that targeted particular social groups marginalized by poverty, sickness, and age. Jewish communities had offered hostels to house the poor and sick travelers, and their healers were obligated to treat the sick poor. Houses were even set aside for lepers. Now Christians adopted similar responses to protect their own brethren.[27]

In Christian doctrine, God's own sufferings provided both meaning and reassurance to the dispossessed.[28] Agricultural failures and commercial downturns impoverished many Byzantine citizens, who suffered frequently from famine, warfare, and new diseases. At the same time, food shortages tended to benefit the rich landowners, who were not above profiteering by selling their grain at exorbitant prices. In effect, as in other Near Eastern civilizations, the rich grew richer while the poor became poorer. However, Christ's power and promise to offer each person a heavenly existence in another life inhibited the greed of the rich while providing consolation and hope to those whose wretched earthly existence generated only despair. Once launched as a religious system, Christianity proved successful. A strong sense of group solidarity and voluntarism strengthened the religious commitment. The rewards of membership were tangible, mitigating social inequities and promising greater security to vulnerable sectors of the population.[29]

From its earliest days, Christianity demanded that all of its adherents aid needy and sick people. In his vision of the Last Judgment, Christ had linked an obligation to visit the sick to the essential good works needed for salvation. The six acts of Christian mercy were based on the Scriptures, notably the Gospel of St. Matthew, composed in Antioch. The original concept of a "visitation" of the sick may have been designed to convey solidarity and empathy, thus helping the sick overcome their isolating experiences. As such, visitations presumed the existence of a home and some familiar caring context. They often included gifts, food, and the performance of informal caring chores. However, when extended to provide lodging and aid to strangers, the New Testament recommendations promoted the need for a special communal shelter and nursing services.[30]

Based on scriptural injunctions, charitable Christian institutions were designed for such multiple functions as sheltering and feeding the poor, providing clothing, and performing other caring functions. Poorer members of a Christian congregation were to be cared for through voluntary and concerted efforts under the supervision of clerics and deacons. While committed to charity, however, early Christian communities also attempted to set limits to their endeavors and curb abuses. In a letter to the Thessalonians (2 Thess. 3:6–10), Paul warned his brethren about Christians who refused to work, urging churches to release quickly those who were not willing to participate. After all, poverty was a condition to be endured, not abused. Before offering material support, some Christian groups required strangers to present episcopal letters to verify their status as members of other communities. Less suspicion was displayed toward widows, orphans, and the sick.[31]

A powerful force in spreading the new Christian attitudes toward welfare and the care of the poor and sick throughout the Eastern Empire was the ascetic and monastic traditions. In his *First Principles*, Origen, (ca. 182–251), an early Christian philosopher and ascetic living in Alexandria, had insisted that all humans were originally created equal as "angelic" spirits intended by God to contemplate his glory. After the Fall, God in his divine mercy had allowed each spirit to descend into a particular physical body. Each person's flesh and blood were particular to that person, and the body henceforth would function as a limiting frame for the spirit and become its source of temptation and frustration. Bodies were the vehicles through which individual spirits were forced to interact with the earthly environment. At the same time, the body was seen as a "temple of God," a sparring partner for the spirit, not necessarily its prison, a mate to be tamed and adjusted for the particular needs of its soul. In its quest for healing and liberation, the spirit needed to return gradually to its former existence, pressing against the limitations imposed by the material body. Origen saw this spiritual transformation as a remolding process whereby the physical body, like a vessel of clay, could be rebuilt into a "holy tabernacle" to be "offered up" and "made holy" for God.[32]

Such ideas concerning the discipline and transformation of the human body were central to the emergent ascetics. Since the body was involved in the soul's transformation, it could not be ignored but rather had to be humbled by a strict regimen of fasting, vigils, and even physical labor. The heart was believed to be the center of a person, the meeting point between human body and divine soul. Since the body displayed a certain autonomy and inner heat, reduction in food intake was seen as the most effective weapon for avoiding physical corruption and achieving spiritual changes. It was therefore critical to master the "struggles of the belly" through fasting and vigils. To implement this agenda, Christians selected deserts in Egypt, Syria, and Palestine, zones deprived of means to produce enough food.[33]

Christian views concerning the relationship between the soul and the body produced two separate currents of asceticism: the eremitic and the monastic. Within the former framework, individual Christians voluntarily withdrew from society and went to live in desert caves and crevices. The goal of the hermit was to master his passions and control his desires through solitude, fasting, and prayer designed to ensure his soul's salvation. Ascetic life also included voluntary chastity. Among the most famous hermits was St. Anthony (ca. 251–350), who gave away his worldly goods and went into seclusion in Egypt. Soon he attracted a veritable colony of hermits, a development that led to the creation of a cenobitic community sharing meals and prayers under St. Anthony's rule.

The *coenobium* or monastery par excellence developed in Egypt at the same time as eremitic life. The first fully communal monastery was founded by a former pagan soldier, Pachomius (ca. 292–346), an Egyptian who had converted to Christianity, around 320. His complex, containing 11 separate houses laid out as a legionary camp, was located near Thebes on the Nile River and eventually housed over 1,000 monks. Soon other Pachomian monasteries were founded as alternative villages in the midst of the settled world, thus blurring the boundaries between desert and world.[34] Given his military background, Pachomius devised a number of rules to regulate life in his monastery. The head of the community was to be the general superior of all houses, and members owed him complete obedience. Although monasteries depended for food on the surrounding settlements, leaders devised a system of daily work and worship adjusted to bodily needs for food and sleep. Monks were also grouped according to their artisanal skills. A guest house became available for the comfort of visitors, including pilgrims and hermits. During the ensuing centuries, such ascetic and cenobitic traditions diffused rapidly throughout Palestine, Syria, and eventually the Byzantine Empire. Many monasteries located away from deserts became self-sufficient units, even producers of foodstuffs such as corn, wine, and oil, as their patrimony expanded through donations of cash and land. Their integration into the official church occurred through links of local patronage with the ruling bishops.[35]

Basil of Caesarea (ca. 330–379) was one of the bishops who played a key role in refocusing Christianity's ascetic idealism and integrating it into the organization of the urban Church. Caesarea was an important city located at the crossing of all major roads in Asia Minor. Following a period of solitary life, Basil, a highly educated individual, had returned home determined to create a model urban Christian community. In his view, cenobitic life was preferable to being a hermit. A solitary life only served the ends of one individual, a somewhat selfish approach. To fulfill the Christian commandments, believers had to become social creatures and perform good works that helped other members of a community. The phrase "If you live alone, whose feet will you wash?" pointedly highlighted the distinctions between solitude and collective service, the latter so necessary in an urban setting with its countless needs.[36]

Famine and disease, of course, were then prominent causes for social upheaval. To Basil, these were also symptomatic of a community's moral malaise, which often could be traced to the rich and their greed. Wealthy Christians reveled in "lives of fantasy." Since current well-being was transitory, penance was in order. Basil considered it essential that the wealthy provide some of their assets during emergencies as an investment in future heavenly rewards. As the events of the year 369 attest, this calculated appeal to self-interest seemed quite effective in Caesarea during a catastrophic food shortage, allowing storehouses to be opened. Under Basil, a precedent of collaboration between the ecclesiastical and political leadership of a city to deal with such events was set. Centuries later, a similar situation happened in Edessa, when Eusebius took charge and grain was also released from the public granaries.[37]

Early Christian theology readily accepted the role of medicine in charitable works. The new Christians lived within a world populated by esteemed and well-educated physicians who played prominent roles in Byzantine community life. Closely linked to local ruling and ecclesiastical elites, most practitioners lived in the cities, probably because, according to St. John Chrysostom (ca. 347–407), urban life took its toll, forcing dwellers to frequently seek professional aid. This selective location seemingly created problems for travelers who lived on the road and lacked baths, physicians, and remedies.[38] The *iatros* (physician) could be distinguished from a lay person because of his learning and practical skills—his *techne iatrike*—including employ the employment of *pharmaka* and surgical instruments.

According to Chrysostom, the greatest of the Greek Fathers and briefly patriarch of Constantinople at the end of the fourth century, medical knowledge could only be acquired through a long and expensive course of studies that included reading the books of Hippocrates and Galen and obtaining the necessary skills through apprenticeship with experienced teachers at their houses. When this was accomplished, St. Gregory of Nazianzen (ca. 330–390), a friend of Basil, suggested that young physicians settle in any city and open their practices, treating persons who came for consultation without worrying about honoraria but rather building their reputation.[39] The advice was quite pertinent, since many Greek physicians during the fourth century were still suspected of being pagans. Often, professional honoraria were considered excessive.[40]

Constructing an image of Christ as the Great Physician acknowledged and legitimized physical healing efforts. According to Origen, God was quite aware of the body's physical frailty and predisposition to disease. Thus, in his mercy, He had also furnished mankind with remedies from the earth to alleviate the pains of physical suffering and, through the gift of *logos*, provided the necessary knowledge to use these remedies. In his *Long Rules*, Basil followed the thought of Origen by also affirming that the use of medicines was congruent with Christian piety. God's grace was as evident in the healing power of medicine and the skill of its practitioners as it was in miraculous cures. Indeed, God had endowed particular plants, minerals, and even thermal waters with curative powers. If He willed it, those who could discover and employ these agents could benefit their patients. For Basil, medical practice was therefore in perfect accord with Christian virtue so long as both the sick and their healers never lost sight of the need to please God and place spiritual health on the highest plane. This favorable view of the contemporary medical profession was also reflected in the writings of Basil's brother, St. Gregory of Nyssa (ca. 340–396), revealing their personal experiences with physicians.[41]

Christians were encouraged to recognize the practical roots of the healing art and appreciate the contributions already made to it by practitioners since classical antiquity.[42] After all, in imperial Rome, both pagans and Christians had increasingly concerned themselves with health and healing.[43] Medicine had already occupied an important place among the human arts, exploiting the manifold healing forces of nature enshrined in roots, flowers, leaves, fruits, and metals, as well as developing surgical skills. For Chrysostom, lay physicians were true Christian benefactors fighting against disease. By following the laws of their art, these practitioners displayed genuine *philantropia*, even when they went against the wishes of their charges or paradoxically caused pain and suffering during the performance of their treatments.[44] Origen had gone even further, explaining that lay physicians should not show pity and compassion toward their patients, even when they felt it, if this compromised their healing task and thus ultimately threatened the welfare of a sick person. Those who acceded to the wishes of their patients for useless treatments, particularly when surgery and cauterization were required, placed both healing and their reputation in jeopardy.[45]

A hundred years before the Edessa crisis, Christianity had made the care of the sick a central component of the good works to be performed by all believers. Sermons given by important Church authorities such as St. Gregory of Nyssa stressed the fact that disease was ubiquitous and attacked all ranks of society, robbing the afflicted of strength and causing them in many instances to stop supporting their families. The ensuing misery and suffering called for mercy, and members of a Christian community needed to come to the rescue, sharing their diverse talents and knowledge for the common good. In that quest, Greek Fathers such as St. Basil, St. Gregory of Nyssa, St. Gregory Nazianzen, and St. John Chrysostom thus supported the participation of secular medicine as one of the options for Christians to consider when afflicted with an illness.

However, the notions that the secular medical art was indeed a gift of God and that those who practiced it could be said to dispense philanthropy encountered some theological and institutional opposition. For one, the New Testament did not appear to sanction the use of medicines. Many bishops stressed the sole power of faith, suggesting that recourse to lay healing implied a weakness or even lack of faith. Medicine merely tried to preserve or recover the health of a Christian's body, which was far less important than his soul. In the fifth and sixth centuries, this opposition to secular medicine remained strongest among those who had contempt for bodily well-being and thus supported an ascetic Byzantine monasticism, as well as Christians devoted to the cult of the saints or *anargyroi*. Later, Christian propaganda promoted the stereotype of the careless and unfeeling physician who neglected his patients and prescribed strong or useless remedies in contrast to Christ, the selfless and all-powerful healer.[46] Christian theologians borrowed heavily from the Old Testament and Jewish demonology to construct a scaffolding for epic struggles between the forces of good and evil, God versus Satan, angels versus demons. Demonic possession and sin were considered to be the main causes of disease. Only God's power, transmitted to Christ, his apostles, and the saints, could vanquish the darker forces.[47] In that context, relics of martyrs and saints were said to possess supernatural powers that could drive out sickness. Visitation of their graves was strongly encouraged, and many pious Christians set forth to visit their shrines, collecting dust with healing properties from the vicinity or using water employed in washing the tombs.[48]

To achieve success, Christianity took over a number of functions from the traditional pagan healing cults, especially that of Asclepius. In the first four centuries AD, some of the famous Asclepian shrines continued to attract many people in Asia Minor and Egypt. Even Emperor Julian (331–363), Constantine's nephew, who reverted to paganism, selected the divine figure of Asclepius to neutralize the personal appeal of Christ as a healer.[49] According to St. Gregory of Nyssa, the remaining pagan shrines were now being filled with the dying, who had come to drink from the sacred spring waters near the temples during the severe epidemics of the fourth century. Christians, in turn, often viewed Asclepius as a pagan competitor, the Antichrist to be destroyed. According to St. Athanasius (ca. 297–373), the patriarch of Alexandria, Asclepius' medical knowledge was believed to be limited, since it had been acquired while he was a mere human. The god's subsequent ascendancy to divine status was seen as an example of the nefarious Greek practice of immortalizing selected heroes.[50] Although most pagan shrines were destroyed or converted into churches, language, ceremonial, and imagery were transferred to the emerging *Christus medicus*, a frequent theme in the writings of St. Augustine.[51] As with the pagan cult of Asclepius, secular and religious healing remained linked. Before their veneration as saints, even Cosmas and Damian had been physicians and patron saints of medicine. Cures by touch with relics were often supplemented by the use of medicines, plasters, and surgical procedures.

Christian welfare: Rise of the *xenodocheion*

In Byzantium, prevailing political, financial, and social conditions during the third century had weakened social and political ties at the local and provincial levels. As economic problems mounted, a gradual tendency to bypass the normal fiscal and judicial systems developed. Town councils or *curias* were assemblies of notables, generally local landowners, who regularly met in a rectangular hall, the *basilica*, for governmental actions, business deals, and lawsuits. Villages were governed by heads of households. Faced with problems, the authorities sought the patronage of a wealthy landowner or merchant to provide solutions. This practice now allowed local bishops and their clergy—derived from this provincial elite—to assume a new role within the civic system, including the task of caring for the *demos* or mass of poor people now populating their cities. This new construction of a Christian bishop as a patron of social welfare schemes within his own city is exemplified by Basil at Caesarea, who focused his religious community on the performance of good works in the city as a proper model for the fulfillment of Christian obligations.[52]

Since their early days, Christian communities had been allowed to manage their own affairs, but progressive inclusion in the state's political structure created overlapping systems of authority. Ecclesiastical jurisdiction tended to conform to existing political boundaries. In the ensuing confusion, bishops such as Basil in Caesarea and later Eusebius in Edessa began taking over functions previously held by the local aristocracy. Unfortunately, the Scriptures furnished no practical guidelines for organizing charitable programs. In the early centuries of Christian rule, the so-called Apostolic Constitutions, a collection of rules reflecting established charitable practices in churches from Syria to Rome, became the compass of social welfare schemes. In their dioceses, bishops and their deacons were told to collect alms from wealthy Christians and redistribute them to the poor. To fulfill Christ's command, bishops were also told to look after the sick. Rules formulated in Rome in the year 215 obligated the bishop to seek out the sick in their own houses. A dramatic example of this duty occurred during the reign of Emperor Gallienus (259–268) as the local bishop Dionysus, with help from local Christians, led an extensive door-to-door relief operation in Alexandria during a plague epidemic.

Why were the authorities, lay and religious, so eager in the 300s to create institutions for sheltering the poor and treating the sick? Given the scope and frequency of the social problems, the classical pagan models of a personal, individualized *hospitalitas* were clearly inadequate. A greater and persistent burden of disease linked to widespread poverty, social dislocation, and warfare created desperate situations, exemplified by the plight of Edessa. Paradoxically, theological disputes among Christian factions after the Nicene Council of 325 provided further impetus for the foundation of philanthropic institutions. In their quest for further members, rival Christian congregations became pawns in a contest for control of charitable works. All local welfare schemes, in turn, became targets of an increasingly competitive patronage that featured the Byzantine emperors, bishops of the Christian Church, monastic leaders, lay aristocrats, and even some physicians.[53]

Not to be ignored in the spread and practice of Christianity were prominent women who played key roles. Prohibition of abortion and female infanticide, both prevalent among pagans and a major cause of the gender imbalance existing at the time, created an oversupply of marriageable Christian women, leading to unions with pagans who converted to the new religion. Many of these women enjoyed great freedom and exercised considerable power, assuming positions of honor and authority, such as serving as deacons in many congregations. Their willingness to nurse fellow Christians as well as some unbelievers during epidemics— a fact attested to by Galen—became a cornerstone for conversion, as well as an important factor in the recovery of countless victims of disease.[54]

By the third century AD, the Christian Church had become the most important patron of charitable works. Its rapid diffusion throughout the Roman Empire created a vast organizational network of dioceses with strongholds in Rome, Antioch, Alexandria, and later Constantinople. Donations and legacies from the faithful were critical to consolidate the growing economic power of the Church, although the administration of its property continued to be controlled by imperial regulations. The earlier provision of shelters for visitors from other churches at bishops' residences or nearby guest houses proved insufficient. In urban settings flooded with refugees from the countryside, Church officials, providing mutual help and hospitality through the use of their deacon system, were quickly overwhelmed by the magnitude of the problems facing their brethren.[55]

One must also consider the Byzantine state and its ruler, the emperor, as an important patron of all charitable institutions, including the hospitals.[56] By the 390s, Constantinople had become the center of social and imperial life in Byzantium. Constantine's Christianity and his Roman heritage fused to establish a close understanding between church and state. Within that framework the emperor became Christ's vice-regent, with supernatural qualities and the source of all authority. Thus, the Christian church came under the general care of the emperor, who played a vital role in the most important organ of church government, the General Council. As in earlier times, the nation's wealth was primarily based on agricultural surpluses first employed for the needs of the court, army, and bureaucracy and then distributed to other members of the ruling class. As God's representative on earth, however, the emperor had an obligation to perform works of mercy for his suffering subjects. This duty made him de facto a critical player during hard economic times, as he could shift revenues from imperial estates to help the needy, and it compelled him to become an important patron in the establishment of shelters. In times of crisis, direct appeals to the emperor, as in the case of Edessa's famine, often bypassed the bureaucratic barriers.[57] In the fourth and fifth centuries, the bigger and wealthier foundations serving the poor and sick were located in or near the capital city, including the Sampson, Isidor, and Euboulos *xenones*.[58]

During the so-called golden age of the urban episcopate in Byzantium, which stretched from the fourth to the sixth centuries, the promotion and expansion of Church activities led to the gradual development of a welfare state, including the foundation of a wide range of charitable institutions including churches, almshouses, hostels, orphanages, and hospitals. The usual place for treatment of illnesses remained the home, but those who were homeless, lacked caring family members, or were traveling needed alternative facilities. Among those caring for the sick of their parish after hours were the *philoponoi* (lovers of labor) in Egypt and *spoudaioi* in other parts of Byzantium. These men and women were usually located in contemporary large cities on the eastern Mediterranean. In Alexandria, they combed the baths and streets of the city in search of the poor stricken with disease, perhaps conveying some of them to established hostels. Their principal function was to bathe and anoint the sick.[59] Given the availability of Christianized physicians together with Church leaders who themselves possessed medical knowledge, free medical advice in the care of the sick poor was always an option.

Before the year 330, for example, the Christian Church in Antioch and its daughter churches in the Syrian hinterland had already set up hostels or guest houses for the poor that they called *xenodocheia*.[60] While based on the tenets of Christian solidarity, these institutions were also designed to restore social order. In time, numerous *xenodocheia*, *xenones*, and *katagogia* (lodges) to house and feed the poor sprouted throughout the land, with devout widows and celibates of both sexes playing important roles in their foundation. By the 340s, the Church of Antioch under the leadership of Bishop Leontios had already begun to operate a number of hostels described as *xenodocheia* or *xenones* to feed and shelter the poor. One was located at Daphne, a spa outside of Antioch, where the wealthy repaired when in poor health. Another "house to nourish the poor" was described in Sabasteia, Armenia, founded by the local bishop, Eustathius (356–380). Despite their relative economic weakness in Byzantium, monasteries also became sites of care for the poor, guests, and the sick who came for help. *Xenodocheia* were frequently attached to monasteries in towns and in the countryside. In the 450s, for example, the monk Theodosius founded such an institution near Jerusalem, with three separate buildings to house monks, the poor, and wealthier individuals in need of medical attention. The sick monks were usually attended by some of their brethren in a separate infirmary.[61]

The basic goal of a shelter was the protection and social control of its inmates. Services were provided with an emphasis on togetherness in a dormitory-type environment. Harsh punishments were recommended for those breaking the rules, including exclusion from religious ceremonies or even excommunication. In addition to shelter, order, and discipline, these "hospitals" offered spiritual care, taking advantage of the inmates' fears, dependencies, and piety. As an adjunct to churches and monasteries, the institution was clearly identified as a religious space, with ceremonies and routines designed to reaffirm the Christian faith. Architecturally, a *xenodocheion* consisted of a square or rectangular complex with a central courtyard. Rooms were arranged around the perimeter and linked by a covered arcade for circulation.[62] Courtyard gardens were ideal for prayer, meditation, and work, thus performing an important restorative and redemptive function.[63]

One of the first institutions providing specific medical attention developed when Aetius, a sectarian Syrian with medical knowledge, and his followers began to treat the sick among hospice guests in Antioch in the 340s. Aetius and his followers may even have established a more specialized institution for those stricken with disease, a *nosokomeion*, described by Chrysostom for Antioch in 381. From the available evidence, there seems not to have been a clear, consistent line of separation between a *xenon*, primarily a hostel basically providing shelter and food for the needy and strangers, and a *nosokomeion*, established for the specific purpose of rendering care to the sick. More homeless migrants than travelers and pilgrims were among the inmates. Their average life expectancy was less than 25 years. Many of those seeking shelter were discovered to be also malnourished or sick, and therefore probably received advice and medicines from clerics with medical knowledge or from consulting lay physicians. Besides medical attention, those

admitted to the *nosokomeion* with presumed illnesses or injuries probably benefited primarily from a regimen of rest, food, and good nursing.[64]

Since both the *xenodocheion* and *nosokomeion* developed side by side with
churches and monasteries, they probably shared common building plans, perhaps
simple basilican buildings gradually modified due to the exigencies of patient care.
Certainly many early shelters must have been makeshift, temporary structures,
sometimes simply a few rooms adjacent to a church, while others were located in
remodeled houses, or, as in Edessa, placed in existing bathing facilities. In larger
urban centers, medieval Byzantine houses were two- or three-story buildings
arranged, like their Roman counterparts, as a rectangular or square building with
central patios or gardens. Additional administrative facilities and baths were placed
in separate buildings.

Each shelter operated under the supervision of clerics, deacons, and deaconesses, with a staff of lay volunteers. At the time of the Edessa disaster, the caring personnel were lay persons, often urban ascetics or *parabalaneis*, bathing and
anointing the sick, feeding them, and carrying them around, as well as changing
and mending their clothes. According to Chrysostom, women were already assigned to bear the major burdens of physical care, with one of the greatest advantages of marriage being the care of illness by wives.[65] Medical treatment could
be furnished by local physicians. Physician-clerics were quite popular in the early
Byzantine Empire. Even Basil is said to have had some medical knowledge. He
and his brother Gregory certainly belonged to the contemporary Greek aristocracy and had close relatives and friends among the prominent physicians of the
day. As mentioned earlier, for leading bishops, medical practice by lay physicians
was not only acceptable, it was a necessary and appropriate approach in case of
sickness, a fundamentally different view from that prevailing in the Western Roman Empire.[66] Within the framework of classical medical ethics, however, physicians were excused from continuing their healing tasks if the patient's illness was
deemed incurable, especially in cases of cancer and "elephantiasis" (a term for
leprosy) since the expected death could be detrimental to their professional reputation.[67] Under such circumstances, even the administration of *pharmaka*—
largely herbal preparations—was reduced since the practice was considered wasteful.[68]

"Slash and burn": Caring for the sick

How did affected Byzantine cities such as Edessa cope with famines and epidemics? Each disaster created a crisis of faith as people pondered the reasons for
these scourges. Pagans, who had self-interested individual exchange relations with
an array of deities, lacked a comprehensive religious doctrine that could energize
and compel them to consider collective charitable actions. Asclepius, for exam-

ple, only provided health advice to individuals who sought him out, worshiped him, and made offerings. He did not offer escape from mortality, nor did he promise eternal salvation. Destitute of a socially relevant ideology to counter mass disease and death, pagans yielded to flight or despair, unable to confront the crises. Often they avoided all contact with the sick, refusing to nurse them. Some escaped from their homes, even leaving their dead unburied. By contrast, as Joshua the Stylite reveals in his chronicle, local Christian congregations, including Edessa's, were highly successful in mobilizing their members, running a "miniature welfare state" within the empire.[69] Their revolutionary beliefs in mutual love and sacrifice, as well as eternal salvation, became the linchpin for communal actions.[70] Charitable work, however, attracted even more needy refugees, "for a report had gone forth throughout the province of Edessa, that the Edessenes took good care of those who were in want; and for this reason a countless multitude of people entered the city."[71]

A somewhat similar event had occurred earlier in the city of Caesarea, located deep in the interior of the empire. Traditionally, agricultural pursuits in the surrounding province of Cappadochia were precarious since farmers had to rely on poor, sandy soils. Periodically threatened with blight and famines, Cappadochia and Caesarea depended on the leadership of its bishop—Basil in the fourth century—to persuade wealthy landowners to open their storehouses and distribute food. In addition, Basil took the first steps toward setting up several hostels outside the city's gates. The *Basileiados* or *ptocheion* was designed to serve the destitute, strangers, and sick poor while keeping the city free of beggars, homeless, and dying people. As St. Gregory of Nazianzen described it, "he [Basil] assembled in one place those afflicted by the famine, including some who had recovered a little from it, men and women, children, old men, the distressed of every age. He collected through contributions all kinds of food helpful for relieving famine. He set before them caldrons of pea soup and our salted meats, the sustenance of the poor."[72] Nazianzen went on to describe this shelter and soup kitchen as "a new city, the storehouse of piety . . . there sickness is endured with equanimity, calamity is a blessing, and sympathy is put to the test."[73] Around 370, this complex started to attract the attention and patronage of Emperor Valens. To serve the needy, Basil hired attendants, physicians, escorts, and pack animals.

Basil was quite proud of his "new city." He frequently visited it and personally greeted the sick as brothers, insisting on dressing some of their wounds. The complex consisted of a church, a residence for the administrator, and quarters for his subordinate assistants, together with a *xenodocheion* for strangers and visitors on a journey. The *Basileiados* was conceived as a religious center as much as a refuge, soup kitchen, and medical institution for those in distress. As in similar establishments elsewhere, the lines remained blurred between welfare, social control, and spiritual care, as well as the specifically medical assistance furnished by physicians. *Xenones* became representative features of Byzantine urban life and therefore hallmarks of the new Christian polis.[74]

Although no contemporary account of life in an early Byzantine shelter, hospital, or monastic infirmary survived, most of the prominent Church fathers described the *xenodocheion*'s rites of passage. Admission rituals emphasized that care was to be primarily directed toward the soul. Cleansing the soul through confession of sins was to precede any efforts to care for the body.[75] Besides staging religious ceremonies, the shelters established an internal order and discipline essential in the midst of terror and chaos produced by famines, epidemics, and wars. Each establishment insisted on the strict separation of men and women. Rituals of prayer and vigils may have aided the management of institutional death. Bishops were aware of the difficulties surrounding the management of a *xenon*'s inmates, revealing the presence of some unruly and even insufferable brethren, who, tired of lying in bed, refused to comply with the physician's orders, threw away their food, and tore at the clothes of their caregivers.

Besides prayer and penance, rest, diet, and nursing were the mainstays of the regimen offered in a *xenodocheion*, *nosokomeion*, or monastic infirmary.[76] To feed the "brothers in Jesus Christ, the needy poor," attendants provided the standard Byzantine fare of bread, wine, and dried or fresh cooked vegetables dressed with olive oil. Barley soup was also typically served, as was honey boiled in water. Monks received dispensation from fasting and were given a better than usual diet to aid recovery. However, they were discouraged from demanding food items not normally available under a so-called antigluttony formula.[77] As always, the boundaries between caring and curing remained blurred, but the salutary effects of rest, diet, and nursing must have been significant.[78]

If the organism's own natural healing forces proved incapable of expelling the presumed poisons or corrupt humors from the sick body, physicians were called on to imitate them. The principal therapeutic strategy, as in Aristides' time, was to extract the spoiled humors with the help of *pharmaka* and physical methods. Emetics and purgatives, expectorants, diuretics, and sudorifics, together with bloodletting, were employed. In theory, this depleting scheme, based on classical humoralism, was to be followed with great caution, letting nature at every step do most of the work in fighting off a disease. Thus, physicians provided little symptomatic relief for employing mandragora and opium for excessive pain. They also withheld most nourishment in febrile cases.

In addition to drugs, a number of counterirritation procedures—notably scarification, the production of blisters and small burns—attempted to expel the noxious humors from the vicinity of vital organs such as the lungs, heart, stomach, and liver and displace them toward the surface of the body. Once diverted to the skin, they were to be herded into discrete but far less dangerous patches, pustules, and abscesses capable of being drained through wet cupping, surgical incisions, or cauterizations. Consulting or attending lay physicians were thus often feared and even despised as "fathers of pain"—a label employed by Origen—because of their frequent use of the scalpel and the cautery.[79]

Although noninvasive, topical surgery and localized hemostatic burns often produced favorable results in the management of wounds; they also seem to have been employed with some frequency in the treatment of internal ailments by practitioners disparagingly called "cutters" by St. Gregory of Nazianzen.[80] Here the religious notion of fire as a purifier melded with practical experiences acquired in wound healing. When it came to cauterization, patients were expected to submit willingly to this procedure and tolerate the pain inflicted by the burning but cleansing iron. This suffering was considered redemptive, in imitation of Christ's own agony. However, the religiously sanctioned stoicism apparently was rare. One writer, Palladios, observed that only a saint would willingly and quietly tolerate the hurt inflicted by the physician's scalpel and cautery. St. Gregory of Nazianzen reported loud cries and screams following the placement of red-hot irons on a number of body areas. According to Eusebius of Caesarea, most patients begged their physicians to prescribe bitter and more gentle *pharmaka* rather than attempt to heal them with sharp knives and fiery irons.[81]

Unfortunately, in times of crisis, many of the emaciated individuals brought to a *xenodocheion* for care were beyond help. However, to die in the shelter nursed by fellow Christians and with the spiritual assistance of clergy was considered quite reassuring. Communal prayer and religious rituals such as the provision of sacraments helped those who were suffering to look forward to their eternal salvation and to die in relative peace, away from the turmoil of social dislocation, terror, and rampant disease. Free burial in consecrated soil attended by the local congregation was another anxiously sought benefit. As Joshua recounted in Edessa, "the bath too that was under the Church of the Apostles beside the Great gate was full of sick, and many dead bodies were carried forth from it every day. All the inhabitants of the city were careful to attend in a body the funeral of those who were carried forth with psalms and hymns and spiritual songs that were full of the hope of the resurrection."[82]

In the end, Joshua also tells us that in Edessa, "nothing could be heard in all the streets of the city but either weeping over the dead or the lamentable cries of those in pain. Many too were dying in the courts of the Great Church and in the courts of the city and in the inns, and on the roads as they were coming to the city."[83] Although public prayers on behalf of the original city dwellers were said for their protection from the epidemic, still "the pestilence began among the people of the city and many biers were carried out in one day. And not only in Edessa was this sword of pestilence but also from Antioch as far as Nisibis the people were destroyed and tortured in the same way by famine and pestilence. Many of the rich died who were not starved, and many of the notables too died in this year."[84]

Thus, in the early Byzantine Empire, the new tenets of Christianity based on traditional Near Eastern welfare concepts gave prominence to the care of the needy, poor, strangers, and the sick. Such religious agendas created a set of overlapping goals to provide shelter, rest, food, and medical attention within segregated guest houses variously called *xenodocheia*, *xenones*, and *nosokomeia*.[85] The primary emphasis was on solidarity with the needy. As Jerome wrote, "He whom we look down upon, whom we cannot bear to see, the very sight of whom causes us to vomit, is the same as we, formed with us from the selfsame clay, compacted of the same elements. Wherever he suffers we also can suffer."[86] Life was but a brief pilgrimage full of hardships, the shelters a welcome pause on the journey. As Basil himself remarked, "There is only one way leading to the Lord and all who travel toward Him are companions of one another and travel accordingly to one agreement as to life."[87] Forged in part under the dramatic circumstances of famine and epidemics afflicting the urban centers of Byzantium, these new healing spaces became the forerunners of a Christian tradition of caregiving that extends to our own day.

HEALING AT ST. GALL:
THE GOLDEN AGE OF BENEDICTINE MONASTICISM

We are about to found a school for the Lord's service, in the organization of which we hope to set down nothing harsh and burdensome. . . . As one's way of life and one's faith progresses, the heart becomes broadened, and with unutterable sweetness of love, the way of the mandates of the Lord is traversed. . . . Continuing in the monastery in His teaching until death, through patience, we are made partakers in Christ's passion, in order that we may merit to be companions in His kingdom.

St. Benedict of Nursia (480–547)[88]

The abbot of St. Gall takes a fall

Almost half a millennium after Joshua's harrowing account of events in Edessa, an accident on the western fringes of the Roman Empire allows us to gauge the status of institutional Christian hospitality and healing. Around the year 968, Purchard I, the ruling abbot of the monastery of St. Gall, happily accepted a present from his niece, Hadwig, the daughter of Duke Henry I of Bavaria and widow of the duke of Swabia. Young and attractive, Hadwig had previously visited the monastery and charmed Purchard into "lending" her his *portarius* (doorkeeper), Ekkehard, to give her private lessons. Moreover, her intrigues at the imperial court had ignited a fierce competition between the monasteries of Reichenau and St. Gall for Emperor Otto the Great's favor. Perhaps feeling guilty after providing

Abbot Rudmann of Reichenau with a sizable donation, Hadwig had decided to present the St. Gall abbot with a purebred horse in full knowledge of Purchard's love for hunting and horse riding, a passion he shared with Otto I, the leading monarch of Europe.[89]

To take possession of the noble beast, Purchard left the monastery for the nearby town of Rickenbach. After his arrival, and to demonstrate his appreciation for Hadwig's gesture, the abbot had the horse immediately saddled and decided to mount it. This gesture by the diminutive monk failed to impress the somewhat fiery animal. Without warning, the horse immediately jumped and threw its new rider to the ground of a courtyard, where he landed against a doorpost. At a time when horseback riding was one of the more common modes of transportation and recreation of the upper classes, such accidents were common, and the assembled dignitaries must have rushed to the abbot's aid. To their horror, Purchard seemed in great pain and was totally unable to move his right leg.[90]

By all accounts, Purchard was considered one of the pillars of St. Gall's monastery, the famous Benedictine institution located in the diocese of Constance, south of the city on the lake with the same name. The institution traced its origins back to a seventh-century Irish missionary effort, having been established by an itinerant monk, Gallus, presumably from Ireland and a follower of St. Columban's rule. Around 612, Gallus withdrew into the wilderness in the valley of the river Steinach near Lake Constance with a dozen companions. Practicing a rigorous Celtic monasticism, Gallus' simple hermitage served as a base for the conversion of local Alemans living at the lake and beyond. After the death of these missionaries, however, the hermitage decayed, although it continued to be a place of pious pilgrimage.[91]

In 719, a converted local Aleman named Otmar founded a new monastery at the site and governed it for 40 years under Benedictine rules. From its early years, the complex contained an infirmary as well as lodgings for the poor. Amply endowed with gifts of land from as far away as Breisgau in the upper Rhine and Thurgau, St. Gall flourished. Otmar's early successors, however, struggled with the Alemannic bishops at Constance, who were their titular heads and envious of their new wealth. The monastery's golden century spanned the years 818–926, following Emperor Louis the Pious' grants of tax immunity and the right to hold free elections for abbot. With the last obligations to pay tribute lifted in 854, the institution gained great prestige and became the destination point of numerous pilgrims who venerated the relics of St. Gallus and the recently canonized St. Otmar. At the same time, St. Gall's productive *scriptorium*, or writing room, had begun expanding the institution's library holdings. Among the treasures was a copy of St. Benedict's original rule made by Carolingian scholars.[92] By the early tenth century, St. Gall had forged ecclesiastical and cultural ties with many other European monasteries, including its nearby rival, the abbey of Reichenau. Both St.

Gall and Reichenau entered into an alliance for purposes of prayers with groups of monks at other monasteries in southwestern Germany and Switzerland. A period of institutional consolidation and reform was at hand.

The injured Purchard had been elected abbot by his congregation at a young age in 958, following a series of incidents and debates at St. Gall concerning monastic discipline. The decades preceding Purchard's ascension had been quite eventful, punctuated by a Magyar incursion in 926. The invaders plundered the monastery but spared the valuable library, which was temporarily removed to the abbey on the island of Reichenau. Eleven years later, an accidental fire virtually destroyed the monastery, but it was rebuilt. In Purchard's time, St. Gall sponsored two separate schools of high standing: an internal one for novice monks and an external school for lay persons, some of whom became prominent ecclesiastical figures.[93]

During Purchard's period as abbot, St. Gall returned to its previous prominence and material prosperity, with the monastery's granaries filled to capacity. His brethren frequently praised their loving father's altruism and easygoing manner. He apparently was well known for his generosity, often providing alms to pilgrims and the poor. Purchard's aristocratic ancestry featured Count Ulrich V of Buchhorn, his father, and Wendilgart, his mother, a granddaughter of King Henry. After Ulrich was taken prisoner by the Magyars in Bavaria and removed to Hungary, Wendilgart promised not to remarry, and with the permission of St. Gall's current abbot, Salomon (890–919), she went to live at the monastery in a separate hermitage. However, Ulrich's unexpected release and safe return to Buchhorn a few years later prompted Wendilgart to petition the local bishop to release her from her previous vows. Soon with child, she and her husband visited the monastery to give thanks to St. Gall and offer their future child to the monastery to be raised as a monk.[94]

Purchard was born around 925, two weeks before term because of his mother's sudden sickness and death. Delivered from her womb by cesarean section, the newborn was wrapped in fat obtained from a freshly butchered pig, ostensibly to protect the delicate wrinkled skin. Following his baptism, the "unborn" Purchard—as he was to be known—was cared for by a wet nurse and, after being weaned, was brought to the monastery's church by his father, who placed him on the altar and officially bestowed him on the monastery together with some property and money. Reared in the monastery by the brothers, the boy turned out to be an easy bleeder, a condition the other monks blamed on his prematurity. Even simple fly bites were said to cause profuse bleeding.[95] He spent a great deal of time in the novitiate's sick ward and was prevented from joining other children of his age. Purchard's story was not unusual, since so-called child oblates—persons solemnly devoted to a monastery—were quite common at the time, and those who were sick were even considered to be closer to God than other members of the monastic community.[96] Although small in stature and of delicate health, the good-looking Purchard grew up to be a kind and well-liked member of the St. Gall monastery. Unlike the situation of other child oblates, monasticism became his true way of life. Given his physical frailty, however, he was exempted from some of the more rigorous monastic routines and allowed to eat meat at the suggestion of Bishop Konrad of Constance.

After the death of St. Gall's abbot, Craloh, in 958, Purchard was sent to the court of Otto the Great (912–973) with a delegation of other monks to discuss the succession. German kings exercised this power of appointment to employ bishops and abbots as their agents throughout the land.[97] Otto, who had returned to Mainz after his victory over King Knut, was told that the members of St. Gall's monastery, as was their right, had already selected Purchard to be their next abbot but needed imperial confirmation. This did not, at first, sit well with Otto. The St. Gall monastery and the founder of the Holy German Empire of the German nation already enjoyed a somewhat rocky relationship, thanks to the monastery's attempts to free itself from feudal entanglements entered into in the turbulent years of the early 900s. At that time, the need for protection from civil wars and barbarian invasions had led the higher monastic clergy to play an active role in worldly politics to protect their institutions and the economic assets underlying them.

The result of that involvement in feudal politics was that bishops and abbots such as Purchard's predecessors had become pawns of the increasingly militant local nobility, who encroached on ecclesiastical lands and continued to impose a number of obligations on the monasteries in the form of revenues and even military service. Within the walls of these increasingly wealthy monasteries, meanwhile, life had become soft, with a decline in discipline and abundant food and drink. A nefarious process of secularization had begun to corrupt all levels of the religious hierarchy, including the papacy.[98] To cope with these developments, a contemporary wave of monastic revival spread from Cluny (911) in Burgundy to Gorze (933) in Lorraine and Brogne (920) in Italy. The goal was a return to the original eremitic ideal of prayer, penance, solitude, poverty, and hard work. On the political front, monasteries sought greater independence, attempting to free themselves from the local episcopate and demanding the free election of their own abbots. The Cluniac reforms aimed to elevate the moral standards of the clergy and restore monastic discipline.[99]

As king of the Franks, "elected" in Charlemagne's own seat at Aachen in 936, Otto was anointed with both royal and priestly authority, including control over the monasteries in his realm.[100] When the emperor's son Liudolf rebelled against his father in 953, however, the St. Gall monastery and its members found themselves among the former's allies. Internal challenges to the rule of their abbot, Craloh (942–958), and further threats from the Magyars ended only after Otto the Great's victory in 955 returned the famous abbey to the imperial fold.[101] At the imperial court, meanwhile, faced with Purchard's boyish appearance and youth, Otto at first refused the monks' demand to ratify their choice of abbot. The emperor may have suspected that the selection was inspired in great part by the monks' desire to retain their soft lifestyle and continue indulging in highly developed liturgical worship, with its ceremonies and processions, under the rule of a more pliant and gentle superior.[102] St. Gall's monks, however, stood their ground, and Otto I finally relented, letting Purchard, then presumably in his early 30s, become the new abbot. If monasteries sought imperial protection, emperors such as Otto I needed the support of wealthy prelates and the resources of their abbeys to assert their political and economic power. Poorly run monasteries, however, could jeopardize their income and diminish local and imperial revenues. Still concerned about the potential disciplinary problems, the emperor later sent a visiting commission to check on Purchard and introduce a number of monastic reforms based on the statutes of Abbot Kerbodo of Lorsch and Cluniac principles. At the time of Purchard's riding accident, relations between St. Gall and the imperial court were the best in a generation. By 962, the empire seemed complete. In that year, Otto I was crowned by the pope and appeared to be on his way to succeeding Charlemagne.[103] An imperial visit to St. Gall in 972, during the feast of the Assumption of the Virgin Mary, featured both Otto the Great and his son Otto II, now co-emperor. With much pomp and ceremony they lodged at the monastery with their wives.[104]

In Rickenbach, meanwhile, Purchard I was probably placed on a table or bed following his equestrian accident. The disabled leg would have been carefully bandaged with woolen rags before his immediate transport back to St. Gall. The impression was that Purchard had suffered a fracture of the thigh bone together with a dislocation of the hip. A messenger may have alerted the current *hospitalarius* and future abbot, Notker II (ca. 905–975), about the seriousness of Purchard's accident given his bleeding tendencies. The early prognosis must have been guarded.[105]

Benedict's monasteries: *Ora et labora*

As in other parts of the medieval world, care of the sick remained an important opportunity for Christian good works. Matthew's six acts of mercy retained their validity and served as a compass for charting the charitable agenda. Healing their sick brethren in spirit and flesh constituted an important function of all monasteries. As noted before, the ideals of monasticism were first articulated by St. Anthony (ca. 251–356), who left for the desert to escape popular religion and persecution. Radical asceticism promoted contempt for the body, and physical suffering was an important means of attaining spiritual purity. Within this ideology the world and the human body were quite corrupted since the Fall, and mortification was necessary to achieve the "perfect life." Thus, monastic life was originally conceived as a series of physical endurance tests and battles fought with tempting demons. However, grafted onto this ideal, Pachomius' rules provided strict norms of collective behavior and an organizational framework designed to ensure the long-term survival of a given community of cenobites, including efforts to restore health. Existing European monasteries followed the example of early cenobitic communities in the Egyptian desert during the increasingly disorganized and violent third and fourth centuries. As public order collapsed, people fled from the cities to build alternative communities, which they organized by establishing a series of rules or *regulae*.

Another important figure in the development of European monasticism was Augustine of Hippo (354–430), who converted to Christianity in 386. Surrounded by devout and intellectual fellow ascetics, Augustine created his famous rule in 397 after setting up his own monastery. This rule, articulated in a series of conferences with monks and nuns, was based on the Scriptures and early Christian religious life. Obedience, poverty, and chastity constituted the requisite triad for membership. Like Basil before him, Augustine tried to deemphasize asceticism, stressing its selfishness and lack of resonance with the natural social tendencies of humankind. Stressing the need for interaction and love, Augustine proclaimed the importance of Christian community life and the performance of charitable acts during one's lifetime as the essential good works necessary for redemption and eternal salvation. During the following centuries, the Augustinian rules were widely circulated both in the West and in the East and were applied to a great number of religious groups, including communities of women, especially wealthy widows and those of noble birth.[106]

In Europe, the *monasterium* rapidly became a new form of social organization composed of a community or brotherhood, initially no more than a dozen people, drawn from circles of family and friends. All members were responsible for each other, often living under the direction of a religious leader or priest, providing the sacramental life, together with another lay superior in charge of internal organization. Subjected to a process of resocialization within the walls of a monastery, these new Christian "families" prayed, worked, and lived together, praising God and ensuring the spiritual salvation of their members. Obedience to superiors was structured as an act of mercy and respect.

The most important figure in the history of medieval monasticism was Benedict of Nursia (480–547), whose model contributed decisively to the organization of all subsequent monastic life. Following his liberal Roman education, Benedict had lived briefly as a hermit north of Rome during Theodoric's rule in Italy and the Gothic Wars against Justinian. In the year 529, he started a monastery at Monte Cassino, south of Rome. Living in a period of rapid economic decline, Benedict aimed to create a small monastic order that, in addition to living a chaste, spiritual life, could also achieve economic self-sufficiency through daily work routines.

Based on traditional Roman family patterns, written in an anonymous "Rule of the Master," Benedict devised a series of common living habits that included prayers, liturgical activities, and readings, as well as agricultural chores.[107] Benedictine regulations represented a compromise between the community orientation of Augustine and the emphasis on isolation and solitude of Cassian (360–435)—a monk from Provence. A common dormitory replaced the smaller separate cells. Food and drink were to be consumed in moderation, and there was to be less corporal punishment.

With some variations, the *Regula Benedicti* governed all monastic life for over six centuries. The rule was based on two key principles: the *conversio morum* or moral conversion of the candidate and *abrenuntiato* or renunciation of worldly goods. The goal was to carry out *opus Dei*, the work of God, by socially disparate groups of individuals. Many monks came from minor noble families or, as in the case of Purchard, were products of the practice of child oblation. Total lack of privacy, uniformity of dress, and emphasis on communal activities sought to obliterate all distinctions. Although monastic life was to be austere, Benedict's rule was much more moderate than that of earlier cenobitic communities and was clearly adapted to his more sophisticated urban contemporaries. Like others before him, Benedict paid considerable attention to the governance of his monastery, granting either an abbot, such as Purchard, or an abbess the powers and responsibilities previously accorded to the Roman *pater familias*. In return for total obedience, the superior was responsible for the monks' welfare until Judgment Day, and he was encouraged to seek the counsel of the whole community on crucial matters regarding monastic life.

Numerous authors have stressed the unique lifestyle prescribed by the Benedictine rules, as well as their emphasis on the rhythmic staging of rituals such as prayers, music, chants, meals, and other routines of work, study, and healing. These practices, including gestures and signs, encompassed all possible human interactions and emotions, creating an intensely regulated life that was predictable, balanced, and secure. Guided by the periodic ringing of bells, the abbey's membership—on average less than 100—submitted to a tightly structured daily schedule that began in the middle of the night and stretched to the evening, with slight variations imposed by the seasons.[108]

Because of their regimented lifestyle and complete devotion to God, members of a monastery were believed to have an excellent chance of securing individual salvation. Because they were perceived as holy people outside the monastery's walls, their prayers and chants were deemed important and useful for avoiding worldly evil and guaranteeing the spiritual salvation of their founders and patrons, including bishops and kings. Thus, in Carolingian times, a symbiotic relationship developed for the mutual benefit of the symbols of both spiritual and earthly power. Monasteries became recipients of generous endowments of land and rents, while rulers hitched the monasteries' rising status to their growing imperial prestige and moral leadership. Finally, while ensuring an inner-directed life of meditation, study, and prayer, Benedictine rules also allowed monks and nuns to relate to the outside world and carry out works of charity. In the example of Christ, involvement with the poor and pilgrims, the homeless, and the sick was an essential part of their monastic existence. Moreover, as their endowments of landed estates grew and as the fame of their libraries converted them into cultural icons of the day, monasteries became closely involved with the secular world.

Monastic caring spaces: Infirmary and hostel

From the start, providing hospitality and healing the sick became key responsibilities of European monasteries, reflective of both the inward and worldly missions they had assumed. As in the East, early Christian welfare in Europe targeted voluntary and structural paupers—there were few distinctions between them—as well as pilgrims. Many were rural peasants, legally free, possibly even owners of small plots who had suffered hard times. As early as Merovingian times, local bishops had been charged with assigning one-fourth of their revenues for the needs of the poor, whose names were kept on special lists, a third in rural parishes. Many were fed, clothed and sheltered in the poorhouse or *mansio pauperum* adjoining the church. Another frequent recipient of Christian charity was the stranger, a rather broad category that included jobless wanderers or drifters as well as errant knights, devout pilgrims, traveling scholars, and merchants. Some had voluntarily separated themselves from their communities and lived as hermits or perennial pilgrims in an effort to ensure their spiritual salvation. Yet, according to canon law, strangers were not considered members of established political and religious communities, and their outsider status began to generate occasional fear, suspicion, and distrust. The Church, however, backed by the Scriptures and still in a proselytizing mode, extended its hospitality to all poor persons and strangers, who were temporarily accepted into the Christian community, housed, and fed in makeshift or permanent guesthouses.

The foundation of *xenodocheia* in the West had followed St. Basil's model of community sponsorship of a "new city" capable of receiving people in need. However, given the prevailing political and economic conditions in the Western Roman Empire, the extensive Byzantine network of *xenones* and especially *nosokomeia* never materialized there. In the first place, these institutions arrived somewhat later in the less urbanized Latin West, with a *xenon* erected in Rome around 397 followed by another at Ostia a few years later.[109] In 399, St. Jerome attributed the foundation of the Roman shelter to one of his disciples, a woman named Fabiola: "She was the first person to found a hospital into which she might gather sufferers out of the streets and where she may nurse the unfortunate victims of sickness and want. Need I speak of noses slit, eyes put out, feet half burned, hands covered with sores? Or of limbs dropsical and atrophied? Or of diseased flesh alive with worms? Often did she carry on her shoulders persons infected with jaundice or filth. Often too did she wash away the matter discharged from wounds which others, even though men, could not bear to look at. She gave food to her patients with her own hand, and moistened the scarce breathing lips of the dying with sips of liquid."[110]

In contrast to conditions prevailing in Byzantium between the fourth and seventh centuries, the German invasions in Europe accelerated the decay of urban life and contributed to the depopulation of the existing cities. Only larger centers in the Italian peninsula, including Rome and Ravenna, retained their late imperial medical structures, including the existence of lay *medici*. As administrative chaos ensued, the former empire broke into small, economically self-sufficient units including manors, villages, and districts. In sharp contrast to the more populous and urbanized Eastern Empire, this process led to the establishment of a rural civilization. After 500, the first *xenodocheia* were established in Gaul in response to a widespread need for assistance of travelers, the poor, and the sick. Whether they were ecclesiastical or privately sponsored, their location at the entrance gates of towns became a boon for the weary seeking help.

Most initial Christian charitable institutions in the West were local foundations established by ruling bishops or private individuals in response to particular needs in their respective dioceses. To reform this decentralized and inefficient network, the Church attempted after 800 to create a European system of social welfare more responsive to the new political conditions created by Charlemagne's empire. At the synods of Aachen in 816 and 817, the assemblies of abbots espoused a comprehensive program of reform and standardization. The principle of monastic hospitality was strongly reaffirmed, and existing *xenodocheia* or *hospitalia* were linked to canonical life and cathedral chapters. Bishops remained responsible for administering the funds earmarked for the care of the poor and sick.[111] Monasteries rather than decaying episcopal cities assumed the greater role in dispensing welfare.

Thus, following the fall of the Roman Empire, monasteries gradually became the providers of organized medical care not available elsewhere in Europe for several centuries. Given their organization and location, these institutions were virtual oases of order, piety, and stability in which healing could flourish. To provide these caregiving practices, monasteries also became sites of medical learning between the fifth and tenth centuries, the classic period of so-called monastic medicine. During the Carolingian revival of the 800s, monasteries also emerged as the principal centers for the study and transmission of ancient medical texts. By this time, the earlier intolerance toward lay medical practices had waned in the writings of influential authors such as the Benedictine monk and historian Bede (673–735) in England. While disease still was a divine visitation attributable to sin, empirical measures to ameliorate physical suffering could also be sought.[112]

As at St. Gall, each institution's *scriptorium*, engaged in the preservation and pro-duction of manuscripts, targeted a number of medical texts for its monks to copy and make available.

The foundations for a recovery of classical knowledge had already been laid by the Gothic historian Cassiodorus (490–585). After his retirement, he estab-lished a monastery with a large personal library in Calabria. Cassiodorus was es-pecially interested in the transmission of Greek ideas and literature to the West, and he gathered in encyclopedic form the best surviving examples of ancient learn-ing. He also sought to rescue the system of Roman education, which included grammar and rhetoric. Monks thus spent their leisure time copying old manu-scripts, including those dealing with topics affecting the "health of the brethren."[113]

In the eighth century, Ravenna took the lead in the translation of Greek med-ical texts, including the writings of Hippocrates, Galen, and Dioscorides. Gradu-ally, most monastic libraries obtained copies of several medical books from which the monks could learn the rudiments of classical healing. Most abbots thus be-came familiar with this literature and often became authors themselves, further expanding the assembled information and creating practical manuals. By the ninth century, Abbot Bertharius at the Benedictine monastery of Monte Cassino had compiled two medical works containing information about antidotes and healing herbs, including their names and synonyms, as well as tables with weights and measures. Well-endowed monasteries such as those at Gorze, Reichenau, and St. Gall possessed several medical manuscripts, most of them practical in orienta-tion.[114]

Caring for fellow monks was traditional in Christian monastic life. The earli-est rule of Pachomius, the Egyptian ascetic (ca. 292–348), had proclaimed that "if anyone is ill, he must go to the house of the praepositus (prior), if ill, let him be led by the prior into the sickhouse." Early monastic rules, including that of St. Benedict, also stressed the care of the infirm and sick monks as one of the im-portant activities of cenobitic life in a monastery. Disabled (*in-firmi*) members of the monastic community sought exemptions from the austere monastic living con-ditions and assistance. Chapter 36 of Benedict's rule proclaimed that "before all things and above all things (*ante omnia et super omnia*) special care must be taken of the sick or infirm so that they may be served as if they were Christ in person; for He himself said 'I was sick and you visited me,' and 'what you have done for the least of mine, you have done for me.' "[115]

As in the East, however, tensions and sometimes open hostility between reli-gious and lay healing persisted. The former continued to focus on supernatural saintly interventions, including prayers, angels, and the use of relics, while the lat-ter was based on diet, surgery, and herbs. Gregory of Tours' opinion that illness was God's punishment, and that no remedies of this world were effective against serious illness, was widely disseminated and led health seekers to scour the countryside in search of holy shrines and miraculous cures. For its part, the lay medical profession survived the fall of the Roman Empire but was largely confined to larger urban centers of the Ostrogothic empire in Italy and the Merovingian kingdom in Gaul. Municipal *medici* were much in evidence during the 400s and 500s in Marseilles, for example. The tradition of *archiatri* physicians continued, but unlike their Byzantine counterparts, these men became mostly court physicians, since they lacked high status and a secure economic position. During the tenth century, instruction in classical medical theory for both lay persons and clerics occurred as part of liberal arts studies at cathedral schools such as those at Rheims and Chartres.[116] Given their small number and few opportunities for training, however, lay healers were clearly overshadowed by well-educated monks such as St. Gall's Notker II, practicing in monastic infirmaries. Medicine was still not institutionalized, and most health-related activities took place in the domestic realm.

Monastic hostels played increasingly important roles in providing charitable aid to the poor and needy. Since Benedict had encouraged hospitality for all, monasteries increasingly welcomed guests and separated them according to class. Poor wanderers found shelter in the *hospitale pauperum*, while the traveling wealthy were received and cared for in better quarters. Further distinctions were attempted between the monasteries' hospitality and the provision of medical aid at its infirmaries devoted to the monks or nuns living in the institution. Poverty, malnutrition, and exhaustion, however, often led to illness, and hospitality blended with medical attention, prompting transfers to the infirmary or consultations with the *infirmarius*.

Benedict may never have envisaged his community as a source of medical care for lay persons, but by the tenth century the increased size of the existing monastic communities and complexity of their multiple activities had created additional needs. Moreover, the monastery's gradual involvement with the surrounding world must have brought additional individuals—mostly laborers working the monastic lands and their families—to the attention of the *infirmarius*. Given the nature of agricultural chores carried out by the peasants, trauma in the form of lacerations, contusions, fractures, and dislocations would have been frequent.

Monasteries were usually built near streams so that water could be diverted to feed their fountains, provide for drinking, bathing, and washing, and flush the sewers. A Benedictine monastery complex was deliberately arranged to ensure the separate existence of two worlds: a spiritual realm involving the church and its adjacent structures, and a worldly sphere dominated by the hostel and necessary support facilities such as granaries and workshops. Such arrangements can be clearly observed on a detailed monastery plan created in 830 by Abbot Heito of Reichenau for the 100–150 monks of St. Gall. Modeled on a Roman villa, this surviving plan of Carolingian architecture, although never implemented, became influential in the development of similar monastic institutions. Here the sacred domain occupied the eastern half of the complex, with the church located at the center. In addition, there were the monks' living quarters, sometimes consisting of a simple dormitory. In the St. Gall plan, three double-storied structures enclosed a cloister with a warming room, dormitory, refectory, vestry, cellar, and larder. This arrangement derived from the open-galleried courts of Roman houses, attached to the church to complete the inner square. The plan featured another building reserved for novitiates.[117]

The monastic infirmary[118] was usually a separate structure and a smaller replica of the monks' cloister houses. It was reserved for sick, dying, or convalescent monks, although permanently enfeebled residents could also reside there. Most plans also show a separate kitchen and bath in an adjacent building. The central courtyard was surrounded by rooms for patients with different degrees of disability. In the St. Gall plan, the infirmary itself faced a separate building, located between a bloodletting house to the west and an herb garden to the east. This structure was reserved on one side for a monk/healer or *mansio medici ipsius*. It had a central room with a fireplace employed for drug compounding and connected to a storage closet for drugs called the *armarium pigmentorum*. On the opposite side was another room—the *cubiculum valde infirmorum*—for critically ill monks who required constant supervision.[119]

Other infirmary models featured a barrel-vaulted basilica built like a Romanesque church. Here each inmate could be placed next to a window, and the alcove would have contained at least two beds ranging from straw pallets to featherbeds with coverings of wool, fur, or down. A chest of drawers at the foot of the bed held personal belongings and a portable tray for eating in bed. Often, all beds were visible from any point in the hall and faced a central altar or separate chapel. This allowed ailing monks to hear and participate in the religious ceremonies. Heating of many infirmary halls was accomplished through the Roman system of pipes leading from the furnace, the *hypocaustum*, and placed below the floors.[120]

At the proposed St. Gall monastery, all health-related buildings stood together at the northeast quadrant. The house for bloodletting had a fireplace at each of its four corners for extra warmth together with the traditional central opening for ventilation. At the extreme corner of the complex, planners had envisioned a garden, the *herbarium* or *hortulus*, usually planted with medicinal herbs employed by the *infirmarius* to compound poultices, purges, and infusions. Here the monks would have grown roses, lilies, sage, rosemary, fennel, iris, opium, watercress, pepperwort, and mint.[121]

The plans called for the western side of the St. Gall monastery to be reserved for worldly activities, ensuring the privacy of resident monks and reached through a gate. Here a porter or *portarius*, who usually controlled a tenth of the monastery's revenues, screened those who asked for shelter and sent them on to the *hospitale pauperum*. Instead of lodging, the needy often received food and clothing. On major feast days, food and wine were distributed, even banquets held for some high-ranking guests such as bishops and the emperor himself. Visitors often sought a temporary shelter to rest in and recover for the weary journey ahead. Regular, nutritious meals were eagerly welcomed by the famished. Often peasants and their families working for the monastery came in search of care. As elsewhere in Europe, health conditions in the Otonian empire were precarious, especially among the poor, because of chronic malnutrition and lack of collective and personal hygiene. As in other parts of the former Roman Empire, the average life expectancy continued to hover at around 25–30 years, lower for women than for men because of the hazards of childbearing.

Monastic guesthouses could be large, able to care for several hundred individuals and their families. The rationale for this charitable activity stemmed from Benedict's original rule in which he stated, "let all guests who arrive be received like Christ for He is going to say 'I came as a guest and you received me.' And to all let due honor to be shown, especially to the domestics of the faith and to pilgrims," adding that "in the reception of the poor and of pilgrims the greatest care and solicitude should be shown because it is especially in them that Christ is received."[122] Thus, Benedictine monasteries traditionally allowed thousands of individuals through their gates for shelter, rest, and nourishment. Welcoming ceremonies included the traditional washing of the feet (*mandatum*) and food offerings.[123]

The St. Gall hostel for pilgrims and paupers could have housed 15–30 individuals. Its urban counterpart, the *xenodochium* or *hospitale*, usually had an average capacity of 20–30 inmates. The St. Gall plan shows a rectangular building, featuring a central hall and fireplace surrounded by benches, connected on both sides to separate dormitories with large beds. A hole in the roof would have allowed the smoke to exit. This building had a supply room, cellar, and servants' quarters and was linked to a separate kitchen consisting of a bake and brew room.

Monastic hostels operated with funds specifically provided by abbots such as Purchard, usually supplemented by private donations of money or land. At Cluny in the 900s, a large guest house for socially prominent travelers was located just west of the church. These facilities were reserved for traveling rulers, knights, and other important persons, and were provided with servant quarters and kitchen facilities. Eventually, the house for distinguished guests experienced further expansion in Spain, as in Poblet (1149) and later El Escorial (1563), where the rulers built small palaces to live out their last years within the monastic walls.

Healing in monasteries: A community approach

Following the accident at Rickenbach, Purchard must have been hurriedly returned on a stretcher to his own quarters in the monastery, but we have no further details about the management of his injury except the fact that he came under the care of Notker II, St. Gall's *infirmarius*, poet, and painter, whose monastic career spanned more than 50 years. Although this monk had acquired a reputation as a skillful diagnostician in the tradition of Hippocratic healers and was knowledgeable regarding drugs and antidotes, his practice was never formalized or institutionalized beyond the broader duties of a self-made monastic *infirmarius*.[124] He not only took care of his brothers but also attended the sick poor and pilgrims who sought hospitality at the monastery. Of noble origin, Notker II would eventually become himself abbot of St. Gall from 971 until his death in 975. Unlike Purchard, he was characterized by his contemporaries as a strong disciplinarian, widely known by his nickname "Peppercorn."

Benedict's original rule ordered that "for these sick brethren let there be assigned a special room and an attendant who is God-fearing, diligent, and solicitous."[125] This monk or nun attending the sick—the *infirmarius* was usually selected because of personality and practical healing skills. The latter were acquired informally through experience, as well as through consultation of texts, medical manuscripts, and herbals available in the monastery's library or elsewhere. Since the time of Cassiodorus, monks elected to care for the sick were supposed to learn the nature of plants and their mixtures, as well as read Hippocrates, Galen, and Dioscorides. At St. Gall, for example, the library held copies of manuscripts by Boethius (480–524), Cassiodorus, and Isidor of Seville (570–636) dealing in part with medical matters. In most instances, the role of *infirmarius* combined nursing functions, such as providing food and clothing, with diagnostic medical procedures and administration of drugs. Monastic routines prescribed two daily visits to the sick, early in the morning and following evening prayer. The *infirmarius* usually talked with patients and asked questions, checked on the food, compounded medicinal herbs, and comforted those in need. According to Benedict's rule, "the abbot shall take the greatest care that the sick be not neglected by the cellarers or the attendants; for he also is responsible for what is done wrongly by his disciples."[126]

Since its foundation, St. Gall had possessed a reputation for extensive medical knowledge. Many monks studied medical subjects as part of their general education, and many of St. Gall's abbots gained great renown as healers. Otmar, the monastery's founder, was canonized in 864 for his care of local lepers and became a patron saint for the sick, especially children suffering from wasting diseases. Another well-known St. Gall abbott and healer was Iso (830–871), whose special ointment found great favor with lepers and the lame, and was even believed to restore sight to a child rendered blind by an infectious ailment. In the same century, Abbott Grimaldus composed a medical manuscript containing a compilation of classical medical treatises and a collection of remedies. Notker II, Purchard's *infirmarius* and successor, spent time as consulting physician at the court of Otto the Great and his son, a common practice whereby monk-practitioners consulted in exchange for an honorarium or gift. As abbots such as these became prominent healers within their institutions, their fame often drew them away from the monastery and put them in contact—as well as conflict—with the contemporary secular powers.[127]

An immediate examination of Purchard's foot should have disclosed the direction of the hip dislocation, but the fractured bone would have obscured such a diagnostic marker. Here Notker faced an immediate dilemma: should he attempt to reduce the dislocated hip even though the thigh bone was fractured? Since antiquity, most practitioners had advised stretching the leg with the help of straps, often placing the patient on planks, benches, and ladders, even upside down with the ankles firmly held in place by foot straps. At other times, assistants would pull the leg and upper body in opposite directions, with a third operator seated on one side who pressed the hip, allowing the thigh bone to slide back into its socket. Because of the fracture, however, there was great danger that during such a manipulation the ends of the fractured bone would damage the leg's vessels and nerves or even protrude through the surface of the skin. The risks of hemorrhage, infection, and paralysis could lead to amputation, gangrene, and death.[128]

Notker's likely conservative strategy was simply to achieve a sufficient extension of Purchard's thigh to align and bring both ends of the bone together through slow, painful manipulation. In most instances the thigh bone would never return to its former state, and a shortened leg might force the sufferer to walk on his toes. A tight set of bandages—sprinkled with warm oil and wine to deal with the local swelling—would have been applied from the waist down to well below the knee joint. The outer layers were usually covered with wax to hold the dressing together. Solid wooden splints extending from the hip to the heel ensured complete immobility, especially preventing the knee from bending. Practitioners were aware that the long leg bones healed rather slowly and had to be kept at rest for at least 40 days. Some adjustment of the bandages would have been done after the local swelling subsided. These necessary steps to deal with the fracture probably came at the expense of Purchard's hip dislocation, which had to be left in its abnormal space long enough to become unreduceable.[129]

One can only surmise that the injured abbot, like other members of his congregation, was subjected to the usual religious ceremonies governing all monastic infirmaries: confession, prayers, and reception of the sacraments. Questions about the meaning of this accident would have been raised by both the patient and his brethren. Was the episode God's punishment of an abbot who craved worldly luxury and entertainment and involved himself in political intrigues? Was this a bad omen, a divine warning from an angry God offended by Purchard's relationship with a beautiful woman?[130] Was the monastery being collectively punished for its lax discipline? One can easily picture the suffering abbot, surrounded by members of his congregation, engaged in penitential supplications.

During the first 10 days after the accident, the danger of infection and prospects for a life-ending amputation were great. The classical regimen included control of food, drink, sleep, exercise, and other lifestyle factors—as well as drugs—probably some opium preparations to fight excessive pain. To forestall inflammation, patients with fractured bones were subjected to a brief fast, followed by a more liberal diet but abstinence from wine. After the initial danger of infection had subsided and amputation became unnecessary, the limb was usually subjected to fomentations with hot water to keep the muscles from stiffening.[131]

Guiding all healing practices in monasteries during Purchard's time were basic notions of classical humoralism, systematized by Galen and subsequently summarized by Byzantine as well as Islamic encyclopedists. Illness reflected states of humoral imbalance, and this pathology was popularly linked to the seasons. Practical problem solving derived from both humoral practices and folk healing traditions and included recipes based on herbal ingredients together with magical procedures such as incantations, laying on of hands, and use of relics. The presence of crypts with the remains of St. Gall (835) and St. Otmar (867) together with the new arrival of relics from John the Baptist made this monastery a popular destination for supplicants. Prayers therefore played a key role in monastic healing. Such religious practices coexisted with natural healing efforts at the infirmaries based on a regimen of diet, drugs, and even surgery.

The illness displayed by a sick monk was checked through an examination of pulse, urine, stool, and blood to determine the trouble and formulate a prognosis.[132] Uroscopy in particular remained a popular system of medical diagnosis and prognosis, derived from the Hippocratic treatise on *Prognostics* but also based on subsequent tracts on urine available in manuscript form.[133] Its rationale was derived from the notion that human urine was an image of the body's blood. Therefore, variations in color, cloudiness, surface scum, and sediment were useful in predicting crisis, recovery, or death. The procedure consisted of a visual inspection of the urine in a graduated glass jar with a wide mouth and rounded body called a *matula*. The jug initially simulated the shape of the human bladder but was soon believed to represent a vertical image of the entire body. Each sediment layer corresponded to a particular body part, and practitioners carefully examined the fluid by holding up the jar against a light source.

Uroscopic skill was a key to a practitioner's reputation. The story was told, for example, of Notker II that he was called to the court of Henry I of Bavaria, who sought to test the monk-practitioner's highly touted abilities by offering him a flask of his urine for examination. However, instead of his own, the aristocrat provided a sample from a young chambermaid in his service. Notker is said to have promptly diagnosed a pregnancy, a miracle he proclaimed as a sign of God's powers to have a man deliver a child in due course. Deeply embarrassed, the duke, who wanted to stay on good terms with the monk, offered his excuses and provided lavish gifts to the convent while his supposedly virginal servant, as predicted, promptly went on to deliver a baby.[134]

Sick and injured monks like Purchard were usually excused from all routines and duties and allowed to rest and sleep for longer hours in the infirmary. Like the rest of the abbey's community, the sick usually received two meals per day, with extra dishes or "pittances" added on Sundays and feast days if they could tolerate them. The staple food in the monastery was bread, generally made from wheat and rye flour, and the most common drink was ale brewed from barley and fruit juices. Wine, however, gradually became a popular restorative, often produced by the monastery's own vineyards. If available, milk was valued for its butter and cheese. Eggs, fish, beans, and honey remained quite popular. A Benedictine rule indicated that "the use of meat be granted to the sick who are very weak for the restoration of their strength."[135]

In most monasteries, the *infirmarius* made extensive use of herbal preparations in his treatments. Since the 700s, a basic group of 71 such medicinal herbs had been known in Europe through abridged editions of the work of Dioscorides, supplemented by additional plants from Germanic and Celtic folk healing practices.[136] Purchard's extremely painful injury may have prompted the use of traditional painkillers, probably mandragora or opium extracts administered orally or by enema, although suffering was considered good for the body and the soul.[137] As in other parts of the world, cinnamon, sugar, ginger, nutmeg, anise, and licorice were employed to make the bitter extracts more palatable. Many of these ingredients could probably be obtained from monastic herb gardens such as the one depicted in the St. Gall plan. At this time, herb collecting was still associated with ideas of magical powers since these plants embodied specific principles of action. Their use in ointments, lotions, and poultices was widespread both inside and outside monasteries.[138]

A rudimentary practice of surgery ("touching and cutting") at the monastic infirmary was usually linked to the management of trauma, including lacerations, dislocations, and fractures. Although these were daily occurrences, the *infirmarius* may not have always been comfortable practicing surgery on his brothers, for it was always a source of considerable pain, bleeding, and infection. Complicated wounds or injuries may have forced some monks to request the services of more experienced local bonesetters or even barber surgeons. Purchard's accident may well have been such an occasion since internal bleeding was always feared. In spite of the agony, occasional amputations of limbs must have been carried out, followed by the use of the cautery iron or *ustio*, still a popular hemostatic and prophylactic for wound infections. As in Roman times, most wounds continued to be irrigated with wine or vinegar and sutured with silk threads. Indications for cauterization continued to include the relief of certain general internal conditions, especially in the chest.

A presumed excess of corrupted humors, such as was believed to occur in fevers, could be removed by bloodletting and collected in cups from the superficial veins at the elbow, ankle, neck, and temples. Most early medieval compendia contained explicit instructions concerning places and methods for venesection. In weaker persons, wet cupping was used to remove smaller amounts through scarifications of the skin made with ivory or bone instruments. Inspection of the blood's color and consistency served as a prognostic guide. At St. Gall's library, a copy of the *Epistula de phlebotomia*, a standard guide to therapeutic and prophylactic bleeding in monasteries dating back to the early 800s, explained the ideal bodily sites for bleeding.[139]

Preventive bloodletting was also a very popular purification ritual deeply embedded in medieval culture. As a universal purge, the practice usually began at puberty and occurred at least two or four times a year during the first days of a waning moon and the changing seasons until the age of 50 in men and 60 in women. It was considered necessary to cleanse the body of old blood in danger of being corrupted by disease and thus to restore vitality. In the plan for St. Gall's new monastery, the architects proposed a separate house reserved for bloodletting, to be located across from the monastery's infirmary. Monks and visitors usually spent three days convalescing after the procedure and were provided with a substantial diet under the supervision of the *infirmarius*. In other establishments the monastic infirmary had its own bleeding room. Even paupers coming to the monastic shelters were offered a cleansing regimen of purges, bleeding, and rest lasting for almost a month in May and September.[140]

Following Roman traditions, bathing was considered necessary for health in the Augustinian rules, with encouragement to visit the available public baths not "for simple pleasure" but based on medical advice and on orders of the superior, and always accompanied by other community members. In contrast, the Benedictine rule, in attempting to chart a more ascetic lifestyle, restricted such activities: "Let the use of baths be afforded the sick as often as may be expedient; but to the healthy and especially the young let them be granted more rarely."[141] Extra soaking, possibly with steam, as well as massage was allowed in case of illness, again strictly for therapeutic reasons and only with permission from the abbot. Purchard's leg may have been subjected to such practices following removal of the splints.

One of the most important functions of the Benedictine monastery was the preparation for death, involving sick brethren who failed to recover.[142] When a member of the monastery's community became seriously ill, all others, at the ring of the bell, assembled to visit the sick and pray. Usually, the gravely ill monk or nun was placed in a separate room. We can be certain that this event took place at St. Gall in the case of Purchard, especially after the abbot had been returned to the monastery from Rickenbach. First, the dying person confessed and then received the sacrament of extreme unction from the cleric who had heard the confession and had absolved him.[143] The administration of holy oil occurred on the traditional places of the five senses and the other bodily areas considered to be suffering. It was repeated for seven consecutive days if the individual continued to survive. After this ceremony, the entire community went to the church and prayed for the dying.[144]

Periodic visits to the sick by members continued. Some brethren remained with the dying inmate throughout the day and night, praying and reading from the Scriptures by candlelight. The point of this vigil was to ensure "proper passing"; nobody should be left to die alone. If death became imminent, the whole monastic community was summoned and the monks congregated around the sick on both sides of the bed alternately to pray and sing, using music to "unbind" the pain and thus provide the departing with spiritual nourishment for the journey to the beyond. Death was usually announced by the clapping of boards or ringing of bells, with burial in the monastic cemetery after elaborate funeral ceremonies. The deceased monk's name and date of death were inscribed in a memorial book, and he was henceforth included in all intercessionary prayers.

At the hostel, meanwhile, the Benedictine rituals of prayer, rest, food, and the administration of sacraments were also believed to be conducive to the recuperation of exhausted pilgrims, the poor, and sick guests housed in the monastery's *hospitalium*. According to Benedict's rule,

> as soon as a guest is announced, let the superior or the brethren meet him with all charitable service. And first of all let them pray together, and then exchange the kiss of peace. . . . After the guests have been received and taken to prayer, let the superior or someone appointed by him sit with them. Let the divine law be read before the guest for his edification and then let all kindness be shown him. Let the abbot give the guests water for their hands and let both abbot and community wash the feet of all guests. After the washing of the feet let them say this verse: "We have received Your mercy, o God, in the midst of Your Temple."[145]

Resting on straw-covered floors, some of the guests must have felt protected behind the monastery's walls and reminded of their Christian identity and the redemptive quality of their suffering. Acceptance and understanding were important. At a minimum, these routines would have had a calming and reassuring effect as the visitors socialized with each other and with members of the caring monastic community. Whether they stayed in the infirmary or the hostel, life in the monastery was fostered by a unique therapeutic environment.

Finally, we can assume that Notker II saved his superior's life but evidently could not restore the leg to full motion. In spite of frequent bandaging and massage and perhaps months of immobilization, the leg either healed imperfectly or suffered extensive muscular atrophy and joint stiffness. After recovery, all sufferers lost their temporary dietary privileges and returned to their spartan life lest they become "slaves of their own desires."[146] If the abbot's hip dislocation had been external, he could have borne his body weight better and with less pain.[147] Henceforth, Purchard walked only with two crutches and was soon forced to delegate most of his duties to an assistant.[148] The result was a further deterioration of monastic discipline, cut short by the crippled leader's resignation in 971, followed by the elevation of Notker II, to the abbotship. When both rulers, Otto the Great and his son, Otto II, visited St. Gall with much pomp and ceremony a year later, the now nearly blind Notker II shared in the honor of the emperor's table. Purchard, however, kept busy. With his previous project completed—a chapel to house the relics of John the Baptist brought from Rome—he was directing the construction of another chapel dedicated to St. Gall. Four years after his resignation, Purchard I ended his days in a small adjacent hermitage, having survived his healer and successor.

THE TWILIGHT OF WESTERN MONASTIC SUPREMACY

Until the time of Purchard's rule at St. Gall, hospitals in the West had been mostly small shelters established mainly for the homeless poor and travelers, including pilgrims. Some were located in cities, attached to a bishop's palace; others operated near major roads, on mountain passes, or in monasteries alongside infirmaries restricted for sick monks. Hospitals comprised a lodging hall with 12–15 beds, an attached kitchen, and a chapel. Dormitories featured suspended mattresses filled with straw, pillows, bed sheets, and blankets. The large beds held two or three inmates.

All hospitals were sponsored by the Church, primarily to achieve the goals of physical segregation, spiritual salvation, and physical comfort. Although often brought together by the vicissitudes of human suffering, hospital inmates were viewed primarily as members of a new spiritual community, temporarily living in a *locus religiosus*. This idea was compatible with the concept that such institutionalization was a form of penance. Those housed in hospitals hoped to achieve redemption through their suffering. Moreover, like monks, martyrs, saints, and finally apostles, the sick could function as mediators between God and His people. Their intercessional prayers on behalf of patrons and caregivers were believed to be valuable. Chronically in short supply, Western lay medical professionals were only minimally involved with these institutions since many monks were skilled healers.

Another ideological component influencing the early rise of such hospitals was the traditional concept of poverty as a voluntary condition providing grace. Traditional links to hermitism and monasticism gave poverty a sterling image and reputation, and many of the most educated lay persons selected a life of want in the belief that it would bring them closer to God and salvation. Besides hermits and monks, some of "Christ's poor" preferred to live an itinerant existence, shuttling between cities, monasteries, and shrines in search of knowledge and grace. Often referred to as "personalized" poor because they could be readily identified by caregivers, they and other needy individuals were admitted to the existing shelters in monasteries, the countryside, or outside city walls and provided with food, clothing, and care.

Because of their religious character, hospitals remained under strict clerical authority, staffed by administrators, priests, and caregivers who had received canonical instruction. Most of the latter were required to be healthy, stay celibate, take vows of poverty, and pass a probationary period. Regarding administrative matters, the supervising bishops expected a full and honest accounting since institutional success was closely linked to the good management of grants and endowments. Service to the sick was structured as another penitential existence: a life of discipline, hardship, silence, and prayer. The hospital's religious status also ruled the behavior expected of inmates. Rituals were designed to control them, as well as to provide reassurance and protection. Like poor people, the sick could be instrumental in providing their sponsors with means of salvation.

Such a state of affairs changed a century after Purchard's rule at St. Gall. Benedictine monasteries throughout Europe ceased to play their hitherto prominent roles in the provision of social welfare and medical care. For almost a 1,000 years, almshouses and hospitals had been organized and run in accordance with highly successful monastic models of prayer and work. Now, in the face of rapid population growth and urbanization, these establishments became inadequate purveyors of traditional charitable assistance. An increasingly urban economy based on commerce that demanded markets, contracts, and currency loans rapidly became the instrument and measure of work. Just at the time their own incomes started to decline, the monasteries' almonries were overwhelmed by the growing influx of needy individuals, a reflection of new and more complex social and economic conditions affecting the European population.

At the monasteries, further reforms beyond the Clunian movement were now pioneered by Stephen, abbot of Citeaux (1099–1109), together with hermits at Burgundy. Cistercianism sought to break away entirely from feudalism and bypass the manorial system, perceived as a pernicious source of monastic involvement with the political and economic world and therefore antithetical to the pursuit of spiritual ideals. Based on Benedict's rules, the Cistercian *Carta Caritatis* (1119) recommended the return to a simple, ascetic lifestyle, including the ideals of monastic solitude, greater seclusion, and renunciation of worldly goods. Gone were the days of study, teaching, and manuscript transcription. The new communities of monks were told to perform heavy farm labor, thereby restoring the traditional self-sufficiency of an abbey. Ideally, monasteries were to be isolated from population centers and their worldly temptations. To fulfill the new rules, such monasteries needed autonomy, exemption from episcopal control and supervision. Under Bernard of Clairvoix (1118–1153), this Cistercian movement of the "white monks" successfully spread to various countries, thus

ending an era during which Benedictine monasteries had been the cultural leaders of Europe and the most important sources for Christian charity, including
caregiving.[149]

In earlier times, monasticism had been compatible with a closed European
economy based on the self-sufficient estates of an agricultural society, the so-called
villa economy. From 500 to 1100, monasteries indeed played a complex role vis-
à-vis the surrounding lay communities and cities. As lords of valuable land parcels,
they were part of the feudal economy. To administer and exploit gifts from the
pious and the wealthy required an army of workers, serfs, and tenants. By the
twelfth century, however, many of these same monasteries had lost some of their
lands to nearby secular lords anxious to test newer farming techniques and improve agricultural yields to feed a growing population. The older manorial system
of self-sufficient villas began to break down throughout Europe, giving way to local urban markets that later became important commercial centers.[150]

A century earlier, cathedral schools of northern France had already began to
replace the monasteries as centers of intellectual culture. Rheims, Chartres,
Poitiers, and Amiens now taught medicine alongside the liberal arts to an expanding audience that included monks, secular clerics, and lay persons. Tensions
between religious and secular healing, however, persisted, as evidenced by the
opinions of Bishop Fulbert of Chartres, who wrote that "as Christians we know
that there are two kinds of medicine, one of earthly things, the other of heavenly
things. They differ in both origin and efficacy. Through long experience, earthly
doctors learn the powers of herbs and the like, which alter the condition of human bodies. But there has never been a doctor so experienced in this art that he
has not found some illnesses difficult to cure and others absolutely incurable. . . .
The author of heavenly medicine, however, is Christ, who could heal the sick with
a command and raise the dead from the grave."[151]

Before the year 1000, several Benedictine healers came to publicize their medical achievements as contributions to their own social status. By the time of the
Council of Clermont, in 1130, this activity had so far transcended the boundaries
of convents and churches that the Church authorities decided to curb it. Frequent
contacts of monk-healers with the outside world became problematic, since they
were seen as interfering with monastic duties. Life needed to be devoted to con-
templation and meditation. Therefore, canon 5 of Clermont, canon 6 of the Council of Rheims (1131), and canon 9 of the Second Lateran Council under Pope Innocent II (1139) stated that "the care of souls being neglected and the purposes
of their order being set aside, they promise health in return to detestable money
and thus make themselves physicians of human bodies, . . . we forbid of our apostolic authority that this be done in the future." In 1163 monks were forbidden to
leave the monastery to study medicine for more than two months.[152]

In the 1050s, Salerno, in cooperation with the Benedictine monastery at Monte
Cassino in southern Italy, emerged as a center of theoretical learning based on

Greek and Roman medical sources. The growth of this lay medical center constituted a tentative first step in the direction of formal medical training through its loose arrangement of individual instructors. However, without a formal faculty, curriculum, or academic degrees, requirements were set by imperial edicts, with examiners appointed by the king testing the students. The Salernitan arrangements, however, led to new efforts in collecting a greater body of medical knowledge contained in Greek and Latin manuscripts, and later to the translation of Arabic texts, especially by Constantine the African (1020–1087), a monk who translated from Arabic at Monte Casino in the 1150s.[153]

By the late eleventh and twelfth centuries, Matthew's six merciful acts, including visitation and care of the sick, had transcended the strict frontiers of ecclesiastical and monastic activities to become important guidelines for lay behavior. Together with a seventh, burying the dead, their inclusion in catechisms and devotional guides characterized them all, albeit stereotypically, as the accepted boundaries of Christ's charitable work. Given the simultaneous and rather dramatic rise in poverty in the eleventh century, lay persons were now invited to join the clergy in performing these functions. Up to this time, the Church had successfully dealt with traditional poverty—usually at a personal level—but the presence of thousands of refugees crowding the new cities demanded greater participation by other sectors of the population. Working together with episcopal and monastic authorities, urban parishes and confraternities slowly began the institutionalization of social welfare in the cities. This task was based on the traditional Christian premise that such assistance was still part of a religious ritual and an important means for acquiring spiritual salvation. In fact, visiting the sick could bring plenary indulgences furnished by the pope. After 1300, such lay participation increasingly dislodged the original charitable Christian guesthouse or *hospitium* from its hitherto exclusive connections with monasteries and cathedral chapters. The stage was set for other actors to participate in the development of the hospital system.

NOTES

1. Matthew 25: 34–36, New Catholic Bible.
2. Judah Ben Segal, *Edessa, "The Blessed City,"* Oxford, Clarendon Press, 1970, pp. 147–48. Today Edessa is the Turkish provincial capital of Urfa.
3. William Wright, *The Chronicle of Joshua the Stylite*, Amsterdam, Philo Press, 1968, p. 28.
4. One recent author has estimated this growth to be 40 percent per decade. See Rodney Stark, *The Rise of Christianity*, Princeton, NJ, Princeton Univ. Press, 1996, pp. 3–27.
5. See, for example, R. J. and M. L. Littman, "Galen and the Antonine plague," *Am J Philol* 94 (1973): 243–55, and T. L. Bratton, "The identity of the plague of Justinian," *Trans Stud Coll Phys Phila* 3 (1981): 113–24 and 174–80.

6. This is certainly the hypothesis of William H. McNeill in his *Plagues and Peoples*, Garden City, NY, Anchor Press, 1976, especially pp. 77–147.

7. A. Scobie, "Slums, sanitation, and mortality in the Roman world," *Klio* 68 (1986): 399–433.

8. See J. Stannard, "Diseases of Western antiquity," in *The Cambridge World History of Human Disease*, ed. K. F. Kiple, Cambridge, Cambridge Univ. Press, 1993, pp. 262–70. Lack of information and difficulties in interpreting ancient sources make all retrospective diagnoses tentative.

9. For studies about the impact of famine, consult Robert I. Rotberg and Theodore K. Rabb, eds., *Hunger and History: The Impact of Changing Food Production and Consumption Patterns in Society*, Cambridge, Cambridge Univ. Press, 1985.

10. Phillip Whitting, *Byzantium, an Introduction*, new ed., New York, St. Martin's Press, 1981, pp. 1–14.

11. See John E. Stambaugh, *The Ancient Roman City*, Baltimore, Johns Hopkins Univ. Press, 1988.

12. Consult Tertius Chandler and Gerald Fox, *Ten Thousand Years of Urban Growth*, New York, Academic Press, 1974, and M. I. Finley, *Atlas of Classical Archeology*, New York, McGraw-Hill, 1977.

13. Wright, *Chronicle*, p. 30.

14. Ibid., p. 31.

15. For details, see M. Yanagi et al., *Byzantium*, trans. N. Fry, Secaucus, NJ, Chartwell Books, 1978.

16. For information about Edessa's role in the story of the famous shroud of Christ, see Holger Kersten and Elmar Gruber, *The Jesus Conspiracy: The Turin Shroud and the Truth about the Resurrection*, Rockport, MA, Element, 1992, especially pp. 109–11.

17. Segal, *Edessa*, pp. 71–73.

18. Wright, *Chronicle*, p. 32.

19. Ibid.

20. Ibid.

21. Ibid.

22. Ibid.

23. Ibid.

24. Details are provided in Wayne A. Meeks, *The First Urban Christians: The Social World of the Apostle Paul*, New Haven, Yale Univ. Press, 1983.

25. Stark, *The Rise of Christianity*, pp. 73–94. Stark echoes previous statements made by William H. McNeill in his book *Plagues and Peoples* and in his lectures.

26. K. H. Leven, "Athumia and philanthropia: Social reactions to plagues in late antiquity and early Byzantine society," *Clio Med* 27 (1995): 393–407.

27. H. Koester and V. Limberis, "Christianity," in *Civilization of the Ancient Mediterranean, Greece, and Rome*, ed. M. Grant and R. Kitzinger, New York, C. Scribner's Sons, 1988, vol. 1, pp. 1047–73. For more information consult Ramsay MacMullen, *Christianizing the Roman Empire (A.D. 100–400)*, New Haven, Yale Univ. Press, 1984.

28. G. B. Ferngren, "Early Christianity as a religion of healing," *Bull Hist Med* (1991): 1–15.

29. Peter Brown, *Power and Persuasion in Late Antiquity: Towards a Christian Empire*, Madison, Univ. of Wisconsin Press, 1992, pp. 71–117.

30. Good works may have improved the quality of life for Christians and even extended their life expectancy. See A. R. Burn, "Hic breve vivitur," *Past & Present* 4 (1953): 2–31. For more information, see Raymond F. Collins, *The Birth of the New Testament: The Origin and Development of the First Christian Generation*, New York, Crossroad Pub. Co., 1993.

31. For a useful summary, see Darrel W. Amundsen, "Medicine and faith in early Christianity," *Bull Hist Med* 56 (1982): 326–50, and his collection of articles in *Medicine, Society and Faith in the Ancient and Medieval Worlds*, Baltimore, Johns Hopkins Univ. Press, 1996.

32. Peter Brown, *The Body and Society*, New York, Columbia Univ. Press, 1988, pp. 160–65.

33. Owsei Temkin, *Hippocrates in a World of Pagans and Christians*, Baltimore, Johns Hopkins Univ. Press, 1991, pp. 149–80.

34. C. H. Lawrence, *Medieval Monasticism*, 2nd ed., London, Longman, 1984, pp. 1–18. For background reading, see Derwas J. Chitty, *The Desert a City: An Introduction to the Study of Egyptian and Palestinian Monasticism under the Christian Empire*, Crestwood, NY, St. Vladimir's Seminary Press, 1977.

35. Consult Phillip Rousseau, *Ascetics, Authority, and the Church in the Age of Jerome and Cassian*, Oxford, Oxford Univ. Press, 1978.

36. Brown, *Power and Persuasion*, pp. 96–103.

37. For details, see Alexander Kazdhan and Giles Constable, *People and Power in Byzantium*, Washington, DC, Dumbarton Oaks Center, 1982, pp. 37–58.

38. Herman J. Frings, "Medizin und Arzt bei den Griechischen Kirchenvätern bis Chrysostomos," Ph.D. diss., Univ. of Bonn, 1959, pp. 29–32.

39. Ibid., pp. 32–37. See also M. E. Keenan, "St. Gregory of Nazianzus and early Byzantine medicine," *Bull Hist Med* 9 (1941): 8–30.

40. F. Kudlien, "Medicine as a 'liberal art' and the question of the physician's income," *J Hist Med* 31 (1976): 448–59, and O. Temkin, "Medical ethics and honoraria in late antiquity," in *Healing and History: Essays for George Rosen*, ed. C. Rosenberg, New York, Science Hist. Pub., 1979, pp. 6–26.

41. M. E. Keenan, "St. Gregory of Nyssa and the medical profession," *Bull Hist Med* 15 (1944): 150–61.

42. For an overview see Vivian Nutton, "From Galen to Alexander: aspects of medicine and medical practice in late antiquity," in *Symposium on Byzantine Medicine*, ed. J. Scarborough, Washington, DC, Dumbarton Oaks Research and Library Collection, 1985, pp. 1–14, and more recently "Medicine in late antiquity and the early Middle Ages," in Nutton et al., *The Western Medical Tradition, 800 BC to AD 1800*, Cambridge, Cambridge Univ. Press, 1995, pp. 71–87.

43. G. B. Ferngren and D. W. Amundsen, "Medicine and Christianity in the Roman Empire: Compatibilities and tensions," in *Rise and Decline of the Roman World*, ed. W. Haase and H. Temporini, Berlin, W. de Gruyter, 1996, part II, vol 37.3, pp 2957–80. See also Ramsay MacMullen, *Paganism in the Roman Empire*, New Haven, Yale Univ. Press, 1981, and Howard C. Kee, *Medicine, Miracle, and Magic in New Testament Times*, Cambridge, Cambridge Univ. Press, 1986.

44. Frings, "Medizin und Arzt," pp. 40–43. The issue of medical philanthropy is also discussed in D. W. Amundsen, "Philanthropy in medicine: Some historical perspectives," in *Beneficence and Health Care*, ed. E. E. Shelp, Dordrecht, D. Reidel, 1982, pp. 1–31.

45. Frings, "Medizin und Arzt," pp. 42–43. See also D. W. Amundsen, "Evolution of the patient–physician relationship: Antiquity through the Renaissance," in *The Clinical Encounter: The Moral Fabric of the Patient–Physician Relationship*, ed. E. E. Shelp, Dordrecht, D. Reidel, 1983, pp. 3–46.

46. A. Kazhdan, "The image of the medical doctor in Byzantine literature of the tenth to twelfth centuries," *Dumbarton Oaks Papers* 38 (1984): 43–51.

47. L. D. Hankoff, "Religious healing in first-century Christianity," *J Psychohistory* 19 (1992): 387–407.

48. P. Horden, "Saints and doctors in the early Byzantine empire: The case of Theodore of Sykeon," *Stud Church Hist* 19 (1982): 1–13.

49. Polymnia Athanassiadi, *Julian: An Intellectual Biography*, London, Routledge, 1992, pp. 167–69, and E. Kislinger, "Kaiser Julian und die christlichen Xenodocheia," in *Byzantios, Festschrift für Herbert Hunger*, ed. W.v. Hoerandner, Vienna, E. Becvar, 1984, pp. 171–84.

50. Frings, "Medizin und Arzt," p. 11.

51. R. Arbesmann, "The concept of 'Christus medicus' in St. Augustine," *Traditio* 10 (1959): 1–28.

52. Philip Rousseau, *Basil of Caesarea*, Berkeley, Univ. of California Press, 1994, pp. 139–44. For more background see A. H. M. Jones, *The Cities of the Eastern Roman Provinces*, 2nd ed., Oxford, Clarendon Press, 1971.

53. For an overview see Timothy S. Miller, "Byzantine hospitals," in *Symposium on Byzantine Medicine*, pp. 53–63. For more details consult the author's *The Birth of the Hospital in the Byzantine Empire*, Baltimore, Johns Hopkins Univ. Press, 1985.

54. Their higher fertility is said also to have contributed to the rise of Christianity. See Stark, *The Rise of Christianity*, pp. 95–128.

55. J. Herrin, "Ideals of charity, realities of welfare: The philanthropic activity of the Byzantine church," in *Church and People in Byzantium*, ed. R. Morris, Manchester Press, Univ. of Manchester Press, 1986, pp. 151–64.

56. P. Horden, "The Byzantine welfare state: Image and reality," *Soc Social Hist Med Bull* 37 (1985): 7–10, and Evelyne Partlagean, *Pauvrété économique et pauvrété sociale à Byzance*, Paris, Moutin, 1977. Another useful collection of papers is *City, Town and Countryside in the Early Byzantine Era*, ed. R. L. Hohlfelder, New York, Columbia Univ. Press, 1982.

57. Kazhdan and Constable, *People and Power in Byzantium*, pp. 19–36.

58. A. Philipsborn, "Der Fortschritt in der Entwicklung des byzantinischen Krankenhauswesens," *Byzantinische Zeitung* 54 (1961): 338–65.

59. G. Ferngren, "Lay orders of medical attendants in the early Byzantine empire," in *Proceedings, XXXI International Congress on the History of Medicine*, ed. R. A. Bernabeo, Bologna, Monduzzi Ed., 1988, pp. 793–99.

60. U. B. Birchler-Argyros, "Byzantinische Spitalgeschichte, ein Überblick," *Hist Hosp* 15 (1983–84): 51–80.

61. E. Kislinger, "Xenon und nosokomeion-Hospitäler in Byzanz," *Hist Hosp* 17 (1986–88): 7–16.

62. For details see Richard Krautheimer, *Early Christian and Byzantine Architecture*, 4th ed., New York, Penguin Books, 1986.

63. M. E. Sullivan, "Horticultural therapy: The role gardening plays in healing," *J Am Health Care Assoc* 5 (1979): 3–8.

64. This blurring of the distinctions between these institutions is supported by the findings of Michael W. Dols. See his "The origins of the Islamic hospital: Myth and reality," *Bull Hist Med* 61 (1987): 371. For Coptic Egypt see P. van Minnen, "Medical care in late antiquity," *Clio Med* 27 (1995): 153–69.

65. Frings, "Medizin und Arzt," p. 85.

66. Temkin, *World of Pagans and Christians*, pp. 109–45.

67. See D. W. Amundsen "The physician's obligation to prolong life: A medical duty without classical roots," *Hastings Center Rep* 8 (1978): 23–30, and "The liability of the physician in classical Greek legal theory and practice," *J Hist Med* 32 (1977): 172–203.

68. These views were primarily expressed by John Chrysostom. See Frings, "Medizin

und Arzt," pp. 44–47. Regarding ethical issues in antiquity see F. Kudlien, " Medical ethics and popular ethics in Greece and Rome," *Clio Med* 5 (1970): 91–121.

69. Paul Johnson, *A History of Christianity*, New York, Atheneum, 1976, p. 75.

70. Stark, *The Rise of Christianity*, pp. 73–94.

71. Wright, *Chronicle*, pp. 32–33

72. St. Gregory Nazianzen, "On St. Basil," in *Funeral Orations by St. Gregory Nazianzen and St. Ambrose*, trans. L. P. McCauley et al., New York, Fathers of the Church, Inc., 1953, p. 58.

73. Ibid., p. 80.

74. Demetrios J. Constantelos, *Byzantine Philanthropy and Social Welfare*, 2nd ed., New Rochelle, NY, A. Caratzas, 1991, pp. 113–62.

75. See F. Kudlien, "Beichte und Heilung," *Medizinhist J* 13 (1978): 1–14.

76. Ralph Jackson, *Doctors and Diseases in the Roman Empire*, Norman, Univ. of Oklahoma Press, 1988, pp. 32–55.

77. See Robert Volk, *Gesundheitswesen und Wohltätigkeit im Spiegel der Byzantinischen Klostertypika*, Munich, Institut für Byzantinistik u. neugriechische Philologie, 1983, pp. 42–44. This publication studies the rules of 37 Byzantine monasteries.

78. Stark estimates that "conscientious nursing without any medications could cut the mortality rate by two-thirds or more." Since epidemic disease generated mortality rates of 30%, Christians should have sustained only a 10% loss, a differential that may have contributed to the growth of Christian communities. See Stark, *The Rise of Christianity*, pp. 88–91.

79. Frings, "Medizin und Arzt," p. 44.

80. Ibid., p. 48.

81. Ibid., p. 79. See also Temkin, *World of Pagans and Christians*, pp. 223–27.

82. Wright, *Chronicle*, p. 33

83. Ibid.

84. Ibid., p. 34.

85. For a comparative view see N. Allan, "Hospice to hospital in the Near East: An instance of continuity and change in late antiquity," *Bull Hist Med* 64 (1990): 446–62.

86. Letter quoted in Brown, *Power and Persuasion*, p. 153.

87. Rousseau, *Basil*, p. 259.

88. St. Benedict, "Prologue," *The Rule of St. Benedict in Latin and English*, ed. T. Fry, Collegeville, MN, The Liturgical Press, 1981, p. 12.

89. Horses were important symbols of rank and office, especially high-priced, purebred ones. See Heinrich Fichtenau, *Living in the Tenth Century: Mentalities and Social Orders*, trans. P. J. Geary, Chicago, Univ. of Chicago Press, 1991, pp. 66–67.

90. Ekkehard IV, *Casus Sancti Galli*, German trans. by H. F. Häfele, Darmstadt, Wissenschaftliche Buchgesellschaft, 1980, p. 199.

91. W. Vogler, "Historical sketch of the abbey of St. Gall," in *The Culture of the Abbey of St. Gall: An Overview*, ed. J. C. King and W. Vogler, Stuttgart, Belser Verlag, 1991, pp. 9–23.

92. Johannes Duft, *The Abbey Library of St. Gall: History, Baroque Hall, Manuscripts*, trans. J. C. King and P. W. Tax, St. Gallen, Verlag Klostehof, 1985.

93. For details see James M. Clark, *The Abbey of St. Gall as a Centre of Literature and Art*, Cambridge, Cambridge Univ. Press, 1926.

94. See Penelope D. Johnson, *Equal in Monastic Profession: Religious Women in Medieval France*, Chicago, Univ. of Chicago Press, 1991, p. 19.

95. Ekkehard, *Casus*, pp. 175–77.

96. Fichtenau, *Living in the Tenth Century*, p. 264.

97. Robert S. Hoyt, *Europe in the Middle Ages*, 2nd ed., New York, Harcourt, Brace & World, 1966, pp. 196–201.

98. More detail can be found in John J. Gallagher, *Church and State in Germany under Otto the Great (936–973)*, Washington, DC, Catholic University of America, 1938. See also Gerd Tellenbach, *The Church in Western Europe from the Tenth to the Early Twelfth Century*, trans. T. Reuter, Cambridge, Cambridge Univ. Press, 1993, pp. 1–21.

99. For parallel developments in Burgundy see Constance B. Bouchard, *Sword, Miter and Cloister: Nobility and the Church in Burgundy, 980–1198*, Ithaca, NY, Cornell Univ. Press, 1987.

100. Further details can be found in H. Zimmermann, ed., *Otto der Grosse*, Darmstadt, Wissenschaftliche Buchgesellschaft, 1976, and Timothy Reuter, *Germany in the Early Middle Ages, c. 800–1056*, London and New York, Longman, 1991.

101. Additional information is presented in Christopher Brooke, *Europe in the Central Middle Ages, 962–1154*, rev. ed., London, Longman, 1975.

102. For a discussion of the rationale and effects of monastic ritualism see Fichtenau, *Living in the Tenth Century*, pp. 70–90. For a medical view of the reforms see D. Bell, "The English Cistercians and the practice of medicine," *Citeaux* 40 (1989): 139–74.

103. Hoyt, *Europe in the Middle Ages*, pp. 172–83. For a biography of the emperor, see Ernst W. Wies, *Otto der Grosse: Kämpfer und Beter*, Munich, Bechtle, 1989.

104. Johannes Duft, *Notker der Arzt, Klostermedizin und Möncharzt im frühmittelalterlichen St. Gallen*, St. Gallen, Verlag Ostschweiz, 1972, p. 53.

105. For more information see Luis Garcia Ballester, *Practical Medicine from Salerno to the Black Death*, Oxford, Oxford Univ. Press, 1994.

106. A collection of articles on this subject can be found in Peter Brown, *Religion and Society in the Age of St. Augustine*, London, Faber & Faber, 1972.

107. C. H. Lawrence, *Medieval Monasticism: Forms of Religious Life in Western Europe in the Middle Ages*, 2nd ed., London, Longman, 1989, pp. 19–40.

108. See Esther de Waal, *Seeking God: The Way of St. Benedict*, Collegeville, MN, Liturgical Press, 1984. Current interest in the therapeutic aspects of monastic music and chanting has produced an extended literature. See John Beaulieu, *Music and Sound in the Healing Arts*, Barrytown, NY, Station Hill Press, 1991, and Randall McClellan, *The Healing Forces of Music: Healing, Theory and Practice*, Amityville, NY, Amity House, 1988. An excellent account of monastery life is provided by Richard Selzer in his essay "Diary of an infidel: notes from a monastery," in *Taking the World in for Repairs*, New York, Penguin Books, 1986, pp. 13–79.

109. Hans C. Peyer, *Von der Gastfreundschaft zum Gasthaus*, Hannover, Hahnsche Buchhandlung, 1987, pp. 116–38.

110. Jerome, *The Principal Works of Jerome*, trans. W. H. Fremantle, Oxford, J. Parker, 1893, p. 190.

111. R. Greer, "Hospitality in the first five centuries of the Church, *Medieval Studies* 10 (1974): 29–48.

112. For more information see Henry Mayr-Harting, *The Venerable Bede, the Rule of St. Benedict, and Social Class*, Jarrow-on-Tyne, United Kingdom, Rector, 1976.

113. More detail is contained in articles published by G. Baader and G. Keil, eds., *Medizin im mittelalterlichen Abendland*, Darmstadt, Wissenschaftliche Buchgesellschaft, 1982. For Cassiodorus, see his *Cassiodori Senatoris Institutiones*, ed. R. A. Mynors, Oxford, Clarendon Press, 1963. It contains lists of medical texts available in monasteries.

114. See K. Figala and G. Pfohl, "Benediktinische Medizin," *Studien u. Mitteilungen Gesch Benediktinerordens* 98 (1987): 239–56, and K. Park, "Medicine and society in me-

dieval Europe, 500–1500," in *Medicine and Society: Historical Essays*, ed. A. Wear, Cambridge, Cambridge Univ. Press, 1992, pp. 59–90.

115. St. Benedict, *Rule*, chap. 36, p. 54.

116. Details are provided in Loren Mackiney, *Early Medieval Medicine with a Special Look at France and Chartres*, Baltimore, Johns Hopkins Univ. Press, 1934.

117. The blueprint for a new St. Gall monastery has received considerable attention. See Walter W. Horn, *The Plan of St. Gall: A Study of the Architecture and Economy and Life in a Paradigmatic Carolingian Monastery*, 3 vols., Berkeley, Univ. of California Press, 1979. For a more recent revisionist view see W. Sanderson, "The plan of St. Gall reconsidered, " *Speculum* 60 (1985): 615–32.

118. P. Jung, "Das Infirmarium im Bauriss des St. Gall," *Gesnerus* 6 (1949): 1–8.

119. H. Horat, "The medieval architecture of the abbey of St. Gall," in *The Culture of the Abbey*, pp. 185–95.

120. D. Jetter, "Klosterspitäler, St. Gallen, Cluny, Escorial," *Sudhoffs Arch* 62 (1978): 313–38.

121. Lorna Price, *The Plan of St. Gall in Brief*, Berkeley, Univ. of California Press, 1982, pp. 40–50.

122. St. Benedict, *Rule*, chap 53, pp. 72–73.

123. Ibid., p. 74.

124. For another notable display of Notker's diagnostic skills see Duft, *Notker*, chap. 2, pp. 45–51.

125. St. Benedict, *Rule*, chap. 36, p. 55.

126. Ibid.

127. The abbess, Hildegard von Bingen was another example. See P. Dronke, *Women Writers in the Middle Ages*. Cambridge, Cambridge Univ. Press, 1984, pp. 144–202. Among some recent publications are Sabina Flanagan, *Hildegard of Bingen*, London, Routledge, 1987, and Barbara Newman, *Sister of Wisdom: St. Hildegard's Theology of the Feminine*, Berkeley, Univ. of California Press, 1987.

128. "Fractures," in *Hippocrates*, trans. E. T. Withington, Loeb Classical Library, Cambridge, Harvard Univ. Press, 1968, vol. 3, pp. 149–69.

129. "On joints," in ibid., vol. 3, pp. 313–21.

130. J. Kroll and B. Bachrach, "Sin and the etiology of disease in pre-Crusade Europe," *J Hist Med* 41 (1986): 395–414.

131. For details see also Celsus, *De Medicina*, trans. W. G. Spencer, Cambridge, MA, Harvard Univ. Press, 1961, vol. 3, pp. 539–49 and 577–81.

132. Heinrich Schipperges, *Die Benediktiner in der Medizin des frühen Mittelalters*, Leipzig, St. Benno, 1964 , especially pp. 37–59. Recent archeological excavations of a medieval infirmary near Soutra, southeast of Edinburgh, are beginning to provide material confirmation for many of the healing activities ascribed to these establishments. Soutra was under Augustinian rule from 1164 to 1464 (personal communication from Dr. Brian Moffat, Scotland).

133. Among them was a treatise on urines and pulses originally written by Alexander of Tralles (525–605) of Constantinople. See Alexander von Tralles, *Original Text und Übersetzung*, trans. T. Pushmann, Amsterdam, A. M. Hakkert, 1963.

134. Duft, *Notker*, p. 45–46.

135. St. Benedict, *Rule*, p. 55. See K. L. Pearson, "Nutrition and the early medieval diet," *Speculum* 72 (1997): 1–32, and for more details see Melitta Weiss Adamson, *Medieval Dietetics: Food and Drink in Regimen Sanitatis Literature from 800 to 1400*, Frankfurt, Lang, 1995.

136. J. Stannard, "Greco-Roman materia medica in medieval Germany," *Bull Hist Med*

46 (1972): 455–68. For more information see Annette Niederhellmann, *Arzt und Heilkunde in den frühmittelalterlichen Leges: eine wort- und sachkundliche Untersuchung*, Berlin, W. de Gruyter, 1983.

137. For details see Marie-Christine Pouchelle, *The Body and Surgery in the Middle Ages*, trans. R. Morris, New Brunswick, NJ, Rutgers Univ. Press, 1990. pp. 13–36.

138. For details see John M. Riddle, *Dioscorides on Pharmacy and Medicine*, Austin, Univ. of Texas Press, 1985, especially pp. 1–24. See also J. Stannard, "The herbal as a medical document," *Bull Hist Med* 43 (1969): 212–20, and by the same author "Medieval herbals and their development," *Clio Med* 9 (1974): 23–33.

139. Linda E. Voigts and Michael R. McVaugh, *A Latin Technical Phlebotomy*, Philadelphia, American Philosophical Society, 1984, pp. 1–11.

140. For more details about the significance of blood, see Piero Camporesi, *Juice of Life: The Symbolic and Magic Significance of Blood*, trans. R. R. Barr, New York, Continuum, 1995.

141. St. Benedict, *Rule*, p. 55

142. F. S. Paxton, "Signa mortifera: Death and prognostication in early medieval monastic medicine," *Bull Hist Med* 67 (1993): 631–50.

143. F. S. Paxton, "Anointing the sick and dying in Christian antiquity and the early medieval West," in *Health, Disease, and Healing in Medieval Culture*, ed. S. Campbell, B. Hall, and D. Klausner, New York, St. Martin's Press, 1992, pp. 93–102, and P. J. Toner, "Extreme unction," in *New Catholic Encyclopedia*, New York, McGraw Hill, 1967, vol. 5, pp. 716–30.

144. For details see Frederick S. Paxton, *Christianizing Death: The Creation of a Ritual Process in Early Medieval Europe*, Ithaca, NY, Cornell Univ. Press, 1991, and Philippe Ariès, *Western Attitudes Toward Death*, trans. P. M. Ranum, Baltimore, Johns Hopkins Univ. Press, 1974.

145. St. Benedict, *Rule*, p. 73.

146. Details are provided in St. Augustine, *The Rule of Saint Augustine*, intro. and commentary by T. J. van Bavel, trans. R. Canning, London, Darton, Longman & Todd, 1984.

147. "On joints," in *Hippocrates*, vol. 3, pp. 335–41.

148. Duft, *Notker*, pp. 48–49.

149. For details see Constance Bouchard, *Holy Entrepreneurs: Cistercians, Knights, and Economic Exchange in Twelfth-Century Burgundy*, Ithaca, NY, Cornell Univ. Press, 1991, especially pp. 1–32.

150. For an overview see Constance Bouchard, *Life and Society in the West: Antiquity and the Middle Ages*, San Diego, Harcourt, Brace Jovanovich, 1968.

151. As quoted in Park, "Medicine and society," p. 64.

152. D. W. Amundsen, "Medieval canon law," *Bull Hist Med* 52 (1978): 22–44.

153. P. O. Kristeller, "The school of Salerno. Its development and its contribution to the history of learning," *Bull Hist Med* 17 (1945): 138–94.

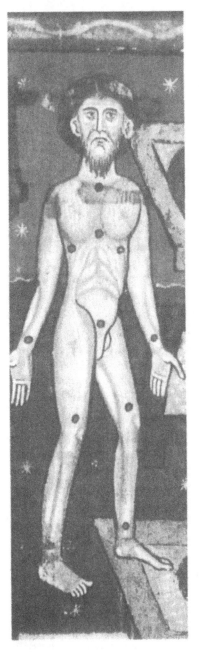

3

CHURCH AND LAITY

Partnership in Hospital Care

THE PANTOCRATOR XENON OF CONSTANTINOPLE

Those communal homes and hospitals for the poor [living] in sickness and penury it is not so much the external appearance of the buildings that is to be commended as the display of compassion, the philanthropeia of both kinds: towards the treatment of sickness through medical help and toward the alleviation of hunger.

Theodoros Metochites[1]

Tales of a feverish poet

In the year 1140, Theodoros Prodromos, royal poet to the court at Constantinople during the reigns of Alexius Comnenus (1081–1118) and John II Comnenus (1118–1143) and a well-respected philosopher and theologian, suddenly became dangerously ill with a fever.[2] In a personal letter composed during the early stages of his illness, the 40-year-old Prodromos shared his troubles with a friend, the provincial bishop Stephanos Skylitzes of Trapezus, an ancient port on the Black Sea. "God hit me with a painful sore throughout the whole body," he wrote, adding that " I say this for I have now been thrown into the most disgraceful condition to look at and suffer pestilence." He went on to observe that "for three days, horrible flames and fiery rivers consumed me, and then there followed vomiting, so much that I feared I might loose all of my bilious humors and afterwards be like the stags who have none."[3] The affliction seemed to spread to his throat and vocal cords, causing his voice to sound weak and thin. In a later poem, Prodromos pronounced his ailment to be a "catarrhus," defined as a disease caused by vapors in the brain and lungs but also affecting the entire body.[4] In this work directed at his "heroic illness," Prodromos characterized the so-called catarrh as a "great and powerful sickness; it flows from the head, [causing] profound pain and unending torture. The forest's mist sends a chill through my brain, colder than the sacred grove of olives and rain comes down from the mountain clouds."[5]

Confronted with such serious symptoms, Prodromos summoned "an inexperienced physician who increased the illness which had been of a nature called atomic by Democritus by speaking of many things." The private practitioner took Prodromos' pulse, "touching with his hands my entire body, until he decided on the nature of my disease." The verdict, he complained, was a "tertian fever and a plague! Such are the physicians of great Byzantium."[6] Given his somewhat uncertain financial condition—his access to the court was unsteady, and he was forced to rely on friends and generous patrons for occasional commissions of poetry—the sudden and violent illness was certainly a most untimely development.[7] It is not surprising that Prodromos blamed his physician for his illness. He had never been a great friend of medical people. Although at times Prodromos grudgingly praised a few individual practitioners for their skills, his work contained more lampoon than homage to the profession, characterizing physicians in one of his writings as vultures in search of honoraria. Instead, Prodromos preferred the "unadorned healing of the Savior," contrasting it with the complex and ineffective ministrations of those who followed Hippocrates and Galen. In one of his satires titled "Executioner or Physician?" he vividly described a personal visit to a surgeon to have a painful tooth extracted. Armed with a gigantic tool, the clumsy man only managed to break off the tooth, thus compounding the poet's sufferings.[8]

In an account to his former teacher Stephanos Skylitzes—he had studied grammar, rhetoric, and philosophy with him at Constantinople's Patriarchal School—Prodromos then related that "on the fourth day, small reddish bumps appeared all over my body which grew quickly and by the seventh day became horrible pustules. Besides being unable to eat or sleep, I had terrible stabbing pains throughout and know that my hair fell entirely out."[9] With growing concern, Prodromos wrote a note to Alexius Aristenos, a high-ranking imperial official in charge of public welfare, indicating that he was upset about the medical diagnosis, presumably just a type of rash.[10] He explained "the so-called pestilence, which though abominable in all ways, men are used to calling by a good name so that because of its name it might be more palatable to the sick in the same way that physicians put a nice name to bitter medicine or call the fiery cautery 'cold,' or the bone on which we sit 'sacred.' "[11] To set the record straight, Prodromos announced that he was calling his disease "the seventh plague which Moses sent to Egypt, which mixed fire and hail, so my body from head to toe was hit by hail. Yes, I do call it hail because it is white and round."[12]

Unfortunately, the fire created by the fever seemed unable to extinguish the widespread skin eruption, and Prodromos grew worse. By the seventh day, the vesicles had completely covered his body. In a second letter to Skylitzes, he asked: "Have you ever seen a violent shower of rain coming down on a lake, how the entire surface of the lake swells up on account of the closely packed bubbles? Such at this time has my wretched flesh become."[13] As the affliction appeared to be reaching its climax, the poet became increasingly apprehensive about the outcome. Nothing was reported about further medical visits. Perhaps the patient had become skeptical about the diagnostic skills of his young physician, but most likely he simply could no longer afford him. Contemporary Constantinople was the center of lay medicine in the empire, but private practice flourished only among those who could pay their healers' rather extravagant honoraria. If Prodromos was suffering from early symptoms of smallpox, as a conjectural diagnosis from the distance of nearly 1,000 years would suggest, his was certainly not an isolated case. The disease had already appeared centuries earlier in Byzantium and the Middle East, most likely as a consequence of new contacts between the European and Asian disease pools. One epidemic had been reported in Syria by Eusebius during the year 302, and the typical clinical manifestations were described during the ninth century in a celebrated book by the Muslim physician al Rhazi (865–925).[14]

In another literary interpretation, Prodromos characterized his illness as vile and demonic, invading his body, binding his chest, pulling hair from his head, and polluting his skin with blotches and pustules.[15] The ugly pustules made him feel like a leper, a person disgraceful to look at. Borrowing from the tenets of classical humoralism, the sick man envisioned a struggle taking place inside him between an ice-cold stomach and red-hot liver. The culprit was a "bearer of thunder who comes holding a grudge against me, besetting me with boils encircling the Achilles tendon of my foot, sapping my mind's strength, for he had dominated all of the earth beneath his fierce fire, engulfing it for seven days in flames and misery without end." Of course, sinful behavior was the cause. "Let us give up impious acts in order to cast evil out of this life," Prodromos wrote, "let us give up stupidity and the hatred of wisdom and proclaim the Logos, the Word of God whose name brings good fortune."[16] Unfortunately, he felt too weak to visit a church and pray for his recovery. In his despair the poet finally pleaded: "O my feet, awaken, go quickly, quickly race to the canopy of the Saviour, Lord, upon my forehead place a kiss. May the kiss which once broke apart deep misery once again reduce the sorrow which I feel."[17]

Miserable and worried, Prodromos decided to enter one of the local hospitals for treatment. Perhaps lack of money for private medical advice was not the issue driving this decision, but rather the fact that Prodromos lived alone and had no one to care for him. However, even wealthier patients were known to enter *xenones* occasionally or to send family members to them.[18] In any event, Prodromos went to the establishment adjacent to the famous, newly endowed Pantocrator monastery. The term "Pantocrator" literally meant supreme ruler, an attribution usually reserved for Christ.[19] Funded by the emperor John II Comnenus around 1136, this monastery quickly became one of the most splendid architectural landmarks of Constantinople. Like most institutions of its kind, the complex featured two separate healing facilities: the *triclinon* or infirmary for sick monks, located inside the monastic compound, and a new *xenon* or hostel for the care of the sick poor, located outside its walls. Prodromos was probably familiar with the Pantocrator. Earlier, he had written an epigram celebrating the icon of Christ, an image placed in one of the monastery's churches.[20] For its part, the institution's hostel had a charter or *typikon* indicating the existence of a special ward with eight beds for "those suffering from illnesses of the eyes and of the intestines and other severe ailments."[21] Perhaps this section was the poet's final destination.

Post-Justinian Byzantium: Society, medicine, and *xenones*

A few decades after the dramatic events in Edessa, the Eastern Roman Empire under Emperor Justinian (527–565) witnessed a series of reform efforts, including a failed attempt to restore the previous imperial unity.[22] Many provinces were devastated by raids and invasions. As in Edessa, successive famines and epidemics strained the resources of local municipalities, forcing Church authorities to create makeshift shelters and hospitals. Yet, in spite of his military burdens, Justinian managed to carry out a vast building program, especially in Constantinople, where the new and spectacular domed church of St. Sophia was erected. The loss of the Western territories, however, created a gradual state of financial bankruptcy, internal upheavals, and external invasions after the year 600, plunging the entire empire into crisis.

As a consequence of erratic tax policies, excessive demands from landowners, wars, and pestilence, a veritable tidal wave of peasants fled to the large cities, especially Constantinople. As earlier in Edessa, the new arrivals were severely malnourished and sick, many victims of leprosy and plague. Not surprisingly, plague broke out in the capital during the year 542, severely straining the local welfare system. In addition to public distributions of food and clothing, the homeless were herded into temporary shelters located in the atriums of churches and monasteries.

Byzantine philanthropy was strikingly ineffectual, however, despite its generous support by a broad spectrum of the population. Bread and money were often distributed without an effort to examine and ameliorate the political and economic conditions contributing to poverty and homelessness. There were no concerted efforts to develop a coherent social health policy or even an attempt to provide adequate medical care to the inhabitants of Constantinople. Instead of developing policies to protect the lower classes from excessive taxation and loss of land, the collective charitable efforts concentrated more on individual assistance in a crisis and the rewards of spiritual salvation for both donor and recipient.[23]

The loss of Alexandria, Antioch, and other cities following the capture of Jerusalem by the Persians in 614 contributed to the rapid imperial decline. In the years 636–638, the Moslems occupied Palestine and Syria, then Egypt in 640, drastically reducing in size the once proud empire. Only the Greek-speaking, religiously orthodox regions surrounding Constantinople remained. Still, the capital endured as an active commercial center at the crossroads of central Asian and Far East trade, continuing to supply wealth and education for its upper and middle classes, encouraging art, literature, and scholarship. Conscious heirs of Roman learning, these elites—Prodromos' patrons—stressed literacy and laid the foundations for primary educational schemes as a first step toward special studies in rhetoric, law, philosophy, medicine, arithmetic, geometry, astronomy, and music. In medicine, systematic instruction in theoretical and practical issues occurred within naturalistic frameworks largely untouched by religious concerns.[24] The teaching stressed the usefulness of compendia and synopses. Greek physicians had always taught their trade as part of their activities, and the evolving *xenon* may have become another site for the informal teaching of practical medicine.

The first important compiler had been Oribasius (325–403), a pupil of Zenon of Cyprus and his famous Alexandrian school and court physician to Emperor Julian the Apostate. In creating an encyclopedia, Oribasius summarized classical medical knowledge, as expressed in the extant writings of the Hippocratics and Galen.[25] In the 500s, Aetius of Amida (500–560) composed his *Sixteen Books on Medicine*, summaries of gynecological and obstetrical works written by Soranus and Rufus of Ephesus. Aetius was a Christian who had studied at Alexandria and became court physician in Constantinople during the reign of Justinian I.[26] His younger contemporary was Alexander of Tralles (525–605) from Lydia, also a Christian living at the imperial court. Alexander added his own observations, including novel pharmacological treatments and the importance of spa baths. Later *xenon* manuscripts revealed the popularity of his works.[27] The last compiler was Paul of Aegina, (625–690), a physician of high repute, who lived far away from the court in Alexandria during the seventh century. Paul's books followed closely the ideas of Galen and Oribasius, and he authored an *Epitome of Medicine* in seven books.[28]

After the 700s, the lay medical profession in Byzantium temporarily lost its social standing, as popular sentiment—shared by Prodromos—came to view many physicians as greedy and incompetent. Without colleges or guilds before 1100 to prevent fragmentation, except for the *archiatroi*, individual medical professionals retained their status and income according to their roots within the urban elites.

The resulting stratification ranged from wealthy court physicians in Constantinople to lowly country practitioners eking out a living in the towns and districts of the vast hinterland. The adverse portraiture was part of the contemporary hagiography that relentlessly rejected secular medicine, targeting the high honoraria and tax exemptions demanded by its practitioners. Another frequent motif was the comparison of healing saints to physicians, with the healing efficacy attributed exclusively to the former.

These tensions between secular healing and Christian care were, of course, not new. One seventh-century document, the *Miracula Sancti Artemii* accused physicians of callous profit making from the exorbitant payments some of them demanded. This picture contrasted sharply with the miraculous cures performed for free by the saints. Even classically educated physicians such as Aetius expressed a belief in miraculous cures, blurring the lines between the supernatural and natural. A mixture of prayer, classical herbal preparations, and local folk healing traditions, as well as the employment of amulets and charms, became socially acceptable remedies, and in the seventh century, popular sentiment continued to stress the role of the Church as the Christian's only hospital and Christ as the Great Physician.

Following Justinian's reign, new *xenones* or hostels were founded with imperial assistance in the most important cities of the empire. Two, the Panteleemon and the Christodotes, were erected in Constantinople before the year 600, and similar arrangements took place in other urban centers such as Alexandria and Antioch. After this time, the word *xenon* came to refer generally to institutions for the poor and sick. The first primarily medical institution was built during the rule of emperor Heraclius (610–641), although the Church retained administrative control. The term *nosokomeion* was also specific to medicalized establishments, but caring functions of one sort or another occurred in all other contemporary welfare institutions. As noted before, the close linkage between poverty, malnutrition, and illness continued to blur the lines between welfare and medical agendas in most charitable Byzantine institutions. Local conditions, including famines and epidemics, and the presence of hostels, monasteries, and leper houses, as well as lay medical professionals, shaped the particular mix of inmates. Whether provided with medical caregivers or not, Byzantine hospitals remained essentially religious institutions within the Christian welfare system.

During the seventh and eight centuries, little information about Byzantine *xenones* is available, although larger institutions in the capital must have remained open to cope with the swelling numbers of sick poor. Those directly sponsored by the emperor and his court may have had to worry less about survival and continuity of service. Their endowments grew from continuous gifts in property and cash contributed by the faithful and their ruler, as well as from tax and lease revenues extracted from landowners. Since ecclesiastical property was inalienable and could not be transferred, long-term leases promised stable income, especially after Byzantium's renewed prosperity in the 850s. Building more shelters became an imperial practice. Emperor Theophilos (829–842) endowed another *xenon* in Constantinople that had beautiful views and was exposed to sea breezes. Imperial generosity was often matched by that of wealthy Christians who built monasteries, orphanages, and hospices. One example was the work of Philentolos from Cyprus, who around the year 850 erected a *xenon* to care for the sick poor. Later, Emperor Lekapenos (920–944) established a *xenon* in conjunction with a palace in the capital. In the 1050s, Constantine IX built his residence with a monastery, a palace, and a *xenon* designed for his own care.

In addition to public displays of personal charity, the donors expected to obtain heavenly rewards through the prayers of the sick but grateful inmates. St. John the Compassionate established seven lying-in hospitals in Alexandria for destitute mothers. When Comnenos established the *xenon* at the Pantocrator monastery—Prodromos' destination—his expressed hope was that his *philanthropia* in founding this institution would provide forgiveness for his sins. Hospital foundations remained individual monuments to the emperor's charity and concern. As the New Moses or God's representative on earth, he was expected to perform works of mercy for his suffering subjects. But a coherent plan of welfare was not in his vision.

At the same time, traditional monastic structures dealing with sick and elderly monks flourished. Surviving rules or *typika* of such monasteries reveal the existence of infirmaries—like that at St. Gall—where the sick cenobites could be temporarily housed and treated. Here the Euergetis *typikon* (ca. 1000) served as a model for a series of monastic regulations. As in most infirmaries, it was a square building with four central columns supporting a central cupola, with a capacity of four to eight beds. This vaulted roof, with its central opening, served as a fireplace surrounded by four aisles where the sickbeds could be placed in eight separate sections. Adjacent to this building was a small chapel, traditionally devoted in Byzantium to St. Cosmas and St. Damian. Baths were often nearby.[29] Most rural religious houses possessed similar infirmaries.

Since the time of Justinian, the administration of *xenones* had remained in the hands of pious Church members. However, physical and staff expansions demanded more administrative skills from abbots, priests, or deacons—*xenodochoi* or *nosokomoi*—in charge. Their roles, outlined in the Justinian reforms, included control over admissions and responsibility for supplies, expertise in Roman law, and understanding of rules governing ecclesiastical property. A chief administrator called *xenodochos* headed the Christodotes *xenon* in Constantinople during the 650s, even supervising the chief physicians. His low pay may have been linked to other court duties and positions with substantial yearly salaries. Monks, former army officers, courtiers, and physician-administrators gradually came to dominate hospital management. Ecclesiastical codes emphasized moral rectitude and administrative ability as the most important qualifications. By the end of the ninth century, the emperor controlled all hospital resources and for this purpose appointed his own official, the *nosokomos*, as was the case at the Pantocrator *xenon* in Constantinople. By the early 1100s, cultural trends in Byzantium allowed lay medical professionals to achieve a status similar to that of bureaucrats and literary figures. By then, all *iatroi* had to pass an examination and receive a license before working in a *xenon*. In Constantinople and other major urban centers, monasteries and ecclesiastical schools, with their abundant libraries, were the main teaching centers of theoretical medicine. Practical matters were usually learned through apprenticeship with more senior physicians.[30]

Like Notker II at St. Gall, monks with medical knowledge were probably the primary caregivers in their monastic infirmaries, while more lay persons, including physicians, would have staffed the urban *xenones*. The first official visits by a physician or *iatros* to a *xenon* were allowed around the year 1000, as noted in the rules of the Euergetis Monastery in Constantinople. This small infirmary had eight beds, a kitchen to prepare food and medications, and two servants or *hyperetai*, presumably laymen, as assistants. After the sixth century, professional physicians and a lay support staff of nurses had begun to replace the corps of urban volunteer caregivers. In Constantinople, the monks also assisted with funerals. By the 650s, the presence of the *hypourgoi* or male assistants together with male servants (*hyperetai*) signaled the gradual shift. The *hypourgoi* performed essential nursing functions such as the administration of medicines and the supervision of patients while physicians were absent. The *hyperetai* were "unmarried, moral workers for the service of the sick" assisting in the performance of all institutional chores. Separately identified were cooks or *mageiroi*. During the seventh century in Alexandria, and perhaps also in Constantinople, the *hypourgoi* formed their own guilds.

The text *Miracula Sancti Artemii*, written shortly after 650, contains two stories that suggest the existence of *xenones* with more elaborate medical services in Constantinople: the Sampson Xenon and the Christodotes Xenon. The former seems to have had practitioners with special surgical skills on its staff; the latter was supervised by *archiatroi* or chief physicians, successors to the traditional city-appointed healers of ancient Greece. In addition, one of the stories reveals the existence of regular physicians, *mesoi* or *iatroi*, and a lower-ranked individual or *teleutaioi*, perhaps a medical apprentice. This suggests a more complex organization of sick care with a hierarchically organized staff. The *archiatroi* apparently worked in monthly shifts at the Christodotes Xenon, a system of rotation that was still in use at the Pantocrator 600 years later. While on duty, the *iatroi* made rounds every morning to visit patients.

By the 800s, the larger hospitals had begun to develop a new category of chief physicians, the so-called *protarchoi*—later called *primmikerioi* in the Pantocrator hierarchy. After 900, the *archiatroi* were also called *protomenites*. During both the seventh and eighth centuries, physicians staffing *xenones* formed a professional pyramid with the *protarchoi* at the top, followed by *archiatroi*, *mesoi*, and junior *teleutaioi*. The plethora of titles may reflect the gradual bureaucratization that infiltrated all offices of the Byzantine government. Perhaps more important, these titles also suggest a gradual fragmentation of the medical profession into distinct levels of knowledge and training. At the top were now the court physicians, whose influence and power made them highly respected emissaries of the emperor.

Whether hospital work contributed to the social and professional standing of the Byzantine physician remains unclear. In spite of low salaries, the opportunity to participate in the activities of a charitable institution such as a *xenon* may have been tempting. The inherent prestige of hospital work as a barometer of munificence and an antidote for perceptions of selfishness and greed could advance private practice. At the same time, many of the Byzantine physicians, like their Islamic counterparts, must have realized that caring for *xenon* patients significantly expanded their clinical knowledge and skills.

Islam's *bimaristan* and Christianity's Pantocrator *xenon*

Apparently the first prominent Islamic shelter or hospital was established in the capital city of Damascus, Syria, around 707 under the Umayyad Caliph al-Walid (705–715).[31] It was founded with support from Syrian Christians, who constituted the bulk of the population and already possessed their own charitable organizations, including leper houses. The new institution was undoubtedly modeled after *xenones* and *nosokomeia* built centuries earlier throughout the urban centers of the Byzantine Empire, including Syria. Moreover, following the expulsion of the Nestorians from Edessa in 489, these shelters had become a popular feature of Christian communities in the Sassanian Empire before their conquest by Arabs in the early 600s.[32]

Several decades later, in 750, the Abbasid rulers moved to the new imperial capital in Bagdad. Here Caliph al-Mansur summoned a Nestorian physician, ibn Bakhtishu, to his court, thus providing a prominent place for Syrian Christian elites, especially those concerned with medicine. Then, under Caliph Harun ar Rashid (786–809), a royal *bimaristan* was founded in Bagdad in the early 790s, apparently located in the suburb of Karkh.[33] While wealthy Christians, including physicians, may have been instrumental in planning and fund-raising for the new institution, it is possible that this *nosokomeion* may have been initially oriented toward Persian and Hindu therapeutics, given the strong influence of the non-Christian Barmakid family at court, including ar-Rashid's tutor and wazir, Yahya ibn Khalid ibn Barmak. Certainly, the Persian term *bimaristan*, ("place for the sick"), employed to designate Islamic healing institutions, implies such a tradition.

Following the fall from power of the Barmakid clan and the ascension of al-Mamum (813–833) as imperial ruler, Hellenistic influences engulfed scientific learning and medical activities at charitable institutions such as Baghdad's *bi-*

maristan. Sponsored by the caliph, translation projects from Greek to Arabic and a vast effort to find extant Greek manuscripts provided a critical mass of scientific and philosophical knowledge. Christian scholars used such activities to preserve professional authority and prestige with their Islamic masters, and the ensuing process of appropriation brought the central tenets of Hippocratic-Galenic medicine to the attention of Muslims who aspired to learn classical medicine.[34]

Although Islam lacked the broad spectrum of charitable institutions first created by Christians in Byzantium and the Latin West, Muslims actively engaged in almsgiving. In addition, the *waqf* system provided pious gifts as part of a voluntary contract between Allah and a potential donor or *waqif*. Religiously sanctioned, this practice played an increasingly important role in furnishing property and cash endowments for the poor and needy. Whether private donors were genuinely motivated by charity or simply desired to avoid taxation, payment of debts, or contested inheritance claims, their gifts provided significant resources. These donated assets, given in perpetuity to a public trust, paid for welfare services no longer available as the Christian population and influence slowly waned, especially in the growing urban centers.[35]

Under such circumstances, hospital foundations became an attractive option for prominent Muslims, rulers, and princes interested in emulating their Byzantine rivals by displaying legitimacy, prosperity, and benevolence. Rather than numerous small shelters, Islam chose selected metropolitan areas to build larger and more elaborate establishments. Limited in number, these imperial showcases had little impact on the health of their cities. Symbols of political and economic power, *bimaristans* carrying the name of their princely patrons flourished after the ninth century in some of the most important Islamic cities, such as Cairo (874), western Baghdad (918), eastern Baghdad (981), Damascus (1156), Cairo (1284), and finally Granada (1366).[36] They followed the rationale that sick Muslims should be sheltered, attended, and treated by physicians. Early institutions to house the insane were also created.[37]

Unlike their Christian counterparts, *bimaristans* were strictly private imperial foundations liberated from religious agendas. In contrast to Christianity, the human body in Islam was an important component of a person and thus greatly valued. Hospitals, moreover, fulfilled the tenets of Islamic religion that stressed the value of personal health.[38] Without a priesthood in control of these establishments to enforce religious orthodoxy, *bimaristans* were more congenial to medical objectives. These included the control of admissions, medical management, therapeutic experimentation, and clinical teaching. Apparently physicians were often consulted during planning and construction of these facilities. Splendid establishments—plans for Cairo's 100-bed Mansuri Hospital founded in 1284 have survived—were likened to royal palaces, with giant columns and numerous pavilions arranged around a central courtyard.[39] Their wards, gardens, and pools were supplied with fresh water from adjacent streams. In fact, *bimaristans* primarily reflected the wealth and will of their imperial patrons, who appointed high court officials—often a relative of the ruler—to administer the institution and its growing endowments, as well as to appoint all personnel.

Such secular direction fostered the creation of specific triage systems based on medical criteria to screen out those who could be attended on an ambulatory basis. Potential patients were examined in an outside hall or room before being assigned to specific wards. These included rooms for fever patients, surgical and traumatic cases, eye diseases, and even intestinal ailments. Patients were not only segregated by sex but gradually differentiated by disease. Criteria for recovery included the patient's ability to resume eating. Discharge procedures could involve a final bath and new clothing. Apparently even money was dispensed to finance home convalescence.[40] Lest one consider hospital life in Islam as proceeding entirely along secular lines, physicians invariably explained their activities as being guided by divine will, especially introducing their prescriptions with the formula "in the name of the Merciful, the Compassionate."[41]

Given its size, the *bimaristan* required a large hierarchy of caregivers and assistants. After opening its doors, the Adudi in Bagdad apparently had 25 physicians on its roster. In an attempt to protect people from inferior practitioners, prominent court physicians were empowered by the rulers to examine those who wished to practice medicine in a city or hospital.[42] Christian and Jewish physicians were allowed to practice together with their Muslim colleagues. In the beginning, the availability of a well-educated, socially prominent medical profession in Syria composed of Christian and Jewish practitioners became the critical factor allowing the relative medicalization of these Islamic institutions. Hospital practitioners were often required to obtain a certificate of good conduct from the police, although personal connections or outright bribes could replace this provision.[43] Later, some of the most prominent physicians joined the medical staffs of such institutions, including al Razi (865–925), who worked at Baghdad's al Muqtadiri.

Routines included rounds with members of the medical staff two or three times per week, and orders were written for dietary items and drugs. Bedside events were recorded, and such progress reports were consulted as clinical management of the patient unfolded before the eyes of medical staff members and perhaps some students. Given the availability of good paper and skilled copyists and binders, some institutions possessed a separate library of medical books and manuscripts. The Islamic world had a well-developed book market, and collections were available in palaces, libraries, and private homes. Finally, most *bimaristans* apparently had their own pharmacy containing an ample supply of drugs together with a compounding facility. Many remedies were chemically prepared[44]; others were available from local herb gardens. Imported medicinals were common, since the Near East was the point of convergence of an active spice and drug trade linking it with Persia, India, and China.[45] Compounding was extremely popular, as physicians hedged their bets by reinforcing the presumed therapeutic qualities of one medicinal plant with those of another obtained from Persian, Hindu, or Chinese sources.

The success of Islam's *bimaristan* may have influenced contemporary Christian healing institutions like Prodromos' destination. In Constantinople, Emperor John II Comnenos and his wife, Irene, established and endowed before 1136 a monastery in honor of Christ, the healer. Dedicated to God by a grateful ruler for military victories in Armenia, southern Russia, and the Balkans, as well as suppressions of internal insurrections, the Pantocrator became associated with a famous icon of Christ.[46] This monastery became part of a large and beautiful complex of buildings that included two churches, north and south, together with a domed mausoleum dedicated to St. Michael that became the resting place for all members of the Comneni dynasty.[47] According to a surviving *typikon* or rule book, there were two separate healing facilities: the traditional *triclinon* or infirmary for sick monks and, outside the walls, a large *xenon* for treatment of pilgrims and the city's sick poor. The monastic infirmary had only six beds and was under the supervision of the Pantocrator's abbot, who was responsible for its supplies, especially bread and wine. Medical care was provided by a lay physician usually assigned to the *xenon*, who upon notification also visited the sick monks. Those with mild illnesses were attended in their own cells. All drugs and medical supplies also came from the *xenon*. Bathing took place at the monastery's *balneum* or bath.[48]

For its part, the Pantocrator *xenon* seems to have been a U-shaped structure open toward the adjacent monastery, with its three wings and central courtyard. If its construction had been as lavish as that of the surrounding churches, the hospital could have boasted windows with stained glass set in lead as well as mosaic floors. A number of accessory structures, arranged around the wall encircling the entire perimeter, contained living quarters for the caregivers, a pharmacy, outpatient room, kitchen, bakery and storage facilities.[49] Like Islamic *bimaristans*, the Pantocrator *xenon* was said to possess a library and lecture hall, as well as the usual administrative quarters and laundry services. Separate facilities to house lepers were also available.[50] An adjacent chapel provided liturgical services. The Pantocrator also boasted its own cemetery, and a special fund was available to pay for the burial costs of those who died in the institution.

Perhaps inspired by contemporary Islamic models, the healing space apparently was arranged in five separate sections or *ordinoi* "for the repose of sick people" of the city. It featured a main dormitory with a capacity of 50 beds divided into separate areas, with about 10 beds "for those with disturbances from wounds or crippled limbs" and another 8 "for those suffering from illnesses of the eyes and of the intestines and other severe ailments." In addition, "for the women who are ill," the charter stated that "there will be set aside twelve beds and the reminder shall be given over to those sick who are simply recovering." Men and women remained segregated. To provide some flexibility in admissions, the hospital's *typikon* suggested that "if there is often a lack of injured or of those with eye diseases or those afflicted with very serious diseases, then the number [of beds] shall be filled with other such persons, those having any kind of illness."[51] Moreover, the rules prescribed extra cots for emergency patients or particularly severe cases, to be available in all wards that "when these fifty beds are divided into five sections, there shall be in each ward an extra bed in which there shall be placed one of the sick who cannot be moved at all, either because of the acuteness of the illness, or because of great weakness, or sometimes even because of the severity of the wounds he has suffered."[52]

As a recent imperial foundation, the Pantocrator may have had more resources than similar establishments in Constantinople and elsewhere. The city in 1140 had close to 300,000 inhabitants, but its hospitals played only a minor role in the provision of care. Among the 32 administrative and religious employees called for by the rules, we can identify 5 administrators, 10 priests and monks, 8 cooks, and 9 servants, all serving under the direction of a *nosokomos*. This manager was not only responsible for the hospital's supplies of food and medicines, but also ensured institutional discipline through his dealings with caregivers and patients. The caregiving personnel consisted of 73 persons, including 21 physicians, 46 nursing assistants, and 6 pharmacists, an impressive ratio for an urban *xenon* with a capacity of only 50 beds that could perhaps house up to 150–200 inmates. Whether such an institutional scheme and volume of patients ever became a reality is unknown. To reassure potential patients, the institution's charter prescribed that "each bed have one blanket with pillow and coverlet but in the winter also with two heavy ones." Institutional clothing was also provided.[53]

A further breakdown of the postulated 21 physicians reveals the presence of 1 supreme teacher and 2 chiefs or *primmikeros*—presumably one for medicine and another for surgery—at the top of the hierarchical ladder. They were to work in shifts of six months each year. Practicing under the chiefs of service were two supervising physicians and an equal number of surgeons, followed by four regular physicians, two additional ones exclusively attached to the women's ward, and two assigned to the monastic infirmary. Four physicians worked in the Pantocrator's ambulatory facility dispensing drugs and carrying out minor surgery. The probable presence of an outpatient room or building staffed by physicians and nurses may have constituted an innovation. This may have replaced a previous scheme whereby groups of nurses or physicians roamed the streets of the imperial city offering assistance to the poor and homeless and bringing some of them into the hospital. Also listed were two additional practitioners—one a female, probably working in the women's ward, and another a surgeon specializing in the treatment of hernias. Hospital physicians apparently controlled the admission of all new patients.

According to the rules, each of the four wards devoted to male patients had three "ordained" medical assistants (*hypourgoi embathmoi*), two "extra" medical assistants (*hypourgoi perissoi*), and two servants or *hyperetai*. Similar staffing occurred in the female wards. Eight additional individuals, including four *hypourgoi* and two *hyperetai*, were assigned to the ambulatory facility and the monastic infirmary. All seem to have been members of a particular guild and were required to undergo a course of basic education and training before passing an examination. As revealed by its complex administrative organization, the Pantocrator Xenon with its extensive and specialized staff was probably meant to be an imperial showcase.[54] Traditionally, however, the expectations of founders and patrons of hospitals—enshrined in detailed regulations—were rarely executed faithfully because of political upheavals, financial difficulties, administrative irregularities, or other problems.[55]

Apart from practical apprenticeships, there is no evidence of formal clinical lecturing before the charter of 1136. The institution's *typikon* stipulated that the hospital should hire a respected physician to instruct students in the basics of the healing art. This task was to be performed "conscientiously," suggesting that it may have been neglected earlier or given lower priority by physicians attending the hospital's patients. The individual entrusted with the teaching, however, held the highest rank in the Pantocrator's hierarchy, a development suggesting that the authorities clearly recognized the advantages of hospital settings for practical medical training. However, those in charge may have preferred a rather informal scheme, perhaps to protect inmates from unnecessary monitoring and experimentation.[56]

Theodoros Prodromos and life in the hospital

Constantinople's public *xenones* probably housed a great variety of sick individuals with a mixture of acute and chronic conditions. Nearby monasteries without infirmaries would send sick monks for treatment, but ill local city dwellers as well as traveling pilgrims must have constituted the bulk of the hospitals' admissions. Unfortunately, we only have very sketchy impressions from Prodromos' own hospital experiences, since his poems only focused on selective aspects of his medical treatment. One can assume, however, that after his arrival, the decision to admit him was left to the chief physician on call assigned to gatekeeping duties. All applicants were screened, and those found worthy of admission were issued a pass to enter. Since the Pantocrator and all Byzantine hospitals were still considered religious institutions, Prodromos first would have been subjected to the traditional admission ceremonial, including prayers and confession, and perhaps the traditional washing of feet also widely practiced in the West. Each newcomer was to be placed in a single bed. Given his febrile condition and noticeable skin eruption, Prodromos may have been taken to the separate ward for serious—mostly infectious—ailments. Here colder air circulated on the medical assumption that such an environment would prevent further debility.

Since medical practice at the Pantocrator *xenon* was essentially Hippocratic and Galenic, the first procedure of the attending physician must have consisted in interrogating, inspecting, and examining the new patient, as well as taking his pulse, actions designed to establish the state of the bodily system and the presumptive cause of the sickness. Diagnosis and prognosis were intimately connected, and uroscopy may have provided important clues.[57] These acts were traditionally followed by a regimen composed of diet, drugs, and surgery. To aid recovery, *xenones* as well as monastic infirmaries dispensed with the religiously sanctioned fasting periods, although avoidance of gluttony remained a concern, expressed in a number of regulations.[58]

Meals were usually served twice a day. A normal Byzantine diet was meatless and consisted of bread, vegetables, and wine. Bread was the staple food, combined with dried or fresh cooked vegetables dressed with olive oil. The most common liquid served was water, sweetened with wine to preserve the body's moisture and sustain its internal heat. A popular component of the regimen, wine helped restore the appetite of emaciated patients and imparted a good color to their skin. The expectation was that wine could help the stomach contract and thus promote its activity, especially good digestion.[59] Boiled honey was believed to be equally nutritious. Meat, poultry, and fish were very seldom served, except to convalescents, together with thick red wine mixed with honey or resins, given with the intention of building up the patient's blood.

In all acute diseases, barley water was freely offered, mixed with juice from the opium poppy if the patient had difficulty sleeping. Purgatives were generally unnecessary since the bowels were often loose. Since sick bodies were usually considered to be moist, pale, and fleshy, a general cooling and drying regimen was prescribed that included drinking grape and pomegranate juices. While feverish patients such as Prodromos were usually made to fast or kept on a liquid diet, those with some appetite would receive barley soup, sour buttermilk, and biscuits for sustenance.

All skin diseases, including smallpox, were viewed within the humoral framework. Physicians reasoned that a faulty fermentation or putrefaction of the blood caused its impurities to be projected toward the skin. Skin eruptions with their multiple pustules were interpreted as successful efforts to rid the body of decomposing humors. Smallpox and other skin rashes were explained as the effects of unripe blood that had failed to undergo the slow and necessary cooking process. Under such circumstances, patients had to be kept warm so that the pores of the skin would remain open and allow sweat to flow freely.

To accelerate skin eruptions, patients such as Prodromos were exposed to hot water vapor, then rubbed and wrapped in blankets or clothes to stimulate further sweating. Here administration of warm drinks with decoctions of figs and raisins was indicated. If the Byzantine physicians were aware of the Islamic experiences with smallpox, they would have provided the special care recommended for the eyes, nose, and throat by dropping rose water into the eyes and using cold water for periodic face washings. The frequent throat involvement could be ameliorated with pomegranate juice gargles to avoid suffocation. For hair loss, purging and friction with nut oils would have been employed.

Standard nursing procedures at that time, as earlier, not only included feeding the patients, administering oral medications, and applying salves and massages, but also bathing them twice a week and carrying out bloodletting. Performed by lancet or with cupping glasses by a special attendant, the *phlebotomoi*, bloodletting was still quite popular, especially in febrile conditions or when symptoms were quite violent. According to most medical authors, however, persons with reduced strength and no one under age 14 or over 70 should be bled.[60] Bleeding was usually achieved by lancing a full vein, preferably at the elbow and following digestion to ensure a full supplement of blood in the liver. Venesections were commonly carried out until the patient fainted. Before the ordeal, the bowels were cleansed with the help of an emollient clyster that, in the physicians' view, prevented intestinal veins from absorbing additional putrid fecal matter.

Medical theory explained skin eruptions or *exanthemata* as the result of thick, faulty humors now impacted in the skin's cuticle. Therefore, they all had to be removed, either through sweating or by the use of local drying agents, including fomentation and cataplasms made of bay leaves, frankincense in honey, and beet.[61] If the lesions were painful, poppy seed juice was sprinkled on them. In the event of smallpox, practitioners waited for the formation of pustules, considered the most critical stage of this disease. Patients covered with such pustules were placed in beds stuffed with rice meal to provide a soft surface. When these lesions gradually turned black, yellow, or green, a more malignant form of the disease carrying a poor prognosis was expected. If nature could not spontaneously rid the body of its morbific matter and death was expected, the medical art took over and practitioners attempted to extract fluid from large pustules by scarification and with the help of soaking rags.

Meanwhile, Prodromos' chest complaints, his difficulty breathing, and perhaps a cough became the target of another common but unpopular therapy: cauterization. In one of his poems, our author vividly described his experiences with this procedure. He compared himself to the three young men from a story in the Book of Daniel, who, thrown into a furnace, were spared from burning to death because they sang a hymn praising God as the supreme creator of all things. Prodromos tells us that "from the midst of another piercing iron oven, not a Chaldean one nor one from Babylon but one of Galen and Hippocrates," he observed a "trio of blazing irons." Instead of facing an evil arsonist, Prodromos encountered what he described as a "dear caretaker" (he who sets sickness in order) who was absolutely determined to apply these cautery irons to his body. Shoveling new heaps of coals to feed the flames around a frying pan, the physician's attendants were characterized by Prodromos as "insufferable flame-throwers, eager as a mob of holy executioners," who not only fanned the blaze but also undressed him from the waist up, as was the practice with condemned criminals.[62]

In Prodromos' time, surgical procedures were limited. Although steady advances had been recorded since Hellenistic times at Alexandria and no separation from medicine had taken place, surgery remained restricted to the care of trauma and the excision of polyps, tonsils, and bladder stones. However, employment of the cautery was common in many medical conditions. Possibly a folk remedy employed in basic wound healing to stop bleeding and prevent infection, the practice can be traced to ancient Egypt and pre-Islamic populations of the near East.[63] In fact, according to the Moslem author Albucasis, it was of "universal application" and "suitable at all times."[64] Rational medical theory categorized the cautery as being hot and dry, to be employed primarily in moist and cold conditions. Here again, the ultimate goal was the extraction of morbific poisons from the body's interior.

Pain and swelling were considered signs of local humoral excess and deterioration, with cauterization recommended since antiquity as one option for prompt drainage. The incandescent iron employed in such a procedure burned the skin to form a coin-sized, black ulcer usually not allowed to heal until the harmful humors were discharged and the presenting symptoms had been relieved. Medical indications for this form of treatment, especially chest conditions, also abounded. If the disease was diagnosed as "phthisis," the burns were made in the form of geometric patterns with one spot under the chin, another on the neck, and finally two on the front chest, as well as two below the shoulder blades.[65] That cautery treatments were popular is attested to by the *Miracula Sancti Artemii*, which depicted a deacon from the Hagia Sophia, Sergios, with a groin swelling being treated by a practitioner with the cautery iron in the Samson Xenon of Constantinople. Only 20 years earlier, the dying Emperor Alexios I had been subjected to a similar cauterization performed on his abdomen.

Prodromos later dramatically related his medical encounter: "On top of everything, the sweet, dear caretaker, the best among physicians and fairest at his craft, my penniless healer of illnesses, grinning and smiling at me, chuckling 'friend' as if applying a medication for my inner labors with sporting words, pleasing utterances."[66] Touching our patient, but not to reassure him, the doctor proceeded to make some measurements from the chest to the eye. Marking a middle spot on the skin with a reed, the practitioner placed the tip of one cauterizing iron on the skin surface, creating a local burn. The black, charred ulcers were not allowed to heal until the cough stopped or became productive and breathing appeared easier.

The effects of such an excruciatingly painful therapeutic session were vividly described by Prodromos: "Oh the misfortune then, oh the suffering then!" he commented. "This fire from the medical treatment has caused a conflagration in me, all the way to my belly and cold stomach, all the way to my bowels and veins, arteries and cartilage, all the way to my bones and marrow, all the way to my very heart and all the way through my entire inner constitution, and it has completely parched me and destroyed me by fire."[67] Restrained, probably by nursing assistants, he was returned to his hospital bed to recover. Pain was often believed to have invigorating qualities and to rally the body's healing forces. But "how," Prodromos wondered, "shall I withstand the piercing of this suffering, the magnitude of this misfortune, the weight of the pain?" In his poem, he moaned: "How I was burned to ashes from the fire! How I roasted on the coals! Backed through by the fire I was being sacrificed to God, not like a blameless lamb—for who am I and from where? But like a black ram cursed for my sin."[68]

We have no clear sense of how long Prodromos remained in the Pantocrator *xenon*. Upon his eventual discharge, he may have written again to some of his friends, sharing more of his impressions and feelings concerning the effects of his fever and the draconian medical treatments he endured, but no documentation exists. Early on in his illness, the poet already appeared to anticipate the disfiguring sequel. "When you see my face, [it will be] full of scars like the faces of blacksmiths who have been burnt by their fires, or like the skin sloughed by snakes or like Jacob's marked and mottled flock. My head [is] bald, without a single hair." In the end, however, no detailed letters or poem could do justice to Prodromos' sufferings. He anticipated telling his story in person, with all the self-pity he could muster, and probably venting his sarcasm about the bungling medical profession. The poet had already asked Stephanos Skylitzes, "When shall I come and see your face? When will I be able to tell you with my lips of this terrible illness? When will I mix with you a glass of tears and laughter?"[69] His pilgrimage to the Pantocrator was over. Whether he ever dared to show himself again to friends and mentors we do not know. Following his illness, Prodromos sought out a rest home affiliated with the St. Peter and St. Paul Church. He died there in 1156.

"OUR PATIENTS, OUR LORDS":
THE CARE OF PILGRIMS IN JERUSALEM

There are three acts in a man's life which no one should advise him either to do or not to do. The first is to contract matrimony, the second is to go to the wars, and the third is to visit the Holy Sepulcher. These things are all God in themselves, but they may turn out ill, in which case he who gave the advice will be blamed as if he were the cause of it.

Eberhard of Wurtemburg[70]

A pilgrimage to Jerusalem ca. 1172

About 30 years after Prodromos' experiences in Constantinople, Adolf of Cologne, a pilgrim companion of Theoderic (Dietrich) von Würzburg (ca. 1147–1224), and others arrived in Jerusalem around 1172. Together with thousands of their fellow Christians, the men were eager to celebrate Easter at the Holy Sepulcher. Presumably, Adolf and his friends had undertaken this journey by crossing the Alpine passes into Italy well before the winter, then heading toward Venice, a favorite port of departure for the *passum vernale* (spring voyage) to Palestine. Weeks later, after landing at Acre (Ptolemais), they proceeded to Jerusalem. Unfortunately, Theoderic, the German cleric from the Rhineland, announced in his *Description of the Holy Places* that by late March, just before Holy Week, Adolf died in Jerusalem. On Palm Sunday, he was laid to rest by his comrades in the field of Aceldama, located outside the city gates and a traditional burial ground for pilgrims.[71]

Nothing more is known about Adolf of Cologne. Perhaps he was one of the hundred knights who in 1166 had crossed the Alps to participate in the Italian campaigns of Cologne's archbishop, Reinald von Dassel, that had allowed Emperor Frederick I Barbarossa (ca. 1123–1190) to enter the Holy City and install his own pope, Pascal II, on the throne of Peter. Alternatively, Adolf and Theoderic may have belonged to a small group of clerical advisers attached to the imperial household. Provided with funds from their respective cathedral cities, these individuals were being groomed for a bishopric.[72] In any event, the companions must have viewed their pilgrimage to Jerusalem either as a penitential voyage to obtain peace of mind and absolution for sins or as a stepping stone to advance their ecclesiastical careers. The former was as likely as the latter. Since the 800s, pilgrimage had become an increasingly common form of atonement, a penance now increasingly imposed even during ordinary confessions. Although such voyages could be made by proxy if one provided the necessary funds, most penitents undertook the journey personally. Expensive and dangerous, travel could also be an exciting and liberating experience, a legitimate excuse to escape from one's parish, family relationships, and other burdensome responsibilities.

A century later, these journeys became even more attractive after the Church decreed that punishment to be suffered in purgatory could be transcended only by becoming a mendicant friar, retiring to a hermitage, or going on a pilgrimage. Pilgrims were even exempted from ordinances against begging. Thus, masses of Europeans sold their property and belongings, bade farewell to family and country, and trekked to Christian shrines in search of pardon, grace, and adventure. Christ and places that had witnessed the events of his life, especially his final suffering, death, and resurrection, were at the top of a hierarchy of holy locations to be visited by the faithful. Jerusalem thus unquestionably became the top destination for Christian pilgrims, the highest-ranking relic of them all.[73] By 1172 the city had around 30,000 permanent inhabitants, but it could experience a 10-fold increase from visitors during the Easter celebrations.

We can suppose that Adolf of Cologne and his clerical companions went aboard a large, oared galley ship owned by enterprising Venetian merchants, although a common trade route also led from Genoa or Pisa to Acre. With the Byzantine navy firmly in control of the seas, at least twice a year large fleets of ships headed across the Mediterranean to the Near East. Even before the First Crusade, maritime commerce between Greeks, Italians, and the Levant had been frequent. Although more expensive, sea voyages on galley ships were considerably safer than the smaller boats advertised by the Neapolitans and Sicilians. These vessels tended to overturn and sink during storms. Sporting warmer clothes, clutching Bibles, and perhaps carrying a barrel of wine for medicinal purposes, penitents embarked on risky journeys marked by boredom and seasickness. Both conditions were mitigated by drinking wine mixed with pepper, saffron, and other spices to settle the stomach.[74]

Voyages in overcrowded ships must have been particularly dangerous ordeals, as one Dominican priest, Felix Farber of Ulm, recounted upon his return to a Swabian convent. Focusing on the imperatives of human digestion, Farber painted a tragicomic picture of the unfortunate passengers lining up in the morning along the spit privies located on either side of the ship's prow. This was especially dangerous during bad weather, when the facilities were periodically inundated by waves. "The pilgrim," he wrote, "must be careful not to hold back on account of false modesty and not relieve the stomach, to do so is most harmful; at sea it is easy to become constipated. At sea, moreover, it is not safe to use pills or suppositories because to purge oneself too much can cause worse trouble than constipation."[75]

Perhaps Adolf, like many undertaking such a voyage, felt equally seasick. The food on board was generally sparse and spoiled, one reason alert travelers carried their own supplementary provisions of cheese, biscuits, and fruit syrups, further sources of constipation. Lying below deck on lice-infested mats helped travelers to endure the frequent nausea, but here they were often visited by the ship's ubiquitous rats. On deck, the pilgrims were assaulted by fiery, unsolicited sermons delivered by idle clerics or forced to join in communal singing. In the meantime, antsy brethren eager to keep in shape and dissipate some of their excess energy kept running around the decks, jumping over the ropes, or lifting weights.[76]

The long-anticipated landing in the harbor of Acre always created some additional anxieties due to its difficult access under windy conditions. Not surprisingly, Theoderic tells us that there were already around 80 ships at anchor there when his ship entered the harbor, a reflection of the enormous popularity enjoyed by the yearly Easter Week pilgrimage.[77] New arrivals were eagerly welcomed by swarms of local vendors, who considered them essential for the economy of Palestine. Chroniclers had already warned about the dangers of unclean water and raw fruits. For personal safety, women, many of them widows, joined some of the existing groups. Walking past stately houses built by the popular Templar and Hospitaller Knights, pilgrims such as Theoderic and Adolf must have suppressed their lingering distress—some even carried wooden crosses over their shoulders—to press forward to their long-awaited destination: Jerusalem.

Due to changes in climate, diet, and the vicissitudes of the sea or overland voyage, many pilgrims became debilitated and malnourished. Multiple sores often covered the feet of overland travelers, part of the desired mortification of the flesh associated with a penitential journey. A large grove of palm trees near the Mediterranean shore provided leaves traditionally carried by pilgrims or "palmers." Bathing in the Jordan River at Jericho, by tradition a "second baptism," was recommended as a purification ceremony to cleanse one's sins, as well as to improve the condition of lepers.[78]

Often brought back from Jerusalem to Western Europe, a palm leaf from Jericho became the symbol of an expected moral rebirth, the formal sign that a pilgrim's vows had been fulfilled. As they hobbled on, observing the coastal plain with its many deserted cities and castles destroyed by Romans and Turks, the pilgrims' anticipation grew. At last, they caught sight of the Holy City. At a village named Mahumeria, a great cross of stone stood on a lofty platform. According to Theoderic, many set down their own crosses, took off their shoes, and ascended the steps to see the tower of David on Mount Zion, as well as the outlines of the walled city. Finally, this alien, exciting world stood before their eyes, and besides the prospect of their pious visits, many a pilgrim like Adolf looked forward to the adventures and dangers lurking in the miraculous city. All were keen to shop, ready to haggle with Arab traders and purchase trinkets, exotic spices, jewelry, and silk at stalls surrounding the church of the Holy Sepulcher.[79]

Near the western entrance to Jerusalem stood the Tower of David, and as our pilgrims walked eagerly toward the Holy Sepulcher, they could not help but admire the large complex across the street occupied by the hospital of the Knights of St. John the Baptist, an internationally famous hostel.[80] The complex was located to the south of the church of the Holy Sepulcher, occupying the western part of an area now known as the Muristan, site of a ruined Byzantine monastery. The initial convent had been built atop the old structure, with a hospice for the poor and the pilgrims located immediately to the north. Initially, this hospital had been just another monastic infirmary like the one at St. Gall, with a number of heated rooms, a kitchen, and an adjoining garden or lawn for the recreation of the sick. Its eventual expansion created an imposing building 230 feet long and 120 feet wide, with 18-foot arches and even higher ceilings, a structure admired by many visitors for its great beauty.[81]

A contemporary description by John of Würzburg, a German priest and pilgrim, confirms this impression: "Next to the Church of the Holy Sepulcher, on the opposite side towards the south, is a beautiful church erected in honor of St. John the Baptist," he wrote. "The hospital is next to it, in which in various houses a great crowd of sick people is collected, some of them men and some women. They are cared for and every day fed at vast expense. When I was present, I learned from the servants that their whole number amounted to two thousand. Between night and day there were sometimes more than fifty corpses carried out, but again and again there were new people admitted."[82]

This German visitor also tells us that although the hospital's average capacity may have been smaller, its cloistered courtyards and small gardens between the buildings became enormously overcrowded with pilgrims on special occasions such as Easter. The establishment was equipped with baths, rooms for bloodletting and shaving, and several kitchens, and was even provided with animal pens. Wrote John of Würzburg: "The house feeds so many individuals outside and within, and it gives so huge an amount of alms to poor people, either those who come to the door, or those who remain outside, that certainly the total expenses can in no way be counted, even by the managers and dispensers of this house."[83] We do not know whether Adolf's party merely walked through the hospital or brought him there for admission, but Theoderic in his book observed that "going through the palace we could in no way judge the number of people who lay there, but we saw a thousand beds. No king nor tyrant would be powerful enough to maintain daily the great number fed in this house."[84]

Jerusalem and the Hospital of St. John: Mission and patronage

To understand the role of this institution in the life of countless Christian pilgrims, we must briefly look back at the evolution of Jerusalem as Christendom's most sacred destination. Before the first century, the city already had a tradition of sponsoring Jewish hospices, and that tradition was eventually taken on by Christians to house and serve their own pilgrims who began flocking to Jerusalem, especially after the legalization of Christianity within the Roman Empire. In the centuries that followed, Jerusalem became an important destination point for travelers who visited the various holy places, reading aloud passages from the Scriptures in their respective locations. This reenactment of the dramatic events in the life of Christ—*imitatio Christi*—eventually became the ceremonial of the stations of the cross, with special status accorded to religious services during Holy Week. It was a truly mystical experience to be at the very site of the Lord's final sufferings and to visit the empty tomb, the visible testimony of His resurrection.[85]

After the year 529, Peter (524–544), the patriarch of Jerusalem, requested funds from Justinian to have "a hospital constructed for the care of the sick from abroad." Whether such aid was forthcoming, Pope Gregory I in 603 seems to have founded a hospice in Jerusalem south of the Holy Sepulcher to provide for poor and sick pilgrims. However, in 638, Jerusalem fell into Arab hands, with Caliph Omar entering the city and visiting the Christian shrines. The resident patriarch, Sophronius, was allowed to retire with his Christian officials and their families to Caesarea. The fall of Jerusalem and the subsequent conquest of all the coastlands of North Africa by the year 700 profoundly shocked all Christian countries. Still, the ruling caliphate of the Ommayad dynasty, with its capital in Damascus, accepted religious minorities, ensured freedom of worship, and encouraged a tolerant attitude toward the vanquished. From the beginning, their rulers employed Christians in their administrations and construction projects, as well as in teaching the sciences and arts. Meanwhile, many of the inhabitants of Palestine either converted to Islam or remained Christian. In Jerusalem, orthodox Christians continued to outnumber Moslems in an atmosphere of prosperity and tranquility. For more than 200 years, access to the city of Jerusalem was made easier by the good will of the Moslem rulers.[86]

Under the patronage of Charlemagne (747–814), a church dedicated to Mary, the Mother of God, was established near the Holy Sepulcher, to be administered by Benedictine monks who had moved from their original monastery on the Mount of Olives. The conversion to Christianity of the duke of Hungary in 985 following Basil II's overthrow of the Bulgarian Empire in 976 and the conquest of Antioch by the Byzantine emperor created an overland route to Jerusalem. Although cheaper and safer than a sea voyage, the new course was slower and had its own hazards, including bad trails, poor weather, ruthless innkeepers, tolls, and roadside bandits. However, some pilgrims could count on hospitable treatment from Byzantine peasants, and many took advantage of shelters along the European route as well as in Constantinople, where the Samson Xenon was reserved for the use of Western pilgrims.

The initial trickle of pilgrims became a raging flood after the tenth century as belief spread in the West that pilgrimage possessed a definite spiritual value and that visitors to the shrines would be granted special indulgences. Protected by armed escorts, travelers to particular places such as the Holy Sepulcher received an automatic remission of all their sins, but they were not normally permitted to touch the relics.[87] However, some of the penitents collected soil from the Holy Land, checking for Christ's own footprints. The destruction of the Holy Sepulcher in 1009 by Caliph Hakim came as a shocking but temporary setback for those planning a voyage to Jerusalem. In 1027, the Byzantine emperor signed another treaty with members of the Fatimid caliphate allowing mass pilgrimages to the Holy City before the year 1033, a date believed to represent not only the first thousand years since Christ's death but also the end of the world. Eventually, the treaty between Byzantium and the caliphs was renewed in 1036, restoring to the Christians all their property and privileges. With permission from the Fatimid authorities, work on the restoration of the Holy Sepulcher proceeded during the 1040s, financed by tolls extracted from pilgrims. At the same time, Palestinian trade began once more to prosper, especially with Christian countries across the Mediterranean Sea. In the year 1048, the Fatimid Caliph al-Mustansir granted permission for a group of merchants from Amalfi to restore a small church and convent, Santa Maria, located south of Jerusalem's Holy Sepulcher. Another daughter convent devoted to Santa Magdalena, later known as St. Mary the Great, was erected to shelter female travelers.

Another setback occurred in 1071, when Jerusalem was overrun by Turkish invaders who occupied all of Palestine. Many pilgrims, however, managed to escape and return to Europe. Five years later the Fatimids recaptured the city, but roads were infested with bandits and local lords extracted further tolls, thus reducing the pilgrim flow from the West. Finally, in 1099, Godfrey of Bouillon led the First Crusade into Jerusalem, killing most of the remaining Moslem and Jewish population. Based on the Holy War Council of Clermont in 1095, the crusade had been defined as another pilgrimage, a key vehicle for individual salvation. The concept that God had invented the crusade as a new way for knights and the masses to atone for their sins spoke eloquently to the same ideology motivating pilgrims and hermits, who could now receive a measure of salvation in exchange for their oath to fulfill the goal of liberating the Holy Land from infidels.[88]

During the eleventh century, the steady increase in European pilgrims and merchants and their plight in an alien land had prompted the Amalfian sponsors of the St. Mary of the Latins monastery to also build and administer a hospice dedicated to St. John the Baptist. This institution, presumably founded around the year 1080 and staffed by Benedictine monks, was to be reserved for "Latins, Italians, and Lombards," according to a later papal bull. Working under the direction of the abbot of St. Mary's, Brother Gerard—probably an Amalfian layman—was appointed administrator. Like similar monastic hostels in Europe, its mission was to provide shelter and security for local and traveling Christians. The brothers servicing this *xenodochium* or *nosocomium*, modeled after other Syrian guesthouses, called themselves "the poor brethren of the Hospital of St. John."[89] They pledged to help the poor and receive needy pilgrims with the aid of alms collected from Amalfian merchants.[90]

Before the triumphal entry into Jerusalem of the forces of the First Crusade, Brother Gerard was accused by the Turkish rulers of Palestine of hoarding money as well as helping the crusaders. Although arrested and tortured by Jerusalem's Islamic defenders, Gerard was saved by the prompt arrival of the Europeans, and he quickly took advantage of his position by persuading the new Frankish rulers to contribute to the endowment of his institution. Indeed, Godfrey of Bouillon granted some landed estates and city properties to Gerard and his brotherhood, thus allowing for a substantial expansion of charitable operations at the hostel. Among those selected for care at the hospice were knights and soldiers wounded in the siege of the city. These activities mirrored contemporary Christian hospitality and charity prevalent in all of Europe and Byzantium.[91]

In 1100, Baldwin of Lorraine succeeded his brother Raymond as Defender of the Holy Sepulcher but also assumed the title of King Baldwin I of Jerusalem. After his victory over the Egyptians a year later, Baldwin I presented a tenth of his spoils to the hospital. With the Holy Sepulcher safely in Christian hands and both pilgrimages and European colonization of the Holy Land unimpeded,[92] the hospital was well positioned to compete for additional donations. Through word from the numerous pilgrims who had received aid there, its fame quickly spread to

Western Europe. In fact, Gerard and his hospice received a foundation charter from Pope Paschal II issued on February 15, 1113, in a bull creating the new St. John Order of the Hospital and placing the institution under papal protection. It also allowed the Hospitaller brothers to elect their own master and stipulated that all property and income provided to the establishment would be used for the benefit of pilgrims and the poor. The bull also confirmed the extensive properties already donated to the hospital in Jerusalem and Western Europe and subordinated the European estates to the master in perpetuity. At the same time, the patriarch of Jerusalem exempted the institution from the payment of tithes.[93] The growing fame of the institution and papal protection even motivated some of the crusaders to organize hospital service in various locations in Europe.

Following Gerard's death in 1120, the Hospitallers elected Raymond du Puy as his successor. Whereas Gerard's institutional rules may have been Benedictine in origin and geared toward an independent monastic community in a city governed by Moslems, the new political and social circumstances created by the First Crusade demanded a total reconstruction of the hospital's mission. Foremost among the reforms was an official shift in attitude toward the sick admitted to the hospital. While traditionally all monastic hostels had stressed the dignity of any fellow Christian, article 16 of Raymond du Puy's new statutes written during the 1150s went further: subordination of the staff to the wishes of the sick. Entitled "How Our Lords the Sick Should Be Received and Served," the rule stated that "in that obedience in which the master and the chapter of the hospital shall permit an hospital to exist when the sick man shall come there, let him be received thus: let him partake of the Holy Sacrament, first having confessed his sins to the priest, and afterwards let him be carried to bed, and there as if he were a Lord."[94]

This characterization of the sick as masters of their aristocratic caregivers was unprecedented but largely symbolic, turning the traditional healing relationship on its head. Reflecting contemporary rules of feudalism and chivalry, inmates of this hospice, rich or poor, nominally acquired the enhanced social identity of Frankish knights. Under such a system, the caregiving Hospitallers—nominally their vassals—were ethically bound to provide faithful service regardless of the risk and expense. In part, this distinction reflected perhaps the needs and special character of the international population living in and visiting Jerusalem. Indeed, a mixture of sick poor and wealthy pilgrims, sick and wounded knights, and affluent traveling merchants made up the Hospital of St. John of Jerusalem's population.[95] As a model for both charitable service and unconditional devotion to the sick, du Puy's decree became a milestone in the development of the hospital.[96]

Not surprisingly, the new stream of pilgrims to the Latin Kingdom of Jerusalem and their testimonials concerning the charity of the Hospitallers of St. John spread rapidly throughout Europe, including England. The existence of a religious order that strongly expressed its fealty to the sick inspired the creation of a network of similar institutions, especially at ports of embarkation in Italy and southern France where pilgrims assembled. At the same time, grateful ex-inmates, charitable nobles, and royals from one end of Europe to the other provided substantial land donations. In 1131, King Alfonso of Aragon bequeathed one-third of his realm to the Hospitallers, and they, in turn, negotiated with representatives of the king of Navarre. By 1141 the order was empowered to receive portions of the customs and duties levied in that kingdom after their recovery from the Moorish wars. Indeed, the hospital's endowment was so greatly enriched by donations of land and manors, both in Palestine and in Europe, that the Order of the Hospitallers became one of the most powerful political and economic forces in the medieval world.[97]

By 1154, and in acknowledgment of the Hospitallers' role in preserving the kingdom of Jerusalem for Christianity, Pope Anastasius I granted further privileges to the order and placed the mother house hospital in Jerusalem under his personal protection. Hospitallers were now also exempt from the Church's tithe. They were also allowed to build their own churches in their domains, hold religious services, and organize the burial of their members, thus operating entirely outside regular ecclesiastical jurisdiction. In addition, they also received protection for their alms collectors and the right to award indulgences not only to their brethren, but also to the tenants, serfs, and servants living on their estates and in other hospices located in the Latin Kingdom.[98] Even hospital patients received such privileges. This drastic move, however, was opposed by the Palestinian bishops and led to a rift between the kingdom's church and the Hospitallers. In response, the latter defended their newly acquired authority and renewed their vow to care for the pilgrims and the poor.[99]

The issue of social control—in this case, the protection of Christian pilgrims while in the Holy Land—was inextricably linked to the Hospitallers' mission. Under the leadership of Raymond du Puy, a strong leader and deft politician, the Knights thrived. Acquisition of estates and a building program of fortresses and castles in Palestine only reinforced their political prominence. Always eager to defend the interests of his order at the very heart of Christian rule, Raymond spent considerable time away from Jerusalem consulting with the pope in Rome. In the meantime, he ruthlessly exploited the existing Hospitallers' privileges. Inevitably, Christian charity and hospital care came to be neglected as political intrigue, military operations, and the complex administration of the vast hospital endowment took precedence, a phenomenon not uncommon elsewhere in Europe at this time. Shortly after the ill-fated pilgrimage of Adolf of Cologne, further concerns about the Hospitallers' growing power were voiced at the Third Lateran Council of 1179, presided over by Pope Alexander III. Some Eastern bishops charged that the order had abused its privileges and failed to follow its vows.

In spite of its international reputation, however, the Hospital of St. John failed to monopolize the care of pilgrims. In response to complaints from German pilgrims about their difficulties in the new French-speaking kingdom of Jerusalem, a German couple established a small shelter in their Jerusalem house during the 1130s. Encouraged by Jerusalem's patriarch, an oratorium devoted to the Virgin Mary was added and the institution placed under her protection. The new hostel was quite successful, and its fame attracted poor and noble German pilgrims alike. By about 1143, some of the Teutonic knights established a separate brotherhood under Augustinian rules: the Brothers of the St. Mariae Alemannorum Hospital. However, this development was not viewed kindly by the existing Hospitallers, who felt that this foundation undermined their own efforts. To avoid dissension, the pope placed the new brotherhood under the supervision of the Hospitallers in exchange for providing the hospice with experienced nursing personnel. A papal bull of Innocent III in 1199 officially sanctioned the statutes of a German Order of Hospital Knights, the *Deutsche Orden*.[100] On this occasion, the pope praised the fact that, in harmony with regulations approved by the Hospitallers, the statutes of this fledgling Teutonic knighthood also focused on care for the sick poor.[101]

Feudal loyalty: Caring for "Our Lords the Sick"

Raymond du Puy's hospital regulations resembled Augustinian monastic regulations. They were much more suitable than Benedict's rules for a congregation having multiple contacts with the outside world, especially Palestine's larger populations of pilgrims and warriors. These changes reflected similar shifts already occurring in Europe during the late eleventh century. Within the new framework, the Hospitallers were to be an order of clerics and lay brothers primarily devoted to the care of indigent travelers and the sick. Like other monasteries in Europe and Byzantium run by an approved brotherhood, the institution was usually headed by an abbot, prior, or headmaster. This elected individual, in turn, appointed administrators or "commanders" in charge of various institutional operations. By 1182, new hospital statutes enacted by Raymond's successor, Roger des Moulins (1177–1187), prescribed that "the Commanders of the houses should serve the sick cheerfully, and should do their duty by them, and serve them without grumbling or complaining, so that by these good deeds they may deserve to have their reward in the glories of heaven."[102] In addition to the new social status accorded to inmates, the rules also reflected a definite European influence in their involvement of knights and other lay personnel in the service of the sick.

Another fateful decision made during Raymond du Puy's tenure as master gave the Hospitallers an additional military role. At first glance, hospital work and military service would seem to be quite dissimilar. However, these new extramural duties can also be interpreted as an extension of the Hospitallers' institutional protection and caring for pilgrims and soldiers. After all, earlier pilgrimages to the Holy Land had been launched with heavily armed escorts that engaged in battle with hordes of bandits. With the prevailing use of military metaphors, Pope Eugenius III observed in 1152 that the Hospitallers were "fighting in the service of the poor" and that this stance could certainly be extended to protect Christians from the onslaught of the Moslem invaders. The involvement with military affairs possibly began as early as the 1130s. Thirty years later, John of Würzburg commented that the order of St. John "maintains in its various castles many persons trained to all kinds of military exercises for the defense of the land of the Christians against the invasions of the Saracens."[103] By 1181, Roger des Moulins' new hospital statutes insisted that fighting was just another charitable activity. In the beginning, however, the only division among Hospitallers was between clerical and lay brethren, and the military obligation seems to have been fulfilled by hiring mercenaries.[104]

Another possible reason for Raymond du Puy's decision to militarize the Hospitallers was the emergence of a new military order in 1128. Established by King Baldwin I with the support of Popes Honorius II and Eugenius III, this militia was devoted to defense of the Holy Land and protection of traveling pilgrims.[105] Further participation of the Hospitallers—depicted as charitable tasks—was observed during the battles at the northern frontier in 1144 and the siege of Ascalon in 1153. Raymond du Puy's involvement of the Hospitallers in these enterprises reflects the emergence of a new ideal of Christian knighthood during the Crusades, cast in a heroic and moral role of fighting in the service of God. This involvement would also bring considerable administrative turmoil and debt to the Order.[106]

As brethren-in-arms, most Hospitallers identified themselves as "soldiers of Jesus Christ" subject to the king of Jerusalem. Their organization now codified an aristocratic form of government with three levels of membership. First-class members or knights belonged to the young European gentry. They pledged to defend the faith and administer the vast estates willed by grateful patients and admiring rulers. The second class was composed of clergymen and brothers entirely devoted to spiritual matters and the physical care of the sick. Both groups wore black robes adorned with the eight-pointed white cross on the chest. At first, military missions appeared to be limited. An internal struggle among the Knights suggests that one faction opposed this extension of duties from their traditional role of protectors and guards. Indeed, on the 20-mile trip from Jerusalem to the Jordan River, our pilgrims, including Adolf of Cologne and Theoderic von Würzburg, had been escorted by a contingent of Hospitallers providing security from marauding Saracens, an intermittent threat in the area even though the territory adjacent to Jerusalem was in Christian hands.[107]

The Augustinian *regula* promoted by Raymond demanded that the hospital staff—including the knights—be bound by the three customary monastic vows of chastity, obedience, and poverty. After the fall of Jerusalem, a new sisterhood came to work at the hospital to care for female patients. Also following Augustinian rules, the Sisters of the Order of St. John of Jerusalem were housed at the St. Mary Magdalene convent and wore red habits with the white eight-pointed cross. Third-class members of the Hospitallers consisted of serving lay brothers and sisters who carried out the necessary menial hospital tasks of cooking, washing, and cleaning.[108]

From the start, Brother Gerard had decreed that physicians could be provided for the sick brethren. Later, Raymond's rules also favored the addition of physicians to the staff. Raymond's rule was confirmed by a bull of Pope Eugenius III in the early 1150s and later by Anastasius IV. The documents confirmed the full-time employment of four lay *medici* (physicians) and four *chirurgici* (surgeons). The practitioners had to live on the premises and take an oath of allegiance to their feudal superiors, the Hospitallers, although they had a higher status than brothers and were allowed to dine at the knights' table. Additionally, des Moulins' rules called for "physicians who have the care of the sick and who make syrups for the sick," a reference to pharmaceutical compounding. These statutes indicated an even greater degree of medicalization than had previously existed, reflected in the rule that "firstly the Holy House of the Hospital is accustomed to receive sick men and women."[109] The institution thus officially shifted its admission priorities from simply housing needy pilgrims to solely selecting those who were clearly sick. The approval of Rogers' statutes by Pope Lucius that same year ratified the greater role of medical care in the institution: "it is decreed with the assent of the brethren that for the sick in the Hospital of Jerusalem there should be engaged four wise doctors who are qualified to examine urine and to diagnose different diseases and are able to administer appropriate medicines."[110]

Unquestionably, the statutes of the Hospitallers reflected a trend toward more professional medical treatment, which can also be observed in contemporary Byzantine *xenones* and Islamic *bimaristans*.[111] These regulations reflected the continued availability of medical knowledge and personnel in Palestine and Syria. Whether under Byzantine or Moslem rule, Antioch, Tripoli, and Jerusalem remained centers of Greek learning, including medicine. It can be argued that one of the reasons for the medicalization of the Hospital of St. John during the 12th century was the presence of both Christian and Moslem physicians, who were officially licensed by local bishops after the conquest of the Holy Land based on the traditional Arab *muchtasip* system employed in the certification and regulation of local craftsmen, including surgeons, oculists, and scarifiers. St. John's also owed much to earlier Islamic hospitals that had flourished in the Near East since the eighth century.[112] By contrast, Frankish healers were rare.

As noted, the Hospital of St. John of Jerusalem was initially devoted to needy Christian pilgrims, but Jews and Moslems could also be accepted.[113] As in other Christian institutions, the admission ritual simulated an act of induction into a new brotherhood of hospice inmates with a significant addition: crossing the institutional boundary now symbolized an important change in social position. We could thus imagine the arrival of Adolf of Cologne accompanied by his fellow pilgrims, perhaps already spiritually cleansed in the Jordan River but becoming progressively ill and incapable of further travel. After confession and reception of Holy Communion, Adolf, like others, would have been escorted to a bed. Because of his social status and illness, he may have been assigned to a single bed in a separate section of the institution devoted to the care of sick knights. Most other beds accommodated two or three individuals. The rules demanded that "the beds of the sick should be made as long and as broad as is most convenient for repose, and that each bed should be covered with its own coverlet and each bed should have its own special sheets."[114] Since new arrivals usually surrendered their own clothing—it was cleaned and mended, to be returned at the time of discharge—they slept naked. However, regulations requested that each sick person "should have a cloak of sheepskin, caps of wool and boots for going to and coming from the latrines."[115]

Beds were meant primarily for rest, one of the key components for restoring health. Sick knights were allowed to remain in their beds or chambers for three days, a disposition copied from traditional monastic rules for sick monks who remained in their separate cells. For their confinement, some soldiers actually brought their own bed and armor to the hospital. Pregnant pilgrims seeking shelter for their deliveries could expect "little cradles for the babies born in the House, so that they may lay separate and that the baby in its own bed may not be in danger from the restlessness of its mother."[116] Many unwed mothers were married in the hospital; others simply abandoned their offspring in the wards, to be cared for by the nursing brothers and sisters.

As in similar institutions of this size, care of the patients' physical and spiritual needs was labor intensive. Benedictine rules emphasized the spiritual welfare of the feeble and sick, with masses and communion celebrated early each morning before a candle-lit altar by the prior dressed in colorful vestments. Frequent prayers during the day, especially Our Fathers and Hail Marys, were part of the routine. At the end of the day, the last religious act was another set of prayers and then each inmate was sprinkled with holy water. "You, Our Lords the Sick!," demanded the Hospitaller on call, "pray for yourselves and for all Christians who are ill in the world, that Our Lord will give them health. Our Lords the Sick!, pray for all members of the hospital fraternity and all other members as well as all men and Christian women who provide charity in the holy house of the hospital, so that the Lord will give them a good death."[117]

The growing status of the Hospitaller order, with some aristocratic members perhaps participating in personal caring activities, gave nursing considerable prestige, although knights were not involved in routine chores. For this purpose, the 1181 regulations demanded that "in every ward and place of the hospital nine servants should be kept at their [patients'] service, who should wash their feet gently and change their sheets, and make their beds, and administer to the weak necessary and strengthening food, and do their duty devotedly and obey in all things for the sick."[118] A female staff washed clothes and bed linens.

Another important therapeutic tool was diet. The two main meals were usually served at 11 AM and 6 PM. Those too weak and sick to get up were fed by aides, while ambulatory patients joined the communal table. All patients had to be fed before the caring personnel could eat, another gesture of humility and subservience. Raymond's eighth rule dictated that "the sick and feeble are exempted from the common dietary rules,"[119] an important directive that freed them from the usual fasting routines prevailing in all monastic institutions. This would have been especially important for patients such as Adolf of Cologne, hospitalized toward the end of the Lenten season, when the official directive proscribed all meat on Wednesdays and Saturdays.[120]

Surgery was mostly restricted to wound-healing measures, with special attention paid to the sores and infections pilgrims had developed on their feet and legs during their journeys.[121] As in other contemporary institutions, bloodletting remained a universal remedy and preventive for all inflammatory diseases, notably fevers.[122] Like other monks, the Hospitallers may have also demanded to be bled as a health preservative at special times of the year, including April, May, and September, to purify their bodies and improve their appetites and sleep.[123] The hospital may also have provided a number of traditional drugs based on the teachings and practices of local Christian and Moslem physicians. Syrups and electuaries containing a number of medicinal herbs were basic therapeutic agents. In fact, Roger des Moulin's regulations of 1181 stipulated the shipment of 200 pounds of sugar from Tripolis for compounding them. Use of the *Regimen Sanitatis Salernitarum*, an anonymous twelfth-century compendium in verse based on practices at the school of Salerno, gave additional popular guidance for those familiar with European healing strategies.

In the wards, physicians usually scheduled two daily visits—morning and evening—always accompanied by a black-robed knight-*infirmarian* with the white starlike cross on his chest and back.[124] The sick not only received medical visits, but the *infirmarian* was also obliged to check them twice each night. Rest and nourishment in this institution during the Lenten season and participation in its routine ceremonies, with their formality and pomp, could only have strengthened patients' faith in the redemptive quality of their sufferings. To the extent possible, spiritual purity was supplemented by physical cleanliness. Bathing, usually in wooden vats filled with warm water, also came under the Augustinian and Benedictine rules and was therefore reserved for the sick, thus forestalling any bathing for pleasure. Although anguish and hope may have alternated, the exhausted and sick pilgrims would have appreciated this attention after their travel ordeals. With their sores healed and their bodies fortified, many were discharged to face the long return voyage. For those like Adolf who would not recover, preparations were made to surround them with caregivers and friends and thus ease their final dying moments.

Instead of being resigned to their fate, some patients must have continued to have great confidence in the possibility of miraculous cures. Suggestion and faith probably were powerful tools in creating an atmosphere of optimism. The proximity of the Holy Sepulcher—indeed, the entire religious atmosphere in Jerusalem—had a profound impact on the sick. Pregnant with religious meanings, the Hospital of St. John was located literally, at the center of the Christian world.

At St. John's, the sick temporarily entered a structured environment of rituals—a journey within their pilgrimage—and if recovery was not possible, they could expect a good death and burial in consecrated soil.[125] In the end, we can presume that Adolf of Cologne succumbed to his ailment while at the hospital following a vigil organized by its caregivers. As for all Christians, Adolf's last wish had been granted. In imitation of Christ, dying in Jerusalem was one of the highest blessings to be bestowed on a believer, the perfect fulfillment of Adolf's pilgrimage and spiritual rebirth. Institutional rituals had structured this passage to eternal life and eventual resurrection. Burial at Aceldama—a field in the valley of Ennon, south of the western city gate—had the advantage of keeping his remains in close proximity to the site already selected for Christ's Last Judgment. Here, according to Theoderic, "simple-minded" pilgrims were already busy erecting vantage points from which to witness the long-awaited proceedings.[126]

St. John's Hospital: Model for the world

In 1187 Saladin recaptured Jerusalem, ending 88 years of Christian rule. He allowed the Hospitallers to leave a small number of their order behind to care for their wounded until they were able to travel under escort to Tripolis. Saladin enlarged the physical plant of the hospital, now named after its new patron, al-Salihani, and appointed a new staff of Moslem physicians. The complex also housed a new teaching center for Islamic religion. Unfortunately, the building was destroyed by an earthquake in 1458.[127] The Hospitallers, in turn, established a new hospital in Acre after its recapture in 1191 by Richard the Lion-Hearted during the Third Crusade.[128] For the time being, lands and manors located in Tripolis, Antioch, and the kingdom of Armenia remained in Hospitallers' hands. Then, after the fall of Acre to the Moslems in 1291, the Hospitallers retreated to Cyprus, where another hospital had already been founded in 1220 near Limassol. In 1306 they captured the island of Rhodes, then under Byzantine sovereignty, and placed it under the command of the Grand Master Foulques de Villaret. An extensive construction program of fortifications began, funded with resources from both the Hospitallers and the former Knight Templars, an order abolished after the loss of the Holy Land.[129]

Since there was no strong tradition in the West for the support of charitable shelters, the Hospitallers, with their new quasi-religious order, were able to encourage European rulers and noblemen to sponsor more establishments for the poor and sick. Emperor Frederick I Barbarossa praised St. John's for its extraordinary works of mercy.[130] The Church strongly encouraged such efforts, and even Pope Celestine III (1191–1198) linked the original hospital in Jerusalem with Christ's own good works, arguing that it was a miraculous gift for all mankind. From the twelfth century on, the St. John's model inspired the creation of similar institutions throughout Europe. They ranged from small shelters housing a handful of persons in villages or on roads to medium-sized establishments in cathedral cities with a capacity for 25–50 individuals. Even larger hospitals housing 75–150 inmates were located in key urban centers.[131] Along the Rhone River alone, one of the main European routes taken by pilgrims to the Mediterranean, the Hospitallers by the thirteenth century were sponsoring about 20 hospices and leper houses. Capable of caring for several thousand people, these houses near Arles were but one example of the early influence exerted by this knighthood in various European regions.[132]

Survival of such hospitals, however, depended on sustained local support and sponsorship, especially after the appearance of the Black Death. Patronage and involvement of private individuals and small groups was essential. Inspired by the example of the Hospitallers, other lay guilds or confraternities founded similar hospices for the benefit of their members. For example, the Order of the Holy Spirit, a group without military obligations founded by Guido of Montpellier, was approved and placed under papal protection by Innocent III (1198–1208) in April 1198. It promoted the same concept of service to the needy espoused by the Hospitallers. Members were exempted from episcopal jurisdiction and taxes. The same congregation helped found the Roman Ospedale di Santo Spirito in Sassia around 1204. In time, however, the various orders experienced the same financial abuses that affected all other charitable European institutions. Bitter disputes arose concerning opposing claims from two Holy Spirit mother houses—Montpellier and Rome—regarding the collection of tributes from affiliated institutions.[133]

In the ensuing two centuries, the model of organization and service provided by the Knights of St. John changed significantly as a result of critical shifts in political, economic, and social power. Beginning in the thirteenth century, rapid population expansion and urbanization together with fundamental economic changes enhanced the importance of hospitals in society and dramatically expanded the range of its patrons. A new cast of lay sponsors, including kings, hospital orders, confraternities, private individuals, and finally municipalities, began a fundamental shift of the hospital's social mission based on new ideologies and the realities of urban life, including transformations in the European causes of disease.

The transition from feudal to burger life was associated with widespread poverty and periodic famines that weakened people's resistance to disease.[134] Diets devoid of vegetables and fresh fruits prompted the appearance of land scurvy during winters. Spoiled grain was responsible for ergotism, the feared St. Anthony's fire. Urbanization, with its higher population density and lack of sanitation, facilitated contagion. In turn, massive migrations and religious pilgrimages imported scourges such as smallpox, influenza, and plague from distant disease pools into the heart of Europe, and others, including leprosy, appeared to increase in frequency. Finally, the discovery and use of firearms after the 1330s became a new source of warfare-linked trauma that would require radically novel surgical approaches.

A new condition, involuntary pauperism, appeared, forcing a reevaluation of charitable giving and its consequences. While the Church had previously coped with voluntary poverty, such as that displayed by hermits, wanderers, pilgrims, students, and apprentices, its welfare instruments were soon overpowered as the ranks of the structurally poor—incapable of earning a living by reason of age, illness, and physical or mental disability—swelled dramatically. Those in need included unskilled laborers—the crisis poor—and often the occasional poor—nearly half of the rural and urban workforce—subject to agricultural failures, military incursions, and epidemics. The increasing presence of idle beggars and vagrants in the urban landscape generated apprehension and eventually fear among established residents.[135]

Royalty increasingly sought to assist or even replace the Church as the premier sponsor of hospitals. Alone or in partnership with religious organizations, wealthy individuals—aristocrats and merchants—founded new hospitals and composed their own statutes. Moreover, an ever-expanding sector of urban middle-class dwellers, generated by the new commercialism, took their place alongside traditional sources of hospital patronage. Many institutions were organized as confraternities, originally groups of lay people linked to monasteries by prayers and privileges but now reorganized as urban associations of mutual assistance because of similar occupations or as members of distinctive parishes. As penitents or *conversi*, many had already received recognition for their charitable work from ecclesiastical and civil authorities. Married, with families, some men and women established these nonmonastic fraternities for the purpose of providing financial support and caregiving to existing or newly founded hospitals. Widows created by the Crusades joined in communities offering assistance.[136] Even the poorer sectors of society, more frequently recipients than givers of charity, gladly offered their voluntary labor. Indeed, all levels of medieval society followed the traditional Christian call of providing charity within the hospital framework, and the institution became deeply embedded in community life.[137]

According to tradition, hospital revenues belonged to the founder or his heirs, and the conditions of their disposition were usually inscribed in a deed of foundation. Besides having the power to nominate beneficiaries, including communities or brotherhoods, founders directly oversaw the administration of endowments and make provisions for their continuance after death. Founders also appointed a hospital's chief administrators and were obligated by law to provide sufficient funds for the establishment's charitable activities. Larger land gifts could be leased or cultivated with the help of volunteers. Houses were rented out. Thus, rents and tithes provided the main income, supplemented by periodic parish collections and in-kind offerings of food, bedding, and furniture, as well as revenues from fairs and festivals and the voluntary participation of local sponsors as caregivers. All private donors, royal officials, and bishops had the right to make periodic visits to check on the activities of their hospitals and decide on the use of funds and the level of care to be provided.[138]

Since religious ceremonies continued to be paramount in hospitals, the Church was able to retain a measure of control over all of these establishments, although the existence of various sponsors and their interests became a source of protracted jurisdictional disputes and legal challenges. During the twelfth and thirteenth centuries, dispensing charity to the needy became a central function of medieval society and its lay authorities. In larger European cities and smaller towns, many of these charitable hospital functions were carried out in the name of the Holy Spirit, the symbol of Christian love.[139] The exalted identity of hospital patients—stressed by the Hospitallers—was increasingly more symbolic but sufficient to ensure that their spiritual and corporal needs would be addressed. Donors, for their part, were driven by personal motives, especially the traditional Christian premise that dispensing charitable assistance was a religious act and a means of acquiring spiritual salvation.[140] In return for such generosity, inmates and caregivers needed to pray daily for their patrons and supporters, helping to guarantee their salvation. Visiting the sick and providing gifts or money for their needs in a hospital—still a *locus religiosus*—generated indulgences.

Larger institutions, especially in Germany, France, and England, preferred to divide their caring space into smaller partitions or rooms with walls, portable panels, or curtains to afford privacy. In many cases, these barriers could be removed to allow all patients a chance to participate in the daily mass through visual contact with the altar and the priest celebrating the Eucharist.[141] During winters, fires were lit in the center of each ward. Often heating was provided by iron baskets filled with coals that could be moved up and down the aisles between the beds. In summertime, pulleys and ropes opened the high windows for ventilation. Most hospitals retained spartan interiors, with crucifixes on the walls to provide believers with courage and strength derived from the sight of Christ's sufferings.[142]

As before, rules and laws were necessary to regulate the organization, management, and economy of these institutions, as well as to ensure hospital discipline. Distrusting lay motives and anxious to preserve the religious character of the newly founded establishments, the ecclesiastical authorities insisted that hospital statutes be based on provisions established by the Council of Paris (1212), the Council of Rouen (1214), and the Fourth Lateran Council (1215). Regardless of their origin, hospitals remained under ecclesiastical protection and sponsorship, and the Church appointed the priests who performed all religious rituals and led the traditional celebrations. These included mass in the memory of hospital founders and benefactors, as well as special watches over gravely ill patients in isolation rooms. A rather large proportion of the hospital's revenues were earmarked for the personal needs of chaplains and to defray expenses for decorating the hospital's chapel. Spiritual life was to be governed mostly by the rule of St. Augustine, and caregivers were persuaded to take vows. Moreover, episcopal authorities authorized hospitals to have their own cemeteries, a very important component of every institution since it allowed burial in consecrated ground for those who died in the house.[143]

Church authorities insisted that the internal organization of the house should follow the model created by the Hospitallers. Thus, the hospital chief administrator or *magister*, rector, or governor played a critical role. If not directly selected by the founder or by the local bishop, he could be elected by a majority of the caregiving members. Appointed for life, these magistrates were invariably consecrated priests or individuals who had received canonical instruction. Only in exceptional cases could lay persons assume these posts, including celibate or married men and even women or couples. To avoid conflicts and legal entanglements, their election had to be confirmed by the pope.[144]

The hospital's principal caregiving functions were executed by a group of primarily lay brothers, sisters, and servants. By the twelfth century, a new division of labor had already assigned the physical care of the sick, as well as cooking and washing, to women. Men still did the heavy lifting chores but otherwise retreated to assume administrative and ceremonial responsibilities, just as the Hospitallers had embraced military careers. Perhaps this shift was part of the process of marginalizing women in society.[145] In any event, all hospital staff members still functioned as a disciplined quasi-monastic community, their often hard and exhaustive caregiving framed as penance. Long hours, frequent night shifts, and little recreation made for a life of sacrifice and monotony. The only breaks in their routines occurred during celebrations of the liturgical year's cardinal feasts, when the rules were suspended, the wards decorated, and special meals served to the inmates, often in the presence of prominent visitors, including donors.[146]

In return, the caregivers "belonged" to the institution; their jobs were secure and their old age protected, especially in cases of sickness and disability. A good death and burial in hallowed ground followed. These factors attracted many younger, unattached women to monasteries and hospitals. However, there was often a ban on hiring them, particularly if they were attractive. Sexual tensions remained a perennial issue for monastery and hospital personnel, as attested to in the statutes of numerous institutions. Monks were prohibited from talking to nuns and female servants, except briefly in public and only if it concerned matters about the internal management of the house. Nurses were included in the prayers of the sick, and if the institutional revenues permitted, they were given *prebends* or stipends, often in the form of money, in apparent violation of their poverty vows. With sick inmates equated with Christ, caregivers considered the hospital as a substitute monastery where they performed their service to God.

HOSPITAL AGENDAS IN PERIL: CORRUPTION AND EARLY MEDICALIZATION

Monastic healing officially ended after the Council of Clermont in 1130, when monks were enjoined from practicing medicine since it was believed that this activity detracted from their stated spiritual goals. By 1219 canon law again prohibited religious persons from practicing medicine because of the monetary gain it brought, a rule confirmed by the Fourth Lateran Council of 1215.[147] However, severe shortages of trained medical professionals in Western Europe continued to foster the activities of monks who possessed medical knowledge. In addition, although officially barred from practicing, a large group of empirics, Jews, herbalists, barbers, and midwives joined in caring for the bulk of the population.[148]

After 1050, a gradual process of formal stratification and exclusion led to the emergence of a relatively well-defined medical profession in Western Europe. Urbanization created an expanding medical market, both public and private, a phenomenon witnessed first and most clearly in northern Italy. During the thirteenth century, universities replaced former cathedral and monastic schools in providing medical education, teaching a wider range of subjects and establishing a standardized curriculum that culminated in a set of degrees. Ratified by ecclesiastical authority, Bologna, Padua, Montpellier, and Paris became the main centers of academic study. Medical practitioners with official credentials and ecclesiastical permission acquired great professional status and social prominence, charging high fees to the wealthy who could afford their services.[149] Yet the Church continued to emphasize the primacy of spiritual over corporal healing. Indeed, the Fourth Lateran Council forbade physicians to visit patients for a second time unless the priest had first been called to attend to all spiritual matters because all bodily ailments resulted from sinful behavior.[150] Surgeons, by contrast, remained within an amorphous group of individuals who shaved and cut hair and performed cupping, leeching, and bleeding, as well as pulling teeth and treating wounds, sores, and traumatic injuries. Their hands-on approach was perceived as less prestigious than and socially inferior to that of physicians. Their training was less systematic and mostly by apprenticeship outside of the new academic frameworks.

Given such professional divisions and the chronic shortage of personnel, Western European hospitals had largely omitted physicians and surgeons from their staffs until the thirteenth century, in contrast with traditions at similar establishments in the Middle East. For one, most institutions retained their original religious character and satisfied their medical needs because members of their caregiving staffs already had significant medical training.[151]

Following in the footsteps of the Hospitallers in Jerusalem, lay physicians and surgeons began to be drawn increasingly into hospital service by the thirteenth century. They attended sick monks in monastic infirmaries and served as consultants in the care of sick poor inmates at existing hospices, eventually becoming regular staff members.[152] At the Hôtel-Dieu of Paris, surgical services had been provided since 1221 and medical ones from 1231 on. In 1328, King Charles IV (1346–1378) decided that patients would thereafter be entrusted to surgeons receiving a daily salary from city funds.[153] In Milan by the 1280s, physicians and surgeons became active caregivers in local hospitals. In 1331, the Holy Spirit Hospital in Marseilles began providing the regular services of a surgeon and barber, adding a physician in 1338. Finally, there was the gradually increasing medical presence at the Santa Maria Nuova Hospital in Florence, founded in 1288, which employed a physician and a surgeon in 1350. Larger hospitals also hired barbers, apothecaries, and midwives.[154]

In view of the blurring distinctions concerning the character of the poor—the previous voluntary–involuntary dichotomy became less relevant—and the greater need for charitable assistance in general, admission to hospitals became more selective after 1300. While the broad categories of poor and sick, pilgrims and strangers, generally characterized those brought into these institutions, restrictions were applied to individuals who had leprosy, suffered from presumably contagious diseases, or were pregnant, crippled, or insane. Moreover, hospitals were now forced to ration their caregiving through better screening of applicants and thus prevent the admission of malingers and freeloaders. Age limits were frequently imposed, often excluding children and the elderly. If pregnant women were allowed in to give birth, they did so in special rooms and had to leave the premises within a few weeks. Unless they were sick, some of the poor, including needy travelers, received lodging only for a night and a meal before being discharged the following morning. As with other shelters, many homeless individuals tried to return every night since the hospital was essentially their only shelter. Convalescents were allowed to linger for only a week following the remission of symptoms.[155]

Throughout Europe, hospital authorities now worried about admitting too many poor people with chronic conditions who would occupy most beds for long periods of time—a costly proposition—and thus prevent others, who had a better chance to recover, from being admitted. One way out of the dilemma was to expand the financial base of hospitals by accepting so-called "given" individuals—who usually lacked family and friends and who entered an institution for the rest of their lives, willing all their possessions to the establishment in return.[156] In countless small hospitals, these pensioners made up the bulk of the inmates, spending their last years of life there, often administering their own endowments and periodically even collecting stipends.[157]

In the fourteenth century, hospital services remained largely traditional and thus custodial: religious ceremonies, rest, warmth, food, and perhaps some medications.[158] The rules insisted on a strict separation of men and women. Those who refused to accept an assigned bed companion could be expelled. As before, liturgical matters remained at the center of hospital life. Special death watches were conducted by those guarding patients at night, with the assistance of the hospital chaplain. Following death, the caregivers prepared a shroud, the priest celebrated a special mass for the departed, and burial followed, witnessed by all personnel, in the adjacent cemetery. As before, for a pauper to receive the last rites and to die in a hospital was considered almost a privilege.[159]

The beginning of the Hundred Years' War between France and England in 1337 signaled the end of many charitable establishments in Europe. In a sense, the hospital movement had become a victim of its own success. Dependence on private donors with their personal motives and agendas tended to result in specific and targeted bequests, which became smaller and incidental and were also diminished by inflation. Increasingly, the result was a segregation and thus fragmentation of the hospital's financial base, complicating management and fostering administrative irregularities. Waste and greed became rampant, with embezzlement and diversion of resources fairly common. Already in the twelfth century, some administrators had begun to perceive the hospital as a source of personal gain. Some overseers of a hospital's revenues now viewed their tasks as an ordinary business instead of a charitable, spiritually rewarding enterprise. They engaged in frequent travel to attend meetings and supervise the hospital's estates while underlings carried on, usually to the detriment of patient care. One author, Jacques de Vitry, had commented in 1226 on the corruption of the religious staff in hospitals. Under the pretext of hospitality and piety, administrators and caregivers had become stone-hearted business people, bartering their meager caregiving and letters of indulgence for more alms and bribes. Vitry denounced this widespread hypocrisy and breakdown of discipline that transformed houses of mercy into "lairs of thieves and houses of prostitution."[160]

By the early 1300s, awareness of abuses had become frequent, and the problem was discussed at the Councils of Ravenna (1311) and Vienna (1324).[161] Pope Clement V explicitly prohibited clerics from profiting personally from hospital business unless this was the intent of the hospital's founders. Periodic inventories and frequent reports, even visits by ecclesiastical overseers, were demanded to curb potential abuses. Since most original foundation deeds were no longer available, it was assumed that ultimately all hospitals had been created to achieve a profit for the benefit of patient care. New institutions continued to be founded and operated under such premises. A founder's wishes may have been based on the tenets of Christian charity but, in time, the financial success of the endowments created temptations difficult to resist. Even the pontiff coveted such revenues for his own treasury. Following the Hospitallers' fate, this development repeated the typical cycle in which the acquisition of power and wealth for these charitable organizations and religious orders became its own raison d'être at the expense of the hospital inmates with whose care they had been entrusted.

At the same time, a decline in charitable giving linked to unfavorable economic and social conditions in Europe created fierce competition for patronage. Local interests, especially the emerging municipalities, tried to channel and control private resources going to hospitals by placing many of them under the secular jurisdiction of their magistrates.[162] Finally, as the concept of indulgences became discredited, the importance of a prior covenant between hospital patrons and the sick, who through prayers contributed to their benefactors' salvation, declined. With the status of the hospital as *locus religiosus* in jeopardy, the poor and sick inmates lost their status as agents for ensuring eternal life. The spread of leprosy and plague in Europe reinforced the role of existing hospitals as tools for social control. Segregation of individuals suspected of suffering from these contagious diseases created specialized institutions: leper houses and lazarettos.

The Hospitallers, meanwhile, were now primarily European landlords instead of healers, deeply involved in politics and warfare. Their main activities increasingly centered on the military defense of the Holy Land and its sacred places of worship. This also applied to the Knights of St. Lazar, who earlier had concentrated on the care of lepers. Engaged in a power struggle with the papacy, the last Knight Templars were arrested in 1306, and by 1312 their entire property had been transferred to the Hospitallers. Thus concluded the competition between these two political and economic powers.[163] After 1349, the Hospitallers' financial status suffered greatly from the impact of the bubonic plague as most land holdings were hit by widespread depopulation, high labor costs, and economic recession. At Rhodes, construction of the Hospitallers' famous hospital was completed around the year 1440. At the new location, the order rapidly became a formidable naval power in the Mediterranean Sea. Rhodes eventually fell to the Turkish sultan Soliman in 1522, prompting the Hospitallers to retreat first to Crete, then to Messina, and eventually to Civita Vecchia in Naples. Finally, in 1530, Emperor Charles V officially ceded the island of Malta to the Hospitallers, ending their successive retreat from their original showcase shelter in Jerusalem. Another important chapter in the evolution of hospitals had ended.

NOTES

1. Metochites was a fourteenth-century scholar and statesman. See Deno J. Geanakoplos, *Byzantium: Church, Society, and Civilization Seen Through Contemporary Eyes*, Chicago, Univ. of Chicago Press, 1984, p. 316.

2. For a recent and readable history of the period see Michael Angold, *The Byzantine Empire, 1025–1204, A Political History*, 2nd ed., London, Longman, 1997, and John J. Norwich, *Byzantium: The Decline and Fall*, New York, A. A. Knopf, 1996, especially pp. 63–95.

3. Letter VI can be found in *Patrologiae Graecae*, ed. J. P. Milne, (1857–64) reprint, Turnhout, Belgium, Brepols Ed., 1983, vol. 133, pp. 1253–58. I am grateful to V. Sweet for her translation. The text is also mentioned by Wolfram Hörandner, *Theodoros Prodromos, Historische Gedichte*, Vienna, Verlag Oesterr Akad Wissenschaften, 1974, p. 30. See also the translated excerpts in P. S. Codellas, "The case of smallpox of Theodorus Prodromus," *Bull Hist Med* 20 (1946): 212.

4. Hörandner, *Prodromos*, p. 544.

5. Poem LXXVII ("Concerning the Heroic Illness") in Hörandner, *Prodromos*, pp. 545–46. I am indebted to Dr. Donald Zukin for this partial translation from the Greek.

6. Letter VI, *Patrologiae Graecae*, vol. 133, p. 1256. See also Codellas, "Smallpox," 213.

7. Hörandner, *Prodromos*, p. 30.

8. A. Kazhdan, "The image of the medical doctor in Byzantine literature of the 10th to 12th centuries," in *Symposium on Byzantine Medicine*, ed. J. Scarborough, Washington, DC, Dumbarton Oaks Research Library and Collection, 1985, pp. 43–51.

9. Letter VI, *Patrologiae Graecae*, vol. 133, p. 1256. See also Codellas, "Smallpox," 213.

10. The Latin term *variola*, meaning a "rash," had been employed since the sixth century.

11. Letter IV, *Patrologiae Graecae*, vol. 133, pp. 1249–50.

12. Ibid., p. 1250. See also Codellas, "Smallpox," 213.

13. Letter IV, *Patrologiae Graecae*, vol. 133, p. 1250. See also Codellas, "Smallpox", 213.

14. al-Razi (Rhazes), *A Treatise on the Smallpox and Measles*, trans. W. A. Greehill, London, Sydenham Society Publications, 1858.

15. Poem LXVIII to the Lord Logothete Stephanos Meles, Hörandner, *Prodromos*, p. 508, also translated by D. Zukin.

16. Poem LXXVII, Hörandner, *Prodromos*, p. 545.

17. Poem LXVIII, p. 508.

18. A text, the *Miracula Sancti Artemii*, composed shortly after 650, mentions a deacon of the Church who was brought to the Samson Xenon of Constantinople for treatment.

19. See Jane T. Matthews, "The Pantocrator: Title and Image," Ph.D. diss., New York Univ., 1976, especially pp. 21–48.

20. Ibid., p. 44.

21. An English translation of selections from the Pantocrator's charter can be found in Geanakoplos, *Byzantium*, pp. 314–15.

22. Philip Whitting, *Byzantium: An Introduction*, New York, St. Martin's Press, 1981, especially pp. 83–110. Another useful source is George Ostrogorsky, *History of the Byzantine State*, rev. ed., New Brunswick, NJ, Rutgers Univ. Press, 1991.

23. This topic is addressed in Demetrios J. Constantelos, *Byzantine Philanthropy and Social Welfare*, 2nd rev. ed., New Rochelle, NY, A. D. Caratzas, 1991, especially pp. 113–39 and pp. 141–62. Consult also the material in Angeliki E. Laiou, *Gender, Society, and Economic Life in Byzantium*, Brookfield, VT, Variorum Reprints, 1992.

24. For more information see Joan M. Hussey, *Church and Learning in the Byzantine Empire, 867–1185*, New York, Russell & Russell, 1963.

25. See B. Baldwin, "The career of Oribasius," *Acta Classica* 18 (1975): 85–97.

26. Consult J. Hirschberg, ed., *Die Augenheilkunde des Aetius aus Amida*, in Greek and German texts, Leipzig, Veit, 1899, and J. Lascatos et al., "Ophthalmology according to Aetius Amidenus," *Doc Opthalmol* 74 (1990): 37–48. A translation of his gynecological and

obstetric texts can be found in Aetius of Amida, *The Gynecology and Obstetrics of the VIth Century AD*, trans J. V. Ricci, Philadelphia, Blakiston, 1950.

27. Alexander of Tralles, *Oeuvres Medicales*, Paris, P. Geuthner, 1933–37. See also J. Scarborough, "Early Byzantine pharmacology," in *Symposium on Byzantine Medicine*, pp. 213–32.

28. Paulus Aegineta, *The Seven Books of Paulus Aegineta*, trans. from the Greek, 3 vols., London, Sydenham Society Publications, 1844–47.

29. Robert Volk, *Gesundheitswesen und Wohltätigkeit im Spiegel der Byzantinischen Klostertypika*, Munich, Institut für Byzantinistik der Universität, 1983, especially pp. 37–61.

30. In this regard, Justinian had already instructed the *archiatroi* to assist in the training of new medical recruits. It is probable that those physicians called to treat the sick in Byzantine *xenones* and *nosokomeia* after the fourth century also brought their students to the bedside and provided them with informal instruction.

31. For an overview see S. Hamarneh, "Development of hospitals in Islam," *J Hist Med* 17 (1962): 366–84. A more critical synthesis is M. W. Dols, "The origins of the Islamic hospital: Myth and reality," *Bull Hist Med* 61 (1987): 367–90. More information can be found in Dols' "Insanity in Byzantine and Islamic medicine," in *Symposium on Byzantine Medicine*, pp. 135–458.

32. Allen O. Whipple, *The Role of Nestorians and Muslims in the History of Medicine*, Princeton, Princeton Univ. Press, 1967. For a recent overview see Lawrence I. Conrad, "The Arab-Islamic medical tradition," in *The Western Medical Tradition, 800 BC to AD 1800*, coauthored by Vivian Nutton et al., Cambridge, Cambridge Univ. Press, 1995, pp. 93–138.

33. Dols, "Origins," 379 and 384. Consult also R. Quadflieg, "Islamische Hospitäler zur Zeit der Omayyaden und Abbasiden," *Hist Hospitalium* 15 (1983–84): 81–96.

34. See A. I. Sabra, "The appropriation and subsequent naturalization of Greek science in medieval Islam: A preliminary statement," *Hist Sci* 25 (1987): 223–43, and L. I. Conrad, "Scholarship and social context: A medical case from the 11th century Near East," in *Knowledge and the Scholarly Traditions*, ed. D. Bates, Cambridge, Cambridge Univ. Press, 1995, pp. 84–100. For details see M. J. L. Young et al., eds. *Religion, Learning, and Science in the Abbasid Period*, Cambridge, Cambridge Univ. Press, 1990. See also *The Classical Heritage in Islam*, trans. E. and J. Marmorstein, London, Routledge & Kegan Paul, 1975. Regarding medicine, see Manfred Ullmann, *Islamic Medicine*, Edinburgh, Edinburgh Univ. Press, 1978, and Muhammad S. Khan, *Islamic Medicine*, London, Routledge & Kegan Paul, 1986.

35. Dols, "Origins," 387.

36. S. M. Imamuddin, "Maristan (hospitals) in medieval Spain," *Islam Stud* 17 (1978): 45–55, and F. G. Irueste, "En torno al maristan de Granada," *Asclepio* 30/31 (1978–79): 223–31.

37. M. W. Dols, "Insanity and its treatment in Islamic society," *Med Hist* 31 (1987): 1–14.

38. See, for example, Fazlur Rahman, "Islam and medicine: A general overview," *Persp Biol Med* 27 (1984): 585–97, and his more extensive *Health and Medicine in the Islamic Tradition*, New York, Crossroads, 1987.

39. Quadflieg, "Islamische Hospitäler," 83. See also D. Jetter, "Zur Architektur islamischer Krankenhäuser," *Sudhoffs Archiv* 45 (1961): 261–73.

40. Some routines were described by ibn Abi Usaibi as taking place at the new Nur al-Din hospital in Damascus, a near contemporary of the Pantocrator (Rahman, *Health and Medicine*, p. 68). Details on the medical profession in medieval Islam are furnished in

Michael W. Dols, trans., *Medieval Islamic Medicine*, Berkeley, Univ. of California Press, 1984.

41. S. D. Goitein, *A Mediterranean Society*, Berkeley, Univ. of California Press, 1971, vol. 2, p. 254. See also C. Bürgel, "Secular and religious features of medieval Arabic medicine," in *Asian Medical Systems: A Comparative View*, ed. C. Leslie, Berkeley, Univ. of California Press, 1976, pp. 44–62.

42. G. Karmi, "State control of the physicians in the Middle Ages: An Islamic model," in *The Town Physician in Europe from the Middle Ages to the Enlightenment*, ed. A. W. Russell, Wolfenbüttel, Herzog August Bibliothek, 1981, pp. 63–84.

43. Goitein stresses the popularity of practicing physicians among the secular elites of many Muslim communities during the ninth and tenth centuries. See his *Mediterranean Society*, especially 249–51. For the medieval appointment of one practitioner in Cairo see D. S. Richards, "A doctor's petition for a salaried post in Saladin's Hospital," *Social Hist Med* 5 (1992): 297–306.

44. S. Hamarneh, "Ecology and therapeutics in medieval Arabic medicine," *Sudhoffs Archiv* 58 (1974): 165–85.

45. Goitein speaks of 3,000 items contained in an Arabic handbook written in about 1150; see *Mediterranean Society*, p. 253. Details can be found in Martin Levey, *Early Arabic Pharmacology: An Introduction Based on Ancient and Medieval Sources*, Leiden, E. J. Brill, 1973.

46. Matthews, "The Pantocrator: Title and Image," pp. 41–46.

47. Cyril Mango, *Byzantine Architecture*, New York, H. N. Abrams, 1974, pp. 243–46.

48. For a summary see P. S. Codellas, "The Pantocrator, the imperial Byzantine medical center of XIIth century AD in Constantinople," *Bull Hist Med* 12 (1942): 392–410. A more recent synthesis is Timothy Miller, *The Birth of the Hospital in the Byzantine Empire*, Baltimore, Johns Hopkins Univ. Press, 1985, pp. 12–29.

49. This tentative plan was prepared by an Athenian architect. See Codellas, "Pantocrator," 399.

50. A. Philipsborn, "Special-Anstalt des Pantokrator Krankenhauses," *Byzantion* 33 (1963): 223–30.

51. Geanakoplos, *Byzantium*, pp. 314–15.

52. Ibid., p. 314.

53. Ibid., p. 315.

54. E. Kislinger, "Der Pantokrator-Xenon, ein trügerisches Ideal?" *Jahrbuch der Oesterreichischen Byzantinistik* 37 (1987): 173–79.

55. Dols states that "even with the typikon, it is quite unclear how the Pantocrator worked." See his "Origins," 371.

56. A comparison with nineteenth-century Parisian teaching hospitals suggested by Timothy Miller in *Birth of the Hospital* is forcefully rejected by Vivian Nutton in "Essay review—*Birth of the hospital*," *Med Hist* 30 (1986): 218–21.

57. At this time, uroscopy reflected professional competence. See S. G. Marketos et al., "Limits in the studies of the art of uroscopy: The Byzantine example," *Am J Nephrol* 14 (1994): 239–45.

58. Volk, *Gesundheitswesen*, pp. 271–80.

59. Paulus Aegineta, *Seven Books*, vol. 1., p. 172, and vol. 2, pp. 36 and 102.

60. Ibid., vol. 2, p. 316.

61. Ibid., vol. 2, p. 37.

62. Poem XLVI, Hörandner, *Prodromos*, pp. 430–31, transl. Karen Veit.

63. S. A. Ghazanfar, "Wasm: A traditional healing by cauterisation," *J Ethnopharm* 47 (1995): 125–28.

64. Albucasis, *On Surgery and Instruments*, trans. and commentary by M. S. Spink and G. L. Lewis, Berkeley, Univ. of California Press, 1973, Book 1, p. 8.

65. Paulus Aegineta, *Seven Books*, vol. 2, p. 331.

66. Poem XLVI, Hörandner, *Prodromos*, p. 432.

67. Ibid.

68. Ibid., p. 433.

69. Letter V, *Patrologiae Graecae*, vol. 133, p. 1251. See also Codellas, "Smallpox," 214.

70. Quotation from Eberhard of Wurtemburg in Jonathan Sumption, *Pilgrimage, An Image of Mediaeval Religion*, London, Faber & Faber, and Totowa, NJ, Rowman and Littlefield, 1975, p. 210.

71. Theoderic, in *Jerusalem Pilgrimage 1099–1185*, ed. J. Wilkinson, J. Hill, and W. F. Ryan, London, The Hakluyt Society, 1988, p. 277.

72. P. Fuchs, ed. *Chronik zur Geschichte der Stadt Köln*, Cologne, Greven, 1990, vol. 1, pp. 133–34. More general information can be found in Horst Fuhrmann, *Germany in the High Middle Ages*, trans. T. Reuter, Cambridge, Cambridge Univ. Press, 1986, and Alfred Haverkamp, *Medieval Germany, 1056–1273*, trans. H. Braun and R. Mortimer, Oxford, Oxford Univ. Press, 1992.

73. For bibliographical details see Linda K. Davidson and Maryjane Dunn-Wood, *Pilgrimage in the Middle Ages: A Research Guide*, New York, Garland Press, 1993, especially pp. 80–127. See also Peter Brown, *The Cult of the Saints: Its Rise and Function in Latin Christianity*, Chicago, Univ. of Chicago Press, 1980.

74. For a useful introduction see S. Runciman, "The pilgrimage to Palestine before 1095," in *A History of the Crusades*, ed. K. M. Setton, 2nd ed., Madison, Univ. of Wisconsin Press, 1969, vol. 1, pp. 68–78. Also consult Marjorie Rowling, *Everyday Life of Medieval Travellers*, London, B. T. Batsford, 1971, and James Martin, *A Pilgrim's Guide to the Holy Land*, Philadelphia, Westminster Press, 1978.

75. Farber traveled to the Holy Land in 1480. See G. Duby and P. Braunstein, "The emergence of the individual," in *Revelations of the Medieval World*, ed. G. Duby, Cambridge, MA, Belknap Press of Harvard Univ. Press, 1988, pp. 587–88.

76. See Farber's descriptions and consult H. F. M. Prescott, *Friar Felix at Large: A Fifteenth-Century Pilgrimage to the Holy Land*, Westport, CT, Greenwood Press, 1967. More information is provided in Donald R. Howard, *Writers and Pilgrims*, Berkeley, Univ. of California Press, 1980, especially pp. 11–52, and Nathan Schur, *Jerusalem in Pilgrims' and Travellers' Accounts: A Thematic Bibliography of Western Christian Itineraries, 1300–1917*, Jerusalem, Ariel Publishing House, 1980.

77. Theoderic, in *Jerusalem Pilgrimage*, pp. 309–10.

78. Ibid., p. 304.

79. Ibid., p. 310.

80. Adolf's companion, Theoderic, later wrote, "I would not trust anyone else to believe it if I had not seen with my own eyes how splendidly it is adorned with buildings with many rooms, bunks, and other things poor people, the weak, and the sick can use. What a rich palace this is." Theoderic, in *Jerusalem Pilgrimage*, p. 287.

81. Another visitor, Nikulas the Abbot, spoke of "the hospital of John the Baptist which is the most magnificent in the whole world." Nikulas of Pvera, in *Jerusalem Pilgrimage*, p. 217.

82. John of Würzburg, in *Jerusalem Pilgrimage*, p. 266. This text is also available in "John of Würzburg, description of the Holy Land (1160–1170)," trans. A. Stewart, in *The Library of the Palestine Pilgrims Text Society*, London, 1896; reprint, New York, AMS, vol. 5, 1971.

83. John of Würzburg, in *Jerusalem Pilgrimage*, p. 266.

84. Theoderic, in *Jerusalem Pilgrimage*, p. 287.

85. Details in E. D. Hunt, *Holy Land Pilgrimage in the Later Roman Empire, AD 312–460*, Oxford, Clarendon Press, 1982, and Joan E. Taylor, *Christians and the Holy Places: the Myth of Jewish-Christian Origins*, Oxford, Clarendon Press, 1993. For a collection of original documents see Francis E. Peters, *Jerusalem: The Holy City in the Eyes of Chroniclers, Visitors, Pilgrims, and Prophets*, Princeton, Princeton Univ. Press, 1985.

86. For subsequent developments see *The Meeting of Two Worlds: Cultural Exchange between East and West during the Period of the Crusades*, ed. V. P. Goss, Kalamazoo, Medieval Institute Publications, Western Michigan Univ., 1986.

87. A frequent practice was to collect dust, stones, or scraps of paper that had been in contact with a saint at a shrine. Relics were also dipped in water or wine to parcel out their miraculous power. Sumption, *Pilgrimage*, pp. 41–53. See also Rosalind and Christopher Brooke, *Religion in the Middle Ages: Western Europe 1000–1300*, London, Thames & Hudson, 1984.

88. For an overview see Jonathan Riley-Smith, *The Crusades: A Short History*, New Haven, Yale Univ. Press, 1987. Also useful is the *Oxford Illustrated History of the Crusades*, ed. Jonathan Riley-Smith, New York, Oxford Univ. Press, 1995. For the First Crusade see John France, *Victory in the East: A Military History of the First Crusade*, Cambridge, Cambridge Univ. Press, 1994, and Jonathan Riley-Smith, *The First Crusade and the Idea of Crusading*, Philadelphia, Univ. of Pennsylvania Press, 1986.

89. See "An account of the location of the places" in *Jerusalem Pilgrimage*, p. 200.

90. I. Sterns, "Care of the sick brothers by the Crusader Orders in the Holy Land," *Bull Hist Med* 57 (1983): 43–69.

91. Consider, for example, the string of hospitals along the road to Compostela. See R. Baltar Dominguez, "Algunos aspectos medicos de las peregrinaciones medievales a Compostela," *Actas del XV Congreso Internacional de Historia de la Medicina, 1956*, Madrid, Instituto A. Vilanova, 1958, vol. 2, pp. 33–52. For a general overview see Marcus G. Bull, *Knightly Piety and the Lay Response to the First Crusade: The Limousin and Gascony, c. 970–1130*, Oxford, Clarendon Press, 1993.

92. The Christian takeover of Palestine during the twelfth century not only reopened the prosperous flow of pilgrims to Jerusalem but also made the new kingdom a favorite destination for many European colonists. Larger population centers near the coast were occupied by merchants and their families. Others eagerly took over ruined villages and wastelands, creating new population centers and, with the help of Syrian peasants, replanted vineyards and orchards near the fertile coast. Within a few years, the kingdom became one of the largest sugar producers of Europe. Cotton and olive oil were also important exports. After barely a century of Christian rule, Latin Syria attracted more than 100,000 western immigrants, and by 1172 it had a total population of about 250,000. See Jonathan Riley-Smith, *The Knights of St. John in Jerusalem and Cyprus, c. 1050–1310*, New York, St. Martin Press, 1967, pp. 17–24. For relationships with the Byzantine empire see Ralph-Johannes Lilie, *Byzantium and the Crusader States, 1096–1204*, trans J. C. Morris and J. E. Ridings, rev. ed., New York, Oxford Univ. Press, 1993.

93. E. J. King, ed., *The Rule, Statutes, and Customs of the Hospitallers, 1099–1310*, London, Methuen, 1934, pp. 16–19.

94. "The rule of blessed Raymond du Puy, 1120–60," in King, *Rules, Statutes and Customs*, pp. 26–27. See also Sterns, "Care of the sick brothers," 50–53.

95. A. F. Woodings, "The medical resources and practice of the Crusader States in Syria and Palestine, 1096–1193," *Med Hist* 15 (1971): 268–77.

96. A. R. Jonsen, "Our Lords, the sick," in *The Persisting Osler II*, ed. J. A. Barondess and C. G. Roland, Melbourne, FL, Krieger Pub. Co., 1994, pp. 3–8.

97. M. Gerves, "Pro defensione Terre Sancte: The development and exploitation of the Hospitallers' landed estates in Essex," in *The Military Orders: Fighting for the Faith and Caring for the Sick*, ed. M. Barber, Brookfield, VT, Variorum Reprints, 1994, pp. 3–20.

98. J. Richard, "Hospitals and hospital congregations in the Latin Kingdom during the first period of the Frankish conquest," in *Outremer: Studies in the History of the Crusading Kingdom Presented to J. Prawer*, ed. B. Kedar et al., Jerusalem, Yad Itzhak Ben-Zvi Institute, 1982, pp. 90–91.

99. See J. Eade and M. J. Sallnow, eds., *Contesting the Sacred: The Anthropology of Christian Pilgrimage*, London, Routledge, 1991.

100. See Franz Meffert, *Caritas und Krankenwesen bis zum Ausgang des Mittelalters*, Freiburg, Caritasverlag, 1927, pp. 187–91. For details see Christian Probst, *Der Deutsche Orden und sein Medizinalwesen in Preussen*, Bad Godesberg, Verlag Wissenschaft Archiv, 1969, and more recently M. Tumler and U. Arnold, *Der Deutsche Orden: von seinem Ursprung bis zur Gegenwart*, Bonn-Bad-Godesberg, Verlag Wissenschaftliches Archiv, 1981. For an English summary see U. Arnold, "Eight hundred years of the Teutonic Order," in Barber, *Military Orders*, pp. 223–35.

101. J. von Steinitz, *Mitteralterliche Hospitäler der Orden und Städte als Einrichtungen der sozialen Sicherheit*, Berlin, Dunker & Humboldt, 1970.

102. "Statutes of Fr. Roger des Moulins, 1177–87," in King, *Rule, Statutes, and Customs*, pp. 35–36.

103. John of Würzburg, in *Jerusalem Pilgrimage*, p. 267.

104. See Alan Forey's collection of articles, especially "The militarisation of the Hospital of St. John," in *Military Orders and Crusades*, Brookfield, VT, Variorum Reprints, 1994, pp. 75–89. See R. C. Smail, *Crusading Warfare, 1097–1193*, 2nd ed., Cambridge, Cambridge Univ. Press, 1995.

105. With lodgings in the area of King Solomon's Temple in the city, a group of knights already protected pilgrims on their way from the port of Jaffa to Jerusalem. These Poor Knights of the Temple or simply Templars soon became a powerful and wealthy group competing with the Hospitallers for royal attention and donations. Their first battle against the Moslems took place in 1129, and they soon began to overshadow the Hospitallers of St. John in prestige and economic power, particularly in Europe. See Barber, *Military Orders*, and B. N. Sargent-Baur, ed., *Journeys Toward God: Pilgrimage and Crusade*, Kalamazoo, MI, Medieval Institute Publications, Western Michigan Univ., 1992.

106. Alan Forey, "Constitutional conflicts and change in the Hospital of St. John during the twelfth- and thirteenth centuries," in Barber, *Military Orders*, pp. 15–18.

107. Theoderic, in *Jerusalem Pilgrimage*, p. 303.

108. For details see Riley-Smith, *Knights of St. John*, pp. 46–54.

109. King, *Rules, Statutes and Customs*, p. 38.

110. Ibid., p. 35.

111. T. Miller, "The Knights of Saint John and the hospitals of the Latin West," *Speculum* 53 (1978): 709–33.

112. Hamarneh, "Hospitals in Islam," 366–84.

113. Riley-Smith, *Knights of St. John*, pp. 246–59. Also see I. Nilsson and H. Sunzel, "The influence of medieval Christian ideology on Western Hospitals: Medical care at the Hospitallers in Jerusalem," *Lychnos* (1992): 9–24.

114. King, *Rules, Statutes, and Customs*, p. 35.

115. Ibid., p. 38.

116. Ibid., p. 35.

117. The prayer started with the invocation: "Our Lords the Sick!, pray for peace, that God shall send it from heaven to earth; Our Lords the Sick! pray for the fruits of the earth,

that God shall multiply them in a way so that they will be sufficient for divine services and the sustenance of Christianity, and also pray for Christian pilgrims on sea or land, that God shall guide them and return their souls and bodies to health, and for all who give us alms, and for all Christians who are in the custody of the Saracens, that Our Lord will free them after our prayer." Personal translations from the German and French versions in Meffert, *Caritas und Krankenwesen*, pp. 282–83. Concerning prayers, see K. V. Sinclair, "The French prayer for the sick in the Hospital of the Knights of Saint John of Jerusalem in Acre," *Medieval Stud* 40 (1978): 434–88.

118. King, *Rules, Statutes and Customs*, pp. 37–38.

119. Ibid., pp. 22–23. See also Melitta Weiss Adamson, *Medieval Dietetics: Food and Drink in Regimen Sanitatis Literature from 800 to 1400*, Frankfurt, Lang, 1995.

120. Hans Karl von Zwehl, *Nachrichten über die Armen-und Kranken Fürsorge des Ordens vom Hospital des heiligen Johannes von Jerusalem*, Münster, Westfalische Vereinsdruckerei, 1911.

121. For descriptions of surgery see S. Edgington, "Medical knowledge in the Crusading armies: The evidence of Albert of Aachen and others," in Barber, *Military Orders*, pp. 320–26.

122. P. Gil-Sotres, "Derivation and revulsion: The theory and practice of medieval phlebotomy," in *Practical Medicine from Salerno to the Black Death*, ed. L. Garcia Ballester, R. French, J. Arrizabalaga, and A. Cunningham, New York, Cambridge Univ. Press, 1994, pp. 110–55.

123. Bleedings were recommended after Christmas, before Lent, after Easter, around the time of the feast of Saints Peter and Paul, and at the time of the Feast of All Saints. See, for example, the statutes of the leper house of Lille, June 1239, in N. Guglielmi, ed., "Estatutos de Hospitales y Leproserias," reprint of texts compiled by Leon Le Grand (1901) and translated by E. Ribe and H. A. Iribar, *Anal Hist Antigua u Medieval* 16 (1971): 175–77.

124. Sterns, "Care of the sick brothers," 53–65.

125. See Victor and Edith Turner, *Image and Pilgrimage in Christian Culture*, New York, Columbia Univ. Press, 1978, especially pp. 1–39, where they frame pilgrimage as a rite of passage.

126. Theoderic, in *Jerusalem Pilgrimage*, p. 305, and Howard, *Writers and Pilgrims*, especially pp. 11–52.

127. Hamarneh, "Hospitals in Islam," 373.

128. Z. Goldman, "The hospice of the Knights of St. John in Akkron," *Archeology* 19 (1966): 182–89.

129. A. Williams, "Xenodochium to sacred infirmary: The changing role of the hospital of the order of St. John, 1522–1631," in Barber, *Military Orders*, pp. 97–102. For details see Anthony Luttrell, *Latin Greece, the Hospitallers, and the Crusades, 1291–1440*, London, Variorum Reprints, 1982, and E. Hallam, ed., *Chronicles of the Crusades: Eye-Witness Accounts of the Wars Between Christianity and Islam*, London, Weidenfeld and Nicolson, 1989.

130. For a discussion of political and spiritual issues see Bernard Hamilton, *The Latin Church in the Crusader States: The Secular Church*, London, Variorum Reprints, 1980.

131. For England see Edwin J. King, *The Knights of St. John in the British Realm*, 3rd ed., London, Order of the Hospital of St. John of Jerusalem, 1967.

132. Cited in A. Luttrell, "The Hospitaller's medical tradition: 1291–1530," in Barber, *Military Orders*, p. 75.

133. Meffert, *Caritas und Krankenwesen*, pp. 211–32.

134. See S. R. Ell, "Disease ecologies of Europe," in *The Cambridge World History of Human Disease*, ed. K. F. Kiple, Cambridge, Cambridge Univ. Press, 1993, pp. 504–19.

135. Michel Mollat, *The Poor in the Middle Ages: An Essay in Social History*, trans. A. Goldhammer, New Haven Yale Univ. Press, 1976, especially pp. 59–65 and pp. 87–107.

136. Raffaele Pazelli, *St. Francis and the Third Order: The Franciscan and Pre-Franciscan Penitential Movement*, Chicago, Franciscan Herald Press, 1989, especially pp. 11–39.

137. Mollat, in *The Poor* (p. 146), refers to the hospital as "the poor man's castle." See also P. Horden's review "A discipline of relevance: The historiography of the later medieval hospital," *Soc Hist Med* 1 (1988): 359–74.

138. Consult Wolfgang Berger, *Das St. Georg Hospital zu Hamburg*, Hamburg, H. Christians Verlag, 1972.

139. Meffert, *Caritas und Krankenwesen*, pp. 233–38, and G. Baader, "Die Entwicklung der Heiliggeisthospitäler in Deutschland," *Der Krankenhausarzt* 44 (1971): 268-276.

140. Mollat, *The Poor*, pp. 154–55.

141. For information on England see M. Carlin, "Medieval English hospitals," and M. Rubin, "Development and change in English hospitals, 1100–1500," in *The Hospital in History*, ed. L. Granshaw and R. Porter, London, Routledge, 1989, pp. 21–39 and 41–59, respectively. Also consult Edward J. Kealey, *Medieval Medicus: A Social History of Anglo-Norman Medicine*, Baltimore, Johns Hopkins Univ. Press, 1981, pp. 82–106. For Spain see Robert J. Burns, *The Crusader Kingdom of Valencia: Reconstruction of a Thirteenth-Century Frontier*, Cambridge, MA, Harvard Univ. Press, 1967, vol. 1, pp. 237–52.

142. Meffert, *Caritas und Krankenwesen*, p. 257. For information on Beaune see E. B. Bavard, *L'Hôtel-Dieu de Beaune, 1443–1880*, Beaune, 1881.

143. For England see Kealey, *Medieval Medicus*, pp. 107–16, and for France see J. H. Mundy, "Hospitals and leprosaries in twelfth and early thirteenth-century Toulouse," in *Essays in Medieval Life and Thought, Presented in Honor of Austin Patterson Evans*, ed. J. H. Mundy, R. W. Emery, and B. N. Nelson, New York, Columbia Univ. Press, 1955, pp. 181–205.

144. The German context has been described by Siegfried Reicke, *Das deutsche Spital und sein Recht im Mittelalter*, Stuttgart, F. Enke, 1932, and for France by Jean Imbert, *Les Hôpitaux en Droit Canonique*, Paris, J. Vrin, 1947, especially pp. 33–54.

145. See Penelope D. Johnson, *Equal in Monastic Profession: Religious Women in Medieval France*, Chicago, Univ. of Chicago Press, 1991, p. 53.

146. Meffert, *Caritas und Krankenwesen*, p. 285.

147. H. J. Schroeder, ed. and trans., *Disciplinary Decrees of the General Councils*, London, B. Herder Book Co., 1937, pp. 236–96, and D. W. Amundsen, "Medieval canon law on medical and surgical practice by the clergy," *Bull Hist Med* 52 (1978): 22–44.

148. See, for example, Tony Hunt, *Popular Medicine in Thirteenth-Century England*, Canterbury, United Kingdom, D. S. Brewer, 1990, and Sheila Campbell, ed., *Health, Disease, and Healing in the Middle Ages*, Toronto, St. Martin's Press, 1992.

149. For England see E. A. Hammond, "Physicians in medieval English religious houses," *Bull Hist Med* 32 (1958): 105–20. Information about France is found in Danielle Jacquart, *Le Milieu Médicale en France du XII–XV Siècles*, Geneva, Librairie Droz, 1981. For the role of women see M. Green, "Women's medical practice and health care in medieval Europe," *Signs* 14 (1989): 434–72.

150. For details see Nicholas Orme and Margaret Webster, *The English Hospital, 1070–1570*, New Haven, Yale Univ. Press, 1995.

151. E. A. Hammond, "The Westminster Abbey infirmarers' rolls as a source of medical history," *Bull Hist Med* 39 (1965): 261–76.

152. M. D. Grmek, "Le médecin au service de l'hôpital medieval en Europe Occidentale," *Hist Philos Life Sci* 4 (1982): 25–64.

153. D. MacKay Quynn, "A medieval picture of the Hôtel-Dieu of Paris," *Bull Hist Med* 12 (1942): 118–28, and Ernest Coyecque, *L'Hôtel-Dieu de Paris au Moyen Age: Histoire et Documents*, 2 vols., Paris, Champion, 1889–91.

154. For information on London see Carole Rawcliffe, "The hospitals of later medieval London," *Med Hist* 28 (1984): 1–21; see also her *The Hospitals of Medieval Norwich*, Norwich, Centre of East Anglia Studies, 1995.

155. For details see Marie L. Windemuth, *Das Hospital als Träger der Armenführsorge im Mittelalter*, Stuttgart, Steiner, 1995.

156. In England a *corrody* was a pension or allowance provided by the house that enabled an inmate or *corrodian* to retire to the hospital as a boarder. A *cremett* was an enfeebled pauper in need of care. See P. H. Cullum, *Cremetts and Corrodies: Care of the Poor and Sick at St. Leonard's Hospital, York, in the Middle Ages*, York, Borthwick Paper 39, 1990; Elizabeth Prescott, *The English Hospital, 1050–1640*, London, Seaby, 1992; and Orme and Webster, *The English Hospital, 1070–1570*

157. For conditions in England see R. L. Goodey, "The Development of the Medieval Infirmary in England," Ph.D. diss., Univ. of London, 1986, and C. Harper-Bill, *Charters of the Medieval Hospitals of Bury St. Edmunds*, Rochester, NY, Boydell Press, 1994.

158. See J. M. Riddle, "Theory and practice in medieval medicine," *Viator* 5 (1974): 157–84.

159. R. Gilchrist, "Christian bodies and souls: The archeology of life and death in later medieval hospitals," in *Death in Towns: Urban Responses to Dying and the Dead, 100–1600*, ed. S. Bassett, Leicester, Leicester Univ. Press, 1992.

160. The quotation is from Jacques de Vitry's *History of the Occident*, chapter 29, reprinted in Guglielmi, "Estatutos de Hospitales y Leproserias," 98.

161. Mollat, *The Poor*, p.181.

162. See, for example, the rules of a hospital in Angers during the early thirteenth century in Guglielmi, "Estatutos de Hospitales y Leproserias," 110–19. See also Johnson, *Monastic Profession*, pp. 257–59.

163. For details see John J. Robinson, *Dungeon, Fire, and Sword: the Knights Templar in the Crusades*, New York, M. Evans & Co., 1991.

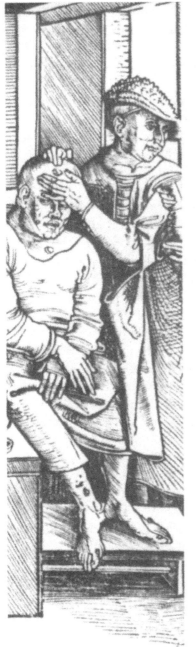

4

HOSPITALS AS SEGREGATION AND CONFINEMENT TOOLS

Leprosy and Plague

LEPER HOUSES

Take this leper lodge for your lovely bower,
And for your bed take now a bundle of straw.
For choice wines and meats you once enjoyed,
Take moldy bread, perry, and cider sour.
But for cup and clapper all is gone. .
      Robert Henryson, *Testament of Cresseid*[1]

A fateful second opinion

In a letter dated June 24, 1492, a panel of seven jurors belonging to the main parish of Diedenhofen, part of the bishopric of Metz in Lorraine, requested the examination of a fellow parishioner. The petition was addressed to the municipal authorities of Cologne. This old Roman settlement on the banks of the Rhine River was an important, large *Reichsstadt* among the patchwork of principalities and free cities comprising the Habsburg Empire under Frederick III. In spite of hefty losses from the plague, the total population, including that of its suburbs, remained at about 40,000.[2] At the time of the request, however, the imperial city was still trying to recover from a severe political and financial crisis that had started in 1473 as a conflict between the local Archbishop, Rupert of the Palatinate, and the city's cathedral chapter and municipal council.[3]

In their message to the municipal council, the jurors demanded that Grette Swynnen Thielen, a housewife and Diedenhofen burgher, be examined once more for signs of leprosy and that a final verdict be officially communicated in writing to the panel reviewing her case. "The reasons for this investigation is that we presume that she had attempted to stop the spread of the disease over her body and hide it with the help of medicines. Therefore, it is necessary that you must precisely examine and observe everywhere," wrote the parishioners,[4] adding that "we trust you completely and want to always show you our good will and appreciation in this matter."[5]

The letter made it clear that Grette was being cruelly harassed and accused of having contracted the dreadful disease. Aware of the allegations, her fellow parishioners had already sent the poor woman for a diagnostic inspection at a leper house in the city of Metz. Here Grette was pronounced leprous, a finding she apparently rejected, demanding a second probe and opinion from the authorities in Cologne. Soon after the receipt of this letter, the presumptive leper was brought to Cologne by Gerhart, a Diedenhofen emissary, to meet with the authorities at Melaten, at the time the most important leper house in the Lower Rhine region. Here the institution's *Probemeister* or chief inquisitor and his panel of lepers were to inspect her body thoroughly, as well as perform a venesection and examine her blood.

As with others before her, Grette's ordeal may have started with a summons to appear before a public tribunal for an examination or a personal visit from a cleric or other Church officials deemed competent to diagnose the disease. Traditionally, the examination of suspected lepers was often performed by parish panels composed of clergy and lay jurors, or sometimes by lepers summoned from the nearest leper house. Although the stakes were very high, the criteria employed in reaching a positive conclusion remained somewhat vague, even arbitrary, ranging from the presence of a red nose and face, strabismus, facial pustules, nasal voice, and hoarseness to the appearance of scabies and other skin rashes. The final assessment or diagnosis was a much feared determination, subject to a wide spectrum of personal intrigues and local manipulations involving competition for love, money, and power. Three judgments could be rendered: healthy, leper, or suspected leper, the last condition to be examined again a year later.

Although the number of certified cases was rapidly declining in Europe, and although less emphasis was placed on contagion, the diagnosis of leprosy continued to have profound legal, social, and religious implications. Those officially branded as sufferers of this disease continued to be forced into isolation. Acceptance of new inmates into a leper house such as Melaten, however, also carried significant financial obligations. Lepers with no funds but clear signs of disease were perceived as unpleasant burdens to share food and shelter. Suspicions were increasingly voiced throughout Europe about the integrity of institutional admission panels, usually appointed by municipal authorities. Given their institutional economic status, many in-house panels of lepers charged with admissions to their houses deliberately avoided distinguishing between true sufferers and pretenders. Prospects of a sheltered, somewhat comfortable life attracted many aged, non-leprous individuals, who were now welcomed if they were wealthy enough to benefit the institution with their mandatory entrance fees.

To create the appearance of a fair process consonant with the original wishes of their founders, leper houses such as Melaten had selected their oldest and most respected inmate as the internal examiner or *Probemeister*. He was asked to conduct his own inquiry into the desirability of accepting specific new lepers. Now, in Grette's time, Melaten had adopted the practice of selecting a six-member commission of inmates or *prebendaries* to carry out such duties after one of their masters was discovered selling a number of falsified certificates of leprosy to healthy applicants. Each panel member took an oath promising to reach a fair conclusion, refuse all gifts or bribes, and keep no secrets concerning the screening procedure. They were not to harm anyone intentionally with an unwarranted diagnosis. All examiners, usually three men and three women, were asked to carry out their inspections of the candidates on clear days one-half hour after dawn or before sunset.

Grette's plight was not unusual in northern Europe. The disfiguring disease was still affecting many people, although the number of those contracting it seemed to be rapidly dwindling. In the Rhineland, for example, one suspected *Aussätziger* (an excluded one), who was also dissatisfied with the verdict pronounced by the inmates at Melaten, demanded in 1447 an examination by physicians. His request, and other similar ones, eventually prompted the medical faculty at the University of Cologne to begin offering in 1455 its own diagnostic services. Founded in 1388, the university had sponsored medical studies for over a century. By the 1470s its medical faculty, composed of 3 professors and about 14 students, enjoyed a certain prominence in the German lands. In 1477, Cologne's municipal authorities approved the right of university members to examine lepers and a year later accepted the validity of a medical verdict or *iudicium*, thus placing it above judgments arrived at by panels of lepers. Soon, the *Leprabeschau* became such a popular procedure that for the year 1492–1493 a total of 21 medical inspections were said to have been performed.[6] The choice of a medical commission to diagnose leprosy reflected the growing availability and prestige of licensed physicians in urban Europe since the fourteenth century.[7] In Cologne the first official examination took place as late as 1486, but soon word spread that, in spite of their cost, such medical proceedings were more rational and trustworthy than those conducted by the laity, a tribute to the growing cultural authority of medical professionals.[8]

In Grette's case, however, the new probe was originally requested from the

panel of lepers but may have been subjected to medical verification. These examinations by the physicians were usually performed under the direction of Dean
Bertram Bau (ca. 1439–1518).[9] Bau was one of the most active examiners in the
college. Between 1491, the date of his first official investigation, and 1516, shortly
before his death, the dean was said to have participated in over 100 such ap-
praisals, which were a good source of additional income for faculty members.[10]
The formal examination usually took place in the dean's house and was attended
by the entire medical faculty, including professors and licentiates. Witnesses
known to be trustworthy citizens of the community or countrymen of the accused
were allowed to be present and explain the reasons for their presumption. Suspects, in turn, could also offer their own witnesses for the defense, including relatives, friends, or co-workers. To begin the ritual, the accused took an oath, touching a crucifix or Bible, or first going to a notary public. Persons like Grette solemnly
promised not to bring any legal complaints or "cause trouble to the masters of
the faculty, either as a group or individually, if [they] received a diagnosis different from the one [they] wanted to hear."[11] Thus, participating academics were to
be protected from lawsuits.

The entire medical procedure was divided into three parts, beginning with an
interrogation of the suspect and other witnesses, followed by a physical inspection, and finally the requested examination of the blood.[12] Since leprosy was assumed to be hereditary or congenital, the alleged victim was asked whether relatives also suffered from the disease. Sexual relations with a leper were also probed,
as well as other habits. The connection between the disease and sexual intercourse
extended to an investigation of the suspect's libido, with increases in the frequency
and intensity of sex considered telltale signs of leprosy's presence. Finally, physicians tried to ascertain a postulated humoral imbalance toward melancholia and
violence that they associated with the disease. Sudden mood swings, anger, violence, aggression, depression, and the frequency of dreams and nightmares were
considered suspicious.[13]

Grette's answers went unrecorded. Like others before her, she was already being subjected to both the marginalization and compassion that characterized Europe's ambivalent response to the disease. Who was she? Her characterization as
a housewife implied that she was married, possibly with children. How did she
discover those fateful manifestations that pointed to the most stigmatized condition in medieval society? Was it a swelling on the forehead, a raspy voice, a numbness in the palm of her hand, or painless bruises on her limbs or back? The letter addressed to the Cologne authorities implied that Grette had desperately tried
to hide the early manifestations of her tragic disease. To cover telltale discolored
skin spots, lepers often employed red dye obtained from madder root and prepared with honey. An astringent ointment was also used to soften some hardening skin patches. Yet, in spite of camouflage, leprosy would inexorably progress
until the ugly and increasingly dysfunctional signs were exposed for all to see and

denounce.[14] After some denial and fear, did a horrified Grette share her findings with her family or keep them to herself? Consistent with social expectations, did she withdraw from her usual responsibilities and routines, terrified of detection and accusation?

After the interview came the physical examination. Individuals subjected to a medical assessment had to wear light clothing and were asked to disrobe in front of the entire panel. A detailed inspection usually started with the face. Six essential signs were sought: changes in the elliptical form of eyes and ears, even bloodshot eyes; the presence of a wild, "satirical" gaze; loss of eyelashes and eyebrows; nasal swelling and deformity, especially narrowing of the nostrils (elicited with the help of a nasal speculum); changes in the color and shape of the lips; and voice changes. A rough, raspy, honking voice suggestive of a palate lesion was always very suspicious and was carefully investigated by having the suspect sing. Muscular weakness could be determined by asking the person to grip a small ball with the thumb and fingers. Among the main bodily signs were changes in skin color, hair loss, and thickened skin patches with no sensation—*signum expertissimum.* These were palpated and pricked with a sharp stylus to elicit a painful response. Scarred, ulcerated, or even mutilated limbs such as the characteristic "bear claw" foot or hand were a *signum malum* that would immediately confirm the presence of leprosy.

Regarding the blood test demanded by the parishioners of Diedenhofen, the *Probemeister*, like the Cologne professors, probably followed a number of procedures used for the past two centuries. A barber performed the necessary phlebotomy and extracted sufficient blood to fill various metal cups. First, the color was observed because suspects with gray or dark blood were deemed leprous. Next came probes of the blood's consistency. Thick, oily blood, detected by rubbing a few drops in the palm of the hand, was suspicious. A grainy, sandy consistency could be another positive sign. As the slowly coagulating blood in a cup was scrutinized, the tester added three grains of common salt to observe its rate of dissolution. If the salt mixed rather rapidly with the blood, the individual in question undoubtedly suffered from incipient leprosy, a test devised by Theodoric of Cervia (1205–1298). This procedure, employed by lay and medical panels, completed the evaluation, and, as was their custom, the examining professors and licentiates would have enjoyed a sumptuous dinner paid for by the persons requesting the examination. In addition, each professor received a gold coin and the licentiates a small barrel of wine. Another fee was requested for use of the University of Cologne's certificate and seal.

Whether by the leper panel alone or in conjunction with the medical committee, the final consensus was that Grette Thielen was indeed significantly "stained" and afflicted with "*mallaitschafft*" (leprosy). An official letter, written in German and dated July 2, 1492, was prepared and signed by the municipal authorities, stressing that those who had taken this diagnostic assignment had proceeded according to established methods. All examiners declared under oath that this was their true verdict. "Now it is up to the church authorities and God to follow through."[15] Over the next century, however, with authority shifting from leper panels to medical boards, such a positive determination became less frequent because university commissions increasingly took an expectant attitude in questionable cases. In many situations, a *sententia suspensoria* (suspended sentence) was followed by another examination after 18 months, with the suspect encouraged to seek medical advice and treatment during the interim. As balneology—the science of bathing—flourished during the 1500s, many suspected lepers were also sent to the thermal sulfurous baths near Aachen to rule out other skin conditions. If a diagnostic error had occurred, there was also the possibility of appealing the final verdict and even requesting release from the leper house if institutionalization had already occurred.[16]

Provided with official documentation of Grette's leprosy, parishioners back in Diedenhofen were now empowered to pronounce the Church-directed official *iudicium* or judgment of moral corruption and recommend her segregation from the community. As a religious device to solemnly ratify the diagnosis and the finality of the subsequent banishment, Grette Thielen's *separatio* ceremony was meant to separate the sick parishioner permanently from community, friends, and family. During a mass attended by all interested members, the leper was made aware of all current proscriptions and given last rites. In fact, some victims were placed briefly in a grave to symbolize irreversible social death. The religious judgment was followed by a loss of civil rights, whereby the newly designated leper was stripped of all ownership or property, with no further rights to any inheritance. In essence, the leper became legally a "living dead" person, to be divorced and driven from home and community. Grette's world was shattered. The most frequent effect of such a separation was the conversion of lepers into unemployed and often homeless members of society, forced to eke out a marginal living by becoming itinerant beggars who survived on alms. Another leper in similar circumstances had commented earlier, "this illness brings poison and wounds; on the one hand sobs and sighs as I wait for the worst, on the other hand I am repaid. God has me serve him with my suffering."[17]

In many places, lepers received special gray clothing, a cape or vestment with a yellow cross, together with a hat and gloves. In addition, they were provided with a warning signal—either a clapper or a horn—to be used whenever healthy individuals approached. At times a long pole was furnished so that lepers could retrieve alms placed in a cup or point out items they wished to purchase. Behaving like a leper reinforced the stigmatized social definition. One possible alternative for Grette was to seek refuge in a leper house. Could she be admitted at Melaten west of Cologne? After all, its *Probemeister* had certified her status after she had been sent to him for a second opinion.

Views of leprosy and the construction of stigma

The beginnings of a disease resembling our modern understanding of leprosy are difficult to pinpoint, especially since, in earlier times, some of its manifestations were confused with a variety of other chronic skin conditions.[18] Whether current patterns of individual immunity and infectivity operated in earlier times is unknown.[19] Yet, if our current typology is any guide, all discussions of a medieval disease called leprosy must correspond to advanced stages of the type now recognized as lepromatous, since the much milder tuberculoid variety would have been confused with other skin ailments. Historically, those persons identified as lepers were easily recognizable by family, friends, and community if they were affected with the severe deformities and progressive loss of limbs characteristic of the lepromatous variety. Their rotting flesh, usually infected and host to worms and insects, constituted a unique and characteristic combination of symptoms in the annals of human disease.[20]

In the Near East and the Mediterranean, traditional references to the Old Testament, especially the Book of Leviticus chapters 13 and 14, merely suggested the presence of a condition (originally identified by Jewish priests as *zaraath*) judged to reflect moral impurity since its victims were cast outside the temple. Whatever the problem, sufferers were seemingly excluded from normal society.[21] When translating this document into Greek around 200 BC, scholars linked the unnamed condition to *lepra*, a term denoting a scaly skin condition in which peeling and flaking skin fragments were compared to falling snowflakes.[22] Henceforth many repulsive dermal discharges occurring with diseases subsequently identified as smallpox, psoriasis, and endemic syphilis were originally grouped together under the generic term *lepra*—meaning "scaly."

This designation stood in marked contrast with another truly deforming condition affecting the face and extremities. The ancient Greeks had called it *elephantiasis* because of the appearance of thick, coarse skin. Others simply named the entire disease complex the *morbus Phoenicus* to reflect its Palestinian origin and frequency during the first millennium BC. Perhaps this condition had already been introduced into the Near East centuries earlier following the campaigns of Alexander the Great. In fact, literary sources including Hindu medical texts suggest the presence of such a disease in the Far East and India around 600–300 BC. Later, this Palestinian connection, highlighted in various Scriptural passages dealing with tainted so-called lepers during Christ's lifetime, prompted another label: the "disease of Lazarus."

As with many other infectious diseases, the incidence of leprosy probably increased in direct proportion to population growth, urbanization, and commerce, especially during the early centuries of the Byzantine Empire.[23] From the scanty evidence, clusters of sufferers seemed to have inhabited virtually all major population centers of the eastern Mediterranean. The grotesque clinical manifestations of advanced leprosy, especially the sights and smells of gradual facial destruction, loss of limbs, and disability—often interpreted as living death—appear to have created sufficient fear and revulsion to warrant physical separation.[24] It is possible that the lepromatous form of the disease was more common in medieval times, a fact possibly associated with the early and ineffective immunological response.[25] Centuries later, it is alleged, gradual resistance followed, thus giving rise to the nondeforming tuberculoid form.[26]

In a sermon given as early as 379 AD, St. Gregory of Nazianzen reiterated earlier views by describing lepers as "men already dead except to sin, often dumb, with festering bodies whose insensible limbs rotted off them, heartbreaking and horrifying spectacles of human ruin, objects of repugnance and terror, driven from the house, the marketplace, the village, and the fountain, and persecuted even by their own parents."[27] Such a view stressed the ghoulish physical characteristics of sufferers, leading to an apparent breakdown of family and community networks that usually provided assistance to the sick. A disease with such abhorrent manifestations was a great challenge to early Christians, who prided themselves on belonging to a religion that included consoling and healing among its good works. Disgust at the sight of infected sores and fear of contagion led to banishment from populated areas.[28] At the same time, incurable lepers with their rotting flesh became powerful reminders of the brief life of suffering and death faithful Christians needed to focus on. Indeed, the lepers' clinical manifestations could be exploited for the work of Christian conversion and redemption. But how could the prevailing social ostracism be justified? In response to this challenge, Christianity constructed a rather ambiguous but nevertheless plausible moral theory based on ideas and practices depicted in the Old and New Testaments.

From the start, two seemingly contradictory views emerged. One was based on the Old Testament disease concepts proclaiming leprosy a divine punishment for sins, with links to other "unclean" bodily secretions, including menstrual blood, and sexual taboos such as intercourse during menstruation, sodomy, and others. Another view considered the disease as a gift of God and labeled its sufferers—pauperes Christi—Christ's special poor. Included in this notion were a series of Scriptural passages wherein Christ healed lepers by touch because they professed faith in the new religion. Singled out for such miracles in the Scriptures of Matthew, Mark, and Luke, lepers came to be regarded as individuals who in spite of their perceived sinfulness were closer to God.

Since the Church became instrumental in upholding a moral definition of leprosy, it also created procedures to officially identify lepers. Based on information provided by family or other community members, ecclesiastical authorities were chosen to make such determinations. As in Grette's case, accusations were combined with physical inspections to reach a verdict. To deal with the common practices of exclusion, the Church at the Synod of Ankyra in 314 established a special religious ritual officially separating lepers from their congregations. Such ceremonies were designed to sanctify the leper's segregation from family and community, thereby condemning the sick to a life of unemployment and poverty often leading to starvation and death. Lest anyone feel too guilty about this religiously sanctioned ostracism, the separation was no longer predicated on the corrupting physical qualities of lepers, but rather on their moral failings. At the same time, the presumed sinners were consoled by the notion that God had marked them in a special way, thus offering opportunities for redemption. Indeed, the leper's horrible condition was eventually conceptualized in the Middle Ages as representing a temporal purgatory on earth. The implication was that, after death, some of these unfortunate individuals would ascend directly to heaven. Separated from society, lepers could therefore contribute to their own atonement and eventual salvation by simply coming to terms with their sufferings and living an exemplary moral life.

During the early Middle Ages, the Church essentially "owned" leprosy. Having defined the character of lepers, the canonical authorities continued to organize their methods of diagnosis and separation while taking responsibility for shelter and care. A papal announcement by Gregory II (726) and a series of stipulations of the Concilium Germanicum (743) insisted on the separation of lepers during the celebration of the Eucharist. Throughout the Carolingian Empire, ordinances were passed forbidding lepers to mix with healthy people as Christian society began to put more distance between the sufferers and society at large.[29]

If public opinion concerning leprosy was based on a hodgepodge of religious beliefs and observations of physical corruption, medical theories about the nature and transmission of this disease were equally inconsistent.[30] A severe ailment suggestive of leprosy had been observed by Alexandrian physicians around the time of Erasistratus (320 BC). Two distinguished medical authors, Aretaeus and Rufus of Ephesus (98–117), both described *leontiasis*, a severely disfiguring ailment that resulted in a lion-like face. Aretaeus linked *leontiasis* with another condition called *satyriasis*, characterized by red cheeks and excessive sexual drive. Galen, in turn, sometimes placed both the Greek *elephantiasis*—with its manifestations suggestive of modern lepromatous leprosy—and *lepra*—a skin disorder—within the same category. Later, Galen's Islamic followers translated the Greek elephantiasis as *Juzam*, eventually known as the *lepra Arabum*, while the name *elephantiasis* was given to another disease with characteristic swellings of the legs.[31]

Galen tried to explain the most typical disease manifestations of *elephantiasis Graecorum* as the result of excess black bile. For all these authors, however, the disease was obviously incurable and fatal, believed to be contracted through the medium of air from some particular miasma or atmospheric poison.[32] The classical humoral verdict that leprosy, like many other skin disorders, was a dry and cold condition, was repeated by subsequent medical commentators such as Oribasius and Paul of Aegina. Later, Constantinus Africanus again stressed the importance of venereal contact or corrupted air, food, or drink, as well as a popular notion that leprosy could result from contact with adulterous females during their menstrual period, an idea in harmony with the Christian construction of sinful behavior as the primary cause of this disease. Medical authors also believed that sustained close contact with those already sick produced contagion through the repeated breathing of air corrupted by the leper. Significant fears of contagion were mostly expressed in relation to illegitimate sexual intercourse. The principal medieval source remained Avicenna and his *Canon of Medicine*, followed by special treatises on the subject such as *Lilium Medicine* (1303), written by Bernard de Gordon, and Guy de Chauliac's *Chirurgie* (1363). All authors tried to link the clinical manifestations with humoral imbalance.[33] However, great importance was placed on an individual's constitution or complexion for possible susceptibility in contracting the disease.

Although subject to wide local variations, the social responses to leprosy in Europe can be divided into three stages: a period before 1100 featuring the separation of lepers from society to protect the healthy; a middle span characterized by stricter isolation of the sick between 1100 and 1350, when the disease was said to have reached its peak; and a final era of lingering stigmatization after 1350, when leprosy seemed to be on the decline. Given the rural nature of early medieval Europe, leprosy initially seems to have been detected mainly in the countryside, moving gradually north from the Mediterranean area. Lepers were first recognized in Lombardy and Gaul during the late 400s and then in England about a century later. Segregation seemed predicated on traditional Christian views of presumed sinfulness and necessary punishment, as well as leprosy's gruesome physical mutilations, which did not respect class or gender. At first, lepers continued to visit their families and participate in the religious life of their parishes. A letter by Pope Gregory II in 726 allowed lepers to join the healthy for evening meals in their communities provided that they refrained from touching others. Some wealthy lepers fashioned their own seclusion on landed estates or in urban houses. Diseased monks, provided with special cells, remained in their monasteries.[34]

Separation created homelessness and unemployment among many sufferers of leprosy, prompting further needs for shelter and assistance. Fortunately, early medieval society continued to hold a favorable view of poverty. As subjects of public sympathy and charitable assistance, lepers were placed in the same category as pilgrims and hermits. The same Church authorities who officially judged lepers and mandated their separation were among their most valuable patrons. At the Council of Orleans in 549 (canon 21) and the Council of Lyon in 583 (canon 6), the Church declared that bishops were responsible for supporting lepers living in their dioceses, supplying them with the basic necessities of shelter—including separate houses—food, and clothing. While this segregation policy appeared to be both cruel and charitable, it created a class of marginalized individuals increasingly subjected to social bias and cultural stigma. Allowed to collect alms in public and to live by themselves just past the town walls or near major roads, lepers occupied a special but widely accepted niche in society.[35]

Judging by the growing number of institutions founded to house its sufferers, leprosy became more prevalent between 1100 and 1350. Such a correlation, however, may be deceiving. So-called hospitals for lepers and the sick poor were often very small establishments housing a handful of inmates in a period when an increasingly broad spectrum of lay patrons began sponsoring charitable enterprises. Perhaps the "epidemic" was simply a social phenomenon, fueled by the awareness that a significant number of prominent persons had contracted the disease.[36] More likely, clusters of newly arrived urban poor streaming from the countryside, among them sufferers of skin diseases, cripples, and children seemed to be affected. Not surprisingly, the presumed epidemic of leprosy occurred during periods of rapid demographic change, frequent and massive human migrations, and severe economic dislocations that produced significant social and cultural flux.[37]

Moreover, both returning crusaders and pilgrims brought disfiguring leprosy to the attention of European society.[38] Indeed, thousands of visitors returning from the Holy Land had witnessed the pitiful sight of begging lepers on the most heavily traveled roads to the Near East. Now their trained eyes seemed to detect similarly affected individuals at home. Given their facial distortions, voice changes, and hand lesions, lepers were quite restricted in communicating with the healthy.[39] Without distinction of class and gender, a new spirit of fear and hostility toward urban lepers gripped the population, fueled by rumors of widespread concealment and deliberate infection of the healthy. Under such circumstances, the religious aspects of leprosy were somewhat downplayed. Instead, the disease was increasingly interpreted as being contagious, and cities began revising their statutes to prevent more than ever before physical contact between the healthy and the sick. Feeding the growing social stigma, urban dwellers were encouraged to ferret out the lepers in their midst and denounce them to the authorities. Laws were passed punishing those who harbored sufferers of the disease.

Provisions of the Third Lateran Council of 1179 reinforced the separation of lepers by banning them from parish churches and burial in their cemeteries. European societies responded by increasing the tempo of Christian charity, which was no longer sponsored exclusively by Church authorities. New legal rules made the religious separation an opportunity for redistribution of landed estates and urban property. Since many aristocratic lepers could no longer remain secluded, some leper houses were now generously endowed by private donors who became inmates. As facilities and staffs multiplied in some establishments, other houses shared the fate of many contemporary hospitals, fighting for a limited share of alms and teetering on the edge of bankruptcy.

To a great extent, therefore, leprosy in the 1200s became the responsibility of a network of religious and lay patrons, including individual donors, confraternities, and municipalities. In earlier times, the most common work of lepers had been to beg for alms in nearby cities and towns to raise sufficient funds for the maintenance of their own hospices. Like other events in their jurisdiction, this activity was now increasingly regulated by burgeoning municipal governments. To avoid all possibilities of physical contact of lepers with the healthy, many cities throughout Europe began imposing stricter limits on the distance to be covered and the times of the day allowed to begging lepers. Although many physicians continued to deemphasize the possibility of contagion in leprosy, popular belief may have suggested otherwise. More ominous was the linkage of leprosy with unemployment and civil disorder. Faced with rapid economic growth and social dislocation, European cities tried to both safeguard public order and protect their healthy citizens. Thus, urban governments in the thirteenth century enforced stricter segregation rules for lepers, often confining them to nearby leper houses or expelling them from their towns together with foreigners and other undesirables.[40]

After 1350, social responses to leprosy in Europe were further influenced by the now centuries-old and well-established cultural stigma of the dangerous, morally degraded, and physically repulsive leper. Ironically, such efforts coincided with the perception that the disease was gradually disappearing. Yet, in a world increasingly burdened by epidemic diseases such as plague, popular fears that leprosy could indeed represent another health menace persisted. Thus, municipalities and parishes made even greater efforts to isolate remaining lepers as potentially contagious individuals, a process that accelerated after the appearance of the Black Death in 1349. Public attention, of course, quickly shifted to this major epidemic killer and may have deprived the "scaly" disease of its previous share of scrutiny and victims. At the same time, leprosy became gradually medicalized, with fateful diagnoses increasingly made by panels of both physicians and lepers. Their objective was the proper identification of true lepers before committing them to lifelong isolation in surviving leper houses. By the late 1400s, when Grette Thielen was sent to Cologne for her second examination, leprosy had become somewhat rare in many parts of Europe, and soon confusion arose between its manifestations and those of an ailment to be known as the "pox," a condition eventually equated with venereal syphilis.

In marked contrast with other infectious diseases such as plague and smallpox, leprosy in Europe never achieved the same demographic, economic, or political importance. Obviously, the disease was devastating to individuals who were discovered and later certified as suffering from the disease. This extraordinary social reaction was based on a complex series of prejudices created by religious judgments, the mutilating physical aspects of the disease, and need for convenient scapegoats in a period of turmoil and rapid social change. Illustrative of this attitude was the notion that lepers, as well as Jews and heretics, were responsible for deliberately poisoning town wells and springs. When in 1321 a rumor started in the Perigueux and Carcassone areas of France that lepers had deliberately poisoned the waters, many were tortured and burned by the enraged inhabitants, reflecting the social anxieties of that age.[41]

Locus of confinement: Anatomy of leper houses

For lepers, the Christian tradition of institutional assistance goes back at least to the reign of Constantine the Great, when an imperial decree had ordered the expulsion of vagabond lepers from the city of Constantinople under the threat of death. The story is told that Zoticus, a high imperial official, defied the order and used public funds to house and care for lepers, an act for which he was supposedly executed. Although Nazianzen in the fourth century supported the central objective of a leper house, to collect and segregate individuals afflicted with that disease, he insisted that they should be well treated and have their souls saved. "This to me is the most wonderful achievement of all, the short road to salvation and the easiest ascent to heaven. We no longer have before our eyes the terrible and pitiable spectacle of men who are living corpses, dead in most their limbs, driven away from their cities and homes, public places, fountains, even from their dearest ones and more easily recognized by their names than by their bodily features."[42] The first leper house in the Latin West was established during the sixth century in Franconia, south Gaul, along the Rhone and Saone waterways, which were important for trade with the East. A typical example was Gregory of Tours' foundation in 560, another in Verdun and in Mastrich in 636, followed by St. Gall in 750. In small villages, the entire institution was under one roof at a stone's throw—about 200 yards—from the population.[43]

When Prodromos was hospitalized in 1140, even the Pantocrator Xenon was reputed to have had a section reserved for lepers. Based on the Byzantine model, many of these specialized shelters in Europe were called "houses of St. Lazar" or "lazarettos" because of their placement under the protection of Lazarus of Bethany. According to the Scriptures, Lazarus, apocryphally considered a leper, had been raised from the dead by Jesus. As noted, the same name was adopted by the original fraternity of monks caring for lepers in Jerusalem, later transformed into a separate order of chivalry, the Knights of St. Lazarus of Jerusalem. They assumed responsibility for a series of leper houses throughout Europe, including Burton Lazars, the chief house in England. Most of these institutions, especially in France, were modeled after the Jerusalem shelter.

Knights and pilgrims visiting Jerusalem were impressed by the care accorded to lepers and the fact that local practitioners seemed well acquainted with the disease. During Adolf of Cologne's visit to Jerusalem, for example, the most famous local leper in that city was none other than the son of King Amalric, Baldwin IV of Jerusalem (1161–1185).[44] In his 1172 *Description of the Holy Places*, Adolf's companion, Theoderic, had also mentioned the existence of a small hospice for lepers outside the walls of the city at its western gate. From the early 1100s on, a so-called Fraternity of Lepers of the House of St. Lazarus of Jerusalem—later known as the Knights of St. Lazarus—operated this institution with the help of generous endowments and a monastic administration.

Following the Knights of St. Lazarus' lead, medieval Europe began to establish a vast network of charitable leper houses during the twelfth century. These initial segregation efforts produced a plethora of individual huts and tents outside city walls and villages that initially were intended to assist poor lepers with food and shelter rather than care. The fact that some prominent aristocrats had contracted the disease, some perhaps during their participation in the campaigns in the Holy Land, must certainly have contributed to this founding impetus. Like other hospitals, individual establishments were granted rights by European rulers to hold fairs, collect tolls, and gather wood in royal forests. Many lepers remained itinerant vagrants living independently off the land in forests or begging near urban centers. Others, however, exchanged a free but lonely life of marginality and homelessness for the safety of a shelter with a highly structured environment. Some individuals even mutilated their skin to gain admission. Since lepers seeking shelter came from different families, parishes, or even villages, the ecclesiastical authorities conceived the notion that they should be organized according to highly successful monastic models of prayer and work. In exchange for room and board, able individuals remained ambulatory, now begging for institutional alms in nearby towns and cities. Others lived in separate huts or small "lazar houses"—known as *maladeries* in France—but shared meals within a greater complex. Their increased numbers did not necessarily reflect a higher frequency of the disease. Scattered over the countryside, these facilities remained the norm in the early medieval period and closely mirrored the proliferation of other charitable shelters outside cities, on roads, and on mountain passes.

Although they needed to be away from settlements and centers of human activity, leper houses were usually placed near well-traveled routes or important crosspoints to make it easier for lepers to move around and beg for alms. In a concession to the prevailing theories of miasma and contagion that were linked to the transmission of leprosy, leper houses were eventually placed downwind from inhabited towns to prevent potential contamination. As with other contemporary hospitals, areas near flowing streams or rivers were selected to ensure a steady supply of fresh water. Like other shelters, most leper houses were of the dormitory variety and averaged fewer than 12 beds, each of them intended to accommodate several persons.

During the twelfth and thirteenth centuries, many larger Lazar houses, as well as other private hospitals throughout Europe, resembled self-sufficient medieval agricultural communities. Supported by a wave of donations, those located near larger towns became veritable monastic estates fenced in by stone walls, complete with a cluster of cottages or a common dormitory supplemented with kitchen facilities around or near a chapel. There were also workshops, granaries, gardens, cattle, and arable land. Here, under ecclesiastical supervision, the administration of the house followed the traditional economy of a medieval abbey. Even its internal organization, formulated in numerous statutes, was modeled after those already operative in monasteries, although perhaps not as closely supervised. As with all charitable foundations, private donors, royal officials, and local bishops had the right to make periodic visits and check on the use of funds and the level of care provided.

Provisions established by the Council of Paris (1212), the Council of Rouen (1214), and the Fourth Lateran Council (1215) demanded that caregivers working in all hospitals take vows and be governed by the rule of St. Augustine. Other regulations followed those originally established by the Hospitallers. Many communities of lepers, therefore, also selected their own superior or *magister*, although later a so-called *provisor*—usually a priest appointed by bishops, rulers, or municipal authorities—was put in charge. Under new rules authorized by the Third Lateran Council in 1179, the Church extended the separation of the lepers from the general population by authorizing the construction of chapels within the confines of a leper settlement, to be independently staffed by priests suffering from the disease. Each leper house was also authorized to have its own cemetery. As the ancillary staff expanded, separate accommodations were made available for priests, nurses, and servants.

In northern France, many Lazar houses consisted of a single large building containing a dormitory, refectory, and kitchen. All accommodations were strictly divided between men and women inmates, including living and food preparation areas. As their endowments expanded, these facilities became larger and less spartan. At St. Denis de Lecheres, in 1336, the principal building was a monastic lodge composed of a refectory surrounded by small individual cells. To ensure agricultural self-sufficiency, adjacent land was made available for farming. The complex at St. Denis had barns, stables, granaries, a pigsty, a root cellar, a wine press, and an oven. The surrounding acreage supplied wheat, rye, barley, and oats for bread, as well as the peas and beans for the inmates' meals. By 1227, the last will of Louis VIII suggested that there were 2,000 leper houses in France alone and perhaps at least as many in the rest of Europe.[45]

Grette Thielen's probable destination, Melaten, near Cologne, was first mentioned in 1180, a few years after the tragic death in Jerusalem of one of the city's sons, Adolf, our faithful pilgrim. Located a mile from the important western city gate on the Roman road to Aachen, this institution was privately funded by donations from wealthy lepers. After the first millennium, when leprosy first appeared there, Cologne had supported a number of small houses outside the city walls.[46] Following its destruction by imperial forces early in 1242, Melaten had risen from its ashes, with a new church consecrated to the Virgin Mary and St.

Dionysius in 1245 and indulgences granted by the archbishop to all who wished to aid this institution.[47]

This new phase allowed Melaten to expand its income and facilities, thanks to support from Pope Innocent IV, who in a series of bulls in 1247 exempted the institution from taxation. In an effort to stimulate the provision of alms, the pope also provided one-year indulgences to all future donors. Another bull placed the Melaten endowment and its inmates under special papal protection. At this point, Melaten began to attract donations of estates, houses, lands, and vineyards from relatives and friends of prominent inmates belonging to the archdioceses of Cologne, Trier, Lüttich, and beyond. Clerics were sent out to carry out further fund-raising, and all parish priests in the Cologne dioceses were empowered to collect gifts during the two consecutive Sundays before Lent.[48]

The initial use of church funds to provide dwellings and supplies was gradually supplemented and even replaced by private donations from local gentry and townspeople. Since Carolingian times, episcopal support had been joined by the collection of alms from local inhabitants. Thus, begging had been a necessary activity for new lepers, and inmates authorized for this purpose were periodically sent out to collect them, always in pairs, to prevent a possible diversion of the collected funds. Almsgiving was still an important charitable activity for all Christians who could afford it, but after 1350 the proliferation of welfare functions and the appearance of mendicant orders substantially diluted this effort. At the same time, the authority of local bishops over the supervision and management of leper houses in Europe was increasingly challenged by nearby municipal authorities, since the collected alms were provided by their townspeople. The result was a sharp decrease in monastic bequests in favor of endowments for chantries with perpetual prayers for the donor and his ancestors, a popular objective linked to the doctrine of purgatory and the need for indulgences.

Beginning in the twelfth century, additional financing for the leper houses derived from the incoming lepers themselves, as their estates were divided and the institutions came to claim a portion of these possessions. Surviving institutions often had generous endowments collected from their deceased inmates. Some persons suspected of suffering from leprosy were barred from entering because of poverty.[49] Under an arrangement, all revenues obtained from the institutional endowment were evenly divided among the inmates and dispensed in the form of an individual allowance called a *prebend*. This share was distributed on particular days to every inmate or *prebendary* in the form of money, food, salt, clothing, and other necessities.

Following the Black Death, revenues from agricultural leases plummeted because of labor shortages and the higher cost of farming. With the perception that many lepers lived in relative comfort in their splendid isolation, previous charitable impulses now often turned into outright hostility and even hate. Under these circumstances, hospitals and leper houses experienced dramatic decreases in donations that often spelled the ruin of smaller institutions lacking solid endowments. Not surprisingly, these financial hardships prompted Lazar houses to exploit the remaining inmates further precisely when their numbers seemed to be dwindling.

New conditions were imposed on those who expected to be admitted, leading to the gradual "gentrification" of leper houses. Gone were the early days when a handful of scattered huts on a roadside near a city or town provided free refuge to wandering lepers begging for alms. Many regulations now specified that the sick had to be from the affluent classes, at least at birth. Not only were incoming lepers often required to provide an admission fee and a number of household goods, including bedding, but many also needed to turn over substantial amounts of property or money from their estates to the institution's endowment. Moreover, most inmates dying in these Lazar houses had made out their wills in favor of the institutions. With additional charitable contributions from families and friends of an incoming wealthy leper, larger institutions not only survived the dearth of almsgiving but actually expanded their tax-free resources. These practices alarmed many financially strapped municipalities in the vicinity of the houses and led in the fifteenth century to efforts designed to control them.[50]

At most institutions, lax ecclesiastical supervision, absence of accountability, and sharp economic fluctuations made the role of house master vital to stability. As in other late medieval hospitals, many administrators were no longer in continuous residence and ruled through deputies, creating an administrative vacuum with predictable consequences. Frequent financial irregularities mirrored those of other charitable medieval institutions, notably monasteries and hospitals. Masters of the houses were also no longer bound by their previous vows of poverty, especially if they were laymen, and thus they often diverted institutional funds for personal gain.[51]

By Grette's time, changes in the legal and social status of lepers had led to the destabilizing possibility that certain inmates could recover their inheritance and possessions previously donated to leper houses. This was especially true of individuals who had entered without medical certification and were now able to convince a medical panel that they were not lepers This financial threat struck at the very heart of the institutions' previous endowment policies and further imperiled projected income. Without new recruits and with populations depleted by death, leper houses were often abandoned, casualties of a new era of modernity in European politics and economics. Others were transformed into municipal pesthouses, almshouses, homes for the aged or the orphaned, and even penitentiaries.

In 1385, the municipal leaders in Cologne prohibited the further provision of endowment property from landed estates to city hospitals and the leper house at Melaten because such assets were vulnerable to destruction during regional warfare. This policy created tension with the local archbishop over the legal jurisdiction of the leper house. In other cities, the economically driven power shift was even more sweeping. Responsibilities for gatekeeping functions, bookkeeping chores, visiting rights, and care of the lepers became the responsibility of the local mayor and his aldermen, while bishops were restricted to fulfilling all spiritual needs by appointing institutional chaplains. All these actions occurred at about the time when the number of lepers in such establishments began to dwindle.[52]

Inside Melaten, the traditional administrative structures were also changing in the fifteenth century. Traditionally, Melaten had operated with a *magister* at its helm, originally selected by the entire congregation. By the late 1300s, this man was appointed by a panel of three additional *magisters* or *provisores* who were prominent men of the city, a move that eventually placed the entire administrative and financial control of the Melaten house in the hands of Cologne's municipal government. Although master of a leper house remained an honorary position, city aldermen after 1385 selected their own candidates. Institutional masters were expected to have the rules read in the vernacular at least once a month to the congregation, and at Melaten they were also responsible for recording and reporting all financial transactions.

In truth, the concept of a *locus religiosus*—a religious space—had long ceased to apply to most leper houses, as both administrators and inmates ignored the original intentions of the charitable founders and considered the institution a source of profit and good living. Melaten had had its own brewmeister on board since 1429, plying inmates with his beer. By the early 1500s, this establishment took advantage of its prime location on the road to Aachen by adding a tavern to the complex and hiring an innkeeper. Henceforth, the former isolation facility provided weary but healthy travelers with hospitality in exchange for money. By the late 1400s, few true lepers were left in prominent British, French, and German institutions; the surviving individuals were mostly chronically ill or aged inmates who had made substantial donations to gain admission. This gradual but complete change in function converted the remaining leper houses into lay institutions with a wide spectrum of activities, although many continued to be used as isolation facilities for victims of the plague and the venereal "pox" believed to have been syphilis.[53]

Institutional rituals

Although Melaten's *Probemeister* and his commission had found Grette to be suffering from leprosy, admission to the institution was by no means certain. Payment of a fee was essential, and the candidate either sacrificed personal assets or requested subscriptions from friends and parishioners. No information is available about Grette's financial status or about whether her family or the Dieden-hofen authorities contributed toward her acceptance. Numerous establishments now also required from the leper an oath pledging to pray regularly, attend church, and avoid dancing, gambling, cursing, gossiping, and sexual intercourse.[54] In some houses, those allowed to enter brought their own bed, clothing, and kitchen uten-sils.[55] Although no records survive, we can assume that if Grette Thielen was in-deed admitted to Melaten, this would have occurred around the year 1492.

Recently, the institution had experienced hard times following the destruction of its buildings in 1474 as part of a series of defensive measures enacted by Cologne to stave off a siege by enemy troops.[56] Melaten's census was already down from a previous high of 100 inmates around the 1240s to about 25, brought together from the region around Cologne but also now including "strangers"—lepers from cities such as Mainz, Koblenz, and Frankfurt. In general, both sexes were equally represented, with married people having to make separate arrangements for ad-mission. Strict separation of men and women, characteristic of all Christian shel-ters, also applied to leper houses, and inmates of the opposite sex were never per-mitted to eat together or visit each other's quarters.[57] A fasting penance of eight days was meted out to anyone attempting such a transgression. Once admitted, the individual could not be banished from the house except for violation of in-stitutional rules. In virtually all leper houses, the threat of expulsion was effective in maintaining institutional order, since those who were expelled could be read-mitted only if they provided once more a full entry fee. Male inmates caught mak-ing romantic overtures to a woman were punished for 40 days, and those at-tempting to have sexual relations were expelled for one year. Pregnant lepers were allowed to stay until they gave birth before being permanently banished. Such ex-pulsion as punishment certainly contradicts the notion that European leper houses like Melaten were designed exclusively to prevent the spread of leprosy among the population.

Rituals of admission were patterned after the rites of the novitiate. Newcom-ers had to join the institution's *congregatio* by taking the modified Augustinian vows of obedience, celibacy, and poverty. As in other monastic communities, the titles "brother" and "sister" sought to reaffirm the religious character of the con-finement. Complete obedience to the master also implied acknowledgment of his spiritual leadership. The degree of isolation imposed by the monastic model var-ied considerably in each historical period and geographical location, although new ordinances and the replacement of alms for other sources of income curtailed the traditional forays into the nearby population centers. At Melaten, no member could leave the institution for visits to the city without the master's permission. In some houses visitors were allowed, at least until the mid-1200s, when the idea of stricter isolation became more popular. At that point, outsiders needed special permission to share a daytime meal with an inmate, usually a family member. Stiff penalties were imposed on lepers who left the house without permission, particularly if they stayed out overnight. At Andelys, in France, male lepers who made clandestine visits to their wives were expelled for at least a year, condemned to a life of vagrancy.[58]

Despite the stigma, life in a well-endowed leper house could be tolerable. Conditions, of course, varied considerably, depending on the size of the institution, its income, and the presence of auxiliary personnel, both religious and lay, to attend the sick. Like Grette Thielen, most new admissions with obvious signs of disease may have been resigned to their fate, expecting to spend the rest of their lives in the house and be buried there.[59] A fellow leper had expressed the predicament: "Two thoughts does my heart know: at the same time joy and pain, laughter and sighs, songs and sobs. Both in my sense and in my gaze . . . the body goes, the soul remains, so I dissolve and I remain."[60] At least Grette's daily struggle to deceive friends and parishioners about her condition was over. At the leper house, she could look forward to getting some rest and care without exposing her family members to embarrassment and penalties for harboring a stigmatized sufferer. Surrounded by servants who made beds, cleaned rooms, and cooked food, lepers could be comfortable in spite of the strictures imposed by the numerous regulations. Since leprosy was a chronic and crippling disease, the average institutional stay must have ranged widely, with many inmates remaining fairly active before dying of complications of their disease.

During their confinement, lepers required a great deal of emotional support and terminal nursing care. Indeed, the original function of houses such as Melaten was to address primarily the spiritual wants of their inmates and the salvation of their souls. Over time, in spite of administrative secularization and the progress made by medicine in understanding the disease, leprosy remained an expression of personal sinfulness, a cross to bear. Attendance at daily mass and the provision of sacraments were welcome routines. At religious services, lepers were given special breviaries but forbidden to touch the communion rail and altar. Confessions were heard at least three times a year: before Easter, Pentecost, and Christmas. Guided by priests—often lepers themselves—their special Christian status made intercessionary prayers particularly valuable to the patrons of the house. At Melaten, the officiating priest did not live on the premises but visited periodically from a nearby monastery. A sexton was also among the staff. He was in charge of the church and was responsible for the care of its cult objects.[61]

Regarding social needs, the objective of the leper house was to provide a restful and supportive environment far removed from the taunts and loathing of former neighbors and parishioners. Removal of people like Grette to a leper house reinforced the moral definition and sustained the stigma attached to this scourge among the general population. Bringing consolation and peace of mind to a group of people willfully removed from their society and dispossessed of all worldly goods was critical. In spite of the isolation and loneliness, the trade-offs of institutionalization benefited many of those who entered. At one level, it provided lepers with new opportunities for socialization after a harrowing period of self-withdrawal and rejection by family members. Bound by stigma and suffering, some inmates presumably formed friendships and derived support from each other. In the final analysis, both lepers and leper houses were involved in a never-ending loop that tended to magnify and exaggerate the disease's perceived social threat.[62]

In the beginning, the celibate form of life imposed on lepers, as well as rules for dress and behavior, followed contemporary monastic rules. The daily routine consisted of the traditional seven canonical hours announced at the sound of a bell. True to the wishes of an institution's early patrons, lepers were thus programmed to lead a disciplined and quiet life, but this was probably seldom successful. Unlike monks and nuns, most lepers had no religious vocation, nor had they voluntarily sought out a monastic environment. The meticulousness of the leper houses' rules suggests that rebellions against the stifling routines must have been common. From several accounts, inmates occasionally broke out into quarrels and brawls and challenged the absolute authority of the master. Physical violence, particularly if the attacker drew his adversary's blood, resulted in one year's expulsion. At Amiens in 1305, there was a strict ban against the possession of sharp utensils and potential weapons of all kinds, including wood and iron sticks.[63] Episodes of drunkenness and sexual liaisons between lepers and the auxiliary personnel were also reported. Indeed, sexual transgressions were always dutifully noted since they confirmed the prevailing cultural stigma of lepers as lascivious individuals. Punishments, including penance and fasting through withholding of the usual stipends of money and food, were questionable deterrents, although expulsion and its financial implications may have been more effective.

At the time of Grette's presumed admission to Melaten, the earlier emphasis on spiritual care and chaste living had slowly given way to much less strict regulations. The mundane pleasures of food and drink were assured by the comfortable financial status enjoyed by many surviving leper houses. With regard to diet, earlier religious considerations had restricted the use of meat to certain days of the week and prescribed fasting on holy days in accordance with the monastic regimen; bishops provided exemptions to very weak and ill inmates. Since the thirteenth century, however, the subsistence level at most leper houses was comparable if not superior to that of the poorer or even middling persons living in nearby urban environments.

Lepers traditionally ate two meals daily for which they received half a loaf of bread with half a gallon of beer in most English and German institutions, while the French houses served three pints of house wine. Before eating, a benediction or prayer was said by all those assembled. White, black, or brown bread constituted the main food staple in a leper house, prepared using varying proportions of wheat, barley, and rye. As part of their stipend, lepers also received an allocation of salt, fruits, and vegetables, perhaps half a bushel of peas and beans per month. Meat, especially roasted pork—in Melaten the much revered *Schweinebraten*—mutton, or fish, milk, poultry and boiled eggs, cakes, and sweetmeats could be served, often daily, as inmates were exempted from the usual fasting rules. At the leper establishment in Saint-Omer, near Lille, inmates during the thirteenth century received a "northern" version of the sustenance outlined above without the wine. Those punished for transgressions in Lille around 1239 received only bread and water and were forced to sit on the ground during mealtimes, facing the congregation. After ending their meals, the inmates would again pray—40 Our Fathers and the same number of Hail Marys—for the soul of the hospital's benefactors.[64]

Where lepers lived alone in their huts, they also got allotments of firewood for cooking and heating, candles, salt, and vinegar. At some institutions, the inmates came together only for meals and religious worship. Idleness and boredom may have been frequent problems. For lepers who were not yet physically impaired, the Benedictine injunction to perform physical labor also applied during the twelfth and thirteenth centuries. Thus, light farming or gardening activities were common between prayers and religious services. Others kept busy working in vineyards and olive groves, while some continued to assist in administrative chores linked to the exploitation of their donated lands and estates. All games for money, food, or drink, including dice, cards, and chess, were prohibited, and violations were punished by 40 days of penance.

Many lepers, of course, cared for bedridden inmates, a difficult and repugnant task. Although urban brotherhoods and confraternities functioning nearby often played important roles in the foundation and administration of hospitals and leper houses, they also became frequently involved as caregivers to bolster their own salvation efforts.[65] If present, confraternity members followed Augustinian rules of obedience, poverty, and chastity. Guided by an elder, they supplemented their nursing with Bible readings and the celebration of religious services in the house's chapel. At Melaten and other institutions, the nursing personnel consisted mostly of lay brothers and sisters whose religious devotion justified caring for these *pauperes Christi*. In most instances, they were aided in their work by hired servants. If Grette Thielen did indeed come to Melaten in 1492, she would have encountered a new cofraternity founded by Lentzo van der Wee and his wife, Margareta de Steynbusch, to serve the sick at this institution. These men and women had obtained authorization for their charitable work from the archbishop of Cologne.[66]

Nothing is known regarding the availability of medical treatments at leper houses. Traditional strategies designed to remove offending humors from the body through the use of purgatives and diuretics usually applied to incipient cases of this disease, not the advanced stages represented in a leper house. In most institutions, efforts must have focused solely on spiritual salvation. Corruption and decay were seen as part of life itself.[67] Most contemporary medical authorities stressed the incurability of the disease "once leprosy reaches the manifest corruption of one's form and figure."[68] Without the presence of physicians, care in leper houses must have been limited to dietary prescriptions, fresh air, and the usual bathing and bloodletting routines.[69] Palliation was perhaps attempted, with the use of mercurial ointments and herbal lotions to dress the decomposing flesh.[70] For cases of advanced leprosy, Guy de Chauliac, a French surgeon, had identified three distinct therapeutic objectives: moistening the drying body, strengthening the heart and other vital organs, and minimizing the deformities.[71]

In Grette's time, the selection of specific remedies was still based on principles of signature and sympathy whereby the postulated cure shared some physical characteristics with the manifestations of the disease. The notion, widely accepted since antiquity, was that God had provided humankind with proper remedies that could be discovered through clues or "signatures" pointing to their therapeutic affinity. Since Galen's times, viper flesh had been an important medicinal agent, linking the poisonous character of snakes with the ability to shed their old skins, a hope lepers still entertained regarding their own cutaneous lesions. When available, viper flesh boiled with dill served as a broth and was employed as a powder. Hedgehog meat and cooked nettles in wine were other dietary items based on their similarities with the drying, itching, rough skin of a leper. Another popular signature was the bleeding heart and other herbs from the *fumaria* family, because its purple, red, and black blossoms and ash-gray leaves suggested leprous skin lesions.[72]

Medieval healers used domestic ointments prepared from burdock weed, swallow droppings, stork fat, and sulfur. Corrupted blood was removed by phlebotomy. For progressive hoarseness, rose honey gargles were commonly prescribed. Barber-surgeons were occasionally summoned to burn away infected portions, amputate limbs, or excise dead flesh with razors, taking advantage of the local, disease-induced numbness. In fainthearted patients, caustic chemicals were used to achieve similar effects.[73] If Grette Thielen lived in Melaten, she may have been subjected to such treatments. Less is known about the psychological trauma lepers endured in the final stages of their disease as embodiments of decay and fragmentation, but it may have been severe, as material continuity was considered crucial to personal identity and eventual resurrection.[74]

Death represented the end of God's earthly punishment, the awaited consummation of a terrible ordeal. House rules encouraged the magister to hire servants who would remain at the bedside of those who were dying, changing their clothing and keeping them warm, especially during winter.[75] Perhaps also cared for by the solicitous members of the institution's confraternity, Grette Thielen may have spent several years at Melaten before the complications of her progressive disease proved fatal. At about this time, the average age of death for female lep-

ers was 33 years, a full 6 years sooner than in the population at large.[76] Last rites
and burial in consecrated ground were the last perquisites.[77]

> Here I bequeath my corpse and carrion
> With worms and toads to be rent;
> My cup and clapper, and my ornament,
> And all my gold the leper folk shall have,
> When I am dead, to bury me in the grave.
> Robert Henryson, *Testament of Cresseid*[78]

PESTHOUSES OR LAZARETTOS

Rome has resorted to celestial helpers as well as human aids for its health. At the first signs
of disease, your Excellency has again executed the first steps of the same public health provisions, namely the containment of such harsh pestilence and the reversal of common mis-
fortunes.

Broadside dedicated to Prince Mario Chigi, 1657[79]

Trastevere : Rome's early plague spot

Late in July 1656, four middle-aged women living at the San Salvatore della Corte
tenement near Ponte Rotto came down with headaches and a fever. Both Marina
de Rossi and Catharina d'Uliva were 40 years old, Clementia and Cecilia di Giovanni somewhat younger. Nothing is known about their family status or occupations. Perhaps they were housewives running small boarding houses in the low-
lying, damp slum of Trastevere across the Tiber River from Rome.[80] Normally,
such illness would have been barely noticed in a crowded suburban neighborhood
of poor people where the burden of disease was always heavy. However, this fateful summer, Rome was in the early throes of a plague epidemic allegedly imported
from Naples.[81] Since the spring, a third of the entire Neapolitan population—
about 100,000 people—had already died as the disease raged out of control.[82] If
the fevers afflicting the women were to be linked to plague, forceful removal to a
lazaretto—a segregated, often makeshift facility—was a definite possibility. These
pesthouses, often former leper houses or convents, were widely feared as prison-
like houses of death.

Before the seventeenth-century outbreak in Rome, plague or pestilence had
frequently visited the Italian city-states, as well as the rest of Europe, since the
Black Death of 1348.[83] Originating in endemic areas in central Asia and Africa, a
disease with clinical characteristics suggestive of modern plague first came to the
attention of populations in Libya, Egypt, and Syria during the Hellenistic period.[84]

After an extensive period of inactivity, a second pandemic occurred during the sixth century—the so-called plague of Justinian (531–580 AD), spreading from the Middle East to areas of Western Europe.[85] Successive epidemics followed, affecting the major urban centers of the burgeoning Islamic empire before disappearing again in the eleventh century.[86]

By the thirteenth century, the existence of a network of caravan trade with Asia, as well as military movements across Asian grasslands, may have contributed once more to a westward spread of illness. By 1346, plague had broken out at the Crimean port of Caffa and spilled from there into the Mediterranean Coastlands. By June 1348, all Italian and Spanish ports had been affected. Poor harvests and sporadic famines in Europe had already created overcrowding in many urban centers as rural refugees streamed into cities in search of food. Thanks to an active shipping web connecting the Mediterranean with northern European ports, the plague slowly advanced in that direction, finally reaching the Scandinavian countries in 1350.[87]

Although Europe had already suffered a number of earlier epidemics of infectious disease, the Black Death of 1348–1350 shocked the continent. Its rapid spread left behind a trail of millions of people who quickly perished, causing major social dislocations. In fact, it is estimated that over 25 million people died in Europe alone, about a fourth of the entire population. In a sense, late medieval European cities, like their earlier counterparts in the East, had shaped their own distinctive ecology of disease that now welcomed a new pestilence. Crowding, lack of sanitary facilities, and lack of garbage removal, along with the presence of domestic animals, created extremely polluted urban environments. To make matters worse, city dwellers depended on meager and frequently adulterated food supplies brought from the outside. Under such circumstances, inhabitants frequently suffered from respiratory and gastrointestinal conditions, some of them deadly. With the cities teeming with famished refugees, debilitated residents, and the homeless and sick, plague mortality disproportionately affected the urban poor, although rural areas were also affected, disrupting agricultural work.[88]

For centuries, people believed that plague traveled with people and goods. Following the Neapolitan outbreak in 1656, Roman officials had been quick to patrol their borders, monitoring all movements and inspecting incoming ships for sick crews and travelers. By May, an unknown Neapolitan fisherman had fallen seriously ill in a Trastevere rooming house after receiving a package of silk ribbons from a deceased relative in Naples.[89] Cloth made of wool or silk was traditionally implicated in the transmission of plague since it was assumed to absorb corrupting disease vapors.[90] Soon the fisherman and his Trastevere landlady were both ill, but they tried to remain quiet instead of reporting it to the Roman authorities. Possible reasons for their secrecy were assumptions that, if plague was officially proclaimed, commerce would be abruptly halted and no further grain delivered, depriving dealers of profits, workers of jobs, and innkeepers of customers.

However, when the proprietor of that particular rooming house and her family also became ill, together with others living in nearby houses, the authorities were alerted. After a visit by a city physician, the fisherman was immediately rushed to the nearby hospital of San Giovanni in Laterano. Together with the *Ospedale Santa Maria della Consolazione*, it was one of the first institutions readied to admit plague suspects. The Neapolitan's subsequent death "with evil signs" was confirmed by an expert physician working for Rome's Health Congregation. This event prompted the issuance of a report on May 20 by the city's authorities officially proclaiming the presence of plague.[91] Now Rome's wealthy elite retreated to their mountaintop castles and summer villas. The traditional adage about the most effective plague remedy—to leave swiftly, go far away, and return late—had not lost its popular appeal. Summer was approaching anyway, and many were yearning for the sea breezes.

As expected, trade with Naples was immediately suspended and chains placed across the shipping channel at Fiumicino near the sea, as well as over the Tiber River at Ripa, to interrupt all ship traffic into the city. Land access became restricted to the five main gates. At each gate, temporary wooden stockades were erected overnight to allow only the admission of people, merchandise, and animals certified to be "clean" because of their plague-free origin. Henceforth, authorized supplies of grain, hay, and wine were to be transferred across the fences through pipes and troughs. As was often the case, angry public officials denounced the reporting delay in Trastevere. Their own credibility was on the line, and deceit from the inhabitants of that slum was not to be tolerated. Henceforth, all planned visits outside the district had to be authorized by a magistrate.[92]

According to the Easter census of 1656, Rome had a permanent population of 120,000, with at least as many visiting pilgrims at any time.[93] Like other large European cities at the time, the metropolis remained largely confined within its medieval walls, a densely populated urban center organized into 14 wards or *rione*.[94] Together with the rest of the Papal States, the city was ruled by Pope Alexander VII (1599–1667), formerly Fabio Chigi, of a prominent banking family in Siena. Conscious of his dwindling international status and power, the recently elected pontiff was determined to restore Rome to its previous splendor by ordering the renovation and construction of piazzas, monuments, palaces, and churches, including an arched colonnade on either side of St. Peter's monumental basilica. The city's economy, after all, was strongly dependent on the visits of pilgrims—close to a million per year. In his quest to bolster the image of the papacy, Alexander VII was ably assisted by a number of powerful cardinals who had already served his immediate predecessors, Urban VIII and Innocent X. The Roman curia, in turn, supervised a number of commissions, or *congregations*, as they were called, including one devoted entirely to health issues. The pope and the cardinals combined their religious and political authority to rule a complex bureaucracy with an iron hand.[95]

Thus, the 1656 outbreak of plague in Rome could not have come at a less opportune time. Here, as in other European cities, the poor appeared to bear the brunt of the epidemic and of public health regulations designed to check its spread. Together with the Jewish ghetto on the left bank, the low-lying Trastevere occupied the Tiber River floodplain, a humid and unhealthy area. Along winding alleys, crowded and dilapidated houses—many four stories high—sported holes in the walls and roofs, together with "nests of spiders, mice, scorpions."[96] Because of the perennial shortage of cheap housing, rents were exorbitant and laborers lived in "cubicles, garrets and holes in the wall."[97] Many Trastevere residents were homeless beggars engulfed in the stench of rotting garbage and filth. "What is the use of living in the grandeur of the city?" protested one critic. "Raise, Holy Father, the poor from the excrement, we no longer live in Rome but in a pigsty."[98]

To "snuff out every spark" of plague, the Health Congregation decided in June to quarantine Trastevere.[99] This measure, confirmed by orders of Alexander VII, was immediately implemented over the strong protests of the inhabitants, possibly including our women from the della Corte tenement, whose livelihoods were directly threatened. Accompanied by workers and soldiers, three members of the Health Congregation—Cardinals Francesco Barberini, Lorenzo Imperiali, and Friedrich von Hesse—came to the affected neighborhood at night to supervise the closure of gates, the boarding up of windows, the blocking of alleyways, and the enclosure of the whole area with a temporary wall. In nine hours, this hastily arranged "cage" was designed to prevent residents of Trastevere from escaping. In effect, the authorities admitted that the unlucky inhabitants had been placed in "protective custody" to suppress the feared contagion "in its cradle." To show his appreciation for the work of his Health Congregation, even the pope came to bless the newly erected barriers designed to prevent plague from entering Rome.[100]

For those barricaded in their houses, ventilation or fumigation with aromatic substances was indicated to cleanse the air. People who could afford it sprinkled their rooms with vinegar and fumigated with incense or smoke from sweet-smelling woods. Personal cleanliness was achieved with vinegar washings, and the application of aromatic oils was believed to neutralize the plague-producing miasma and prevent it from entering the pores of the skin. Similar strategies were employed to avoid the inhalation of this poison by placing citrus peels in the mouth under the tongue, carrying fragrant apples in the hands, or placing camphor, musk, sage, or rosemary in small bags hung around the neck. To protect themselves, roving physicians and surgeons not only wore waxed robes, leather gloves, and beaked masks, but also carried sponges soaked in vinegar around their belts. Others lugged large torches of tar, their flames expected to purify the air.

In spite of official pronouncements, the inhabitants of Trastevere remained skeptical about the very existence of plague in their midst. Many grew concerned about the prospect of 40 days of forced inactivity and the inevitable food shortages that promoted widespread hoarding, theft, and eventually famine. Anxious dwellers escaped their newly created prison, trying to elude Rome's multiple block-ades and police patrols. Some of the men may have hidden in their shops outside the district. In the meantime, the proprietor of the ill-fated boarding house and her entire family seemingly succumbed to the pestilence, but not before disobey-ing the new orders of the magistrate and secretly visiting relatives who lived in the heart of the city. Days later, new cases of plague appeared in the adjacent Jewish ghetto across the river and at other points of the city.

On June 27 all city wards, including Trastevere, organized local health com-missions composed of prelates, prominent neighbors, physicians, and surgeons, as well as notaries. Cardinals Barberini and Rivaldi were assigned to monitor Traste-vere, together with two official city physicians and a surgeon. Beggars were re-quired to report to prisons and were employed to keep the city clean. Terrified inhabitants peering from their windows now witnessed a growing parade of offi-cials, policemen, and soldiers, together with physicians, surgeons, and even priests. Rumors flew that the physicians were part of a secret municipal police, ready to extort bribes from dwellers hiding their sick. Quarantine signs went up every-where, placed by the authorities on houses sheltering suspected plague victims. At night, however, the signs were secretly removed and attached to other dwellings housing the healthy. Periodic visits by the pope's brother, Mario Chigi, called to Rome to assist in this emergency, followed. Chigi tirelessly crisscrossed the city in his carriage, inspecting the closed gates and providing alms from Alexander VII's personal fortune to quarantined families. The healthy poor were encouraged to seek assistance at churches and shelters, including a hospital for incurables. By early July the blockade of Trastevere had already created widespread food short-ages, prompting the pope to order immediate delivery of supplies to the starving residents.

Following anonymous tips and notifications, the medical personnel visited peo-ple suspected of suffering from plague and prepared daily reports for their supe-riors. Among the early symptoms considered suspicious were high fever and pros-tration, severe headaches, a white-coated tongue, and bloodshot eyes. By the third day, victims began to notice swollen lymph nodes or buboes in the groin, armpits, and neck. In addition, sufferers exhibited a number of infected, red or black skin sores or carbuncles over various parts of the body, known as "God's tokens." Less frequent were respiratory symptoms such as cough and sputum production. They represented the much more dangerous and contagious pneumonic form of the dis-ease that could potentially wipe out a whole population of lazaretto patients. Ail-ments creating diagnostic confusion with the buboes of plague were hernias and the newly described venereal affliction known as the "French disease." Like the lepers before them, true plague sufferers tried desperately to hide their stigma-tized sickness and especially to conceal the telltale blotches and buboes, hoping to cure them secretly with the help of prayers, relics, and home remedies. Plague also affected pregnant women, who experienced more miscarriages or stillbirths.

Because of the proximity of the groin to the genitalia, females sometimes attributed swellings in the groin to disorders of the uterus. All such symptoms were carefully concealed, given the high rate of illegitimate births and the stigma of venereal disease. Brisk sales of so-called plague preventives dispensed by greedy physicians and apothecaries ensued, generating further anger and anxiety when they failed to stem the progress of the epidemic. Given the widespread fear of forceful removal to a lazaretto, domestic purging and bloodletting remained routine, and antidotes for the plague poison were secretly prepared following popular recipes.[101]

By late July all four women, Martina, Catharina, Clementia, and Cecilia, had developed symptoms suggestive of plague. Both Martina and Catharina had a carbuncle on the thigh, a type of sore domestically treated with lotions and the placement of leeches. Cecilia was reported to have both a carbuncle and a bubo on her right thigh. In desperation, people lanced such swellings with a cutting glass or a hot iron, hoping such telltale signs of disease would disappear. Acting on a tip or on routine patrol, Valentino Honorati or Cinzio Coletti, the two physicians working for the Health Congregation, must have made a sweep through the San Salvatore della Corte tenement. Examining questionable cases, they discovered the four women with their swellings and reported them to the Health Congregation as *sospetti*.

Immediate transfer to a lazaretto was their fate, a measure that only added to the terror they were already experiencing. "People greatly fear being moved to the lazaretto," admitted Geronimo Gastaldi, the cardinal in charge of Rome's network of lazarettos in 1656,[102] although he claimed that such a measure saved lives. The coerced separation from the healthy was said to be justified for the purpose of preventing further contagion and curing the sick. Given the fact that about half of the individuals removed to a lazaretto survived their ordeal, optimism pervaded some of the official pronouncements concerning the management of plague. Escorted by a platoon of armed soldiers, the women were herded into wagons covered with wax cloth, their fellow travelers including not only *sospetti* but also a host of persons suffering from other ailments, often minor, or victims of trauma. Destination: a temporary lazaretto on the island of San Bartolomeo.

Framing and fighting plague: Pestilence and public health

Since the Black Death, religious views of pestilence explained epidemics as God's punishment for the sins of humankind. Unlike leprosy, perceived to slowly attack particular sinners whose fate was inexorable, plague was viewed as a fast-moving mass disease that indicated His displeasure, even anger, with communities at large. In numerous writings and sermons, theologians and ecclesiastical authorities stressed collective and personal guilt, as well as the need for repentance. Moral reform and a restoration of faith were imperative. Following an outbreak, affected communities engaged in a full spectrum of religious pageantry, including frequent church services, penitential processions, pilgrimages, and mass preaching. Gestures of public piety included almsgiving to the poor and support for the sick in isolation facilities.[103]

Prayers were addressed to the third-century martyr Sebastian, formerly a Roman officer of the Praetorian Guard, now a protector of those who suffered from plague. St. Sebastian was said to have been executed with a volley of arrows, the favorite symbolic instrument for divinely delivered pestilence since pagan times. Another popular protector was St. Rochus, a fourteenth-century nobleman from Montpellier, whose pilgrimage to Rome had apparently coincided with a local outbreak of the Black Death. Rochus had provided care to other victims and, after contracting the pestilence himself, was said to have nursed himself to health through divine assistance. He gave away his entire fortune to finance hospital care for those afflicted by the epidemic. Henceforth, St. Rochus was widely venerated. His remains were stolen in the late 1400s from a Montpellier grave by anxious Venetians who brought the relics home and enshrined them in a special church—San Rocco—thereafter devoted to his cult. It was therefore widely assumed that, with God's help and the saint's intercession, there was a chance that the pestilence could be overcome, perhaps even prevented.[104]

Such expressions of religious fervor and penance helped diffuse widespread feelings of panic, fear, and hopelessness that could virtually paralyze the public will. At Rome in 1656, however, the authorities canceled all processions and other religious ceremonies, suggesting instead that the population pray for the sick and dead in the privacy of their own homes. Public gatherings were increasingly at odds with the tenets of public health supported by the authorities. Therefore, each day during the epidemic, at 2 AM, the bells of Rome's major churches rang, summoning the faithful to their private prayer sessions with the promise of an indulgence for those who said three Our Fathers and three Hail Marys.[105]

Even within a belief system that explained plague as a punishment visited by God, however, scholastic authorities argued that divine agency could only be mediated through nature and that therefore the disease behaved in accordance to natural laws. Following the ideas of Avicenna, late medieval scholars considered two types of causes responsible for pestilence: universal and particular. Following tenets of astrology, the former was celestial, linked to the heavens, a result of harmful planetary conjunctions as well as solar and lunar eclipses. The resulting changes in light affected the climate and seasons and thus the air quality. The second cause was terrestrial, linked to particular local geographic conditions affecting the earth and water, such as earthquakes and storms. These factors contributed to the rise of corrupted vapors from decaying organic material or manmade fermentation. Together, cosmic and earthly events polluted the air, diminished the growth of crops, and fostered the appearance of snakes, lizards, frogs, and pestilence.[106]

If a pestilence was the spontaneous product of macrocosmic powers corrupting the air on a vast scale, medical authors relied heavily on the concept of environmental miasma articulated in Hippocratic writings.[107] This term designated a putrefaction of the air associated with a bad odor. Miasma derived from a variety of sources, including decaying vegetable matter and spoiled food, ground exhalations, and vapors from animal and human corpses, as well as from sick persons and their discharges. Such rotting matter could taint the air, making it heavy and humid, especially during summer and early autumn. However, although the concept of ubiquitous corrupted air could explain pestilence in one locality, dissemination at some geographic distance and perhaps from body to body occurred by contagion involving the transfer of seeds or particles. These were cast off into the atmosphere through expired air, sweat, or even direct eye contact. Since Galen's time, this transmission model had explained the spread of other diseases, including ophthalmia, scabies, leprosy, rabies, and ergotism.[108] In the final analysis, both miasma and contagion remained ambivalent and complementary concepts that expressed both environmental and human agency in the spread of pestilence.[109]

After 1348, these concepts were gradually extended to explain the spread of plague and appeared in numerous popular writings. A widespread belief held that those affected by pestilence gave off particular vapors or particles that could be transmitted by contact. This plague contagion was considered a genuine poison that would stick to body hair. It could even penetrate the weave of clothing and other materials, especially feathers, furs, woolens, and rags, unless they were covered with wax or oil. Individuals could therefore inhale disease-producing miasma or touch persons or objects harboring seeds or particles of disease capable of sticking to and penetrating their clothing and skin pores. In the case of pestilence, medical authors explained that the poisonous miasma disturbed the humoral balance of those who fell ill, creating widespread internal putrefaction that could suffocate the heart, liver, and brain. Beware, warned authors, of rotting matter reaching the heart, since its vital spirit would be promptly snuffed out, causing death.[110] Protection from pestilential air was best accomplished through flight from the affected area, a recourse available to the affluent, who went into hiding in suburban villas.[111] For individuals, general prevention stressed the value of managing the Galenic six nonnaturals, including environmental factors such as air, food, and drink, as well as bodily functions including motion, sleep, evacuation, and the emotions.[112]

Based on such contemporary notions of miasma and contagion, plague management—as exemplified in Trastevere—relied on frantic cleansing efforts to purge all corrupted humors, including lancing and draining the dreaded *bubones* and *carbunculi*.[113] As always, whether such agents succeeded in preventing illness was believed to depend on the individual's own physical constitution, a combination of hereditary humoral mix and way of life. Persons of sanguine temperament—with a tendency toward warmth and humidity—were in greater danger, but personal habits, nutrition, and emotions played equally important roles in deciding whether a particular individual would contract the pestilence. Fear of contagion and death, it was believed, could create sufficient anxiety and panic to actually induce disease.[114]

Public policies dealing with plague in Italy and elsewhere evolved gradually, punctuated by greater involvement of local governments in framing a coherent response to the pestilence. In fact, the periodic appearance of plague may have been a catalyst in the formation of the modern European state and its far-reaching administrative institutions.[115] Following the Black Death, the goal of early public health measures in the face of an epidemic was to protect the healthy—whose productivity was increasingly perceived during the Renaissance as a valuable resource of the state—from further onslaughts of poisonous miasma that could potentially overwhelm their constitutions, regardless of virtuous lifestyles and proper nutrition. Such a threat called for basic sanitation in villages and cities to prevent the formation of miasma that could generate pestilence. Given the scope of the environmental corruption in cities, the impact of an epidemic could only be blunted by a series of simultaneous approaches: prevent the entrance of people suspected of having contact with plague victims (sospetti) and their tainted belongings, including cargo—especially pertinent for trading posts around the Mediterranean seaboard—and mount a comprehensive effort to eliminate local sources of filth and poisoning, including the proper burial of the dead. Inside city walls, another series of measures sought to limit human contacts and thus reduce contagion by isolating suspects in their houses. In streets, houses, and churches, the foul-smelling miasma could then be minimized or even eliminated through vigorous municipal cleaning campaigns that removed garbage and manure.[116] Animals were banned from the city center. The stench was neutralized by lighting numerous bonfires with sulfur, making smoke by firing canons, or burning aromatic oils and incense.[117]

After 1400, various northern and central Italian city-states began to appoint special, temporary health commissions to deal with epidemics. In the duchy of Milan, a commisario oversaw all health regulations and sanitation. In addition, he checked food supplies entering the city and screened newcomers, denying access to those who appeared to be sick, especially if they seemed leprous. If an epidemic struck, foreigners and vagrants were summarily expelled, prostitutes monitored, and parish elders empowered to receive official notifications of all illnesses and deaths in the city made by either physicians or heads of households. Moreover, the authorities developed a more efficient form of distribution of alms and food to the needy as the economic consequences of the interrupted commerce became obvious. With wealthy citizens out of town, protection of their property and houses also became an important issue. In Venice, the health authorities accelerated the collection of rubbish by barges and laid sewage pipes to drain into the canals. These canals, in turn, were dredged to reduce the silt believed to be responsible for the polluted water. Considered important plague carriers, pigs, cats, and dogs were prohibited in the city and killed during epidemics.[118]

During the plague epidemic of 1468, the authorities of Milan took advantage of its slow spread to study the transmission mechanisms through careful contact tracing. This work, accomplished through the cooperation of local authorities, health board officials, and medical professionals, confirmed the important role of contagion in the spread of plague among the population. In time, the Milanese insights led to a much more aggressive policy of separating the healthy from the potentially infected, an approach promptly copied by Venetians in the 1470s and throughout the northern Italian city-states therafter.[119] All policies and measures based on miasmatic notions remained firmly in place, but the actual spread of pestilence among the population was increasingly blamed on human agency.[120] This policy phase further stigmatized the poor as bearers of epidemic disease because of their weak bodily constitutions, deficient living conditions, and ignorance of preventive measures.[121] If a threat of plague was imminent, beggars and prostitutes were targeted for expulsion, and the working poor were closely monitored and institutionalized if they appeared to be sick. Implementation of this program often required harsh measures and the use of police and armed forces by health boards and commissions, deepening class divisions, creating further economic hardships, and breaking down family networks through separation and isolation in out-of-town lazarettos. At the same time, the working poor—always an asset to the state—became renewed objects of charitable assistance. They received provisions and alms during periods of quarantine-imposed scarcity, as well as replacement clothing and bedding if theirs were destroyed through fire or disinfection.[122]

As occurred in Rome during 1656, an initial alert could result in a *suspensione* or suspension of free traffic of goods and persons from regions suspected of having plague. All travelers had to be quarantined and their goods subjected to a *purga*, or cleansing procedure, consisting of exposure to fresh air and sunshine. A *bando* or closure was much more radical: it completely interrupted the flow of persons and goods from regions or population centers known to have plague. City gates were closed, and as in Rome, makeshift fences were erected to prevent access except for those who possessed health certificates. Safe-conduct passes were issued for ambassadors, officials, and aristocrats, but the poor, especially vagrants, were kept out. In some cases the borders of an entire province were sealed, creating a so-called sanitary cordon with fences, observation towers, and military patrols to enforce the isolation.[123] This cordon and other measures were quite costly and labor-intensive. In general, compliance with such wide-ranging public health rules remained perfunctory by all sectors of the population, and enforcement continued to be hampered by a chronic lack of resources and personnel.

Inside the cities, temporary and, later, permanent health boards created their own comprehensive systems of information and obligatory reporting of plague cases. Under threat of severe punishment, including public execution, citizens were enjoined to report to a magistrate all individuals with symptoms suspicious of plague, from dark, blotchy faces to open sores. As in Trastevere, whole sections of a city could be fenced in to prevent all movement of people. This system fostered frequent underreporting of cases among those who sought to avoid such quarantines. It also created frequent rifts and confrontations among power groups, including the church, with its pageantry and charitable agenda, the largely absent healthy elite, commercial interests affected by an interruption of trade, and the medical establishment, as well as the sick and their families. In Rome, Church authorities were divided and conflicted between their religious role as providers of charity and their political duty to ruthlessly enforce the quarantine measures. One of the paradoxes of European plague control was that quarantines fostered further economic dislocation, unemployment, and even malnutrition among the very segments of the population already most susceptible to plague. At the same time, it provided new but risky jobs for fumigators, cleaners, and grave diggers.[124]

Like the bodies of lepers such as Grette Thielen, those of poor plague sufferers were perceived to be deadly weapons. Widespread fear that the sick poor would at times deliberately spread their disease among the healthy was common. In the Trastevere episode of 1656, the action of the infected boardinghouse owner who visited relatives in Rome was interpreted as a willful act of sabotage. Such stigmatization allowed health officials to manipulate plague outbreaks and achieve other goals, such as curfews to reduce crime, the expulsion of undesirable vagrants to decrease welfare assistance, or forcible recruitment of beggars for public projects. Like Jews, indigents were often forced to wear special clothing for prompt identification. Soldiers patrolled their neighborhoods with orders to arrest violators of sanitary regulations and punish unreported victims and their relatives, as well as smugglers bringing in supplies. Many were summarily tried, confessions extracted through torture, and the guilty jailed. Others were promptly executed in public places by firing squads or hanged. In a few flagrant cases, the papal authorities in Rome not only killed the guilty but mutilated their bodies and publicly exhibited the severed parts before burning them to terrorize the citizenry.[125]

The conceptual shift to contagionism demanded vigorous and coercive methods of segregation and confinement. Early identification was essential, and Rome in 1656 ordered physicians capable of diagnosing plague to remain in the city under the threat of death. In positions drawn by lottery and with a promise of a generous reward, physicians and surgeons followed up on citizens' reports and rumors and made a professional assessment of each situation. Hiding the sick and dead was widespread. However, not everyone found with plague was sent off to an institution. Many houses belonging to upper- and middle-class families were simply locked up by the health authorities whenever a case of plague was suspected or reported. Those remaining in their homes, including relatives and servants, were revisited periodically as part of the general surveillance scheme. Officials bolted the doors from the outside and marked them with a cross or the sign "*Sanità*" to warn passersby. At night, police frequently patrolled to prevent any escape or outside contact. Trapped inside, residents would frequently appear at the windows to beg for alms, lower baskets to the street to obtain food and supplies, and get priests to give their blessings. In Florence during the 1630 plague outbreak, women abandoned in a quarantined house accused the official visiting surgeons of stealing valuables during their visits. At other times, medical professionals demanded bribes for not reporting possible plague cases. Because of their contact with suspected plague victims, their own "unclean" status lent credence to the widespread belief that they were also instrumental in spreading the disease.

For those who died of plague, either at home or in lazarettos, "unclean" workers were hired to transport the covered corpses in carts to a number of collection points. Given the stigma attached to the disease and the public health implications, deaths were often concealed if they occurred in homes or health professionals were bribed to issue false death certificates. Prompt burial was encouraged outside the city in deep pits to avoid harmful emanations from the decomposing bodies, a practice that denied families the staging of proper funeral rites. Private furnishings of those infected were taken from the homes, inventoried, and carted away for cleansing by sunshine and smoke outside the city limits. Not surprisingly, such official cleansing activities remained perennial sources of blackmail, bribery, and theft.[126]

To prevent the spread of pestilence, governments after 1500 also gathered intelligence about the movements of plague throughout the Italian peninsula and the Mediterranean in general, a feat accomplished by a cadre of informers on a city or government payroll. Such periodic communications were intended to facilitate better sanitary planning and make decisions regarding restrictions in travel and commerce from plague infested areas. In response, cities or neighboring states burdened with epidemic disease suppressed this information in an effort to sustain trade. A world of intrigue, disinformation, and hypocrisy regarding the presence of plague came to dominate the affairs of many northern Italian states, especially after two severe epidemics in 1522–1523 and 1526–1528.

Given the scope of such activities, health boards in northern and central Italy became vast bureaucracies closely associated with ruling elites, along with their police, army, and legal personnel. Indeed, a growing emphasis on law and order tended to displace the traditional Christian welfare schemes and religious coping mechanisms based on elaborate public ceremonies and processions. In Rome, the spiritual capital of Catholicism and the destination point of thousands of European pilgrims, such rituals now clashed with the contagionist ideology that sought to minimize large urban assemblies in order to decrease human contact. Nevertheless, even outside the Papal States, the Church continued to play an important role in the fight against epidemics, providing churches and convents as makeshift isolation facilities and dispatching priests to provide sacramental comforts to the sick and dying at great risk to their own lives.[127]

Lazarettos: Makeshift isolation, cleansing, and treatment

Like other charitable institutions, the pesthouse had its roots in late medieval Christian institutions designed to shelter the needy and sick. In Venice in 1348, the overseers of public health had ordered the detention of potentially infected goods, ships, and persons on a separate island in the lagoon. Pure air and sunshine were expected to purge human bodies and belongings of poison. By 1374, new ordinances forbade the entrance of suspected ships to the harbor altogether and required custody of their crews for 30 days (the *trentina*). Following the massive plague epidemics of 1399–1400, Venice established in 1403 a hostel on the island of Santa Maria not just for the detention of travelers, but also for the internment of local plague suspects. While the rich usually fled town, other inhabitants, especially the employed poor, remained to pursue their livelihood, and they became the usual inmates of the pesthouse, where they were now subjected to a longer isolation period, 40 days or *quarantina*. This waiting period can be seen as a type of ritual purification with clear religious roots, since 40 days carried special significance in Judeo-Christian theology.[128]

In August 1423, the Venetian senate decreed the city's first permanent establishment—Lazzaretto Vecchio—on the small island of Santa Maria de Nasova (Nazareth) in the Venetian lagoon off the Lido. Formerly a hospice for pilgrims returning from Nazareth in Palestine, this 20-bed shelter, known as Nazaretto, was now to be reserved for the detention of foreign traders, together with their goods, who were sick or suspected of carrying pestilence. Here they were to be kept away from the port for the traditional 40 days. To finance this establishment, the Venetian state drew on private charity to supplement its own contribution.[129] In addition to a prior in charge of the institution, the staff consisted of one or two physicians and three servants. During the 1430s, the Lazzaretto Vecchio became an accepted institution to house the sick, expanding its staff to include a priest, male and female servants, boatmen, and gravediggers. With an expanded endowment, even the pope provided a special indulgence for those who financially aided the institution.

Because of their pilgrim origin, similar facilities in fifteenth-century Italy were also first known as *nazarettos*, but the term changed to *lazzarettos* or *Lazar houses* because their new segregating function was equated with that commonly employed with lepers. Indeed, since the admission of lepers had already declined, some larger leper houses were converted into plague shelters. This transformation was due in part to Europe's shifting ecology of disease but also to the result of transformations in society and culture linked to population growth, economic expansion, and especially urbanization. However, given the temporary character of both plague epidemics and health boards, the construction of permanent facilities was often delayed for decades in favor of makeshift arrangements that included former out-of-town monasteries and private estates.

Even before the end of the fifteenth century, many cities in northern Europe began to consider pesthouses or lazarettos as indispensable for the detention and care of all the plague victims, especially the urban poor. Among them were Münster (1475), Frankfurt (1494), and Nürnberg (1498). In Venice, a second establishment—the Lazzaretto Nuovo—had opened in 1468 on St. Erasmo, another lagoon island located five miles from the city. The new facilities were to house *sospetti* taken from a victim's house, as well as convalescents from Lazaretto Vecchio who were required to spend an additional 40 days before being allowed to return to Venice. Similar specialized institutions modeled after the Venetian hospice were also proposed for other major Italian cities such as Mantua (1450), Ferrara (1464), Florence (1463), Genoa (1467), Siena (1478), and Milan (1488).[130]

First to enter the institution were those already sick—*brutti* or *infetti*—followed later by all suspected carriers of epidemic disease who could not be shut in and isolated in their own dwellings. Crowding in slum tenements had made such individualized isolation impractical and ineffective; therefore, lazarettos became a perfect solution for removing those who posed a risk of contracting plague. The purpose of pesthouses was to guarantee physical separation between the healthy and those suspected of having or already afflicted with pestilence while simultaneously ensuring social control. Because of the large number of presumed plague cases, most local sanitary boards also sent some suspected plague patients directly to ordinary hospitals, especially in towns lacking specialized institutions.[131]

Like leper houses, most lazarettos were established outside of towns near crossroads and in downwind locations based on similar considerations of easy access and environmental contamination. Given the prevailing winds in Europe, this meant a southeastern or eastern location at a prudent distance from human settlements. For additional purification and security purposes, locations surrounded by water—especially islands near port entrances—or downstream spaces near a river were preferred.[132] Following the Black Death, their construction occurred mostly in Italian city-states and European trading ports, frequently first in the form of temporary wooden huts. Expropriated with papal consent, monastic buildings in isolated areas were also requisitioned. Among early lazaretto patrons were ecclesiastic authorities, local rulers, municipalities, and parish confraternities. Like other charitable institutions, pesthouses reflected the size and financial status of a community. Since they were often provisional facilities, they lacked endowments and depended on financing by nearby endowed hospitals. Following an epidemic, their furnishings were frequently burned before the establishment was closed or returned to its previous use. From the 1500s on, more permanent isolation hospitals in other European countries demonstrated the willingness of citizens to prioritize the management of plague and provide the necessary funds to erect and manage this type of facility.

By 1503, Venice already boasted four individual lazaretto units, each providing 10 successive days of quarantine to separate groups of plague suspects. If the disease actually broke out among members of one unit, the entire group returned to the first facility to initiate another complete round of quarantine. Fueled by contagionist ideas, the emphasis on isolating people and their property increased. In Venice, the lazarettos not only continued to receive merchandise from various plague-infested areas for disinfection, they also became depots for housewares, furnishings, and clothing removed from the houses of plague victims. During the fifteenth century, all goods deemed infected had been summarily burned and destroyed, but successive epidemic bouts a century later demanded a more conservative approach. The idea behind the 40-day disinfection or *sboro* was that plague-producing particles embedded in textiles could be removed not only through exposure to sunlight and fresh air, but also with cold and hot water washings. Some materials were treated with salt water. By the 1650s, as the Trastevere quartet of suspected plague sufferers made its way to a Roman lazaretto, other Italian cities employed testers called *bastazi*, individuals risking infection by plunging their arms twice a day into separate packages of potentially infected clothing and merchandise.[133]

The best-known Italian example of a permanent institution was the lazaretto of Milan, started in 1488 and completed in 1513. Given the deteriorating economic conditions brought on by the quarantine in Milan, fifteenth-century health commissioners enjoined all existing religious hostels or hospices to accept poor inhabitants during plague epidemics if they were in danger of starving. To enforce a strict segregation of the infected sick poor, officials ordered the construction of temporary shacks or cabins outside the city and assigned some patients to nearby monastic hospitals. By the end of the fifteenth century, however, authorities deemed it necessary to build a single large pesthouse. The sixteenth-century lazaretto was a quadrangular building with 280 single cells surrounding a central courtyard provided with an octagonal chapel. At this point, the Milanese authorities were no longer concerned with pestilential winds and vapors, but considered the plague to be transmitted by contact with sick persons and their goods. With windows placed toward the courtyard and the outside, each cell contained a bed, toilet, and fireplace with its own ventilation chimney to help expel the corrupted pestilential air produced by the inmates. Strict discipline and control of the patients required towers for the guards. Surrounded by a moat of flowing water that also functioned as a sewer, this complex had a separate canal system for washing clothes. Dwarfing both the cathedral and other prominent Milanese buildings, this unique facility combined the functions of a quarantine station for observation of suspected patients, a plague hospital to care for the sick, and a recovery center to house convalescents. During the 1630 plague, Milan's model lazaretto housed more than 16,000 individuals at one time. As in other establishments, there were separate areas, each devoted to a particular category of patients: *sospetti*, *infetti*, and convalescents. Later, to facilitate turnover during severe epidemics and avoid frequent relapses, convalescents were quickly dispatched to other care facilities to complete their recovery.

In wealthy Florence, funds were provided as early as 1464 for a special isolation hospital, but the Ospedale di San Bastiano, with a capacity for 26 beds, opened to plague victims only 30 years later. The building was divided into four separate rooms, two for male and female victims, two for convalescents recovering from the disease. Its staff consisted of a priest, physician, barber-surgeon, and apothecary together with servants. During the 1630 epidemic, the public demanded that all lazarettos be closed and everyone granted permission for treatment at home. This plan favored those who, for a variety of reasons, could not leave the city but had the means to survive in isolation. Although temporarily approved, the order had to be rescinded and the lazarettos reopened because of further spread of the epidemic, inadequate manpower, and the high cost of the new decentralized domestic assistance program. Stigmatized or not, plague houses continued to be the most efficient means of isolating the sick and thus presumably stopping the spread of plague.[134]

Verona built a smaller lazaretto between 1549 and 1592.[135] In the meantime, Venice in 1528 began using the leper island of St. Lazzaro as an additional quarantine center, as the authorities stressed that all plague-infected houses should be evacuated during an epidemic, regardless of class and circumstances. During the epidemic of 1576, close to 8,000 patients were housed at the Lazzaretto Vecchio, creating dreadful living conditions because of bed and staff shortages. The stench emanating from the patients and their groans were said to resemble Dante's vision of the inferno. In Venice, the lazarettos were known for their humane treatment of plague victims.[136] By the time the plague came to Rome in 1656, Europe was witnessing another wave of pesthouse foundations, including facilities in Hamburg (1606), Paris (1607), Ragusa (1628), Amsterdam, Bologna and Cambridge (1630), Westminster (1636), and Genoa (1657).

Like all charitable institutions, lazarettos were increasingly placed under the supervision and administration of municipal instead of ecclesiastical authorities during the early 17th century and thus experienced fierce competition for resources with existing hospitals. Most establishments depended on income from land endowments. In Italy, parishes and city councils headed by leading local families became increasingly involved in their governance. Lay administrators, appointed by municipalities, were usually in charge of running lazarettos and reporting to their respective health boards. As an important arm of the public health bureaucracy, lazarettos were also targets of public discontent. Not surprisingly, corruption was rampant and frequently exposed. Because of their specialized status and intermittent utilization, many lazarettos failed to obtain the funds necessary to sustain their operations. Between epidemics, many of the buildings stood empty or needed repairs, their basic inventory of beds, mattresses, blankets, and clothes burned. Theft of these items by attendants was habitual, with the lazaretto transformed into a factory as blankets were ripped into smaller pieces to make new garments.[137]

The staff closely resembled that of other contemporary hospitals of similar size, except for additional security; guards or porters closely monitored inmates, preventing their flight. In addition to visiting priests, the institutions had a number of male and female nurses, mostly lay persons. In some cases, volunteers from local confraternities, as in leper houses, risked their lives with such hazardous duty. Their selection was influenced by contemporary perceptions of a strong physical constitution and thus possible resistance to plague, a frequently inaccurate and fateful judgment. Additional helpers were involved in washing laundry, although most clothing worn by patients was either burned or sent with other "unclean" sheets, blankets, and mattresses to special facilities outside the institution. In Rome during the 1656 epidemic, both the vineyards of the Villa Sannesia, outside the Piazza del Popolo gate, and the ruins of the Caracalla Baths to the south were destination points for linens and woolen clothing.

Unlike leper houses, lazarettos also had small medical and surgical staffs composed of "plague doctors," usually young physicians and surgeons with no established practices of their own. Their availability was closely linked to the creation of local medical colleges and surgical guilds in the greater urban centers. The secular goal of physical recovery led even pesthouses to accelerate their ongoing medicalization process. In Italy, these men accepted a fixed retainer to visit the sick in homes, prisons, hospitals, and convents, as well as on ships.[138] They also conducted autopsies on victims sent for postmortem diagnoses.[139] Here the plague was instrumental in establishing a new medical deontology. The earlier flight of practitioners from the cities at the appearance of plague followed ancient traditions and devotion to individual wealthy clients who paid retainers. In time, however, late medieval universities and guilds of physicians and barber-surgeons produced a cadre of professionals who owed their allegiance and licenses to particular states, regions, or municipalities. This linkage made flight punishable with loss of citizenship and loss of permission to continue to practice.[140] In Rome in 1656, high fees and special prizes did not attract enough physicians to attend patients in the city's pesthouses. Since there were not enough barber-surgeons to perform this work, the Health Congregation compelled the local medical association to provide a number of "volunteers."[141]

Freed from the social and economic restraints operating in private practice, *medici condotti* (contract physicians) went on to acquire greater clinical knowledge and skills, thus improving their individual and collective reputations and cultural authority.[142] Hospitals and pesthouses added an important educational dimension to their traditional mission as charitable shelters and centers of medical treatment. Teachers such as Taddeo Alderotti in Bologna and Giambattista da Monte in Padua offered clinical instruction in their wards, making rounds with students and organizing lectures to demonstrate particular cases. Most northern Italian universities also began offering doctorates in surgery, and in Florence a school of surgery was created on the premises of the Santa Maria Nuova in the late 1500s.[143] Similar professionalization efforts occurred among pharmacists.

Medical professionals willing to work in lazarettos or visit the sick in their homes were hired primarily for their diagnostic skills. Separating the healthy from the sick, whether suspicious or overt plague cases, lay at the bottom of the elaborate public health scheme. This activity made plague doctors de facto "unclean" and a feared source of contagion. Forced to display a cross that revealed their sospetti status, the men remained under constant scrutiny throughout the epidemic, unable to mingle with the rest of the population. As hirelings of urban public health boards, physicians were distrusted by the population. Like priests, many were accused of spreading the plague to further their own interests. They also took bribes for nonreporting of cases, trafficked in herbal remedies, and were accused of stealing valuables. However, many paid with their lives for providing services, while their senior colleagues, on private retainers, left the city for safer and more salubrious environments. Nonetheless, the "plague doctors' " status was apparently not affected by the obvious failures of treatment. To the contrary, their willingness to assume the considerable risks associated with their professional functions earned them the respect of the authorities, who often awarded them citizenship, a coveted recompense that allowed them to launch a private practice after the epidemic ended. Others signed lucrative contracts with the city—in exchange for such hazardous duties—that guaranteed a good monthly salary or reward, free rent, living expenses, and advanced payments.[144]

The lazaretto was a difficult place both to work in and to be an inmate. Often, in time of severe epidemics, four or five patients were herded together in one bed.[145] Delirious individuals were restrained and strapped to the beds they usually shared with other inmates. Their moaning in a dense atmosphere of sweat and smoke could only enhance the apprehension of the newcomers. The stench of the infected and draining buboes apparently was enough to stimulate frequent attempts to fumigate the premises with fragrant herbs or rose water sprinkled with vinegar. In 1629, one public health official visiting the Milanese pesthouse "went into a dead faint for the stinking smells that came forth from all those bodies and those little rooms."[146] Ventilation was bolstered by the flames of numerous wood fires escaping through existing chimneys. Since the air around the beds was deemed contagious, all caring personnel employed the widely recommended aromatics or vinegar sponges as plague preventives. They also smoked tobacco and protected their mouths by chewing ginger or juniper berries.

Because the urine of plague patients usually appeared turbid and dark, toilets were repeatedly covered with layers of linen to avoid the escape of noxious fumes. According to contemporaries, fleas in the pesthouses—carried by the incoming patients—were pervasive and voracious, harassing both the patients and their caregivers. Their bites occurred most frequently on the legs, and the itching led to scratching, blisters, and more carbuncles. In 1630, a Bolognese cardinal reported his experiences in the local lazaretto, observing that some inmates complained, others cried, and still others became black and deformed, were delirious, and died. "Here you are overwhelmed by intolerable smells. Here you cannot walk but among corpses. Here you feel naught but the constant horror of death. This is a faithful replica of hell."[147] At times, reactions to poor food and strict discipline caused anger and hostility toward the caregivers and administrators. Letters of protest were written to the health boards complaining about poor conditions. Discipline was bound to break down given the paucity of personnel. Escapes were frequent. Terror, however, could strike without warning from an entirely different source. One report by a nurse at the Florentine lazaretto of San Miniato in 1630 concerned the rape of several young women inmates among those suspected of having plague.[148]

From Asclepius to San Bartolomeo: Purification rites

In Rome, the Health Congregation decided in late June 1656 to open another lazaretto on the island of San Bartolomeo, site of a former Benedictine monastery, now the *xenodochium* of the Brotherhood of St. John of God. Located on the Tiber River and linked by bridges with Rome and Trastevere, this complex of buildings stood at the site of a previous temple dedicated to the Greek healing god Asclepius. The legendary arrival of Asclepius was said to have occurred after a pestilence among the Romans about 1,000 years earlier. With the banks reinforced to prevent flooding, the island, with its sacred well, was shaped like a ship in remembrance of the original arrival of the god from Greece. The basilica of San Bartolomeo the Apostle contained the saint's relics and had been a traditional destination for pilgrims.[149] Now the various buildings were divided to house three separate groups: a lazaretto for the admission of *sospetti*, another for the *infetti*, and a collection point for those already dead.

Before the establishment of makeshift facilities, the Roman authorities had sent some *sospetti* and *infetti* to local hospitals such as San Giovanni in Laterano, near a city gate, and the famous Ospedale di Santo Spirito upstream from the island and close to the basilica of St. Peter. Here the Health Congregation installed a temporary *pallazzetto* or big tent to attend some of the victims. Other suspects were sent to the convents of Santa Michelle, Santa Maria de la Consolazione, and San Eusebio. Additional extramural lazarettos were located at San Pancrazio in the hills above the city and at the Casaletto di Pio Quinto. Inside the city walls, more lazarettos were erected in Ripa, Strada Giulia, San Giuliano, and Porta Portese. Months later, their total reached 28, 2 for each district. At the height of the epidemic in the fall of 1656, over 4,000 inmates were detained in Roman lazarettos. The entire bureaucratic apparatus fighting the plague had been placed in the hands of Cardinal Barberini, a member of the Health Congregation.[150]

Access to the dreaded precinct was provided from Rome across the bridge of the Quattro Capi (Four Heads), guarded by soldiers and blocked by two temporary "clean" and "unclean" gates. A similar arrangement was in place on the bridge to Trastevere. As described by an eyewitness, transportation to the lazaretto was accomplished in wagons and covered litters carried by criminals—mostly convicted beggars—who previously had been condemned to the galleys. Forced to work, these men, like the roving physicians, wore a costume of green waxed cloth and black leather gloves, with sponges soaked in vinegar on their belts that they periodically held to their noses. Escorted by soldiers who shouted for the public to get out of the way, the wagons and carts with their human cargoes slowly made their way to the gates, allowed to enter only after their identity had been established. Names were entered on lists posted outside the gates for the information of relatives and friends. The identities of the four Trastevere women can be confirmed by a list of institutional arrivals in a report dated August 4 and prepared for Cardinal Barberini by Dr. Francesco Malvetani, superintendent of the San Bartolomeo lazaretto. The dead were collected at the southern tip of the island and loaded into "unclean" boats by auxiliary personnel for their final voyage downriver to the nearby cemetery adjacent to the church of San Paolo.

After arrival, the *sospetti* were usually subjected to a period of clinical observation, the *purga di sospetto* or cleansing isolation. Their tainted garments were either burned or sent out for washing to a garden at Ripa and possibly returned if the owners survived, since replacement clothing was difficult to obtain. According to the regulations, all belongings had to be exposed to fresh air and sun for up to three days to destroy the feared contagion. The facilities at San Bartolomeo included separate wards for men and women, as well as private quarters for sick noblemen. *Sospetti* frequently resented and protested their protective custody, fearful of catching the dreaded disease from each other or their caregivers. If some of the plague suspects began developing telltale signs within the following 10 days—believed to be the usual incubation period for plague—they were certified as sick and promptly transferred to the adjacent isolation facilities devoted to infectious cases. This was the fate of the foursome from Trastevere.

Admissions classified as infected had typical signs of plague and were brought to separate wards. Since admission of infected patients to a pesthouse was usually delayed until the patients had been medically certified, the *infetti*'s deteriorating physical condition generally created shorter institutional stays and higher mortality. This was particularly true for sick women and children who had hidden in their dwellings, often without food and care. Children under the age of 14 were among those most frequently hospitalized, a measure that often implied their forceful removal from homes and caregiving mothers. During the seventeenth century, various lazarettos reported death rates of about 60%, somewhat higher for urban dwellers than for those arriving from the countryside, perhaps a reflection of the latter's superior physical condition prior to their illness.

At the Lazzaretto de San Bartolomeo, contemporary statistics revealed that between the institution's opening date of June 24 and August 24, 1656, medical officials admitted 542 individuals from Trastevere. Of these, 274 were men and 268 were women. The former had a mortality rate of 53%, the latter 78%.[151] However, institutional mortality remained a questionable index, since inmates frequently perished from other ailments. Even these somewhat favorable odds failed to change the public's perception that pesthouses such as the lazaretto of San Bartolomeo were places of suffering and death to be avoided at all costs.[152] Like earlier epidemics, the plague seemed to be gaining ground as the summer progressed, and Dr. Malvetani's reports noted the arrival of 60 new dead on July 22.

In spite of naturalistic explanations of causality involving miasma and contagion, victims brought to the lazaretto were stigmatized and, like lepers, often blamed for their disease. Like other contemporary hospitals in Counter-Reformation Europe, Roman lazarettos emphasized religious routines. Priests comforted incoming plague sufferers and administered communion to all *sospetti* and *infetti*. If the sick body would not mend, salvation of the soul was always possible, and last rites for the very sick were imperative. Midwives stood by if pregnant plague patients delivered their mostly stillborn babies, ready to baptize them.[153]

Anxiety and fear were bound to increase among the inmates, exemplified by the frequent complaints of abuses perpetrated by an authoritarian staff primarily concerned with social control who ran the lazaretto as a virtual prison. In a replay of previous battles between them since Byzantine times, clashes regarding treatment modalities were reported between the medical and ecclesiastical personnel in lazarettos. At times, physicians complained that the prior in charge of the institution often ordered insufficient medicines.[154] Not unexpectedly, religious health officials such as Cardinal Gastaldi, the General Commissioner for Lazarettos, took a dim view of the efficacy of medical practices. "Writings of physicians on cure of plague produce much smoke and offer little light," he wrote.[155] In his opinion, they were all ineffectual or even dangerous.

Nursing care was placed in the hands of Capuchin friars or lay volunteers, who worked closely with a corps of servants and resident physicians. Sponges or balls soaked in perfume or vinegar hung from their necks, and they all ate sparingly and periodically purged themselves. As physicians made their rounds, dressed in their protective robes, an assistant walked before them carrying a lit candle and a bowl of vinegar. Avoiding the patients' soiled clothes, they took the pulse after dipping their hands in vinegar.[156] When examining patients, physicians and surgeons held sponges soaked in vinegar to their noses to avoid contact with the sick person's fetid breath.

While the medical profession had created a greater role for itself within the new rehabilitative goals of the Renaissance hospital, nourishment and nursing of patients still remained key institutional actions. The humoral balance, disrupted by the offending poison, needed restoration. Unlike leprosy, plague triggered a hot, moist humoral corruption, requiring a balancing regimen of cool, dry foods and medicines. The traditional anti-inflammatory cleansing routines included emetics and purgatives. If tolerated, bread, meat, and wine were the cornerstone of the diet. Humoral purification began with the ingestion of sour drinks, especially lemonade. As one report described, at dawn everyone was given a beverage, either a glass of goat's rue, chickpea water, or pimpernel water. Other options included electuaries of mulberry to be consumed throughout the day, juice of marigolds, syrup of roses and violets, spicy drinks with cinnamon and lavender, and, of course, dry, cooling wine. Meat and eggs were offered, especially during the convalescent period.[157]

Before meals, this liquid diet was supplemented with antidotes designed to neutralize the plague poison. Here physicians selected once more the traditional *theriac* preparations—also widely employed as preventives—made mostly from snake meat on the assumption that it possessed particular properties capable of neutralizing venom. Local variations were prepared by boiling snakes or scorpions in oil—*olio contraveneni*—creating particular brands administered in limited drops mixed with water. In the hope of neutralizing the poisonous humors oozing from the lesions, the same oil was also applied locally to the bubonic swellings, particularly those that were open and infected. Similar anointing of the skin focused on the area over the heart, stomach, and major arterial pulses. In an effort to withdraw the plague poison directly, bloodletting was also performed unless the patient was already considered too weak to tolerate it.[158] The lazaretto's chief surgeon, Giuseppe Balestra, considered these phlebotomies quite dangerous, even fatal.[159]

Special care was devoted to the painful buboes and black carbuncles, which were thought to represent bodily efforts to expel the plague poison through the skin. To prevent a possible flow of poisonous blood to the heart, physicians used tourniquets on arms and legs, hoping to trap the venom in the extremities. Therefore, physicians and surgeons made great efforts to speed up the maturation and eventual draining of such buboes through the use of emollient plasters, scarification, cupping glasses, and irritating ointments—called *rottori* or breakers—containing substances such as mustard, rock salt, and turpentine. After the buboes were fully developed and presumably after the poisoned humor had collected in them, efforts were made to expel their contents. Once the lesions began to drain, they were periodically rubbed with pork fat and dressed with linen pads to draw out the bad fluids—the "fountain treatment." At other times, local applications of pomegranate juice were substituted and cabbage leaves placed over the suppuration. In certain circumstances, an attending surgeon used a cautery instrument made of gold, silver, or preferably iron to speed the drainage or place leeches to withdraw more poisonous fluid. In another strategy derived from folk healing, the flesh of recently killed animals, including pigeons, roosters, and even dogs, was placed over the buboes in the hope that the poison in them could be persuaded to transfer from human to animal flesh.[160]

We can only assume that Marina, Catharina, Clementia, and perhaps Cecilia were subjected to a similar medical regimen, including the care of their buboes mentioned in the medical report. Perhaps they even shared beds and kept each other company. At the lazaretto of San Bartolomeo, nursing care was also provided by pious members of a local confraternity composed of Trastevere parishioners who had volunteered to feed and clean the sick. In spite of the prison-like atmosphere of the lazaretto, there would have been opportunities for the women from the tenement house near Ponte Rotto to establish or renew bonds of solidarity and friendship not unlike those some of their husbands had created earlier by fleeing the houses and holding out in workplaces and stores. Maybe terror and despair were relieved though faith in God and reassurance from other sufferers, and this was the most tangible benefit of a stay in a lazaretto besides nourishment. Perhaps lazaretto life, with all its horrors, could at times overcome the desolation and helplessness felt especially by many female plague victims who were simply abandoned by heartless mates, starving to death in their hiding places.[161]

In the end only Cecilia died, sometime before August 4, in the female ward of the lazaretto of San Bartolomeo.[162] Following contemporary sanitary regulations, her naked body must have been carried on a stretcher to the tip of the island together with other victims of the plague and then loaded onto a barge by a group of "unclean" workers. Piled high with corpses, the vessel—identified by a cross as carrying Christian victims—slowly made its way downriver towed by another "clean" tugboat, while onlookers on both shores watched the grim procession. Another similarly packed boat without markings made its way directly from the Jewish ghetto. Both eventually reached the meadows of San Paolo outside the city walls next to the church, where newly hired diggers were busy preparing new mass graves. The boats tied up near a guard house at the edge of the river and transferred their lifeless cargo to horse-drawn wagons. A short trip through the fields ended with a summary dumping of the bodies into numerous pits.[163] In cities such as Florence and Venice, those who buried the dead were often volunteers drawn from local confraternities. Everywhere this was a repugnant and risky activity, with many of the diggers ripping off all remaining clothing from the corpses, fleeing the scene, and selling their stolen goods. In the end, among Trastevere's nearly 3,000 residents, more than half perished during the plague epidemic of 1656–1657, a mortality rate six times higher than that of the rest of the city.

If life in the lazaretto had any silver linings, they were few. Surviving patients and convalescents appreciated the regular distribution of food and the presence of an institutional patient network providing solidarity. Tedium replaced anxiety. Patients who survived the ordeal of their 40-day hospitalization were transferred to another institution for an additional two- or three-week period of convalescent isolation to avoid the possibility of reinfection and to facilitate turnover in the lazarettos. *Sospetti* who failed to contract the disease were also sent to separate convalescent homes. The authorities also realized that further rest and ample food, essential for recovery, could be better provided away from overcrowded lazarettos. During the 1656 epidemic in Rome, the convent of San Pancrazio and the Casaletto di Pio Quinto were transformed into houses devoted to convalescents discharged from San Bartolomeo. After spending a "clean" quarantine period in the convalescent home, patients were transferred to their final destination: a new, vacant prison built by the previous pope, Innocent XI, on the Strada Julia, where they spent an additional month before returning home.[164]

Nothing more is known about the three Trasteverian women who survived. They apparently recovered from their illness and must have been discharged to the convent of San Pancrazio in the nearby hills outside the city gates for additional quarantine and recovery time. In Rome, the authorities had created a two-tier system of makeshift facilities in monastic hospitals and jails to extend the convalescent period for up to three months, thus effectively preventing a significant portion of the population from returning home before full recovery. Assembled in groups, convalescents such as Marina, Catharina, and Clementia left the island lazaretto on foot or in coaches, again escorted by soldiers and a public health official, often Cardinal Gastaldi himself, to their final "clean" *quarantina*. As processions reached St. Peter, Pope Alexander VII, carried by his guards in a sedan chair, made an appearance, bestowing his blessing on the survivors and cheering them on their journey toward final recovery with a hearty "God be with you!"[165]

By the time London was visited by the plague nine years later, in 1665, the second wave of lazaretto foundations had reached its peak throughout Europe. Even municipalities reluctant to invest in more than temporary isolation facilities had finally relented as the onslaught of the epidemics more than decimated their populations and seriously hampered commerce. Paradoxically, just as the construction of more elaborate and permanent pesthouses ended, plague gradually vanished from Europe.[166] Even the last major outbreak in Marseilles, in 1720, while temporarily filling the local lazaretto and other hospital facilities with suspected and real plague victims, failed to reverse the downward trend. Just as some facilities originally created for lepers came to be used to house plague victims, they were now filled with smallpox patients in the eighteenth century, and later in the

1800s they took in individuals afflicted with typhus and cholera. Others became houses of correction and prisons, and some were transformed into military establishments providing medical assistance to sick and wounded soldiers. A number of lazarettos at Marseilles, Genoa, Naples, Malta, and Venice continued to function as permanent quarantine stations, monitoring the movement of travelers and goods from the Levant. Reports from John Howard (1726–1790), the English prison reformer, who visited some of these institutions in 1785, described the centuries'-old purification procedures still used to fight the plague.[167]

Frameworks for early medicalization

While leper houses and pesthouses functioned primarily as segregation facilities for persons suffering from particular diseases considered contagious, other hospitals during the sixteenth and seventeenth centuries focused on different populations. To be sure, most European hospitals after 1500 continued to provide traditional welfare services—shelter, food, and spiritual salvation—thus remaining depositories for the chronically and hopelessly ill poor. At the Santa Maria Nuova Hospital in Florence at the beginning of the sixteenth century, for example, rules still demanded that the authorities "shelter and tend the sick poor who come to the hospital as they would Christ himself. They must receive them with their own hands, care for them, console them, and warm, feed, and wash them with compassion. They must attend to their needs and treat them with all care and charity."[168] Moreover, hospitalization still contributed to the social control of the sick and increasingly dangerous poor.[169] But thanks to a new economic and social order, many larger hospitals now began to place more emphasis on restoring the physical well-being of those they admitted. With patient populations increasingly composed of younger workers who sought institutional assistance for their ailments with the hope of returning to their previous occupations, hospitals began to function as institutions of first resort for them when they became acutely ill. The hospital was being transformed into a house of recovery.

Tuscany, in fact, was at the forefront of this new development. Originally established in 1288 as a small shelter, Florence's Santa Maria Nuova had 250 beds in 1500 thanks to private bequests and public subsidies. The patient population in the early 1500s consisted mainly of sick townspeople and travelers, especially pilgrims en route to Rome. Even some "nobles, who have decided to come to us for treatment on account of poverty or a religious vow," were cared for, albeit in separate facilities.[170] Others "who cannot afford house calls by a private physician" sought free ambulatory assistance in the form of food and medicine.[171] Based on surviving records, almost half of the incoming patients suffered from fevers, particularly during the summer months. The next most frequent category was skin diseases, led by scabies and followed by herpes and smallpox. The length of stay in Florentine hospitals was brief and the mortality quite low, if the example of the hospital of San Paulo (10 days, 3–10% mortality) is taken as an indicator.[172]

Another medicalizing institution was the *Blatternhaus* or "pox house," first founded in several southwest German cities for the care of local individuals afflicted by a seemingly novel ailment during the summer of 1496 referred to as *morbus gallicus* (French disease) by the Germans and Italians.[173] Like other eruptive diseases during the Middle Ages, including leprosy, this disease—presumably an early and much more aggressive form of syphilis—was suspected of being venereal, with sexual promiscuity blamed for its nearly epidemic diffusion throughout Europe. Acute and highly lethal, this disease presented with high fever, eye infections, and great pain in joints and bones, with occasional paralysis and destruction of the nasal cartilage. Secondary skin eruptions appeared within a matter of days and became infected. Many patients suffered from a "galloping" syphilis, a disfiguring variety with large, ulcerating, stinking sores that even prompted remaining lepers to refuse being placed near them.[174] Perhaps a good number of them around 1500 were former mercenary soldiers, now homeless adventurers and beggars scattered throughout Europe's countryside, spending their idle hours in taverns and bordellos.[175]

Augsburg had one of the biggest municipal hospitals, founded in 1495 for pox sufferers in early modern Germany, with a capacity of 122 beds. In addition, the city featured a private facility, the famous Fugger-financed hospital, the *Holzhaus* (wood house).[176] Prominently involved in founding these hospitals were municipal authorities, private philanthropists, and a new group of specialized healers: the so-called *Franzosenärzte*—physicians devoted to the treatment of the French disease. In marked contrast to the older leper houses and pesthouses, many of the pox houses were located within the urban walls on the fringes of the town, although several cities used abandoned leper houses.[177] A *Blatternhaus* resembled an ordinary town house, with its multiple rooms used for separate male and female wards as well as chambers for the dying and convalescents. A special feature was the *Holzstube* or sauna room, equipped with a big wood-burning stove, where patients were made to to sweat profusely, an important feature of the treatment. Medical personnel, including physicians, barber-surgeons, apothecaries, and empirics, were part of most pox houses' staff from their inception. Contemporary therapies for the disease included the administration of mercury and a decoction from guaiacum wood obtained from a common evergreen tree from the West Indies said to have medicinal properties.[178] Like other isolation hospitals, pox houses lasted into the nineteenth century, specializing in the treatment of venereal diseases.

In the end, these activities owed much to new ideas, derived from Renaissance humanism, that attempted to recast the traditional religious role of the hospital. Here the works of Erasmus and the English statesman Thomas More, chancellor of England under Henry VIII, were quite persuasive. More, for example, argued in 1516 for the care of the sick in hospitals in a popular book entitled *Utopia*. Such institutional attention, in More's polemical fantasy, was to be a rational and routine activity of the community. Just as important, More's utopian hospitals were no longer conceived as shelters for the poor, but rather were designed to be medicalized institutions for the care and isolation of any and all sick citizens.[179]

WELFARE AND HOSPITALS IN EARLY MODERN EUROPE

Even before 1500, as poverty became endemic in many areas of Europe, a more discriminating philosophy regarding society's poor had taken hold. Charity was no longer conceived as either private or religious. Welfare policies began cutting across religious boundaries and followed patterns closely tailored to local urban conditions.[180] Emphasis shifted away from the medieval concept of generalized hospitality broadly dispensed to the "poor of Jesus Christ," which had led to widespread abuse and fraud. The voluntary poor, especially now the mendicant orders, had siphoned off the lion's share of charitable giving, leaving the increasingly involuntary poor with few opportunities to receive aid. With private giving dwindling because of wars and economic crises, social welfare had to be rationed and better targeted, a function increasingly undertaken by the civil powers. Instead of the traditionally individualized relationship between donors and recipients epitomized by almsgiving, charity thus became channeled through existing social structures such as parishes, confraternities, and municipalities to benefit almshouses, schools, and hospitals.[181]

To implement a more restricted form of poor relief directed at particular categories of indigents, welfare reformers employed a number of religious and economic rationales. By attacking begging and the mendicant orders, the Protestant Reformation added emphasis to already widespread concerns about the growing ranks of idle vagrants, with their aggressive demands and threats. For Protestants, a new relationship to both God and the community stood at the center of a profound change in charitable assistance. Divine Providence, not the quest for indulgences, was the path toward salvation, with an emphasis on individual faith and grace, not priestly mediation. Gone was the need for inmates' prayers on behalf of hospital patrons that had driven so many donations to charitable institutions before the Reformation. Gone also was the charitable institution as an instrument of salvation. In addition, living within a Christian community assumed that individuals had a right to charitable assistance together with obligations to

contribute and assist others. Thus, Protestant countries in Europe tried to organize local or national systems of relief financed by subscriptions or taxes.[182]

At the same time, a new work ethic, viewing daily labor as spiritually fulfilling and a communal obligation, was adopted by both Protestantism and the
Catholic Counter-Reformation as the centerpiece of a rational and organized society.[183] Earning one's daily bread fulfilled both moral and civil obligations by
keeping individuals from lust and idleness. In selecting its welfare recipients, modern European society thus sought to identify those it considered *deserving* of assistance. According to newly established moral and economic criteria, these were
individuals who had resided for some time in a parish or community and whose
family or friends could provide necessary references concerning background, character, and behavior. In early modern Europe, most of the deserving poor were
working people, barely above the poverty level but seemingly content with their
status in society as bestowed by Divine Providence. Holding meager artisanal or
service jobs, they were characterized as modest and law-abiding. To determine
their eligibility for aid, communities developed a series of means tests. Those who
passed them were placed under local patronage and included in existing charity
schemes when misfortune threatened.[184]

European society chose to deal differently with individuals who were neither
regular residents nor stable members of any given community. As urbanization
accelerated, a new view of poverty emerged, differing sharply from that prevalent
in previous centuries. Hordes of homeless people and strangers, as well as drifters,
vagrants, and beggars, were identified with social unrest and crime. Broadly characterized as the "poor of the Devil" or the "fifth estate," this group of paupers
included a large number of seasonal, transient laborers. Ignorant and unskilled,
they were often miserable wretches, shunned by a society that no longer favored
almsgiving or tolerated idleness. Painted as potential troublemakers and even criminals and feared as vectors of disease, this "populace" was characterized as *undeserving* of social welfare and was therefore often targeted for coercive reeducation
schemes or forced labor. The establishment of workhouses or "houses of occupation" in Protestant countries, for example, was an attempt to punish and rehabilitate unworthy individuals. Other efforts focused on vocational training and the
education necessary to secure employment.[185]

To fulfill their social contract and remain productive, workers in early modern Europe needed to stay healthy, or, if sick, to be assisted in their recovery.[186]
Rebounding in number in spite of high infant mortality rates and a falling life expectancy, urban populations in the seventeenth and early eighteenth centuries fell
prey to an expanding array of illnesses affecting especially the young and the aged.
Smallpox had supplanted plague as the greatest killer. Townspeople were often
undernourished and sick, suffering from a variety of new fevers (influenza or English sweat, probably malaria), gastrointestinal parasites, and deficiency diseases.[187]
Under the circumstances, efforts at the local level designed to stem such assaults

on health were encouraged and greatly valued. Protestant providentialism conferred an active role on individuals in seeking their own recovery,[188] but help was always near. Outdoor relief in the form of home care by visiting nurses and medicines was furnished to maintain the deserving poor's legitimate status in society until they recovered. To finance it, citizens paid compulsory taxes or poor rates.

Since hospitals were now mostly under civic authority, they thus became enmeshed in such new schemes of social control and assistance.[189] In Protestant countries, institutionalized health care took place in smaller infirmaries and dispensaries supported by local governments or community chest organizations. With the closing of monasteries, monastic infirmaries ceased to be available. However, many Holy Spirit hospitals scattered across Protestant Europe survived. Previously under papal auspices and affiliated with the Ospedale di Santo Spirito in Rome, these endowed institutions continued to care for the poor and sick. After 1600, the modern state sought also to protect, rehabilitate, and retire deserving members of its armed forces, a development that created impressive networks of military and naval hospitals, as well as institutions for those classified as invalids. In all establishments, administrators were empowered to exercise gatekeeping functions in the selection of proper inmates. In turn, belief in Divine Providence encouraged medical activities as another divinely approved instrument to assist in recovery.[190] The hospital could be a place of first rather than last resort, a place offering more than an assurance of last rites, holy burial, and eternal salvation, as it so often had been before the Reformation.

In Catholic Europe, meanwhile, the Council of Trent (1545–1563) had made specific efforts to eliminate widespread administrative abuses by religious personnel, including the excesses of greedy hospital administrators. Corrupt managers and monastic caregivers were dismissed. With rents and taxes declining, lay administrators with business experience were entrusted with the accounts and held authority over the remaining priests, who were now restricted to carrying out religious rituals. Bishops were empowered to visit hospitals periodically, although rulers and municipalities often prevented them from exercising that right.[191] As a result of the Tridentine reforms, the Catholic Church reorganized religious hospitals and closed small, poorly endowed institutions, thus accelerating an ongoing, two-century-old consolidation process.[192] In their place, privately endowed, large general hospitals or shelters, often run by local confraternities, were designed to bring together diverse groups of needy people. These included orphans, chronic sufferers, mentally ill individuals, and the elderly.[193] The sick poor found care in "God's hostels" (Hôtels Dieu) and other infirmaries. Northern Italian cities founded a series of hospitals for beggars or mendicanti in the seventeenth century. In the eyes of the Catholic Church, the distinction between worthy and unworthy poor remained blurred. They were all sinners who should be saved. Indeed, spiritual salvation remained the primary objective of hospitalization, and religious ceremonies continued to be central to hospital life, leading to tensions with medical caregivers.

NOTES

1. This excerpt from Robert Henryson's fifteenth-century poem has been modernized from the Middle English text in Denton Fox, ed., *The Testament of Cresseid by Robert Henryson*, London, Nelson, 1968. For commentary see Saul N. Brody, *The Disease of the Soul: Leprosy in Medieval Literature*, Ithaca, Cornell Univ. Press, 1974, pp. 173–77.

2. Robert S. Hoyt, "Agrarian and urban unrest," in *Europe in the Middle Ages*, 2nd ed., New York, Harcourt, Brace & World, 1966, pp. 590–606.

3. For more information see Ludger Tewes, *Die Amts-und Pfandpolitik der Erzbischöfe von Köln im Spätmittelalter (1306–1463)*, Cologne, Bohlau, 1987, and Brigitte M. Wobbeke, *Das Militärwesen der Stadt Köln im 15. Jahrhundert*, Stuttgart, F. Steiner, 1991.

4. The letter is listed among "Urkunden und Aktenstücke zur Geschichte der Leprauntersuchung in Köln und Umgegend, 1357–1712," collected by Hermann Keussen, *Lepra* (Leipzig) 14 (1914): 109–10. I am indebted to Professor Alfons Labisch for assisting me in obtaining a copy of the original document from the city archives of Cologne, and to Barbara Schürmann, Fritz Dross, Robert Jütte, and Claudia Stein for deciphering the early modern German text.

5. The English translation is mine. I am grateful to Claudia Stein for rendering this document into modern German.

6. Erich Meuthen, *Kölner Universitätsgeschichte*, Cologne, Böhlau Verlag, 1988, vol. 1, pp. 120–25. See also A. Zimmermann, ed., *Die Kölner Universität im Mittelalter: Geistige Wurzeln und soziale Wirklichkeit*, Berlin, W. de Gruyter, 1989.

7. Most of the Cologne faculty were originally from the Low Countries, and some had visited the Italian universities. Details are presented in Marion Wuhr, *Die Apotheken im ehemaligen Oberen Erzstift Köln*, Stuttgart, Deutscher Apotheker Verlag, 1985.

8. See L. Demaître, "The description and diagnosis of leprosy by fourteenth-century physicians," *Bull Hist Med* 59 (1985): 339.

9. This possible dual approach is suggested by the fact that Thielen's documentation was filed together with the official university examinations. Bau had been dean of the faculty since 1478. For an overview of Cologne's documentation see R. Jütte, "Die medizinische Versorgung einer Stadtbevölkerung im 16. und 17. Jahrhundert am Beispiel der Reichstadt Köln," *Medizinshist J* 22 (1987): 173–84.

10. Hermann Keussen, "Nachrichten über die in den Lepraprotokollen gennanten Professoren und Lizentiaten, welche an den Untersuchungen teilnahmen," *Lepra* (Leipzig) 14 (1914): 99–100. For details about contemporary Cologne physicians see M. Bernhardt, *Gelehrte im Reich: Zur Sozial-und Wirkungsgeschichte akademischer Eliten des 14. bis 16. Jahrhunderts*, Berlin, Dunker & Humblot, 1996, pp. 113–34.

11. The oath, written in Latin, was put into writing in 1512 and reprinted in Hermann Keussen, "Urkunden und Aktenstücke," *Lepra* (Leipzig) 14 (1914): 108. I am indebted to Victoria Sweet for the translation.

12. O. von Bremen, "Die Lepra-Untersuchungen der Kölner medizinischen Fakultät von 1491–1664," *Westdeutsche Zeitsch Gesch u Kunst* 18 (1899): 65–77. One of the most popular fourteenth-century manuals for such an examination was written by Arnald de Vil-

lanova of Montpellier, *On the Examination of Lepers*, together with Jordanus de Turre's *Notes on Leprosy*. For details see Demaître, "Description and diagnosis," 334.

13. See A. Homolka, "Die Lebensgewohnheiten der Leprakranken im Spätmittelalter," and G. Keil, "Der Aussatz im Mittelalter," in *Aussatz, Lepra, Hansen-Krankheit, Ein Menschheitsproblem im Wandel*, ed. J. H. Wolf, Würzburg, Deutsches Aussätzigen Hilfswerk, 1986, vol. 2, pp. 85–102 and 152–53, respectively, and S. R. Ell, "Blood and sexuality in medieval leprosy," *Janus* 71 (1984): 153–64.

14. Peter Greave's *The Seventh Gate*, London, T. Smith, 1976, provides an excellent account of the process. See especially pp. 190–217. See also F. Bergman, "Hoping against hope? A marital dispute about the treatment of leprosy in the 15th century Hanseatic town of Kampen," in *The Task of Healing*, ed. H. Marland and M. Pelling, Rotterdam, Erasmus, 1996, pp. 23–48.

15. This document is listed in Keussen, "Urkunden und Aktenstücke," 10. The original is in the city archives of Cologne. Again, I am grateful for Claudia Stein's translation into modern German. No official medical report has survived.

16. Demaître, "Description and diagnosis," 340–44. For a general overview consult Peter Richards, *The Medieval Leper and His Northern Heirs*, Cambridge, Brewer, Rowman & Littlefield, 1977.

17. Bodel wrote around 1202 before leaving his native city of Arras in northern France. See Jean Bodel, "Les conges de Jean Bodel," ed. G. Raynaud, *Romania* X (1880): 235. I am indebted to Victoria Sweet for the translation.

18. For more details see Charlotte Roberts and Keith Manchester, *The Archeology of Disease*, 2nd ed., Ithaca, Cornell Univ. Press, 1995, pp. 142–50, and Robert C. Hastings, ed., *Leprosy*, 2nd ed., Edinburgh, Churchill Livingstone, 1994.

19. See K. Manchester, "Tuberculosis and leprosy in antiquity: An interpretation," *Med Hist* 28 (1984): 162–73, and J. H. Wolf, "Zur historischen Epidemiologie der Lepra," in *Maladie et Société (XIIe–XVIIIe Siècles)*, ed. N. Bulst and R. Delort, Paris, Ed. CNRS, 1989, pp. 99–120.

20. Greave, *The Seventh Gate*, p. 202.

21. See J. G. Andersen, "Studies in the Medieval Diagnosis of Leprosy in Denmark," *Danish Med Bull* 16 (1969): suppl IX, 15–16.

22. E. V. Hulse, "The nature of biblical 'leprosy' and the use of alternative medical terms in modern translations of the Bible," *Palestine Exploration Q* 107 (1975): 87–105, summarized in *Med Hist* 20 (1976): 203. The word *lepra* was also used in the New Testament to indicate skin blemishes that could be cleansed. See F. C. Lendrum, "The name 'leprosy,' " *Am J Trop Med Hyg* 1 (1952): 999–1008. See also P. A. Kalish, "An overview of research on the history of leprosy," *Int J Leprosy* 43 (1975): 129–44.

23. For an overview see K. Park, "Medicine and society in medieval Europe, 500–1500," in *Medicine in Society: Historical Essays*, ed. A. Wear, Cambridge, Cambridge Univ. Press, 1992, pp. 59–90.

24. Aretaeus of Cappadocia (81–138 AD) observed that "when in such a state, who would not flee; who would not turn from them, even if a father, a son, or a brother? There is danger also, from the communication of the ailment. Many, therefore, have exposed their most beloved relatives in the wilderness, and on the mountains, some with the intention of administering to their hunger, but others not so, as wishing them to die." See Andersen, "Medieval Diagnosis of Leprosy," p. 37.

25. D. G. Smith, "The genetic hypothesis of susceptibility to lepromatous leprosy," *Hum Genet* 50 (1979): 163–77.

26. P. A. Kalish, "An overview of research on the history of leprosy," *Int J Leprosy* 43 (1975): 129–44.

27. Quoted in Brody, *Disease of the Soul*, p. 79

28. Andersen, "Medieval Diagnosis of Leprosy," p. 37.

29. R. J. Palmer, "The church, leprosy, and plague in medieval and early modern Europe," in *The Church and Healing: Studies in Church History*, ed. W. J. Shields, Oxford, Blackwell, 1982, pp. 79–99.

30. F. Beriac, "Connaissances médicales sur la lèpre et protection contre cette maladie au Moyen Age," in *Maladie et Société*, pp. 145–63.

31. M. W. Dols, "Leprosy in medieval Arabic medicine," *J Hist Med* 34 (1979): 314–33.

32. Wrote Aretaeus: "Sometimes, too, certain of the members of the patients will die, so as to drop off such as the nose, the fingers, the feet, the privy parts and the whole hands." Andersen, "Medieval Diagnosis of Leprosy," pp. 17–43. See also H. M. Koelbing and A. Stettler-Schär, "Aussatz, Lepra, Elephantiasis Graecorum—zur Geschichte der Lepra im Altertum," in *Beiträge zur Geschichte der Lepra*, ed. H. M. Koelbing et al., Zurich, Juris, 1972, pp. 34–54.

33. Demaître, "Description and diagnosis," 327–44. See also R. H. Major, "A thirteenth-century clinical description of leprosy," *J Hist Med* 4 (1949): 237–38.

34. An important study of this problem is Margaret A. Wheatley, "Leprosy—A Disease Apart: A Historical and Cross Cultural Analysis of Stigma," Ph.D. diss., Carleton University, 1985.

35. See M. W. Dols, "The leper in medieval Islamic society," *Speculum* 58 (1983): 891–916.

36. S. R. Ell, "Diet and leprosy in the medieval west: The noble leper," *Janus* 72 (1985): 113–29.

37. S. Jarcho, "Lazar houses and the dissemination of leprosy," *Med Hist* 15 (1971): 401. Much has been made of the warmer climate since postglacial times in the epidemiology of leprosy. See T. Dunin-Wasowicz, "Climate as a factor affecting the human environment in the Middle Ages," *J Eur Econ Hist* 4 (1979): 691–706.

38. See F. O. Touati, "Facies leprosorum: Reflexions sur le diagnostic facial de la lèpre au moyen age," *Hist scien méd* 20 (1986): 57–66.

39. D. Ploog and F. Brandt, "Die Zerstörung des Antlitzes—eine ethnologische Betrachtung bei Lepra," in *Aussatz, Lepra, Hansen-Krankheit*, vol. 2, pp. 331–37.

40. See H. Hörger, "Krankheit und religiöses Tabu—die Lepra in der mittelalterlich-frühneuzeitlichen Gesellschaft Europas," *Gesnerus* 39 (1982): 53–70. See also Françoise Beriac, *Histoire des lèpreux au Moyen Age: une société d'exclus*, Paris, Imago, 1988.

41. R. I. Moore, *The Formation of a Persecuting Society: Power and Deviance in Western Europe, 950–1250*, Oxford, B. Blackwell, 1987, especially pp. 45–65. See also M. Barber, "Lepers, Jews, and Moslems: The plot to overthrow Christendom in 1321," *History* 66 (1981): 1–17.

42. St. Gregory Nazianzen, "On St. Basil," in *Funeral Orations by St. Gregory Nazianzen and St. Ambrose*, trans. L. P. McCauley et al., New York, Fathers of the Church, Inc., 1953, p. 81.

43. D. Leistikow, "Bauformen der Leproserie im Abendland," in *Aussatz, Lepra, Hansen-Krankheit*, vol. 2, pp. 103–49.

44. P. D. Mitchell, "Leprosy and the case of King Baldwin IV of Jerusalem: Mycobacterial disease in the Crusader States of the 12th and 13th centuries," *Int J Leprosy* 61 (1993): 283–91.

45. For London see M. B. Honeybourne, "The leper hospitals of the London area," *Trans London Middlesex Archeol Soc* 21 (1963–67): 1–61. For England and Wales see David Knowles and R. Neville Hadcock, *Medieval Religious Houses: England and Wales*, London, Longmans, Green, 1953, pp. 250–324.

46. For an overview see W. Frohn, *Der Aussatz im Rheinland*, Jena, G. Fischer, 1933, pp. 117–23. The designation *Melaten* or *Malaten* for a leper house and its inmates was characteristic of establishments in the Lower Rhine region. The name probably derives from the French term *mal ladre* ("illness of Lazarus"), since this sore-covered beggar figure from the Scriptures had become the patron saint of lepers.

47. P. Fuchs, "Die mittelalterliche Stadtbefestigung," in *Chronik zur Geschichte der Stadt Köln*, ed. P. Fuchs, Cologne, Greven, 1990–1991, vol. 1, p. 196.

48. Johannes Asen, *Das Leprosenhaus Melaten bei Köln*, Bonn, J. Bach, 1908, pp. 20–33.

49. See Brody, *Disease of the Soul*, p. 98.

50. R. L. Goodey, "The Development of the Medieval Infirmary in England," Ph.D. diss., Univ. of London, 1986, pp. 261–66.

51. Ibid. pp. 255–63.

52. Asen, *Leprosenhaus*, pp. 33–49.

53. Frohn, *Der Aussatz in Rheinland*, pp. 180–83.

54. This oath was officially instituted in the leper house at Basel after 1533. For details about institutional life see Homolka, "Lebensgewohnheiten der Leprakranken," p. 151.

55. Regulations of the leper house at Andelys before 1380, Bibliothèque Nationale MS, cited in N. Guglielmi, "Estatutos de hospitales y leproserias," *Anales Hist Antigua Medieval* 16 (1971): 187.

56. Asen, *Leprosenhaus*, pp. 49–58.

57. Regulations enacted by the bishop of Tournai for the leper house at Lille and dated June 1239. Available in Guglielmi, "Estatutos," 175.

58. Guglielmi, "Estatutos," 180.

59. For a recent regional study see P. Borradori, *Mourir au Monde: les Lèpreux dans le Pays de Vaud, XIIIe–XVIIe Siecle*, Lausanne, Univ. of Lausanne, 1992.

60. Bodel, "Les conges," 242–43.

61. Asen, *Leprosenhaus*, pp. 83–86.

62. N. Waxler, "Learning to be a leper: A case study in the social construction of illness," in *Social Contexts of Health, Illness, and Patient Care*, ed. E. Mishler et al., Cambridge, Cambridge Univ. Press, 1981, pp. 181–88.

63. Guglielmi, "Estatutos", 181.

64. Ibid., 175.

65. For an overview see V. L. and B. Bullough, "Medieval nursing," *Nursing Hist Rev* 1 (1993): 89–104.

66. Asen, *Leprosenhaus*, p. 83

67. Consult Piero Camporesi, *The Incorruptible Flesh*, trans. T. Croft-Murray and H. Elsom, Cambridge, Cambridge Univ. Press, 1988, p. 78.

68. Quotation from Bernard de Gordon, a fourteenth-century physician of Montpellier. See L. Demaître, "The relevance of futility: Jordan de Turre (fl. 1313–1335) on the treatment of leprosy," *Bull Hist Med* 70 (1996): 29.

69. According to the rules of a French institution in Lille (1250), the bleedings were administered six times a year: a day after Christmas, before Lent, after Easter, around the feast of Saints Peter and Paul, early September, and before the Feast of All Saints. See Guglielmi, "Estatutos," 133.

70. See Camporesi, *The Incorruptible Flesh*, pp. 90–96.

71. Guy de Chauliac, "Chirurgia magna," quoted in Demaître, "Treatment of leprosy," 35.

72. C. Habrich, "Die Arzneimitteltherapie des Aussatzes in der abendländischen Medizin," in *Lepra—Gestern und Heute*, ed. R. Töllner, Münster, Verlag Regensberg, 1992, pp. 57–72.

73. See the recommendations of Henri de Mondeville and Guy de Chauliac in Demaître, "Treatment of leprosy," 37–38.

74. Carolyn W. Bynum, *Fragmentation and Redemption: Essays on Gender and the Human Body in Medieval Religion*, New York, Zone Books, 1992, especially, pp. 239–97.

75. Guglielmi, "Estatutos," 185.

76. These statistics apparently include young children and are therefore somewhat misleading. See Asen, *Leprosenhaus*, pp. 74–75. Leprotic children may have contracted the disease in the leper houses. See S. Jarcho, "Lazar houses and the dissemination of leprosy," *Med Hist* 15 (1971): 401.

77. Authors have stressed the accuracy of medieval diagnosticians of leprosy because of the high proportion of skeletons found with pathological changes suggestive of the disease at cemeteries belonging to leper houses. See V. Moeller-Christensen, "Location and excavation of the first Danish leper graveyard from the Middle Ages: St. Joergen's Farm, Naestved," *Bull Hist Med* 27 (1953): 112–23, and E. Schmitz-Cliever, "Das mittelalterliche Leprosorium Melaten bei Aachen in der Diözese Lüttich (1230–1550)," *Clio Med* 7 (1972): 13–34. The postulated diagnostic accuracy of medieval churchmen and medical professionals must be tempered by the possibility that nonleprous inmates may have contracted this illness after being admitted.

78. Fox, *Testament of Cresseid*.

79. This dedication, dated February 21, 1657, was included in a series of broadsides designed and produced by Giovanni G. Rossi illustrating the contemporary plague in Rome. Photos and Print Collection, History Division, National Library of Medicine, 68–221–23. For a discussion see E. B. Wells, "Prints commemorating the Rome 1656 plague epidemic," *Ann Inst Museo Storia della Scienza Firenze* 10 (1985): 15–21.

80. P. Savio, "Richerche sulla peste di Roma degli anni 1656–1657," *Arch Soc Romana Storia Patria* 95 (1972): 121.

81. G. B. Risse, "Epidemics and history: ecological perspectives and social responses," in *AIDS: The Burdens of History*, ed. E. Fee and D. Fox, Berkeley, Univ. of California Press, 1988, pp. 33–66. For more information see Ellen B. Wells, "The Plague of Rome of 1656," M.A. thesis, Cornell Univ., 1973.

82. K. Park, "Black Death," in *The Cambridge World History of Human Disease*, ed. K. F. Kiple, Cambridge, Cambridge Univ. Press, 1993, pp. 612–16, and G. Calvi, "L'oro, il fuoco, le forche: la peste napoletana del 1656," *Archivo storico italiano* 139 (1981): 405–58. For a popular book on the plague see Philip Ziegler, *The Black Death*, New York, Penguin Books, 1970. For Italy see Alfonso Corradi, *Annali delle epidemie occorse in Italia dalle prime memòrie fino al 1850*, 8 vols., Bologna, Gamberini & Permeggiani, 1865–1894.

83. A. Wade, "Mechanisms of long and short term immunity to plague," *Immunology* 34 (1978): 1045–52; R. R. Brubaker, "The genus *Yersinia*: Biochemistry and genetics of virulence," *Curr Top Microbiol Immunol* 57 (1972): 111–58; and R. E. Lenki, "Evolution of plague virulence," *Nature* 334 (1988): 473–74.

84. J. Norris, "East or West? The geographic origin of the Black Death," *Bull Hist Med* 51 (1977): 1–24.

85. T. L. Bratton, "The identity of the plague of Justinian," *Trans Stud Coll Phys Phila* 3 (1981): 113–24 and 174–80.

86. M. Dols, "Plague in early Islamic history," *J Am Orient Soc* 94 (1974): 371–83.

87. See O. J. Benedictow, "Morbidity with historical plague epidemics," *Pop Stud* 41 (1987): 401–31, and William H. McNeill, *Plagues and Peoples*, Garden City, NY, Anchor Press, 1976, pp. 149–98.

88. M. Silver, "Controlling grain prices and de-controlling bubonic plague," *J Social Biol Struct* 5 (1982): 107–20.

89. Paolo S. Pallavicino, *Descrizione del contagio che da Napoli si comunico a Roma nell'-anno 1656* (1657), reprint, Rome, Colegio Urlano, 1837, p. 10. I am grateful to Ellen B. Wells for providing a copy and a partial translation.

90. J. Henderson, " 'A certain sickness with suspicion of contagion': physicians, plague, and public health in early modern Florence," in *A History of the Concepts of Contagion, Infection, and Miasma*, ed. W. H. Bynum and B. Fantini (forthcoming).

91. Pallavicino, *Descrizione*, pp. 15–17. Recent studies include E. Sonnino and R. Traina, "La peste del 1656–57 a Roma: Organizazione sanitaria e mortalità," in *La Demografia Storica delle Città Italiane*, Bologna, CLUEB, 1982, pp. 433–51.

92. Pallavicino, *Descrizione*, p. 17–18. Daily reports prepared for Mario Chigi during the epidemic are available in MSS Chigiano Codex E III, 62, Manuscript Collection, Bibliotheca Vaticana, Rome.

93. For mortality statistics of Naples and Rome see L. del Panta and M. Livi Bacci, "Chronologie, intensité et diffusion des crises de mortalité en Italie: 1600–1850," in *The Great Mortalities: Methodological Studies of Demographic Crises in the Past*, ed. H. Charbonneau and A. Larosse, Liege, Ordina, 1980, reprinted in a special issue of *Population* (1977): 401–44. A geographical distribution of plague epidemics is presented in L. Del Panta, *Le Epidemie nella Storia Demografica Italiana, Secoli XIV–XIX*, Turin, Loescher, 1980.

94. For more information see Massimo Petrocchi, *Roma nel Seicento*, Bologna, L. Capelli, 1970, and Giacinto Gigli, *Diario Romano (1608–1670)*, Rome, Tumminelli, 1958.

95. For more details see Richard Krautheimer, *The Rome of Alexander VII, 1655–1667*, Princeton, NJ, Princeton Univ. Press, 1985.

96. Lorenzo Pizzati of Pontremoli, an ex-official at the papal court, in a memorandum to Alexander VII, from Krautheimer, *Rome*, p. 127.

97. Ibid.

98. Ibid., p. 130. Also see Fioravante Martinelli, *Roma nel Seicento*, Florence, Vallecchi, 1968.

99. Pallavicino, *Descrizione*, p. 17

100. Ibid., pp. 17–20. For Trastevere see Cesare d'Onofrio, *Il Tevere e Roma*, 2nd ed., Rome, Romana Soc Edit, 1980.

101. M. P. Chase, "Fevers, poisons, and apostemes: Authority and experience in Montpellier plague treatises," in *Science and Technology in Medieval Society*, ed. P. O. Long, New York, New York Academic Sciences, 1985, pp. 153–69.

102. The quotation is from Geronimo Gastaldi's work *Tractatus de Avertenda et Profliganda Peste*, Bologna, 1684. It appears in English translation in Carlo M. Cipolla, *Cristofano and the Plague*, Berkeley, Univ. of California Press, 1973, p. 29.

103. B. Pullan, "Plague and perceptions of the poor in early modern Italy," in *Epidemics and Ideas: Essays on the Historical Perception of Pestilence*, ed. T. Ranger and P. Slack, Cambridge, Cambridge Univ. Press, 1992, pp. 101–04. See also R. Palmer, "The Church, leprosy, and plague," pp. 79–99.

104. L. Clendening, "The plague saints," *Bull Soc Med Hist Chicago* 4 (1930): 133–41.

105. Pallavicino, *Descrizione*, p. 29

106. J. Arrizabalaga, "Facing the Black Death: Perceptions and reactions of university medical practitioners," in *Practical Medicine from Salerno to the Black Death*, ed. L. Garcia Ballester, R. French, J. Amizabulaga and A. Cunningham, Cambridge, Cambridge Univ. Press, 1993, pp. 248–53.

107. For an overview see C. Hannaway, "Environment and miasmata," in *Companion Encyclopedia of the History of Medicine*, ed. W. F. Bynum and R. Porter, London, Routledge, 1993, vol. 1, pp. 292–308.

108. V. Nutton, "The seeds of disease: An explanation of contagion and infection from the Greeks to the Renaissance," *Med Hist* 27 (1983): 1–34.

109. See V. Nutton, "The reception of Fracastoro's theory of contagion: The seed that fell among thorns?" *Osiris* 6 (1990): 196–234, and J. Henderson "The Black Death in Florence: Medical and communal responses," in *Death in Towns: Urban Responses to the Dying and the Dead, 100–1600*, ed. S. Bassett, Leicester, 1992, pp. 136–50.

110. Consult Johannes Nohl, *The Black Death; A Chronicle of the Plague, Compiled from Contemporary Sources*, trans. C. H. Clarke, London, Unwin Books, 1971, pp. 58–72.

111. For Boccaccio's ideas on the pestilence see "Contemporary views of the plague" in *The Black Death*, ed. W. M. Bowsky, Huntington, NY, Krieger, 1978, pp. 7–18. A collection of original documents related to the Black Death, particularly for England, is Rosemary Horrox, ed. and trans., *The Black Death*, Manchester, Manchester Univ. Press, 1994.

112. L. J. Rather, "The six things non natural," *Clio Med* 3 (1968): 337–47, and P. H. Niebyl, "The non-naturals," *Bull Hist Med* 45 (1971): 486–92.

113. H. A. Savitz, "Jacob Zahalon, and his book, *The Treasure of Life*," *N Engl J Med* 213 (1935): 175. See also J. O. Leibowitz, "Bubonic plague in the ghetto of Rome (1656): Descriptions by Zahalon and Gastaldi," *Koroth* 4 (1967): 25–28. An original source of medical advice is Mattia Naldi, *Regole per la cura del contagio*, Rome, 1656.

114. C. Singer, "Some plague tractates (fourteenth and fifteenth centuries)," *Proc R Soc Med* 9 (1915–16): 159–212. For further information see Dominick Palazzotto, "The Black Death and Medicine: A Report and Analysis of the Tractates Written between 1348–1350," Ph.D. diss., Univ. of Kansas, 1973.

115. See M. Dinges, "Pest und Staat: Von der Intitutionengeschichte zur sozialen Konstruktion?" in *Neue Wege in der Seuchengeschichte*, ed. M. Dinges and T. Schlich, Stuttgart, F. Steiner Verlag, 1995, pp. 71–103.

116. More details can be found in Carlo M. Cipolla, *Miasmas and Disease: Public Health and the Environment in the Pre-Industrial Age*, trans. E. Potter, New Haven, Yale Univ. Press, 1992.

117. See the useful comparisons with non-Christian societies in M. W. Dols, "The comparative communal responses to the Black Death in Muslim and Christian societies." *Viator* 5 (1974): 269–87.

118. Girolamo Fracastoro, "Contagion, contagious diseases, and their treatment" (1546), reprinted in translation by W. C. Wright in *Milestones in Microbiology*, ed. T. Brock, Englewood Cliffs, NJ, Prentice Hall, 1961, pp. 69–75.

119. A. Carmichael, "Contagion theory and contagion practice in fifteenth-century Milan," *Renaissance Q* 44 (1991): 213–56.

120. See J. Goudsblom, "Public health and the civilizing process," *Milbank Q* 64 (1986): 161–88. For a possible mechanism of transmission see S. R. Ell, "Interhuman transmission of medieval plague," *Bull Hist Med* 54 (1980): 497–510.

121. Pullan, "Plague and perceptions of the poor," pp. 101–23.

122. For a more complete view see Carlo Cipolla, *Public Health and the Medical Profession in the Renaissance*, New York, Cambridge Univ. Press, 1976, pp. 11–66.

123. S. Jarcho, *Italian Broadsides Concerning Public Health*, Mt. Kisco, NY, Futura Pub. Co., 1986.

124. A. G. Carmichael, "Plague legislation in the Italian Renaissance," *Bull Hist Med* 57 (1983): 508–25.

125. See the contemporary Rossi drawings of the 1656 epidemic. Photos and Prints, NLM.

126. Giulia Calvi, *Histories of a Plague Year*, trans. D. Biocca and B. T. Ragan, Jr., Berkeley, Univ. of California Press, 1989, pp. 118–54.

127. For more information see J. Henderson, "Epidemics in Renaissance Florence: Medical theory and government response," in *Maladie et Société*, pp. 165–86.

128. One must consider the 40 days and nights spent on Noah's ark but, more important, the injunction in Leviticus specifying that women subject themselves to a 40-day cleansing period after childbirth. For Christians, the 40 days corresponded to Jesus' fast in the desert, or the Lenten period, often characterized as the "holy quarantine."

129. Richard J. Palmer, "The Control of Plague in Venice and Northern Italy, 1348–1600," Ph. D. thesis, Univ. of Kent, 1978, pp. 183–210.

130. For a comparative evolution see M. Dinges, "Süd-Nord-Gefälle in der Pestbekämpfung: Italien, Deutschland und England im Vergleich," in *Das europäische Gesundheitssystem*, ed. W. U. Eckart and R. Jütte, Stuttgart, F. Steiner Verlag, 1994, pp. 28–33.

131. See R. Jütte, "Social construction of illness in the early modern period," in *The Social Construction of Illness*, ed. J. Lachmund and G. Stollberg, Stuttgart, F. Steiner, 1992, pp. 23–38.

132. D. Jetter, "Das Isolierungsprinzip in der Pestbekämpfung des 17. Jahrhunderts," *Med Hist J* 5 (1970): 115–24, and by the same author, "Zur Typologie des Pesthauses," *Sudhoffs Arch* 47 (1963): 291–300.

133. Palmer, "Control of Plague," pp. 183–210.

134. G. Calvi, "The Florentine Plague of 1630–33: Social behavior and symbolic action," in *Maladie et Société*, pp. 327–36.

135. L. Camerlengo, *L'Ospedale e la Città: Cinquecento Anni d'Arte a Verona*, Verona, Cierre, 1996, pp. 179–91.

136. Palmer, "Control of Plague," pp. 183–210.

137. R. Minghetti, "I lazzaretti del seicento e loro regolamenti per la disciplina dei ricoverati e del personale addeto," *Congr Europ Storia Ospital Atti* I (1962): 840–50. For an excellent micro study in the Italian town of Pistoia during the seventeenth century see Carlo M. Cipolla, *Fighting the Plague in Seventeenth-Century Italy*, Madison, Univ. of Wisconsin Press, 1981.

138. K. Park, "Healing the poor: Hospitals and medical assistance in Renaissance Florence," in *Medicine and Charity Before the Welfare State*, ed. J. Barry and C. Jones, London, Routledge, 1994, pp. 26–45.

139. C. M. Cipolla, "A plague doctor," in *The Medieval City*, ed. H. A. Miskimin and D. Herlihy, New Haven, Yale Univ. Press, 1977, pp. 65–72.

140. D. W. Amundsen, "Medical deontology and pestilential disease in the late Middle Ages," *J Hist Med* 32 (1977): 403–21.

141. The information comes from Geronimo Gastaldi. See Cipolla, *Cristofano and the Plague*, p. 26.

142. For details see K. Park, "Medical profession and medical practice in the Italian Renaissance," in *The Rational Arts of Living*, ed. A. C. Crombie and N. Siraisi, Northampton, MA, Smith College, 1987, pp. 137–57, and R. J. Palmer, "Physicians and the state in post-medieval Italy," in *The Town and State Physician in Europe from the Middle Ages to the Enlightenment*, ed. A. W. Russell, Wolfenbüttel, Herzog August Bibl, 1981, pp. 47–61.

143. J. Henry, "Doctors and healers: Popular culture and the medical profession," in *Science, Culture and Popular Belief in Renaissance Europe*, ed. S. Pumphrey et al., Manchester, Manchester Univ. Press, 1991, pp. 191–221.

144. Firsthand information from a lazaretto physician in Florence attending the sick in 1630 is provided in Calvi, *Histories*, pp. 184–86.

145. This experience is related for the 1630 epidemic in Florence. See Cipolla, *Cristofano and the Plague*, p. 26.

146. Ibid., p. 27.

147. Ibid.

148. Calvi, *Histories*, p. 181.

149. For details see G. Micheli, *L' Isola Tiberina e I Fatebenefratelli: la Storia dell'Insula Inter Duos Pontes*, Milano, CENS, c. 1995.

150. Pallavicino, *Descrizione*, pp. 23–24. Measures are described in a series of letters written by Gregorio Barbarigo, an official of the Health Congregation: B. Bertolaso, "La peste romana del 1656–57 dalle lettere inedite di S. Gregorio Barbarigo," *Fonti ricerce storia ecclesiastiche padovana* II (1969): 219–69.

151. Savio, "Richerche," p. 132.

152. Cipolla, *Cristofano and the Plague*, pp. 144–47. The data were obtained from the pesthouse of the Tuscan town of Prato during the 1630–1631 epidemic.

153. Calvi, *Histories*, p. 89.

154. Ibid., pp. 181–96.

155. Gastaldi is quoted in Cipolla, *Cristofano and the Plague*, p. 21.

156. Cipolla, *Fighting the Plague*, p. 12.

157. Ibid., pp. 148–51.

158. Cipolla reproduces the treatments reported to the local health department from the lazaretto of Pistoia during the 1630–1631 epidemic in that town in *Fighting the Plague*, pp. 63–64.

159. For details see Giuseppe Balestra, *Gli accidenti piu gravi del mal contagioso osservati nel lazzaretto all'isola*, Rome, 1657.

160. Calvi quotes a representative source, a consiglo by Marcello Ficino (1576) concerning the humoral views of plague and the remedies to be employed in fighting it. See *Histories*, pp. 66–70.

161. The behavior of male workers towards their spouses is attested to in documentation presented by Calvi in *Histories*, pp. 89–97.

162. It is difficult to obtain statistics from lazarettos. In 1630–1631 Cipolla's institution in Pistoia reported a 60% mortality rate for individuals arriving from the town and a 49% rate for those brought in from the countryside. Cipolla, *Fighting the Plague*, pp. 58–60.

163. The transportation from the island of San Bartolomeo to the cemetery at the convent of San Paolo is depicted in a number of Rossi's dramatic broadsides. Photos and Prints, NLM.

164. Pallavicino, *Descrizione*, pp. 28–30.

165. Details are available in MSS Corsiniano 171, Manuscript Collection, Accademia dei Lincei, Rome. All available Rossi drawings depict these public health measures together with a number of explanatory captions. Photos and Prints, NLM.

166. A. B. Appleby, "The disappearance of plague: A continuing puzzle," *Econ Hist Rev* 33 (1980): 161–73, and P. Slack, "An alternative view," *Econ Hist Rev* 34 (1981): 469–76.

167. See John Howard, *An Account of the Principal Lazarettos in Europe; With various Papers Relative to the Plague*, Warrington, W. Eyres, United Kingdom, 1789.

168. Statutes for the Santa Maria Nuova Hospital (ca. 1500), reproduced in K. Park and J. Henderson, " 'The first hospital among Christians': the Ospedale di Santa Maria Nuova in early sixteenth-century Florence," *Med Hist* 35 (1991): 176.

169. For Britain see J. Durkan, "Care of the poor: pre-Reformation hospitals," in *Essays on the Scottish Reformation 1513–1625*, ed. D. McRoberts, Glasgow, Burns, 1962, pp. 116–28, and Felicity Heat, *Hospitality in Early Modern England*, Oxford, Clarendon Press, 1990.

170. Park and Henderson, "The first hospital," 182.

171. Ibid.

172. B. J. Trexler, "Hospital patients in Florence: San Paolo, 1567–68," *Bull Hist Med* 48 (1974): 41–59.

173. R. Jütte, "Syphilis and confinement: Hospitals in early modern Germany," in *Institutions of Confinement: Hospitals, Asylums, and Prisons in Western Europe and North America, 1500–1950*, ed. N. Finzsch and R. Jütte, New York, Cambridge Univ. Press, 1996, pp. 97–115.

174. See J. Arrizabalaga, "Syphilis," in *The Cambridge World History of Human Disease*, ed. K. F. Kiple, Cambridge, Cambridge Univ. Press, 1993, pp. 1025–33, and D. J. Cripps and A. C. Curtis, "Syphilis maligna praecox. Syphilis of the great epidemic. An historical review," *Arch Int Med* 119 (1967): 411–18.

175. Claude Quetel, "The great pox (sixteenth century)," in *History of Syphilis*, trans. J. Braddock and B. Pike, Baltimore, Johns Hopkins Univ. Press, 1990, pp. 50–72, and A. Foa, "The new and the old: The spread of syphilis (1494–1530)," in *Sex and Gender in Historical Perspective*, ed. E. Muir and G. Ruggiero, Baltimore, Johns Hopkins Univ. Press, 1990, pp. 26–45.

176. I am indebted to Claudia Stein for information regarding this institution, the topic of her forthcoming dissertation.

177. A. Kinzelbach, " 'Böse Blattern' oder 'Franzosenkrankheit': Syphiliskonzept, Kranke und die Genese des Krankenhauses in oberdeutschen Reichsstädten der frühen Neuzeit," in *Neue Wege in der Seuchengeschichte*, ed. M. Dinges and T. Schlich, Stuttgart, Steiner, 1995, pp. 43–69, and K. F. Sudhoff, "Vorsorge für die Syphiliskranken in Würzburg und Augsburg zu Ende des 15. und bis ins zweite Viertel des 16. Jahrhunderts," *Derm Wochenschr* 97 (1933): 1431–45.

178. R. S. Munger, "Guaiacum, the holy wood from the New World," *J Hist Med* 4 (1949): 196–229, and O. Temkin, "Therapeutic trends and the treatment of syphilis before 1900," *Bull Hist Med* 29 (1955): 309–16.

179. For details see Thomas More, *The Utopia of Sir Thomas More*, modern text, with an introduction by M. Campbell, Princeton, NJ, Nostrand, 1947.

180. T. Riis, "Poverty and urban development in early modern Europe (15th-18th-19th centuries): A general view," in *Aspects of Poverty in Early Modern Europe*, ed. T. Riis, Florence, Le Monnier, 1981, pp. 1–28.

181. F. Heal, "The idea of hospitality in early modern Europe," *Past & Present* 102 (1984): 66–93. For the role of confraternities see Christopher Black, *Italian Confraternities in the Sixteenth Century*, Cambridge, Cambridge Univ. Press, 1989.

182. See O. P. Grell, "The Protestant imperative of Christian care and neighbourly love," in *Health Care and Poor Relief in Protestant Europe 1500–1700*, ed. O. P. Grell and A. Cunningham, London, Routledge, 1997, pp. 43–65. For a comparative view see J. Henderson, "Charity and the poor in medieval and Renaissance Europe: Italy and England compared," *Continuity & Change* 3 (1988): 247–72.

183. B. Pullan, "Catholics and the poor in early modern Europe," *Trans R Hist Soc* 26 (1976): 15–34. For more details see H. Outram Evennett, *The Spirit of the Counter-Reformation*, ed. J. Bossy, Notre Dame, IN, Univ. of Notre Dame Press, 1970, and Euan Cameron, *The European Reformation*, Oxford, Clarendon Press, 1991.

184. For examples see N. J. Wilson, "Conceptions of poor relief in sixteenth-century Strasbourg," *UCLA Hist J* 8 (1987): 5–24, and S. Macfarlane, "Social policy and the poor in the later seventeenth century," in *London 1500–1700, The Making of the Metropolis*, ed. A. L. Beier and R. Finlay, London, Longman, 1986, pp. 252–77.

185. In London, vagrants in the seventeenth century were housed at Bridewell, lunatics at Bethlehem Hospital. For details see V. Pearl, "Puritans and poor relief: The London

workhouse, 1649–1660," in *Puritans and Revolutionaries*, ed. D. Pennington and K. Thomas, Oxford, Clarendon Press, 1978, pp. 206–32, and P. Slack, "Hospitals, workhouses, and the relief of the poor in early modern London," in Grell, *Health Care and Poor Relief*, pp. 234–51.

186. Details are presented in John R. Hale, *Renaissance Europe: Individual and Society, 1480–1520*, Berkeley, Univ. of California Press, 1978. See also Andrew Wear, "Medicine in early Europe, 1500–1700," in *The Western Medical Tradition, 800 BC to AD 1800*, co-authored with Lawrence I. Conrad, Michael Neve, Vivian Nutton, and Roy Porter, Cambridge, Cambridge Univ. Press, 1995, pp. 215–361.

187. R. Palmer, "Health, hygiene, and longevity in medieval and Renaissance Europe," in *History of Hygiene*, ed. Y. Kawakita, Tokyo, Ishiyaku EuroAmerica, 1991, pp. 75–98, and M. Pelling, "Illness among the poor in an early modern English town: the Norwich census of 1570," *Continuity & Change* 3 (1988): 273–90.

188. D. Harley, "Spiritual physic, providence, and English medicine, 1560–1640," in *Medicine and the Reformation*, ed. O. P. Grell and A. Cunningham, London, Routledge, 1993, pp. 101–17.

189. R. Jütte, "Poor relief and social discipline in sixteenth-century Europe," *Eur Stud Rev* 11 (1981): 21–52. See also his survey *Poverty and Deviance in Early Modern Europe*, Cambridge, Cambridge Univ. Press, 1994, especially pp. 193–200.

190. Harley, "Spiritual physic," pp. 105–07. See also A. Wear, "Puritan perceptions of illness in seventeenth-century England," in *Patients and Practitioners*, ed. R. Porter, Cambridge, Cambridge Univ. Press, 1985, pp. 55–99.

191. Linda Martz, *Poverty and Welfare in Habsburg Spain*, Cambridge, Cambridge Univ. Press, pp. 34–91.

192. In demanding centralization and accountability of poor relief in its American colonies, the Spanish Crown followed developments in contemporary Europe. See G. B. Risse, "Hospitals and society in sixteenth-century New Spain," in *The World of Dr. Francisco Hernandez*, ed. S. Varey and D. B. Weiner, Stanford, CA, Stanford Univ. Press, in press. For France see J. Imbert, "Les prescriptions hospitalieres du Concile de Trente et leur diffusion en France," *Rev d'Hist l'Église de France* 42 (1956): 5–28.

193. "I call 'hospitals' those places where the sick are fed and cared for, where a certain number of paupers is supported, where boys and girls are reared, where abandoned infants are nourished, where the insane are confined, and where the blind dwell." Juan L. Vives, *Concerning the Relief of the Poor*, trans. M. M. Sherwood, New York, New York School of Philanthropy, 1917, pp. 11–12. Vives' description comes from a memorial addressed to the senate of the city of Bruges in 1526.

5

ENLIGHTENMENT

Medicalization of the Hospital

EDINBURGH, 1750–1800

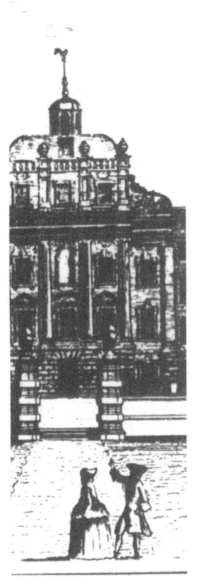

The Royal Infirmary of Edinburgh has been established above seventy years, and during that period it has uniformly maintained its claim to the public favour. By this institution, the Poor under the pressure of disease are provided with everything which can tend to their comfort and relief, and many lives are annually saved to Society through the attention and abilities of the Medical gentlemen to whom the care of Patients is committed.

Royal Infirmary of Edinburgh,
Annual Report, 1801[1]

Wanted: A letter of recommendation

On Sunday morning, December 13, 1772, a young woman, Janet Williamson, came to the gates of the Royal Infirmary of Edinburgh "desirous of accommodation in the house," perhaps accompanied by a relative or neighbor.[2] Tired, restless, and aching all over, she had been battling severe headaches and a fever for about a week. "Fevers" were notorious, especially during Edinburgh's wet winters. Now Janet also felt an "oppression" in her chest, in spite of the fact that someone had bled her three days earlier to ease the symptoms. Directed by the porter, she must have proceeded to the hospital's waiting room, an often noisy and crowded chamber on the ground floor off-limits to medical students. Why would a young woman such as Janet seek admission to the hospital, especially on the "Scotch Sabbath?" Although the Church of Scotland had relaxed some of its rules proscribing most activities, Sundays were still designed for pious reflection, prayer, and church attendance. Contemporaries still spoke of "reverential silence" in the streets. Moreover, most of the poor applying for admission viewed hospitals—characterized as "abodes of sorrow"—with a mixture of fear and hope.[3]

Unlike other British voluntary establishments, the Infirmary admitted sick persons every day.[4] Aged 19 and single, Janet Williamson was listed in the Infirmary's General Register of Patients as a servant. Enjoying considerable freedom of movement, unattached young women had been flooding Edinburgh from the economically depressed Highlands, eager to find work and a suitable husband. Unfortunately, lack of education and illiteracy severely constrained their options. Most of them ended up working as low-paid domestic servants. Contemporary visitors from England, however, praised these helpers, remarking about their openness and friendly manners, their fresh faces free of paint, as they greeted guests with a kiss. Janet, like many other servants in Edinburgh, probably lived with her employers in one of the city's high-rise "land" houses, with low-ceilinged rooms and small windows. Working long hours, receiving little food, and sleeping under the kitchen table or in the lower drawers of kitchen cupboards, Janet may have been eager to find an excuse to get away for a while from her employers.[5]

More likely, however, her master, fearing the spread of this respiratory contagion among his family, had insisted that she seek care outside the home. Faced with sick helpers, kind employers rented separate rooms for them at lodging houses, but many women simply lost their jobs at the first sign of illness. Without resources and family caring networks, Janet and others considered Edinburgh's hospital an appropriate venue in which to seek assistance. Infirmaries were viewed as suitable institutions for indoor medical care if the sick individual seeking it was deemed socially worthy of charity and suffered from a condition considered proper for treatment, taking into account the contemporary limitations of the healing art. This combination of criteria, based on social welfare and medical practices characteristic of Protestant countries, dispelled notions operative elsewhere that hospitals were establishments of last resort. Because of such admission filters, statistics published during the 1760s insisted that nearly 80% of those discharged from the Infirmary left "cured," meaning that the patients displayed subjective or objective signs of recovery.[6]

To screen applicants properly, the hospital needed to ascertain the "deserving" nature of the poor who applied for admission. For this purpose, unless there was an emergency, the Infirmary required a letter of recommendation from known Edinburgh citizens or pastors from other Scottish parishes. These coveted documents were only in the possession of current voluntary contributors to the hospital who regularly paid their subscriptions. In exchange for their gifts, these men obtained the right to sponsor a specific number of patients in direct proportion to the amount of the donation.[7] To streamline the process and provide potential donors with a standardized text, printed copies of such letters were published in local newspapers and mailed to ministers of parishes supporting the hospital. In addition to certifying the deserving status of those they sponsored, the donors were required to assume responsibility for conveying patients to and from the Infirmary, as well as assume burial expenses if the patient died in the institution.[8] After all, the voluntary hospital was a private corporation eager to optimize its charitable mission while limiting its financial liabilities.

For Janet and other potential patients, therefore, the first task was to find a current subscriber provided with valid letters, not always an easy proposition. Persons like Janet were usually lower-class individuals who had been judged by their superiors worthy of charitable support because they demonstrated self-reliance and a willingness to work instead of being idle. The widely accepted social contract, articulated earlier in the century by the Quaker John Bellers, a prominent reformer and typical representative of the British philanthropic movement, insisted that "it is as much the duty of the poor to labour when they are able as it is for the rich to help them when they are sick."[9] From a mercantilist standpoint, Janet was considered an investment, because of illness now in need of assistance lest she slide into total poverty, degradation, and thus become another burden to society. Her employers among Edinburgh's middle and upper classes were expected to provide the necessary help for ensuring Janet's recovery so that she could return to be a productive worker in her community.

In spite of its venerable age—dating from 1575—the old Scottish poor-law system based on parish-centered relief still provided no assistance for those who were unemployed or suffering from temporary sickness. Even earlier, Edinburgh had sponsored a leper house and monastic healing, but by the late sixteenth century, the city paid a surgeon for providing some medical services to the poor.[10] The Presbytery of Edinburgh, like many others in Janet's time, imposed no assessments for the support of the poor, nor did it provide relief, in spite of widespread criticism. The usual response of Church authorities was that this aid would lessen people's self-respect and self-sufficiency and eliminate the legitimate sense of shame felt by those who received it. No one wanted to offend the generous rich by imposing a relief tax on them, thus inviting a severe decline in voluntary donations, the very basis of Edinburgh's welfare schemes. Because of an increase in jobs and wages, poverty in Edinburgh was actually declining in the 1770s. By 1773, the city apparently had only 1,800 registered paupers receiving aid.[11]

By calling the newly medicalized institution an *infirmary* instead of a hospital, British philanthropists eagerly sought to signal that such institutions were meant— like their monastic predecessors—only to treat the sick, removing all stigma from the traditional linkages between hospital and almshouse. Infirmary patients were seen as legitimate recipients of a charitable gift from their communities that entitled them to the privilege of free shelter, regular meals, and medical care. In return for the hospital's "noble and benevolent provision," the givers were entitled "to your best acknowledgments of gratitude and love," according to one medical student's 1772 letter.[12] Eventual admission, while dictated primarily by medical criteria, was also designed to reinforce the patients' morality through a routine of introspection, prayer, and Bible readings. In exchange for the admissions letter, the deserving poor promised to obey unconditionally the strict hospital rules and to follow the doctors' orders, acknowledging gratitude for the donors' interventions on their behalf. Violations of conduct and house rules were immediately punished with expulsion "for irregularities." This social control extended to sufferers of venereal diseases, who were confined in a "locked" ward to enforce therapeutic compliance and thus prevent further spread of their sickness.[13]

Janet's sponsor could not be identified in the General Register—perhaps an omission by an overworked medical clerk. On the other hand, she may simply have carried a certificate attesting to her employment status if her master contributed regularly to the hospital's Servants' Fund. With the participation of Edinburgh's Presbytery, this special endowment had been created during the 1750s, and annual fund drives on "Infirmary Sunday" kept the treasury alive.[14] The appeals for funds were made on behalf of the city's lord provost, magistrates, and council. In the January 1771 request, servants were portrayed as deserving charity recipients, hard workers who, because of illness and after spending all their wages, "sometimes [are] obliged to pawn or sell their clothes to procure lodging, medicine, and advice."[15]

Like other provincial cities in the late eighteenth century, Edinburgh was not a healthy place. According to its general bills of mortality, consumption was the most commonly suspected cause of death, blamed for more than a third of all those registered.[16] Smallpox was also endemic, but in contrast to the ill-defined consumption, it was clinically better recognized and thus more accurately labeled by the public and the authorities. Smallpox epidemics seemed to have raged about every three or four years, and deaths from this scourge made up about another 21% of the total in peak years. Influenza was periodically reported as part of a generalized pattern affecting all of the British Isles. A severe outbreak had occurred in May 1762, and another would arrive in the fall of 1775 from the Continent. Not surprisingly, the incidence of smallpox and respiratory ailments was substantially higher during the winter months. Yet, in spite of such prevalence of infectious diseases, Edinburgh witnessed a sustained population growth, fueled by the constant influx of young newcomers, especially from the Highlands.

Back at the Admissions Room, Janet must have been interviewed after waiting patiently for some time. The hospital's physician-in-ordinary on call usually questioned newcomers before his noon rounds. By now, in medicalizing institutions such as the Edinburgh Infirmary, religious admission rituals had been replaced by bureaucratic and medical ones. Having successfully passed the social filter because of her status as a deserving servant, Janet now needed to pass the clinical test of eligibility. Her history was important for the physicians deciding whether she would be admitted. These encounters could be frustrating and deceptive, as prospective patients tried hard to tell doctors the "right" stories about their sufferings to ensure admission. Physicians, in turn, were on the lookout for symptoms or signs that clearly marked particular diseases, and the applicants went out of their way to provide them.[17] In theory, the Infirmary's statutes allowed "diseased people of all countries or nations" to be admitted, although in practice, most candidates came from the city and its surrounding villages.

The clinical test thus served as a second important screening device to separate those who, in the eyes of the admitting professionals, would probably benefit from institutional care, as opposed to the hopelessly sick or those who feigned illness, who "had been long accustomed to lodge in hospitals and expected to meet with good entertainment and to pass the winter with us."[18] For this purpose, the admitting physicians needed to determine whether the presumed ailment was "proper," meaning not only that it was suitable for hospital management but also that, with adequate treatment, the patient had a good chance to recover. This policy implied that, as a general rule, individuals suffering from acute, self-limited, and benign diseases were admitted. All others, especially the chronically ill and dying, were "improper" candidates for hospitalization and were to remain in their homes or seek attention in hospices. Women made up about 38% of admissions during the early 1770s, and half of them claimed to be unmarried. Most were quite young, with an average age of 25 years. At this time, life expectancy at birth did not exceed 35 years because of very high rates of infant mortality.

Because infectious respiratory diseases frequently affected urban populations, people tended to blame the "contagion of fever" received from family members or co-workers for their complaints. Many also admitted excessive exposure to cold air, especially during the frequent frosty nights of a typical Edinburgh winter. Individuals such as Janet often spoke of falling ill with a fever after drinking cold water while they were overheated and perspiring either in the wake of hard manual labor or after dancing the night away. Others simply attributed their fevers to Edinburgh's most disagreeable smells or "flowers," neutralized by its inhabitants by burning sheets of brown paper in their rooms. From the mid-1760s on, rising living standards caused a greater consumption of coal for heating. Black smoke billowed from thousands of chimneys, transforming the city into the "auld reekie" (old smoky) of nineteenth-century infamy.[19]

Perhaps unknown to Janet, her arrival coincided with an accelerated admission of fever cases to the Infirmary's teaching ward, open during the university's academic year from November 1 until April 30. The physician then in charge of this unit was William Cullen (1710–1790), professor of the theory of medicine at the University of Edinburgh. Perhaps the most accomplished and most famous

English-speaking clinician of his time, Cullen was soon to assume the presidency of the local Royal College of Physicians.[20] He not only managed the 24-bed teaching ward (divided into male and female sections), he was also responsible for a biweekly course of clinical lectures in which he discussed the clinical management of his cases. Since the subject of fevers was traditionally taught at the peak of its appearance during January, Cullen could often be found in the Admissions Room, personally interrogating potential teaching candidates and dictating his findings to a clerk.[21] In December 1772, the word was out that the professor wanted more fever cases for his ward. Four women suffering from this condition had already been hospitalized, but Cullen always aimed at presenting a number of typical cases to his students. By meeting his pedagogical criteria, Janet became the fifth such person within three weeks admitted to the teaching ward.

After the interrogation was completed and the decision to admit Janet reached—perhaps without Cullen's consent since he probably did not make rounds on Sundays—the salaried house physician proceeded with another set of rituals. He signed a paper indicating the patient's destination. Medical clerks, in turn, made an appropriate entry in the General Register of Patients and in a separate Admissions Book, two components of an extensive record-keeping system devised to ensure and document the hospital's social contract with its subscribers. A list was also sent to the matron for the provision of bed clothing and linens, together with a proper diet sheet. Escorted by a nurse, Janet finally went up to the female teaching ward, a 12-bed chamber, 50 by 26 feet long and located in the west wing, now virtually a fever ward, where she would have been greeted by the other inmates. Removal of personal clothing and exchange for a hospital gown, if available, followed. Because of limited funding at the time, the Infirmary filled only 180 beds of the available 228.[22]

Age of Enlightenment: Edinburgh and its Infirmary

At this time, European states were trying to increase their strength by promoting population growth, economic expansion, and military superiority. Since the late seventeenth century, such political and mercantilist goals had underscored the widespread belief that a nation's population was its most valuable natural resource in need of protection. This notion prompted initiatives to enhance the productivity of citizens. Health played a crucial role in this quest. Workers had to be protected from disease or injury, since these conditions represented direct losses to community well-being and wealth. Preventing sickness through traditional dietary and behavioral means[23] lay at the base of a comprehensive program that stressed environmental hygiene and proper lifestyle.[24]

This concern with the health of populations coincided with the expansion of clinical medicine. Before the proliferation of hospitals attended by medical professionals during the Renaissance, most physicians possessed only limited knowledge of clinical matters, including diagnosis and treatment, since they were almost entirely dependent on private consultations with willing patients. Many of these visits remained sporadic, dictated by the whims and financial status of those requesting them. On the whole, most practitioners continued to be exposed to a series of discontinuous and distorted clinical encounters without obtaining the necessary feedback to assess their own diagnostic or therapeutic success.[25]

Within the new Enlightenment framework, the daunting task of bringing illness prevention and medical therapy to the masses represented a dramatic break with previous, less optimistic views of the human capacity to tame diseases. It also represented a significant expansion of the role hitherto assigned to medical professionals in European society. Indeed, society was to become more medicalized, especially in view of the alarming deterioration of health conditions brought on by population growth and urbanization.[26] The underlying premise was that sickness could be controlled, removed, and even prevented by the conscious and deliberate application of enlightened views concerning health and disease. The operative goal was to "defend" the population against society's ills, including those that spawned diseases, while also preserving the social order.[27]

To implement such policies, Britain relied largely on private initiatives instead of the organized schemes developed by national governments in other European countries. Since the 1650s, one approach had depended on the use of vital statistics to propose social and medical reforms. Beginning with John Graunt's *Natural and Political Observations upon the Bills of Mortality*, published in 1662, and William Petty's *Essays on Political Arithmetic* of 1687, Britons gathered demographic data to highlight the deplorable health conditions that prevailed among members of their working class. This information was designed to impress upon the prosperous classes the urgency of reforms.[28] The range of recommended measures included environmental health, infant and maternal welfare, and military and naval medicine, as well as mass treatment of the sick population in dispensaries and infirmaries.[29]

The British hospital movement shared its values and organizing principles with those of other contemporary reforms, including charity schools, orphanages, workhouses, and prisons. Changes were to be made through the actions of voluntary associations rather than being imposed by government. Relief and employment of the poor were linked to their health status and capacity to work. Both traditional religious and secular philanthropic motives merged with practical political attempts to protect the social order and ensure material prosperity.[30] As before, the religious roots went back to Matthew's injunction in the Scriptures to visit the sick. The performance of charitable good works was compatible with Anglican as well as Calvinistic theology, involving bishops, ministers, elders, and parish members. Drawing on time-honored models, infirmaries were places "to reclaim the souls of the sick" while caring for their bodily ills.[31] Qualities such as submission, servitude, discipline, and respect were also expected, especially from female patients, many of them young servants and laborers, whose moral upbringing—in the eyes of the managers—always needed reinforcement within the hospital's structured environment.

Unlike other European countries, Britain, and especially the city of London by the early 1700s, retained only a few establishments primarily devoted to the care of the sick.[32] Given this lack of institutional frameworks and no central governmental agency to provide medical assistance, local and private initiatives prevailed, especially in the larger urban areas, where individual communities could no longer cope with the existing health problems of the poor. While some parishes provided relief and assistance to their paupers in almshouses established under the Poor Laws, this rudimentary welfare system still left significant gaps. Moreover, not all schemes necessarily provided hospital care. Indeed, many cities organized a system of paid home visits by physicians. Others created dispensaries for outpatient advice and medicines.

If the ideology guiding the British voluntary hospital movement represented an "associated philanthropy" based on religious and humanistic values, corporate and professional interests, including the traditional medical and surgical groups, were also important. Those advocating medical reform in the seventeenth century, including William Petty, had already stressed the importance of medicine and the participation of physicians in hospital care. Indeed, hospitals were also to function as veritable clinical research centers, where patient management could yield important new knowledge.[33] By the early eighteenth century, efforts were proliferating in Britain to structure this type of bedside education and thus facilitate the training of greater numbers of competent practitioners.[34] In the eyes of some reformers such as John Bellers, hospitals were to be seen as "great nurseries" that could "breed some of the best physicians and chirurgeons because they may see as much there in one year as in seven anywhere else."[35]

The first voluntary hospital to open its doors was the Westminster Infirmary in London in 1720. It was soon followed by a spate of others: Guy's Hospital in London (1726), the Edinburgh Infirmary (1729), St. George's Hospital in London (1733), the Winchester Infirmary (1736), the Bristol Infirmary (1737), London Hospital (1740) and Middlesex Hospital, also in London (1745). All except Guy's resulted from "alliances against misery" composed of civic-minded businessmen, bankers, lawyers, and teachers, as well as physicians and surgeons.

Such a display of charitable enthusiasm and the creation of patronage networks was not totally disinterested. To heal the sick retained a universal appeal, unsullied by religious, political, and social partisanship. The good will generated by charitable acts also went a long way toward glossing over the inequalities of a slowly industrializing society. Subscribers to these charities acquired status and prestige among their peers and the poor, who depended on their letters of recommendation. Donors were entitled to have their say about the management of a particular charity. Some evolved into efficient governors and directors. Meanwhile, the charitable institutions themselves became sources of civic pride and achievement, visible monuments to a caring citizenry that understood and successfully discharged its social obligations.[36]

Since its union with England in 1707, Scotland, and especially the Lowlands, had undergone a significant transformation from a poor, backward country to a prosperous British province. Although Edinburgh was no longer the seat of royalty, by midcentury the city was dubbed the "Athens of the North," hub of a remarkable social and cultural development known as the "Scottish Enlightenment."[37] With nearly 70,000 inhabitants in the early 1770s,[38] the former capital of Scotland had become the winter quarters for Scottish aristocrats and landowners. Their needs and tastes generated a vast service industry that included artisans, clothiers, jewelers, wig makers, musicians, actors, painters, book sellers and binders, physicians, club owners, and an army of servants that included Janet. A growing middle class sought to imitate the aristocracy and join in their fashionable pursuits, creating a cosmopolitan society. With broad participation from its elite, including aristocrats, literati, philosophers, lawyers, merchants, and medical men, Edinburgh—characterized by Tobias Smollet as a "hot-bed of genius"— played a leading role in the formulation of a new ideology of Scottish self-improvement. From the 1720s on, the city experienced remarkable economic stability and growth that ended only with the war against France in the 1790s.[39]

Guiding this program of agricultural improvement, small-scale industrialization, and educational development was a web of prominent patrons representing the landed and new industrial interests, the Church of Scotland with its kirks and assemblies,[40] the legal and medical professions, and universities. The dominant Presbyterian church system was led by a well-educated clergy strongly supportive of the planned agendas of improvement. Personalities such as the historian William Robertson, leader of the Moderate party and principal of Edinburgh University, as well as Hugh Blair, minister of the High St. Giles Kirk and university lecturer in the 1770s, were examples of the close association between the Kirk and the city's intellectual circles. With this moderate faction dominating the Presbytery of Edinburgh, secular pursuits were placed side by side with the "purpose of eternity." There was little concern at this point with traditional Calvinist theology, now substituted for by a "rational" religion that chose to emphasize good works, kindly thoughts, and social order. Religious toleration and sustained aristocratic patronage were important sources of political and institutional stability protecting the activities of Edinburgh's cultural elite.[41]

Another key player in the implementation of Enlightenment values was the University of Edinburgh. After 1750, this institution became not only a welcome alternative learning center for British students barred from Oxford and Cambridge for religious reasons, but also a prominent international center for individuals from other European countries and America pursuing a medical degree. Its medical faculty was based on plans laid down by John Monro (1670–1740), a surgeon-apothecary, who had attended the University of Leyden. Closely connected to Edinburgh's Town Council, Monro secured a professorship in anatomy for his surgeon son Alexander, known as Alexander Monro, Primus (1697–1767), in 1720. The Council's Act of 1726 established the first faculty of medicine, composed of five professors who had all studied at Leyden and supported the ideas of Herman Boerhaave (1668–1738), the most prominent European physician of the early eighteenth century.[42] A new direction away from the Boerhaavian system of medicine was chartered with the appointments of William Cullen (chair of chemistry) in 1755 and John Gregory (chair of medical practice) in 1766.

Plans for the creation of a voluntary hospital in Edinburgh were also laid in the mid-1720s. The project was supported by the Royal College of Physicians, which had already provided free ambulatory care for the poor, the Incorporation of Surgeons and Apothecaries, and the University of Edinburgh, represented by the newly elected professor of anatomy, Alexander Monro, Primus. "As men and Christians we have the strongest inducements and even obligations to this sort of charity as it is warmly recommended and enjoined in the gospel," Monro and his associates wrote in justification of their efforts. Dominated by its moderate faction, which promoted Enlightenment values, the Church of Scotland remained a powerful and supportive partner in this enterprise. The mercantile angle, moreover, was not forgotten: "as the relief is a duty, so it is of no less advantage to the nation, for as many as are recovered in an infirmary are so many working hands gained to the country."[43]

Finally, in establishing the Infirmary, professional goals were not far behind, as sponsors stressed "that students of physick and surgery might hereby have rather a better and easier opportunity of experience than they hitherto had by studying abroad."[44] Surgeons were particularly conscious that these clinical opportunities would enhance their knowledge and skills while improving their professional status and private income. Thus, from its very inception, the hospital became another participant in the educational program articulated by the Scottish Enlightenment, which also included several learned groups in the city such as the Philosophical Society, the popular Royal Medical Society, and numerous literary clubs. By the early 1770s, the Infirmary and its teaching program were famous throughout Europe and the North American colonies, attracting students from England and other countries. At that time, the University matriculated a yearly average of about 200 students from the British Isles and abroad.[45] Both the University and the Infirmary became important contributors to the conscious local drive toward material improvement and achievement fueled by the Scottish Enlightenment.

The Infirmary plan was implemented in the 1720s, when, at the suggestion of George Drummond, recently elected lord provost of Edinburgh, supporters of the infirmary project contacted a fishery company previously managed by Drummond.

They offered to buy stock as the core of an endowment to finance the hospital venture. With approval from city authorities and the Bank of Scotland, this scheme succeeded thanks to pledges from 352 individual subscribers representing a cross section of the upper and middle classes of Edinburgh. A subsequent meeting of donors, called in 1728, established new procedures to elect annually 20 "extraordinary" supervisory managers and 12 "ordinary" managers, the latter charged with supervising the daily affairs of the planned institution. Both the Royal College of Physicians and the Incorporation of Surgeons negotiated with the managers a system of free attendance at the new facilities. The "Little House," a two-story house in Robertson's Close, opened its doors in 1729 to a total of 35 patients after hiring a housekeeper and a clerk.

The early success of the Edinburgh Infirmary for the Sick Poor encouraged further efforts. Fund-raising efforts in the 1730s and beyond showed widespread community support for the new infirmary. Supporters among city officials remained highly visible,[46] and the Church of Scotland's General Assembly ordered ministers throughout the land to solicit additional subscriptions. "The Lord begs to build him a house to reside in while some of his faithful servants, eminent for their skill in physick, minister to his cure," preached one of them.[47] Other sums came from pledges by prestigious guilds such as the Faculty of Advocates and Writers to the Signet and from a tax that the Edinburgh freemasons imposed on themselves. In 1736 George II signed the charter of incorporation, and a few years later, planners decided to build a new hospital on a well-drained two-acre site overlooking the Cowgate Valley in the southwestern part of the city.[48] After the foundation stone was laid in 1738, construction proceeded slowly over the next decade, although the first patients were transferred from the Little House in 1741. The building was to reflect the new Protestant philanthropy, with its stress on austerity and efficiency, while at the same time creating a home-like "upstairs-downstairs" atmosphere. After its completion, the 150-bed Royal Infirmary became a city landmark, "undoubtedly the most noble of the institutions in Edinburgh reared by the hand of charity."[49]

By 1772, both Janet and her hospital physician, William Cullen, still lived nearby in the center of town, composed of noisy and dirty, tall buildings or "lands"—often 10 stories or higher—located in crowded "closes" or dead-end alleys. Access was possible only along "scale" stairways so steep and narrow that they even precluded the transport of a coffin. These crowded conditions forced residents of all social classes to mingle, creating a vibrant outdoor life. High Street was the axis for a long string of taverns and lodging houses stretching south from the castle toward the abbey and palace of Holyrood. Few wells supplying water were available, and there were no drains to remove waste.[50] However, the winds of change were to radically restructure the character of Edinburgh in the years ahead.[51] In 1772, the North Bridge had been completed over the Nor' Loch, now a filthy ditch, allowing access to a suburban plateau north of the old walled city.

With the physical expansion to the so-called New Town across the loch, proposed as early as 1752, the upper ranks of society were poised to retreat from the crowded central ridge marked by the main thoroughfares of High Street and Canongate. As in other European cities, the flight to the suburbs created a cluster of exclusive Georgian townhouses, shattering the traditional "social mix" between rich and poor that had provided the extraordinary cohesion of community life.[52] Built entirely according to a preconceived plan, the new city tried to express in stone its aesthetic notions of harmony and reason.[53]

For its part, the façade of Edinburgh Infirmary, designed by the famous architect William Adam, resembled a large Palladian stone mansion and represented the block type of hospital that had succeeded the cruciform models popular centuries earlier. Arranged as a central four-story structure, the Infirmary also possessed two attached wings projected forward, creating a U-shaped building, to improve the circulation of air through its tall windows, a feature more compatible with the newer priorities of institutional ventilation and cleanliness based on military experiences. The surrounding grounds featured courts and grass walks, as well as public gardens to be used by ambulatory convalescents. All floors were connected by a large central hall and stairway ending below a domed room or amphitheater with a large skylight for lectures, surgical operations, and religious services. Built as a large house with separate rooms, this hospital type shattered the spatial unity of previous religious institutions in an attempt to achieve a better flow of air. At the same time, the new ward arrangements restricted the flow of inmates and caregivers, thus facilitating institutional control through better supervision and strict compliance with hospital rules. In the 1770s and 1780s this interior design allowed the Infirmary to admit significant contingents of sick soldiers and sailors, who could be placed under guard in separate wards to prevent desertion. These plans also reflected new medical agendas that sought to separate and confine patients according to broad categories of disease.[54]

Given the traditional miasmatic considerations, exposure to the northerly winds ensured greater environmental purity, while larger windows and fireplaces located in the corners of each ward were designed to provide ample ventilation, a goal only partially fulfilled because of numerous closets and partitions. In truth, the Edinburgh Infirmary was planned before many of the newer hygienic principles formulated by John Pringle for field hospitals and army barracks had been properly transferred to civilian use.[55] On the ground floor, the central admissions room was surrounded by a number of vaulted rooms for the hospital's kitchen, pantry, apothecary shop, and living quarters for the matron, porter, and nurses. Each central ward on both sides of the stairs contained 24 single beds, and each wing housed 12-bed wards and extra rooms for the nurses. To discourage cross-infections, beds were spaced six feet apart. Curtains could be drawn around each bed to provide a degree of privacy. To minimize the problem of in-house infections or "hospital distempers," the staff ordered periodic sprinklings of vinegar and fumigations with muriatic acid gas, and the walls and ceilings were subjected to "whitewashing" with lime.[56] However, John Howard, on his visit to the Infirmary in 1785—following his inspection of Continental lazarettos—pointed out the filthy brick floors and dirty patients who were prohibited from using the baths the institution reserved for paying customers.[57]

Hospital patients and their management

Janet Williamson was probably visited the day after her arrival by William Cullen.[58] To navigate the narrow streets and make his house visits, Cullen was usually carried in a sedan chair. Wearing a huge wig beneath his top hat and dressed in a big coat, the professor, with his strange pendulous lips, was a familiar site in the city and its hospital.[59] The expanding medical presence in hospital wards had given rise to institutional rituals designed to enhance the status of the professionals who managed the wards. The routine was for physicians first to contact the nurses and inquire about the state of the patients, then to make rounds. Followed by a "train" of assistant physicians and students, university professors such as Cullen made their entrance at a predetermined hour—usually noon—eagerly awaited or dreaded by the patients, who greeted the procession in silence. Ambulatory inmates were required to stand next to their beds at military-like attention. Because of potential inaccuracies and omissions in history-taking from "vulgar" patients, physical inspection at Edinburgh assumed great importance. Bodily postures and discharges, as well as the gross appearance of the tongue, were always checked and carefully noted. Cullen and Alexander Monro secundus (1733–1817) employed the direct percussion method developed by the Austrian physician Leopold Auenbrugger for the detection of fluid in the abdominal cavity.[60] Bodily functions such as pulse, respiration, appetite, digestion, motion, and excretion were also routinely recorded. At times, the patient's complaints prompted the use of special diagnostic tests, including urethral inspections with probes and catheters. Tubes were employed to check the throat and printed cards to determine visual acuity. When appropriate, a description of sputum, feces, blood, and urine was appended to the clinical chart, relating the physical characteristics and quantities of such discharges.

Although clinical thermometers were already available, hospital practitioners, including Cullen, preferred to distinguish "low," "moderate," and "excessive" heat in managing their patients. Available thermometers were inaccurate, frustrating most correlations between the patient's subjective complaints and the measurements.[61] Cullen did not employ one routinely, guiding his treatment by simply touching the patient's skin and checking for delirium. Janet had no appetite and was constipated; her skin was described as hot. Cullen counted her pulse with his famous hourglass—a fast 120 and full. (Contemporary physicians were aware that the patients' pulse rates accelerated when they approached a bed and pressed the wrist.) Another valuable piece of information in females was the menstrual history, still recorded in Latin for the doctors' eyes only, given contemporary sensitivity regarding all sexual matters. In routine cases, modesty also prevented the examination of any female patient's genitalia by physicians unless the symptomatology pointed to an obvious vaginal or uterine disorder. When necessary, such examinations were often carried out with the assistance of a female midwife, not only to confer propriety to the procedure but also to ensure that the findings were interpreted correctly since most male physicians were notoriously ignorant of women's diseases. In Janet's case, no mention was made of her menstrual status. It is possible that her menarche was delayed, a common occurrence in Scotland among the hard-working, poorly nourished young women Cullen described as of "lean and dry habit."[62]

Provided with the pertinent clinical information, physicians such as Cullen were ready to make their diagnoses, which fearful patients viewed as sentences confirmed by "the judges of life and death."[63] At this time, the term *fever* designated a variety of clinical conditions with symptoms of general malaise and a rise in temperature. "In the language of this country, the vulgar, if they are hot, say that they are in a fever," wrote the contemporary physician George Fordyce (1736–1802) in one of his treatises.[64] Cullen, who in 1769 had published his own classification of diseases, placed fevers under his first class of *pyrexiae*, defining them as "a frequent pulse coming after some degree of cold shivering, considerable heat, many of the functions injured, the strength of the limbs especially diminished."[65] Within that class of diseases, Cullen followed previous taxonomists in distinguishing two basic types "according as they showed either an inflammatory irritation or weaker reaction."[66] In Cullen's own language, true inflammatory fevers were now to be called *synocha*, while the less intense or low "nervous fever" was renamed *typhus* (in Greek, "smoke" or "mist") to emphasize one of its cardinal symptoms: delirium or stupor.[67]

Between these two classes of fevers, Cullen then added a third category he called *synochus*, a hybrid arising from different causes, most notably contagion exacerbated by cold air. According to the professor, synochus was the most common type of fever seen in Scotland during the winter months.[68] Clinically, its early stages resembled those of an inflammatory fever, with high fever, chills, and a frequent, hard pulse; later, its bodily manifestations diminished and it simulated the milder typhus. Although Cullen's nosological distinctions remained somewhat tentative—in his lectures he admitted that "nothing shows so much the deficiency of observation as that this matter is not yet settled upon a tolerable foundation from Galen to Boerhaave"[69]—these categories nevertheless began to shape clinical experience, especially at the Infirmary's teaching ward during Cullen's tenure and Janet's sojourn. They were part of his pedagogical goals to bring order into clinical knowledge and fulfill the professional contract arranged with students who paid him to attend his rounds and lectures.

Disease classifications such as Cullen's were no longer believed to consist of immutable natural species following earlier botanical schemes. Indeed, many contemporary European physicians, including Cullen, had reluctantly concluded that in one sense all disease categories were arbitrary and ephemeral, merely heuristic devices designed to guide physicians and students in their diagnostic and therapeutic efforts. Within this more flexible framework, revisions derived from new clinical observations were always encouraged, and patients such as Janet could prove quite helpful in that quest.[70]

The explanations Cullen offered regarding the genesis and evolution of fevers were intimately linked to his comprehensive system of medicine, then taught at the University of Edinburgh. The theories were articulated in his most important book, *First Lines of the Practice of Physic*, originally published in 1776–1778 and expanded into a new four-volume edition in 1786. According to Cullen, all fevers went through three distinct stages. The initial "cold" phase, dominated by chills and generalized malaise, was ascribed to the impact of causal agents, especially contagion, which created a debility in the nervous system reflected by widespread arterial spasms along the skin surface. In response to such vascular blockages, clinically manifested by goose flesh, the heart and arteries were stimulated into greater action, creating the second "hot" stage of fever, with a faster heartbeat and pulse, hot skin, and greater nervous excitability. Somewhat later, a final phase of resolution ensued, characterized by a lower pulse rate, profuse sweating, and greater urinary discharge, signaling a relaxation of all excretory function and the restoration of normal nervous excitability in both the brain and nerves.[71]

In Cullen's view, a proper degree of tension or "excitement" needed to be present in nerves and the brain for the transmission of impulses necessary to ensure all bodily functions. Such excitement depended directly on environmental and internal stimuli that influenced the nervous system and allowed it to regulate and distribute all vital energies with the aid of a certain "sympathy" or consent of the organs. These ideas were based on earlier investigations dealing with the properties of irritability and sensibility carried out by two famous physicians, Francis Glisson and Albrecht von Haller. Disease occurred when the amount of nervous excitement became abnormal. Cullen postulated that all outside agents—including weather, food, and drugs—could either stimulate or depress the nervous system. In the former state, excessive excitement with increased muscular tone occurred, producing the numerous vascular spasms and chemical abnormalities observed during fevers. The opposite state, insufficient excitement, created muscular debility, vascular paralysis, and eventually total collapse of bodily functions followed by death.[72]

These basic explanations offered by Cullen were part of a new and speculative pathogenesis derived from his vitalistic neurophysiology. It explained the presumed causes and mechanisms of disease through the actions of the nervous system. Cullen's dictum that "almost the whole of the phenomena of fevers lead us to believe that they chiefly depend upon changes in the state of the moving powers of the animal system"[73] pointed to significant changes taking place in medical theory at that time, signaling the shift from traditional humoralism to a new set of explanations that superimposed the actions of "solid" components of the human body, specifically the brain and nerves, on the fluids.

Meanwhile, at the Infirmary's bedside, Janet's clinical history and febrile symptoms suggested a diagnosis of synochus. Although Cullen was prone to speculate about bodily reactions, he also remained the eternal skeptic at the bedside, cautioning students to subject all their ideas and practices to empirical verification and correction. "I am not ashamed to say that I fail in judgment and I shall never hide a doubt with regard to a doctrine I advance or a practice I follow. I think candor requires it," he told them.[74] In Janet's case, Cullen chose to begin a traditional "antiphlogistic" (antifebrile) regimen consisting of a low diet, emetics, purgatives, and bloodletting to "starve a fever." For him and other attending physicians, dietary prescriptions constituted the first line of therapy.[75] During daily rounds, detailed food instructions were issued, with orders for drugs and other procedures. Given their considerable control over the patients and nursing staff, practitioners were reasonably sure that their orders would be followed in spite of the occasional smuggling in of favorite food morsels by visitors. At the same time, to forestall protests and criticisms, hospital authorities repeatedly stressed that meals ordered for the sick were "proper and suitable, keeping in view of the ordinary food of the poor in Scotland."[76]

To illustrate their charitable disposition and impress their donors as well as the general public, British voluntary hospitals frequently published these diets. Since food was considered a general stimulus to the human system, physicians distinguished three types of diets: "low," "middle," and "full." The first, also known as a "fever" diet, omitted all animal products, providing instead bread and milk, porridge made of oats and barley, or a "panada" in which bread was boiled with sugar and nutmeg to form a soup. Febrile patients such as Janet received plenty of water or milk, often acidulated with vinegar. All food was served in wooden "cogs" or cups of different sizes without tableware. Regulations discouraged the medical personnel from carrying out examinations while patients ate their meals.

In general, hospital physicians were cautious about prescribing too much food, fearing that febrile illnesses could thus turn into much more dangerous "putrid" fevers. To preclude such transformations, they withheld all meat and prescribed acid fruit drinks believed to possess antiseptic qualities. Low and middle diets also appealed to frugal hospital managers, especially in times of tighter budgets. If physicians wanted to complain about the quality and quantity of food, they needed to write formal protests to the matron, who usually promised improvements but continued to operate within her budgetary constraints. Beyond tea, jelly, and biscuits, coveted supplemental provisions such as bread, potatoes, and fish were smuggled in by visitors, often after bribing the nurses.[77]

During the 1770s, Edinburgh's teaching ward was staffed by one "ordinary" day nurse and another night nurse. Their low status—they were poor, often illiterate, unskilled servants hired at minimum wages—conspired against the need for persons with more than just cleaning skills since food and drug distributions were now key components of the medical regimen, requiring nurses to have some knowledge of their importance for individual patients. Nurses were kept busy throughout their 10- or 12-hour shifts, assisting at baths, persuading inmates to comply with medical recommendations, and reporting on the changing physical conditions and complaints of their charges. Working under the keen supervision of Elizabeth Paton, the matron from 1770 until 1775, the nurses were also charged with enforcing all regulations, a power that often created conflicts and abuses. Gratuities—commonly provided to all servants in Scotland—could escalate into bribes and blackmailing schemes, contributing to the contemporary nursing stereotype of corruption, ignorance, and brutality. Excessive drinking and cavorting with the medical personnel sometimes led to dismissals. However, in spite of such unflattering portrayals, especially by physicians and administrators, these lowly nurses contributed significantly to patient care. For inmates such as Janet, their common servant status promoted social solidarity and mutual support. By the early 19th century, one Edinburgh professor, Andrew Duncan, Sr., characterized both day and night nurses in the teaching ward as "very attentive and humane."[78]

Besides receiving rest and regular food, Infirmary patients were subjected to treatments with physical methods and drugs. "Nothing is more evident," wrote Cullen, "than that bloodletting is one of the most powerful mean of diminishing the activity of the whole body, especially of the sanguiferous system."[79] Indeed, the withdrawal of blood retained its importance in spite of the significant shifts in medical theory since ancient times. Cullen justified bloodletting because it could lessen the tension and spasms occurring in a febrile body. He had recast the traditional therapeutic strategies designed to restore humoral balances, with the focus now on adjusting bodily excitement through either nervous stimulation or sedation. Among the agents considered stimulants were meat, wine, exercise, fresh air, warm baths, and tonic drugs; the depressant regimen included rest, a vegetarian diet, bloodletting, purging, and antispasmodic and sedative medicines.[80]

To the trained eye, the sudden removal of four to eight ounces of blood seemed indeed to improve several cardinal symptoms accompanying fevers. Pulse rates fell, body temperatures declined, pain sensations lessened, the reddish color of the skin paled, and the patients were overtaken by a feeling of relaxation, even faintness, and sleep. Although temporary, such physiological responses suggested to eighteenth-century practitioners that bloodletting was still a useful measure in all inflammatory states and the keystone of their antiphlogistic regimen.[81] Thus, during her first two days in the infirmary, Janet was bled eight ounces and also given a saline enema. Cullen also ordered ipecac powder, his favorite fast-acting emetic, designed to cleanse the weak stomachs of all fever patients. In a sense, these were traditional measures that most individuals employed under similar circumstances at home. Janet's reaction went unrecorded.[82]

When patients experienced a very high fever and were delirious, infirmary physicians often also ordered fomentations with flannel cloths dipped in hot water, believing that they produced a relaxing and soothing effect. In Janet's case, the nurse fomented her legs and feet hourly while she was delirious, not only to quiet her down but also to allow other patients in the teaching ward to get their night's rest. When her condition worsened, and she began complaining of chest pains and a persistent cough—both signs of a respiratory infection—an expectorant, a mucilaginous mixture, was added to the regimen.

To complicate matters, the surgical clerk found it impossible to locate a good vein in Janet's arms or hands to draw the blood. Therefore, he was forced to obtain blood from a foot and recorded that her symptoms were somewhat relieved. All prescribed venesections were carried out by the students, clerks, or dressers, a practice that drew the ire of attending surgeons such as Benjamin Bell, who in his *System of Surgery* remarked that "I have seldom seen bloodletting with the lancet correctly done."[83] After the vessels were properly engorged through the use of tight ligatures, operators employed a lancet or small knife to make an oblique incision in both the skin and the vein. One of the most common effects of the procedure was patient fainting, caused more by the sight of blood than by the actual amount of the withdrawal. At the Infirmary, venous blood drawn from patients was successively collected in three separate tin platters and allowed to clot. Kept in the ward, the bowls were inspected by Cullen and his entourage of students the next day for the presence of *sizy* blood, a term describing the semisolid, jelly-like surface developed by clotted blood placed in these containers. If present, this surface layer was termed a *buffy coat* because of the light buff or yellowish color covering the more compact portions of the clot, the *crassamentum*, composed of red blood cells.

For 2,000 years, increased siziness of blood indicated a systemic inflammation within the humoral framework. While nervous disturbances now ruled supreme, eighteenth-century practitioners still strongly believed that such a buffy substance was the product of faulty humoral mixes responsible for the incitement and its febrile symptoms. Frequent detection of this layer in bleeding bowls seemed to confirm this relationship, especially after the first blood samples had clotted quickly. The more physicians bled, however, the greater seemed the proportion of serum capable of solidifying into a yellow crust, a potentially dangerous circle tempered only by the clinician's assessment of the whole patient and any progressive weakness and fainting. "I seldom can venture upon a conclusion," declared Cullen with respect to the behavior of extravasated blood, thus providing a needed and moderating influence to counter enthusiastic contemporary blood-letters.[84]

Cullen ordered a second withdrawal of eight ounces of blood from his patient on the evening of her third day. This measure apparently provided more relief of Janet's symptoms. The emetic, too, was finally having an effect, making her throw up several times, as well as causing her to pass several stools. Janet's pulse was still around 120 but softer and regular. Night delirium and sweats continued. Fever patients were ordered to remove their soaked clothing periodically for washing, but if no additional shirts were available, they lay naked under the sheets. Concerned about her recent respiratory symptoms, Cullen now also ordered the creation of a blister on Janet's back between the shoulder blades, not however for the reason that humoral therapeutics suggested such a course, namely to remove harmful substances from the body. Rather, in Cullen's neurophysiological theory, blisters stimulated the body and nervous system and thus neutralized the action of fever-producing substances. According to Cullen's student Thomas Fowler, "blistering plasters certainly constitute one of the most efficacious remedies we have to boast in the practice of physic."[85]

To create such a blister, practitioners usually applied an adhesive plaster or dressing covered with a caustic, irritating substance. The most commonly employed product was an ointment or powder made of Spanish flies or cantharides, a type of Mediterranean beetle used since Roman times. Other dressings contained mustard, onion, and leek. They could all be placed on the shaved crown of the head, the nape of the neck, the sternum, or, as in Janet's case, on the back of the chest after the skin had been cleansed with vinegar and water. The selected site usually "answered" within 12 to 24 hours by "rising" and forming a vesicle that was then pierced with a needle to allow discharge. Henceforth, the blister was kept open and dressed daily with more ointment to prevent it from drying out. This required a "blistering schedule," popularized in Leyden by Boerhaave earlier in the century and adopted by Cullen and his colleagues through the steady application of a paste made with mustard flour, garlic, and sulfuric acid.[86]

Nearly a fourth of all hospitalized medical patients were subjected to this practice, as well as almost half of those suffering from respiratory symptoms. Because of the pain and the danger of secondary infections, most patients dreaded blisters, often refusing them outright or trying to hide any symptoms that could prompt the attending physicians to order irritating plasters. Excessive or repeated use of the cantharides powder also produced severe bladder irritation with painful voiding and even bleeding. Cullen, for his part, frequently used the threat of a blistering schedule to rid himself of unwanted hospital patients feigning illness. Confronted with this order from the professor, many inmates promptly picked up their belongings and bade farewell to the Infirmary.[87]

The problem of feigned complaints was no trifling matter, especially for those who were homeless and faced Edinburgh's cold and wet winters. Cullen seems to have been particularly concerned about this problem, repeatedly telling his medical students how to sharpen their diagnostic skills and uncover the impostors. Cullen employed the nurses as informants, since their common social status perhaps encouraged patients to share their true feelings. The prospect of a painful procedure or a new experimental treatment frequently exposed those who attempted to manipulate the attending physicians and extend their stay to receive the traditional shelter, rest, and food. On the other hand, many patients with real illnesses were in awe of professors such as Cullen, impressed by their social status, professional reputation, and friendly demeanor. For them, blistering rituals, however painful, possessed healing qualities.

On the sixth day of her hospitalization, Janet reached a critical stage in her illness, a subject traditionally debated by practitioners. The fever seemed to abate and her cough was less frequent, but partial deafness was still a problem and the blister had failed to rise. For the first time, however, the patient was able to take some food. Cullen prescribed a powder of golden root or virga aurea, a bitter, astringent remedy designed to counteract systemic debility. To the delight of her attending physicians, she seemed to tolerate this bitter powder. Then, on December 22, Janet became quite nauseated, forcing Cullen to discontinue the medication without telling her that she was experiencing a side effect of the remedy.[88] A day later, she was clearly on the mend, sleeping a good deal and free of delirium, with a lower pulse and more appetite.

At this point, Janet may have been switched to the Infirmary's middle diet consisting of cooked meat and vegetables.[89] Fomentation of her feet and legs continued, as did the administration of an expectorant mixture after her cough became more productive. Following Christmas Day, Janet slowly improved, her pulse now 80. However, part of her arm at the elbow had begun to hurt and swell, a feared complication of an earlier venesection attempt. Contemporary accounts reveal the existence of many such accidents, including punctured nerves in the arm or injury to the biceps tendon. The most common problem, however, was local abscesses produced by dirty skin and instruments. Cullen called a surgeon in consultation, who ordered a poultice of bread and milk.

Spending Christmas in a hospital was unfortunate, but Janet's condition still did not warrant discharge. In fact, if she had no family in the city, being in a ward together with other young women in various stages of recovery was probably more desirable. A visiting program allowing family and friends daily access to the wards may also have contributed to a climate of camaraderie and mutual acceptance so important in ensuring a return to health. At this time, the female teaching ward housed six fever patients ranging in age from 17 to 28, together with three others of about the same age suffering from acute and chronic forms of "rheumatism." The similarity of their sufferings certainly must have promoted some bonding and friendship among them.

Finally, on New Year's Eve, Janet's status was officially changed to that of a convalescent, and she was placed on a full diet. The breakfast remained essentially unchanged, except for additional allowances of light beer, but dinner now included meat—considered a powerful stimulant—in the form of beef tea, a thicker broth, and boiled or roast mutton and chicken. The so-called house beer, brewed near the institution, was usually available in quantities of about a quart per day and was served during both breakfast and supper. If supplies were plentiful in good economic times, nurses carried pieces of raw, "undressed" meat directly into the ward on a board. With extra allowances granted by the professors, patients roasted the steaks in the fireplaces of the teaching ward and presumably distributed some portions to those still confined to their beds. Wine frequently became the ultimate restorative, often mixed with water. Cullen, however, seemed somewhat reluctant to prescribe it routinely, perhaps more aware of its intoxicating qualities and concerned about promoting alcoholism, then rampant in Scotland.

As in earlier times, convalescents were usually pressed into service, assisting with a variety of hospital routines.[90] Feeding other inmates, assisting with housekeeping, and preparing cotton dressings were among the typical chores performed. As the Infirmary statutes indicated, "Patients shall work as the matron or clerks shall desire them." These activities created opportunities for "social chats," possibly trading illness stories for emotional support, and "harmless jest"—the always necessary touch of humor to conquer apprehension and fear. Early bedtime plunged the wards into darkness and silence, interrupted by the whispers of patients engaged in "friendly converse" as part of a resocialization process with its potential for healing. "Grief attracts by stronger bonds than pleasure ever knew," wrote one contemporary eyewitness.[91]

House of teaching: Clinical instruction and research

On Tuesday evening, January 12, 1773, William Cullen inaugurated a series of clinical lectures at the Infirmary. The topic was fever and the nosological label discussed was synochus, featuring the cases of Janet Williamson, Isabel (Bell) Donaldson, and Anne Ross. Bell had been admitted to the teaching ward a day before Janet, while Anne came in on December 14 with similar complaints. All three were 17 years old, and Cullen had subjected them to a nearly identical therapeutic regimen. Before lecturing, Cullen usually made extensive notes about each clinical case based on information contained in the ward journal kept on a desk or table with casters for easy transportation. This large folio was divided into 17 separate columns, listing dates, symptoms and signs, pulse and appetite, bodily discharges, food and drink recommendations, and drug prescriptions. Students were also authorized to make notes about hospital cases selected for discussion by listening to the clerk each Saturday afternoon in the operating theater as he dictated the main facts from the same ledger. This practice had been in place since 1743 and was strongly supported by the professors. Because of their growing popularity, these copy hours were extended, with medical students replacing clerks to continue the dictation. Having invested considerable time and money in attending the infirmary, students were eager to reproduce complete cases, reports, and prescriptions. Some even took down the lectures in shorthand. In time, these casebooks became essential reference tools guiding the practices of young physicians entering the medical marketplace.[92]

Cullen's lectures were part of an official program of clinical instruction organized by the University of Edinburgh in cooperation with the managers of the local Infirmary. Working in concert with local professional associations such as the Royal College of Physicians and the Incorporation of Surgeons, Monro Primus, had first established a system of informal student visits to the Infirmary linked to the traditional surgical apprenticeship. Surgery could not be learned from books alone; competence resulted from observation and practice. Students gained access to the wards of the Infirmary by purchasing admission tickets and following their masters on rounds.

Since the sixteenth century, prominent physicians and surgeons affiliated with hospitals had brought their own apprentices to the institutional bedside for further learning, but most of that instruction had remained informal and unsystematic. In 1539, Giovanni B. da Monte (1498–1561), then professor of medicine at the University of Padua, had taken his students to the local Ospedale di San Francesco to see patients with illnesses on which he was lecturing.[93] Brought to Holland by a number of Flemish disciples, clinical teaching achieved new importance at the University of Leyden under the guidance of Otto van Heurne (1577–1652) and Franciscus de le Boe Sylvius (1616–1672) and was expanded in the early 1700s by Herman Boerhaave.[94] Students followed the attending professionals through ward rounds, observing while their masters interacted with selected patients and prescribed remedies. Because the European nations' armed forces required more military and naval surgeons, hospitals became key training grounds for competent professionals.

This clinical teaching model was brought to Edinburgh by Boerhaave's pupils, and also found wide acceptance among the city's surgeons and physicians.[95] Contemporary European practitioners now readily supported a shift in medical epistemology from theoretical concerns and hypothetical reasoning to expanded empirical bedside observation. Thus, they eagerly wished to offer students a limited sample of clinical reality available at the local hospital. At Edinburgh, John Rutherford (1695–1779), then professor of the practice of medicine, petitioned the Infirmary managers in 1748 to organize a formal course of clinical lectures. Two years later, the financial and professional success of this course led to the creation of a separate teaching ward that was open only during the academic year. By 1756, three other university professors—Monro Secundus, Cullen, and Robert Whytt— began to manage this new unit in two-month rotations, a system modified in the late 1760s to allow only two professors, John Gregory and Cullen, to assume these duties for three months. Following Gregory's death in early 1772, Cullen not only managed all teaching cases for the entire academic year, but also offered a complete series of clinical lectures, a grueling schedule for a prominent consultant with a busy private practice.

Boerhaave's teaching practices at the Caecilia Gasthuis in Leyden, involving 12 patients in a ward specifically set aside for educational purposes, set new standards in practical medical education.[96] Based on the Leyden model, the initial capacity of the Edinburgh unit was also set at 12 beds, but the lure of student fees and, thus, greater hospital revenues prompted lay managers during the 1780s to expand it to 30 and eventually 50 beds. University teachers were authorized to select their own patients for admission from among the socially eligible contingent, as well as to demand transfers of other patients located in other wards to fulfill their pedagogical needs. To supplement daily bedside instruction, the same professors organized a series of biweekly clinical lectures during which the management of the most important cases was presented. Students were also allowed to see all hospitalized patients by accompanying the salaried house physicians on their daily rounds and calling on the sick before such visits. For access to the wards, they purchased a three-month or yearly ticket.

The initial size of Edinburgh's teaching ward conformed to contemporary agendas and the needs of the medical profession.[97] As earlier in Leyden, official teaching was primarily meant to illustrate in greater detail the natural history of specific diseases, together with their current classification and therapeutic management. For the benefit of students, a limited number of patients such as Janet were admitted with already "well-formed" illnesses that were easy to diagnose and treat. The Edinburgh strategy was to select patients for a didactic, in-depth management of common diseases that students were bound to encounter in their private practices.[98] As elsewhere, this move signaled a fundamental change in the patient–physician relationship as the professional focus began to shift toward the common character of inmates' diseases rather than the individuality of the sufferers. A 1791 review in the *London Medical Journal* put it succinctly: "The great advantages derived by medical students at Edinburgh from the clinical ward of the Infirmary have long been deservedly acknowledged. The best marked diseases, such as are the most singular in nature, and the greatest variety of acute as well as chronic complaints are selected for it."[99]

At noon, the professor, accompanied by the medical house clerk and the ticketed students, made daily rounds in the teaching ward. Student contact with patients remained highly regulated, in consonance with the Infirmary managers' fiduciary role in the protection of patients. Medical power bred arrogance and condescension. There was cause for patients to fear harassment and exploitation. Senior attending physicians and teachers were repeatedly urged to "recommend by precept and enforce by example the humane attention here recommended."[100]

By 1778, "a composed and decent carriage" came to be an official requisite for the growing army of ticketed students invading the Infirmary and beginning to interfere with the performance of some hospital routines. Managers warned students to avoid "strolling about in the wards."[101]

Despite the physicians' emphasis on teaching and treating diseases rather than patients, managers believed, and the Infirmary's subscribers certainly expected, that as part of the social contract, the political and charitable objectives of their institution were paramount. Patients thus remained somewhat protected by the "associated philanthropy" of the British voluntary hospital movement, and managers, although aware of the medical needs—especially the educational ones— were keen on maintaining the reputation of their charity. Medical interests, therefore, whether investigative or educational, remained secondary and were a perennial source of tension and even conflict with students and attending physicians.

Physicians, for their part, were interested in expanding their limited therapeutic arsenal. They strongly defended their sporadic experimentation with new drugs, stressing its potential benefits to patients. One of them, Andrew Duncan, tried out new botanicals, including a few sent to him from America and others grown in the university's own medicinal garden. Such plans led to a number of debates regarding the physician's proper role in a hospital: should he simply follow nature or attempt to question previous dogmas and treatments? Hospitals and dispensaries, with their compliant patient populations, were potential sites for therapeutic experiments. In fact, such experiments were not conducted in secrecy; the teaching ward was never shrouded from public view. One of the first steps was to rid traditional pharmacopoeias of their useless remedies. Clinical experimentation was instrumental in reforming the materia medica contained in the Edinburgh's Royal College of Physicians' Pharmacopeia, eliminating many drugs that had proven ineffective while changing the indications for and dosages of others. Reflecting such therapeutic experiences, new formularies appeared, sponsored by local colleges, and older ones, including the official *Edinburgh Dispensatory*, were repeatedly revised with the help of medical luminaries such as Cullen. Even the Edinburgh Infirmary came out with its own in-house dispensatory.[102]

Eighteenth-century physicians also expressed optimism that new cures could be found for hitherto incurable diseases. As new botanical research and classification schemes flourished everywhere in Europe, physicians embarked on a more systematic investigation of plants—many of them exotic—with potential medicinal effects. This work could only be accomplished through empirical drug trials, not by following traditional indications from older medical authorities. Even within the constraints of the British voluntary system, physicians could justify the use of old and new medicinal preparations with the intent of discovering more beneficial ones. Superior efficacy was critical to physicians competing in a marketplace flooded with popular remedies. One compendium with the title *Practice of the*

British and French Hospitals appeared in 1775 and featured successful prescriptions employed in British naval hospitals and Parisian institutions such as the Hôtel Dieu and La Charité.[103]

Surgeons had different professional needs. Hospitals provided them with opportunities to acquire valuable anatomical and pathological knowledge necessary for improving the management of accidents and surgical conditions central to their future practices. However, the creation of a teaching ward devoted exclusively to medical cases tilted the balance of organized instruction toward the more politically and socially powerful physicians and their Royal College. In the 1770s, local surgeons required the consent of physicians to admit their patients, representing about 20% of the total institutional population. Devoid of proper anesthetic agents and faced with the twin threats of circulatory shock and infection, the contemporary keyhole surgery demanded great speed and anatomical proficiency, the latter a rare commodity since traditionally anatomical dissection had been a punishment for deceased criminals and was thus stigmatized. Yet, most surgeons were eager to perform dissections to extend their knowledge and improve their skills, to the point of collaborating with organized gangs of body snatchers.

While hospitals had traditionally created favorable conditions for postmortem examinations, the Edinburgh Infirmary, like other voluntary British hospitals, proved to be less sympathetic to such studies. In an effort to prevent negative publicity that might jeopardize support from their subscribers, the managers severely limited human dissections. Autopsies were not to be performed merely "for the gratification of idle curiosity, or as making the hospital a school and the dead patients the subjects of anatomical instruction."[104] Rules required that attending physicians and surgeons first secure permission from the next of kin or friends of the deceased. If successful, the practitioners then needed to obtain an order signed by at least three current hospital managers before scheduling the dissection. Paradoxically, the only individuals exempted from this last requirement were the university professors, all physicians, but not the surgeons. Together with the low institutional mortality rates previously noted, these rules were responsible for the paucity of autopsies in Edinburgh during the second half of the eighteenth century. "I was desirous to have a dissection but the interposition of his friends was violent and prevented us," explained a frustrated Cullen in another contemporary fever case.[105]

Dissections authorized by the Infirmary were conducted by surgical clerks who had never managed the medical cases. The professional ethos of the British physician as gentleman virtually precluded his hands-on involvement with rotting corpses. It is even unclear whether both students and professors ever congregated around the autopsy table to discuss the anatomical findings and attempt any kind of correlation with the clinical manifestations of the disease. Moreover, dissections seldom disclosed the immediate causes of death, ostensibly the primary goal of physicians. Knowledge derived from pathological anatomy thus provided only supplementary information designed to confirm bedside events. Final reports were understandably brief and fairly ambiguous.

With its claims of greater certainty, rationality, and logic, medical system building enhanced the professional status of Enlightenment physicians. The ability to rationalize the causes and manifestations of disease within a coherent cosmology shared by the educated elite obviously created an aura of certainty that could provide an edge to physicians vying for patients in Britain's competitive medical marketplace.[106] At the time of Janet's admission, Cullen's theories conferred a mantle of intellectual respectability on medical practitioners and students who professed to follow it. However, adherence to his medical system and nosology shaped but also limited the ideas and activities of Edinburgh's medical elite and their students. During the 1780s, the Cullenians in Edinburgh became engaged in a war with the Brunonians, students and physicians influenced by the ideas of John Brown (1735–1788), one of Cullen's former students. In the end, as with all systematists before him, Cullen's medical ideas were abandoned; he was ridiculed as "Old Spasm" (because his physiopathology had been based on vascular irritability).[107]

The educational value of the Infirmary was significant, even though most of the learning was passive. Given the capacity of its institution, social filters, and urban size, the city of Edinburgh could, however, furnish only a selected fraction of its inhabitants for hospitalization and study. Professors teaching in hospitals such as the Edinburgh Infirmary were especially keen to educate gentlemen physicians whose manners and rhetoric would conform to contemporary social norms.[108] Opportunities for closely observing the evolution of acute diseases with experienced clinicians and without the restrictions imposed by private practice were critical. Moreover, the teaching was not exclusively meant to demonstrate, like anatomical theaters, the existing species of disease, but also to advance clinical knowledge and therapy.[109]

Janet Williamson remained in the teaching ward for another week. She was discharged "cured" by Cullen on Saturday, January 9, 1773, after spending four full weeks in the Infirmary, somewhat more than the average length of stay. Professors often delayed the discharge of certain patients because their clinical course had considerable teaching value. In Janet's case, however, the purpose could have been chiefly charitable. As Cullen admitted to students about other patients, he often violated hospital rules by keeping them in the "warmth and shelter of the house in hopes of a better season."[110] Perhaps the professor assumed rightly that his probably now unemployed, homeless patient would quickly suffer a relapse. The grateful patient, in turn, fulfilled her part of the social bargain by helping out with a variety of institutional chores. As a Scottish minister summarized in his fund-raising sermon, "The persons to be received into the hospital . . . want that which makes poverty tolerable. They would want no more but to be re-established in their former health, to return to their labor and industry, and be no further burdensome to the public."[111]

VIENNA, 1750–1800

His Majesty emperor Joseph II asked me whether I was pleased with his hospital. Splen-did, I replied, now I am somewhat reconciled with the concept of a large institution. [He]: 'What criticisms do you have about such an establishment?' [I]: 'As a great clockwork, it seldom tends to function correctly.' [He]: 'It works!' [I]: 'Indeed, as long a such a pow-erful weight sets it in motion!' My audacity did not incur his displeasure.

Johann P. Frank, *Selbstbiographie*, 1785[112]

Seeking care: A tailor's fate

Ending another day's work in early November 1797, Johann Duschau suddenly felt a cold chill sweeping over his entire body together with an oncoming headache. The 27-year-old tailor was probably working in a shop and drawing low wages, since guild control had already ended in Vienna's urban economy. As he climbed the stairs to his small, cold room on the top floor of a house, he tried to ignore the symptoms. After all, winter was on its way and colds were frequent. Sudden overheating from strenuous physical activity followed by exposure to cold was seen as debilitating. Exhausted Viennese even worried that their favorite pastime— dancing the waltz, especially at Fasching time—would land them in the hospi-tal.[113] After surviving the usual childhood diseases, Johann considered himself quite healthy, although an acquaintance later revealed to physicians that he had been nursing a bad cough and had had difficulty breathing for several months. Hope for a spontaneous remission remained. Without appetite and energy, Jo-hann, who seemingly was a bachelor, tried to return to work the next morning af-ter a bad night. Unfortunately, it was not to be. His energy steadily flagging, he was unable to get out of bed. Chills alternated with high fever, and the general-ized feeling of weakness increased.[114]

As he shivered in his lonely abode atop the city's overcrowded rooming houses, Johann may have wished he was back in his native Prague. Vienna, with a popu-lation of close to 300,000, was, of course, the political and intellectual center of the Habsburg Empire. Not only did the ruler live there with his family, but the city also hosted an extensive imperial bureaucracy and was the playground of a nobility not known for frugality. Although most aristocrats had already moved to quieter summer residences in the suburbs—more than 30 new baroque palaces had been built—the demand for luxury goods and services involved a formidable army of architects, builders, decorators, furniture makers, jewelers, hairdressers, tailors, coachmen, and thousands of domestic servants.

Vienna's inner city was a tangle of narrow streets still surrounded by a me-dieval wall. The buildings were old, dark, and tall and emitted a musty, unpleas-ant odor. However, the fashionable commercial center, the Graben, was colorful and busy. All classes mingled and admired the merchandise displayed on stands while indulging in the ices, sweets, and lemonade made from polluted water dispensed by itinerant vendors. The traditional coffeehouses were filled with loafing bureaucrats watching people pass by in the latest fashions. Because of the tall dwellings, the wind converted the dark alleys into veritable wind tunnels, and people blamed their respiratory ailments on this phenomenon. Many wheezed in the heavy dust that rose up in spite of the fact that the streets were sprinkled twice a day.[115]

High rents forced the poor such as Johann to live on the fourth floor or higher in small, dingy spaces without ventilation and sunshine. Entire families crowded into one room. People were afraid to open the windows, lest they waste the little but expensive heat furnished by their landlords. Such conditions helped spread illness and worsen them. Venereal disease and tuberculosis were quite common. The latter was prevalent enough to merit the cynical label *morbus Viennensis*—Vienna's disease.[116] In a 1794 fictional letter written for a satirical Viennese paper, the author focused on the contradictions between medical advances, institutional reforms, and health, observing: "we have also visited the new *Allgemeines Krankenhaus.*" It is really arranged for those who get sick. My cousin, however, tells me that it is really not that large. The real big hospital is the entire city of Vienna."[117]

Recently, however, Vienna had endured a major scare. Napoleon Bonaparte and his troops, fresh from their victorious Italian campaign, had marched on the capital, only to sign the Peace of Leoben in April. This was followed by the Treaty of Campoformio, which temporarily ended Austria's five-year war with France's revolutionary Directory. Following the sudden death of emperor Leopold II on March 1, 1792, of "inflammatory" fever, his 24-year-old son Francis II had assumed the Habsburg throne. The new ruler inaugurated another period of war and political conservatism during which the enlightened policies of the previous monarchs were rolled back.[118] Fear of subversive political activities now gripped the Viennese upper classes, and censorship, police action, and heavy penalties fostered an increasingly repressive political climate. Police searches for French agents and local revolutionaries continued unabated, as public discontent was often misinterpreted as political activism and opposition. This had been illustrated by the highly publicized Jacobin trials of 1793, followed by the arrest of a number of cobblers and Johann's peers in the tailor's trade, accused of "infection" with the revolutionary germ. Now, under the rule of the pliable Francis II, the Austrian nobility strongly reaffirmed its privileges and ended peasant reform, further increasing the gap between rich and poor. As a result, the latter streamed into urban areas in search of work, overcrowding the metropolis with malnourished, sick newcomers who competed with Johann for jobs.[119]

Conditions had been better. Empress Maria Theresa's (1717–1780) long reign had witnessed a welcome 25-year peace between the major European powers following the Peace of Paris. She and her son Joseph II (1741–1790) had inaugurated a period of "enlightened despotism" during which a series of important political and institutional reforms were accomplished. Their aim was to strengthen the Habsburg state and especially rebuild its armed forces so that Austria could once more play a leading role in European geopolitics. Like other enlightened European despots, Austria's rulers also sought to develop state power through demographic growth, economic development, and military supremacy guided by political and mercantilist ideologies.[120] First, however, the monarchy needed to curb its powerful church and aristocracy. In 1782, a wave of closings focused on religious houses, especially the Jesuits. Joseph II followed with other measures to centralize power, a difficult task in a multiethnic empire.[121]

Like other rulers, Joseph II, who presumed to understand his subjects and to know what was best for them, had embraced *cameralism*, a comprehensive and rational framework of administration characterized by a paternalistic and pronatalist approach.[122] The ultimate goal, summarized by the Austrian cameralist and adviser to Joseph II, Joseph von Sonnenfels (1737–1817), was to reform European government and society and create the bases for a modern, efficient state: "Every tradition which has no justifiable basis should be automatically abandoned."[123]

Johann, in the meantime, consulted a local healer, who prescribed a diaphoretic powder to be mixed with tea. Successive cups of the brew, however, seemed ineffective, and he then medicated himself with a potent purgative. The expected effect—more than 10 visits to the latrine—also provided no relief. Dizziness, a sore throat, and difficulty swallowing now joined the previous febrile symptoms together with a persistent, dry cough. Finally, on November 29, Johann ended seven days of suffering by dragging himself to the city's large Allgemeines Krankenhaus or General Hospital located in the suburb of Alsergründ.

Joseph II and Vienna's Allgemeines Krankenhaus

The institution that Johann Duschau entered in November 1797 was an imperial foundation, the outgrowth of the personal vision of the late Emperor Joseph II and already widely admired as one of the best hospitals in Europe.[124] It had its origins in the growing need for institutional care of the sick poor and the centralizing policies of the eighteenth-century Austrian crown. In the early 1780s, with the support of a Bohemian nobleman, Johann N. Buquoi, Joseph II had sought to cut the Gordian knot that had tied poor relief to sick care since medieval times. The need for social reform was urgent. The ranks of the poor had swollen significantly, and the emperor now sought to engage the resources of the Catholic Church in the service of the state. In April 1782, the emperor had ordered the government of Lower Austria to establish a commission to study the future of hospitals and other welfare establishments. His goals were first to preserve the population by protecting mothers, assisting them through childbirth, and caring for foundlings and abandoned children. Second, the sick poor were to be provided with rest, food, and medical aid. Finally, shelter needed to be organized for the old and disabled who lacked families and were too poor to fend for themselves. A year later, the authorities estimated that Vienna had 4,912 poor and ill, of whom 2,100 were eligible for hospitalization.[125]

Not surprisingly, the solution was by now old-fashioned. In the name of administrative efficiency and economy, Joseph II thus quickly decentralized poor relief in the early 1780s and placed it in the hands of local parishes, which were to assess the needs of their members. But who was entitled to what? With begging strictly forbidden, cash distributions were to be made to the deserving poor on Sundays at individual parishes based on charitable donations. New confraternities—now to be called *poverty institutes*—were also to be engaged in providing social services. While the Church was enlisted in these imperial welfare schemes, its religious practices were to be stripped of "superstitious" rituals. Lured by the prospect of cash payments, many of the poor inmates cleared out of the central city almshouse, the Grosses Armenhaus, and other Viennese hospitals. At the same time, the emperor ordered police to begin regular round-ups of beggars, unceremoniously dumping all foreign homeless across the border in Bavaria. After ridding themselves of many chronic and aged patients, hospitals were to offer care only to be truly sick. Conventional wisdom suggested that perhaps less crowded hospitals could now better spend their resources on those who could be rehabilitated and returned to work.[126] In the meantime, Joseph II, the populist and frugal *Volkskaiser*, often roamed through Vienna incognito, visiting taverns and attending spectacles such as buildings on fire, eager to establish personal contacts with his subjects and presumably improve his understanding of their plight.[127]

An enlightened state had to ensure the happiness of its citizens through a healthy, regular life of work and leisure. The intent was perhaps benevolent, but strict rules of behavior, educational requirements, and prescribed age for marriage caused near-universal resentment, antipathy, and distrust. Joseph II's approach was characteristically arbitrary, coercive, and thus often counterproductive.[128] Under the aegis of the term *medical police*, first employed by a German municipal physician, Wilhelm Rau (1721–1772), in 1764, some European governments sought to formulate autocratic cradle-to-grave programs for public health, environmental hygiene, health care, and regulation of the health professions. In contemporary mercantilist ideology, the term *Policey* or police consisted of a state-sponsored administrative apparatus presided over by a wise ruler, who used a number of bureaucratic devices to take care of his people.[129] To implement policies designed to preserve the population, national governments, local authorities, professional corporations, and private philanthropists were enlisted for reforms within the medical profession, affecting its knowledge base and improving its clinical skills.

As part of his program of health reform, Joseph II envisioned the centralization in one institution of all hospital care then distributed among a dozen institutions in the city. All endowments still supporting these institutions were to be transferred to the state. The new institution was to be reserved for sick care, and would be focused primarily on the recovery of physical rather than spiritual well-being and nondenominational in character.[130] The royal plans, however, faced considerable obstacles. In 1781, Vienna had barely 20 institutions with 1,000 beds available for the infirm, with the truly sick concentrated in merely 6 of them. In the tradition of Catholic charity going back to the Middle Ages, most of the metropolitan facilities functioned as shelters and hostels for the homeless and the old.[131]

Vienna had provided charitable assistance in hospitals since the 1240s. Among the most important was the Bürgerspital, the city's oldest such institution, with over 200 beds. Founded in 1257, it functioned as a guesthouse and pesthouse for centuries. Another was the Bäckenhäusel, established as a lazaretto in 1656—the year in which both Rome and Vienna suffered from the plague. Other important establishments were the Holy Trinity and Spanish Hospitals, consolidated in 1754. High institutional mortality, estimated at around 15%, earned them a reputation as gateways to death. This stigmatized status prevented people from seeking admission until they were near death, with the deliberate intention of having the institution cover their burial expenses. Indeed, the crowding and mingling probably generated more sickness than the attending physicians could cure.[132]

During the foregoing two centuries, Viennese hospitals, like their counterparts in Catholic Europe, had suffered from a chronic shortage of funds. Private charitable donations were steadily declining. Quick fixes engineered by municipal authorities in the form of tax exemptions and assessments on profits from tobacco consumption and lottery earnings proved insufficient. At the same time, demand for charitable services including medical care in cities had increased dramatically, far outstripping available resources. As in other spheres of Austrian life, Joseph II now raised questions of economic efficiency and centralization concerning these hospitals. Although the emperor had seen the decrepit Hôtel Dieu in Paris during a visit to his sister, Marie Antoinette, in 1777, he was determined to establish a similarly large 2,000-bed facility in Vienna.[133]

Impatient with the pace of a royal commission studying the problem, Joseph II issued a *Hofdekret* or court edict on September 5, 1782. Funds for construction would come directly from the emperor's private fortune. Instead of new facilities, the frugal ruler suggested that the Grosses Armenhaus at the Alsergasse simply be remodeled into a 2,000-bed general hospital. Established in 1683 by Emperor Leopold I, this central almshouse was located in the Alser Valley next to a creek, and accommodated the poor as well as military invalids from the Turkish wars. By the early eighteenth century, the self-contained complex was a small city just outside Vienna's walls. Over 5,000 individuals lived there by the 1750s. Inspired by earlier monastic plans, the long, three story-buildings were arranged around three successive, gigantic courtyards, with an octagonal chapel located in the center of the first cross structure. This arrangement and the geographic location exposed the almshouse to the presumably cleansing actions of sun and wind.[134]

To accomplish his goal, Joseph II decided to sponsor a contest for designing his new hospital. The winner would be named director. In Vienna, the royal competition generated a heated debate among prominent physicians of Vienna. Most of them, including Johann P. Fauken (1740–1794) and Johann Hunczovsky (1752–1798), the latter a prominent surgeon and head of the military medical academy, suggested a smaller or less centralized facility than Emperor Joseph envisioned. They cited their concern that such a large hospital would fail to provide adequate ventilation, hygiene, and prevention of cross-infection.[135] In fact, Fauken's views generated similar hospital reform proposals in Paris two years later.[136] But Joseph's mind was not to be changed, and the plan he chose in February 1783 was that of his personal physician, Joseph Quarin (1733–1814). This rather undistinguished courtier had merely adopted the ideas of his sovereign and proposed a 1,500-bed facility together with a modest salary for the director. Joseph II responded by ordering the immediate remodeling of Vienna's Grosses Armenhaus. Current residents were given two weeks to vacate the premises. Their ultimate fate was not recorded. The refurbished complex was to feature a general hospital, a lying-in facility, an insane asylum (the only new building), and another establishment for foundlings. The original courtyards lined with linden trees and gardens were preserved.[137] In accordance with contemporary notions of salubrity, each ward was to have upper and lower windows, ventilating chimneys, and even metal floor shafts to allow miasma to clear the premises. Similar vents were placed over all the doors. In the end, the hospital remained a veritable labyrinth of 111 sickrooms—61 for males, 50 for females. Some were private; others were small 20-bed wards. Links between them were cumbersome and travel across the outdoor enclosures was hazardous, especially during winter.

Based on medical criteria, the sprawling Allgemeines Krankenhaus was divided into sections: four medical, two surgical, one venereal, and one contagious. This classification and the assignment of patients to the teaching ward or surgical operating room generated confusing and frequent patient transfers, a feat accomplished with the assistance of six sedan chairs and their attendants. Further communications took place via couriers. Although the primary goal was the physical care of the sick, the emperor did not ignore the religious sensibilities of the hospital population. Although all religious symbolism such as altars and shrines was carefully omitted—the entrance inscription spoke of *saluti* (well-being) and *solatio* (consolation) of the sick—two resident Catholic priests circulated daily through the wards to hear confessions and dispense the sacraments.

Many omissions jeopardized the salutary qualities of this hospital. In their haste, planners forgot to create extra rooms for the nursing personnel, forcing male and female attendants to sleep in the wards they supervised, frequently on the floors. The existing structure of the Armenhaus demanded the alignment of three adjacent wards which communicated freely with each other and thus spread contagion. Corridors were narrow and filled with smoke because of insufficient ventilation from small kitchen facilities placed between rooms. Only a few toilets were located under the stairways, prompting a heavy traffic in bedpans. Moreover, facilities for storage of linens and medications or for examinations and treatments were nonexistent. A board affixed to the bed allowed nurses and physicians to record basic patient information, including name, date of admission, diagnosis, diet, and drugs. A table in the center of the ward had a book containing all dietary instructions. On the wall hung a printed set of management rules for the benefit of all caregivers. It prescribed the daily routines, including pharmacy pickups and laundry disposals.[138]

According to the proposed staff arrangements, Quarin, who reported directly to Joseph II, had the right to appoint four primary physicians (physicus primarius) and five secondary one (physicus secundarius). Two of them were required to live in the hospital and make rounds twice a day. To assemble his medical staff, Quarin drew from a cadre of more than 300 young practitioners, educated since the 1760s at the reorganized local university and trained at the bedside. Since the Habsburg rulers were bent on curbing Church power, many individuals previously destined for the priesthood had shifted careers and became physicians instead. Among the early primary physicians were Bartolomeo Battisti, a student of Maximilian Stoll (1742–1787), the famous professor of clinical medicine and chief physician from the Trinity Hospital, and A. Stragy, who adopted a somewhat passive attitude toward treatment, stressing diet and enemas. Other senior physicians were Sigmund Barisari, a friend and medical consultant to Mozart, and Thomas F. Closset, who looked after the composer's wife.[139]

Quarin also appointed a chief of surgery, three senior and five junior hospital surgeons, and eight additional clerks, many selected from among experienced military surgeons. Surgeons, when not working in a small, dimly lit facility in the main building, performed operations directly in the wards and at the beds of their patients. In the end, the hospital had 15 physicians and an equal complement of surgeons and their assistants to care for 2,000 patients. They instructed the nurses, supervised procedures such as enemas, bloodletting, and blistering, and prescribed drugs.

The nursing staff consisted of 140 lay attendants about equally divided between the sexes. Misgivings had been expressed about hiring religious personnel.[140] Although their caregiving skills were limited and their duties focused primarily on keeping the premises clean, the emperor had insisted that nurses be paid a higher wage—nine florins a month together with room and board—than that routinely offered to ordinary servants. This measure was designed to prevent bribery, which, as we know, was common at the Edinburgh Infirmary. In fact, inmates were encouraged to report nurses who solicited money.[141] The ward nurses saw patients daily and the physicians visited every other day, except for acute cases requiring closer monitoring.

On June 20, 1784, over 6,000 printed brochures announced the impending opening of the Allgemeines Krankenhaus for the "conservation of the population." This *Nachricht* or notice stressed the philanthropic underpinnings of the institution and Joseph II's special premise that a new love of humankind would now permeate charitable activities, thus removing the old religious stigmas that had discredited social welfare.[142] This was to be particularly true in the care of unwed mothers, the mad, and those who suffered from venereal diseases. Persons of all religions were to be admitted. The first patients were admitted on August 16, 1784, and soon all the beds were filled, many with transfers from other institutions. The average length of stay was about 50 days. Quarin quickly developed into an autocrat obsessed with regulations and discipline. He cracked down hard on his staff and tried to imitate his emperor's frugality by cutting bread allowances and establishing an institutional dispensatory, only to find that his medical personnel deviated from it in their daily prescriptions. Joseph II, for his part, was seemingly proud of his accomplishment, although his idea that the institution could quickly become financially self-sufficient was unrealistic, an expression of imperial penury amply displayed in other realms. Nevertheless, the institution was perceived as a monument to his efforts to secularize and centralize the care of the sick according to a rational as well as economical plan. With separate facilities for the insane (the famous circular Narrenturm), pregnant women, and orphans, the Allgemeines Krankenhaus quickly became a tourist attraction and a model for subsequent foundations and renovations elsewhere in German-speaking countries.[143]

By showing his contempt for learned opinion and his general bias against medical professionals, however, the emperor had made a fateful mistake: the hastily remodeled facilities could not be kept clean and properly ventilated, a fact reflected in the high institutional mortality of patients and caregivers. In spite of tireless attempts to keep the antiquated premises scrupulously clean, the sheer institutional size and complexity of the Allgemeines Krankenhaus generated garbage piles between buildings and fostered hospital diseases. Indeed, as predicted by the medical experts, waves of typhus and puerperal fever generated an institutional mortality of nearly 20%, a medical embarrassment in Vienna, where smaller institutions such as the Spanish Hospital had a rate of less than 8%. To fudge the statistics, the administration assigned many deaths to the Alserbach lazaretto administratively linked to the imperial institution but located at some distance from the city.

Despite Joseph's frequent visits to raise staff and patient morale, the hospital increasingly acquired the reputation as another house of death. The severe economic crisis of 1788 resulting from the Turkish War affected both the population and the hospital, curtailing services and creating further deficits. In turn, the crowd of prospective paying patients never materialized. Instead of the anticipated thousands, barely 100 inmates contributed a daily fee and the Allgemeines Krankenhaus became a severe drain on the state treasury. As long as Joseph II was in charge, some of the deficits were made up by drawing on private endowments and the emperor's personal fortune.

Following Joseph II's death, however, his brother and successor, Leopold II, faced growing shortages and unfavorable sanitary conditions at the flawed hospital. Anton von Störck (1731–1803), the emperor's new personal physician, openly expressed the view that the hospital was unfit for its medical mission. There were even rumors that the imperial commission, composed of officials and physicians, had decided to close the Allgemeines Krankenhaus altogether, but the economic and logistic consequences of such an action and lack of alternative institutions precluded it. With his mentor dead, Quarin abruptly resigned the directorship in 1791 to resume his private practice. Quarin's temporary successor, the physicus primarius Ferdinand Melly, was ordered to handle only medical matters. The new emperor decided to consult Johann P. Frank (1745–1821), an internationally famous German physician now in the service of the Habsburg monarchs, before instituting reforms. All administrative powers were transferred to government officials who became responsible for the internal economy of the hospital, including staff appointments and food supplies. Severe budget cuts affecting patient care were introduced, including reductions in nursing personnel and surgical assistants. In the midst of these reforms, Melly, who had been appointed director in 1794, suddenly died. A year later, the emperor finally named a successor. Francis II's personal choice was Frank.

Johann Peter Frank:
Hospital director and Brunonian practitioner

The new director of the Allgemeines Krankenhaus, Johann Peter Frank, was also a patron of the arts and sciences, and he quickly attracted a circle of famous friends that included Ludwig van Beethoven and Franz J. Haydn. Those who knew him stressed Frank's superior clinical skills, his friendly and supportive bedside manner, and the time he spent listening to patients.[144] Frank was the most influential spokesperson for a program of medical police, having published since 1777 his influential *System einer vollständigen medicinischen Policey*.[145] In 1785 he had joined the medical faculty of the University of Pavia and became director of the local Ospedale di San Mateo before moving on to take the post of Director General of Public Health for Lombardy, the northern Italian province then under Austrian control. To the delight of his imperial master, Joseph II, Frank had recommended a host of regulatory functions that intruded into every aspect of life, from birth through childhood and adolescence, education, marriage and occupation, housing, personal hygiene, the management of injuries and diseases, old age, and death. The task was to persuade or even force the lower classes to seek and preserve health.[146]

At the center of Frank's program in Lombardy was the provision of medical care for the poor. This could be accomplished through home care but more importantly at hospitals if they could be transformed into places of rehabilitation and cure. Frank still believed that the sick were better off at home, if attended by loving relatives and visited by district physicians, but such conditions seldom applied in crowded urban environments populated by strangers. Practitioners, in turn, fought hard to ensure that patients were classified and segregated into hospital wards according to their ailments. To avoid the dangers of cross-infection, each inmate at the Ospedale di San Mateo was assigned an individual bed.

In a 1784 publication, Frank had branded most contemporary hospitals as "murderous pits."[147] Both traditional designs and constructions reflected the vanity of their founders, who had squandered enormous resources to build veritable palaces for the admiration of contemporaries. In Frank's opinion, previous medieval courtyard shelters were not suited for medical care; rectangular or square constructions such as that of the Edinburgh Infirmary also failed to meet the new hygienic requirements, since corners and closed-off spaces contributed to air stagnation. Frank warned that the savings in building costs obtained from herding the sick into narrow spaces would come back to haunt patrons in the form of higher mortality rates. In his view, the most efficient plan was to build a 300- to 400-bed hospital in a straight line without lateral wings. More capacity would require separate buildings arranged in rows, the so-called pavilion type of hospital, which became a reality a century later.[148]

In objecting to the establishment of large hospitals, Frank and other contemporary experts stressed the danger of hospital-acquired infections. "Mortality," wrote Frank, is "in indirect proportion to the size of the hospital." Since institutions now selectively admitted sick people suffering from acute conditions, hospitalism was becoming an important issue in any debate concerning hospital architecture and internal management. Frank worried that the earlier dread of crowded almshouses was being replaced by the new terror of hospital contagion. "Can there be a greater contradiction than a hospital disease?" asked Frank. In larger institutions, supervision and enforcement of hygienic principles was extremely difficult. One proposed remedy was that wards, like fields, should be left fallow from time to time, devoid of patients, to allow for proper cleaning and airing out of the premises, supplemented by painting or whitewashing of the walls to rid the rooms of any remaining contagion. When Frank assumed the directorship of Vienna's Allgemeines Krankenhaus in late 1795, he immediately sought to minimize the tangible disadvantages of this mammoth institution and implement some of his previous ideas. For him "a large hospital without disorders is an impossible thing."[149] Weekly meetings with all senior physicians and surgeons were held to coordinate clinical activities. Because of his total administrative control of the institution—he was both the director and chief of the teaching unit—Frank instituted a number of useful reforms. Stables were converted into private and isolation rooms for epileptic patients or those requiring special quiet and rest. A surgical amphitheater was constructed to prevent the performance of surgical operations in the wards in front of terrified inmates. Responding to the needs of a metropolis with its growing burden of trauma, Frank also created a separate emergency room.[150]

Frank's first year in his new position could not have been more tragic. Two of his sons, Joseph and Franz, who were also physicians, had joined their father at the institution. Joseph Frank was a physicus primarius; Franz, a recent graduate from Pavia, was Johann's assistant. On March 19, 1796, however, Franz fell victim to the feared institutional contagion. His father commented years later that the mortality of physicians and surgeons attending the Allgemeines Krankenhaus for the previous decade had been higher than that in all the other important Viennese hospitals combined.[151] This situation similarly affected patients in the lying-in facility who contracted puerperal fever, a condition that drew the attention of the famous Hungarian physician Ignaz Semmelweis (1818–1865) almost 50 years later. More than a third of all the medical patients suffered from tuberculosis, and contagion was rampant in the small rooms that housed them.

As part of his administrative reforms, Frank strongly advocated a revision of the institutional dispensatory, and he forced hospital physicians to limit their prescriptions to items included in it. The substantial savings—almost a 20% reduction in drug expenses—were used to buy additional food, especially for convalescents. Frank was concerned about the role of diet in medical management and placed the hospital's kitchen directly under medical control. He was especially appalled by the meager rations, which jeopardized recovery, the primary goal of a medicalized institution operating according to mercantilist objectives. With the approval of the emperor, daily bread rations were increased. In 1796 the hospital regained control over its supplies, which had previously been provided by private contractors. New regulations about the timing of physicians' visits sought to avoid conflicts between medical functions and the proper distribution of meals.

As for the medical staff, Frank pressed for a fifth physicus primarius, explaining to the imperial administration that the existing physicians could not cope with the large patient population. Calculating that each patient visit would take a minimum of three minutes and that each primarius took care of 150–180 patients, especially during the winter, Frank argued that the clinical rounds would exhaust the physicians already exposed to miasma in the wards and also interfere with patient mealtimes. His argument was accepted, and in 1797 Frank appointed Mathias von Sallaba (1754–1797), who had attended Mozart's final illness in 1791. Unfortunately,

Sallaba, one of the most sought-after practitioners of Vienna, was also felled by a hospital fever just a few months later, another illustration of the lethal risks inherent in hospital service.

Not surprisingly, Frank's reforms at the Allgemeines Krankenhaus created new financial deficits, prompting imperial authorities to appoint a separate hospital director for economic affairs, responsible to the government instead of to Frank. This move was the work of Joseph A. Stift (1760–1836), Vienna's *Stadtphysicus* or city physician and darling of the Viennese nobility, who recently had been appointed court physician of Francis II. Apart from an obvious loss of authority for Frank, this bipartite structure violated his strong belief that all administrators— he was in favor of having someone with business experience in such a capacity— should be subordinate to the medical directorship to ensure the hospital's curative role. Otherwise, Frank predicted that there would be continuous conflict between administrators and physicians. In the name of public order, administrators always wanted to preserve their power and their vision of the hospital as an instrument of social control. Physicians, on the other hand, wished to remake the hospital into a medical institution with outreach functions that included the distribution of medicines and immunization against smallpox.[152]

In 1797, when Johann Duschau sought help at the Allgemeines Krankenhaus, Frank was already at odds with Stifft. The original source of the conflict seemed to have been Frank's insistence that the state assume the additional costs required to provide an acceptable level of hospital care. Stifft took the bureaucratic stance congenial to his royal patrons that the best management of the Allgemeines Krankenhaus was more frugality and discipline. He wanted to return to the moralistic agendas originally formulated by the Church, now staunchly resurrected by the Habsburg monarchy.[153]

Stifft also greatly distrusted Frank because of his expressed interest in Brunonianism, a revolutionary medical system quickly branded in conservative Viennese medical circles as a form of Jacobinism, a characterization bound to inflame both medical and governmental leaders.[154] This reaction was occurring at the same time that the clergy was recapturing Austria's educational system by purging teachers and professors. Brunonianism was based on the ideas of John Brown (1735– 1788)—Joannis Bruno—a Scottish physician and former student of William Cullen. Brown's system, presented in his work *Elementa Medicinae* in 1784, sought to simplify the existing medical theories and practices while also increasing their certainty through measurements of bodily excitability.[155]

Such political and professional divisions were far from the mind of our apprehensive tailor, Johann, as he arrived at the hospital's Admissions Room. Like many individuals residing in Vienna, he was probably a lukewarm Catholic whose routine "*Grüss Gott*" salutations, prayers, and occasional church visits were suffused with the widespread skepticism and natural deism that were partly the legacy of Emperor Joseph II's ecclesiastical reforms. The hospital, in turn, was no longer thought of as merely a charitable shelter, and it certainly had ceased to be a place of required religious worship, although it still featured a small chapel. Its organization and patient classifications revealed a keen concern with costs. Since more than 14,000 patients now came through the Allgemeines Krankenhaus each year, Frank maintained a "prescribed order" of admissions. He hoped to avoid filling the wards with all sorts of complaining persons, especially those suffering from chronic conditions who would remain there for years, thus preventing admission of those with more pressing ills. So far as the teaching ward was concerned, certificates of real poverty and illness alone did not entitle a person to be received there. No longer leased to the university professors, the unit was supported by a separate teaching fund. As Frank indicated, "predominantly curable diseases of poor persons are those that should be accepted at hospitals."[156]

Since its opening in 1784, the institution had accepted four separate classes of patients. Those in the first category paid in advance the sum of one florin per day for a private room, better food, and exclusive nursing services. Forty such rooms had been reserved on the top floor of one wing. A second-class patient paid half a florin daily, a week in advance, before being placed in a smaller ward elsewhere. Those unable to make such payments—Johann included—belonged to the third or fourth class of patients. Third-class individuals received some support from the newly created central relief agency, which turned over this money to the hospital. Finally, the fourth-class patients were mostly jobless and without resources. They were required to present a certificate to that effect, issued by their parish priest and a welfare official.

Since Johann was employed before his illness, he was not registered as a welfare recipient, but he probably lacked funds to pay for his hospital care. In any event, the nature of his illness and an available bed in the male teaching ward must have secured his admission, probably authorized by Frank's assistant physician, Thomas Cappellini, an Italian from Pistoia, who, like his master, had recently arrived from Pavia. Like Cullen in Edinburgh, Cappellini and Frank were careful in making their patient selections. Johann's symptoms suggested that he was an ideal teaching case and a candidate for the Brunonian therapeutic approach being touted by Frank. Johann was officially admitted to the small 12-bed teaching ward on November 29. In theory, the tailor appeared to fit Frank's profile concerning the most common candidates for hospitalization: poor people whose "lack of basic necessities" was responsible for illness. The deserving patient, for Frank, was one who "has spent all day doing heavy labor, has filled his stomach insufficiently with coarse bread, and has warmed his blood with a glass of sometimes adulterated brandy. He does not have enough left to protect his bare body against the cold; he wears his only shirt so long that it drops in rags from his body."[157]

But Frank was also concerned about the admission of patients with contagious diseases like Johann's that could perhaps spread among other inmates. Daily experiences with "improvident blending of contagious diseases with less critical ills" generated the dreaded hospital fever, a major concern of every contemporary hospital director. The pernicious patient mix usually brought birthing women in contact with scarlet fever patients, generating puerperal fever. Wounded inmates placed near those with fevers suffered purulent complications. As in times of the plague, the danger of a deadly miasma emanating from sick bodies was still believed to be quite real, and physicians were anxious to place such individuals in small, well-ventilated rooms to avoid its spread.[158]

After his arrival, Johann gave up his street clothes and was assigned to a single bed outfitted with a straw-filled mattress, a woolen blanket, and a pillow stuffed with horsehair. Unlike the private rooms housing paying patients, no curtains separated the beds. Frank himself had described the admission routine: "his body is cleansed of dirt and vermin, he is revived by a lukewarm bath, his skin is refreshed by a fresh shirt; his tired limbs find rest on a comfortable bed; he is in a warm and friendly room."[159] Like all arrivals, the new patient was also provided with a new pair of pants, a frock, socks, and slippers. As he had done earlier with patients in Göttingen and Pavia, Frank assigned a senior medical student to Johann for history taking and a physical examination. The patient's face was pale, his expression fearful. He complained of intense headaches radiating from the temples to the ears and the back of the neck. When ordered to stand up, he felt quite dizzy. His eyes and throat burned badly, and he could barely swallow. Both tonsils were enlarged. With his nose plugged up, Johann also experienced difficult, painful breathing and developed a dry cough in the stuffy, heated room. He preferred to lie on his right side because of severe pain under his left ribs. A fast pulse, hot and sweaty skin, and general debility completed the initial clinical findings. Johann's case seemed quite ordinary: a poorly managed catarrh transformed into an inflammation of the lungs.[160]

A tentative diagnosis of typhus-like fever and pneumonia was made by the medical student and confirmed by Frank, who came to see him during morning rounds the next day. According to the disease classification then in vogue at the Allgemeines Krankenhaus—which Frank had partially adopted from the tenets of John Brown—the tailor's condition was considered "asthenic." During the 1780s in Scotland, Brown had rejected all conventional classifications of disease, promoting instead the notion that all health problems were simply due to changes in bodily excitability, caused either by excessive stimulation to create *sthenia* or more likely being the result of deficient stimuli ending in *asthenia*.[161] In his writings, Frank had repeatedly defined his own therapeutic approach as one of activism and moderation, in contrast to the traditional and more aggressive antiphlogistic one, with its purging and bleeding routines. Stressing simplicity and economy, Frank argued instead for a supportive regimen that included rest in a warm room, clean clothes, perhaps a lukewarm bath, stimulants, and, if tolerated, good food and drink that included beer and wine.[162]

Consequently, Frank and his assistant, Cappellini, initially prescribed a strengthening regimen of fluids, beginning with beef soup and an infusion of the Angelica tree root, a tonic to be administered in doses of half a cup every two hours. As an antidiarrheal remedy, Frank ordered a decoction of a species of orchid. This therapeutic approach was quite at odds with conventional eighteenth-century treatments of fever and pneumonia that recommended a meager diet and humoral depletion through the aggressive employment of emetics, bloodletting, and purgatives.[163] Unfortunately for Johann, this regimen failed to relieve his symptoms. He kept shivering and sweating, coughed frequently, and experienced ringing in his ears. Sleep was nearly impossible.

In employing this Brunonian approach—the name Brown was frequently Latinized as Bruno in Continental medical circles—Frank had come into open conflict not only with Stifft but also with the majority of Vienna's physicians, including those who practiced in the Allgemeines Krankenhaus. Most of them had been trained under Anton de Haen (1704–1776), a student of Boerhaave's, and Maximilian Stoll and still supported traditional humoralism. An avowed follower of Hippocrates, de Haen had adhered to classical humoral concepts. He repeatedly stressed the empiricism of Hippocrates, Thomas Sydenham, a seventeenth-century English physician, and Boerhaave, based on detailed clinical observations, especially of the quality and quantity of patients' bodily discharges. Unlike other colleagues on the Continent, de Haen was therapeutically very conservative, allowing such discharges to occur freely. He dispensed drugs only if they could help cool and dissolve those corrupted humors, as the alleged healing power seemed unable to dislodge them from the body.[164] Stoll was keen on prescribing emetics and purgatives in the belief that the stomach played a major role in humoral corruption.[165] Moreover, the notion of natural healing powers in the body—traced back to Hippocrates—came into stark contrast with Frank's more interventionist approach.

On December 1, repeated sips of hot milk administered by the nurses helped to ease Johann's sore throat and facilitate swallowing, but the dyspnea and cough became worse, the pulse weaker and faster. Frank now discontinued the previous infusion and replaced it with Seneca snakeroot, the tonic and expectorant introduced from Virginia in the 1730s. He added to it a much more potent drug: an extract of camphor prepared in sugar pills.[166] In general, expensive foreign materia medica was omitted in favor of cheaper domestic equivalents, although for Frank "the best remedy is the one that cures most quickly."[167] To make his case, Frank quoted a study carried out by a prominent German clinician, Ernst Horn, at the Charité Hospital in Berlin. Horn had discovered no decreases in mortality when more costly remedies were used. He also warned of fraud and misappropriations and of the theft of opium and other tinctures. Most eighteenth-century hospitals therefore insisted that their salaried physicians use the institutional dispensatories. Moreover, the cost of a particular remedy was partly related to the time and the method required to prepare it in the hospital's pharmacy. Therefore, powders and tisanes should be employed before tinctures, decoctions, and pills. To avoid waste and soiled bed linens, ointments were to be sparsely applied.

On December 4, Johann remained delirious and his chest pains seemed to abate, but those attending him believed that he had fluid in his chest cavity. Frank therefore prescribed a diuretic drink made of a vinegar extract of squill and honey. For nourishment, Johann received beef broth and wine. Now the camphor dosage was doubled and the painful area on the left chest was treated with an irritating plaster. From subsequent reports, Frank's delirious patient spent another difficult day, restless and at times agitated. The attending physicians discontinued the squill medication and prescribed a cardiac tonic, Kermes, together with the camphor. By December 7, the patient's fever and dyspnea were somewhat diminished, but another crisis forced Frank to prescribe an additional powerful tonic: a syrup of Peruvian bark (containing quinine) prepared with wine, ether, and peppermint water. On December 12, new abdominal pains prompted the prescription of opium.[168] Wine and a diet consisting of soft eggs were also provided to overcome the perceived organic weakness. Frank's liberal prescription of wine caused quite a stir among Viennese practitioners and the public. In a letter written in 1797, an anonymous author sarcastically suggested that people in Vienna would no longer die because the hospital physicians had discovered a universal arcanum: wine. The purported panacea came from Britain and would force the conversion of all pharmacies into *Weinhäusl*, or wine bars.[169]

As the progress notes in Johann's clinical chart reveal, Frank and his assistants were quite aware of the pneumonic consolidation in the left lower lung, and they suspected the presence of pleural fluid, presumably ascertained through diagnostic percussion, since Frank was known to employ the direct method of chest percussion pioneered by the Austrian physician Leopold Auenbrugger (1722–1809), physician-in-chief at the Spanish Hospital, who had developed the technique on the basis of pathological findings.[170] The presence of fluid in the chest prompted a prescription of digitalis in powder form, then considered a powerful diuretic. In spite of tonic medications to spur to body's vitality, the attending physicians also returned to the traditional approach of placing irritating plasters around the ankles and legs. The resulting blisters were expected to divert the inflammation from the affected left lung to the periphery of the body. In spite of this aggressive therapeutic regimen, Johann's condition steadily deteriorated, punctuated by bouts of delirium, dry cough, dyspnea, and pain. On December 20, just a few days before Christmas, all hope for recovery vanished and the patient was switched to a palliative regimen based on periodic enemas containing beef broth as his only means of nourishment. Nauseated from the medicinal powders, Johann could barely swallow the few sips of wine and spoonfuls of warm milk periodically administered by the nurses.

Contrary to Frank's initial expectations, Johann's clinical evolution proved an embarrassment to "the first physician of Europe"[171] and his cadre of young, enthusiastic physicians, including his son Joseph, who all followed the Brunonian approach.[172] The serial introduction of stimulating drugs and the total omission of traditional humoral depletion strategies had not helped this patient. In fact, Johann's condition matched the stereotype of the delirious and drunken inmate of the Allgemeines Krankenhaus that opponents of the Franks and Brunonianism employed in ridiculing the experimental treatments. Finally, on January 8, 1798, the now quite emaciated tailor from Prague died quietly at 1 PM, prompting a ringing of the hospital's bell, a nefarious practice that agitated and demoralized the surviving inmates.

Clinicum practicum: **The patient as teacher**

To implement the broad health policy agenda of the Enlightenment, Europe needed many more competent physicians and surgeons. In Vienna's inner city at the time of Duschau's death, there were only 87 registered physicians and 44 surgeons. This represented an adequate number for a profession hitherto largely dedicated to the care of an elite clientele. The challenge was to organize new forms of apprenticeship and training and expand teaching facilities at universities and hospitals. According to Frank, "well equipped hospitals in large cities are the best school for training skilled physicians and surgeons, because the most widespread diseases and other cases are seen there in large numbers and in the most varied modifications." Frank also observed that "the young physician and surgeon have the excellent and valuable opportunity of observing what he would hardly see in the course of many years of private practice."[173]

Frank's selection of Johann Duschau as a teaching case in 1797 followed a well-established tradition of clinical education in Vienna that had begun decades earlier, long before the opening of the Allgemeines Krankenhaus. In fact, after some informal beginnings, clinical bedside teaching had become a regular academic subject. This followed university reforms initiated in 1749 by Gerard van Swieten (1700–1772), personal physician to the Empress Maria Theresa and a former student of Boerhaave at Leyden. Under van Swieten and with part of the state's efforts to assume greater power through bureaucratic consolidation, the medical faculty lost its traditional autonomy and was forced to accept a new course of studies. With the creation of an anatomical theater and establishment of a chemical laboratory and botanical garden, the school began to shed its medieval character and offer regular courses in the basic sciences and clinical medicine of the day.[174]

Following a directive of August 7, 1753, Anton de Haen was selected to carry out such a *clinicum practicum* at Vienna's Bürgerspital as professor of clinical medicine. The institution housed about 230 poor inmates, many of them old, disabled, and sick. Some females were pregnant; others were mothers with infants. Inspired by Boerhaave's model at Leyden, de Haen gave daily clinical lectures to his students based on patients admitted to a separate teaching ward that consisted of two small six-bed rooms, the St. Sebastian and St. Roche "Stuben." To protect students from contagion, the wards were well ventilated and always kept at 60–65° F for the comfort of both patients and students. To improve his selection of teaching cases, de Haen received authorization to fill the wards with patients from other Viennese hospitals. These institutions would henceforth also be obliged to supply cadavers for postmortem examinations and the study of pathological anatomy. An active outpatient department or polyclinic at the Bürgerspital provided an additional array of ambulatory cases for study.[175]

Not surprisingly, de Haen followed the Leyden model closely, arriving early in the morning to check the patients before lecturing for one hour between 8 and 9 AM. Aided by a young assistant, Störck, de Haen interrogated and examined all the selected admissions himself and barely allowed students to whisper their impressions privately in his ear. As in Leyden and Edinburgh, this routine reduced students to spectators, passively watching the master and absorbing some useful practical knowledge while developing observational skills and learning proper bedside manners.[176] Working in a public almshouse, de Haen became concerned about the reliability of his patients' clinical histories, especially those who had fever. This led him to thermometry and, after 1762, to the routine measurement of his patients' temperatures by placing the instrument in their mouths or under the armpits. In therapeutic experiments to test the Hippocratic "critical days"—crises in the evolution of particular diseases—de Haen also began to employ a thermometer systematically. Because of the type of institution in which he was practicing, de Haen was not afraid to admit patients with very acute diseases to his teaching ward, including some who seemed almost certain to perish, for they could be dissected without authorization. Whenever possible, he used the postmortem findings to illustrate the previous clinical course and confirm the diagnosis.

By the early 1770s, just as Cullen's clinical teaching in Edinburgh was flourishing, enthusiasm among Austrian students for de Haen's teaching waned. For many, total passivity and a restricted number of interesting cases made the experience questionable. However, a new university plan of curricular reforms proposed by Störck, now dean of the medical faculty, went into effect in January 1775, placing the *clinicum practicum* in the fourth year of medical studies as a requirement for graduation. All candidates for a degree were now authorized to visit the various Viennese hospitals on their own and were encouraged to observe the clinical management of patients.[177] With the departure of the ailing de Haen, his successor, Maximilian Stoll, moved the teaching unit to another hospital, the Unierte Spital (United Hospital), a new 178-bed institution created through the merger of the Spanish and Holy Trinity hospitals.[178]

Presiding over another 12-bed teaching ward and a lecture room at the United

Hospital, Stoll made significant changes that soon attracted more medical students from both the city and other areas of the empire. Although he maintained the format of clinical lectures based on patients selected from a much larger pool, Stoll allowed senior medical students a measure of autonomy unknown in the Edinburgh Infirmary. Pending the professor's approval, they handled the clinical histories, progress notes, and prescriptions of hospitalized individuals assigned to them at admission. Like Edinburgh's medical leaders, Stoll believed that clinical histories provided valuable documentation and rules for medical management. Students and physicians were encouraged to record and collect clinical cases by writing daily progress notes and including autopsy reports if their patients died. Such information, Stoll insisted, was necessary to discern the true patterns of disease and make proper nosological distinctions among them. Here the hospital setting became the center of an ambitious program of clinical research into the epidemiology of common illnesses in Vienna. This approach coincided with Frank's notion that hospitals offered the best opportunity for perfecting the art and expanding the science of medicine, in part because the observations were not distorted by disobedient patients who had secretly taken food and omitted their medicines.[179]

The medical faculty in Vienna, like those elsewhere in Europe, was engaged in new botanical research and classifications and was making efforts to upgrade the existing materia medica, simplify it, and weed out ineffective remedies. Unfettered by the strictures affecting British physicians who worked in private infirmaries, Viennese physicians took advantage of their public hospital populations—patients were sometimes characterized by them as *Schlachtopfer* or slaughter victims—to conduct numerous clinical trials.[180] Among those carrying out such human experiments was Störck, famous in the 1760s for his aggressive clinical tests with two toxic substances, hemlock and aconite, in the treatment of incurable cancer patients at Vienna's Bäckenhäusel Hospital.[181]

After the opening of the Allgemeines Krankenhaus in 1784, Stoll's teaching ward at the Unierte Hospital was closed. It reopened a few weeks later in mid-August at Joseph II's new institution. Unfortunately, Stoll's Boerhaavian unit of 12 beds was housed in a separate building used for administrative purposes and located in the first courtyard. Here on the third floor, teaching took place in two small, dark rooms separated by a narrow corridor. Moreover, these facilities were poorly ventilated—with windows on only one side of the room—and were unable to accommodate the 80–100 students and physicians Stoll attracted to rounds and lectures. Nor was there a separate lecture hall or autopsy room in the vicinity. Apparently such conditions were deemed responsible for the problems of 26 physicians and students in late 1786 who witnessed an autopsy and later came down with typhus fever. Half of them died. Operating under strict regulations imposed by Director Quarin, Stoll was now unable to freely select patients from the general hospital population for his teaching. His written requests were seldom granted.

Stoll died in 1787 and was replaced by Jakob Reinlein, a professor of surgery. Under such less than ideal conditions, clinical instruction quickly deteriorated and the class size shrank to fewer than 30 students during the early 1790s.[182]

With Johann P. Frank's appointment in 1795, a new era of clinical instruction began. As he expressed in his work on medical police, "without a practical school equipped like a hospital, no university can succeed in supplying the state with perfectly trained physicians who will be able to practice satisfactorily upon leaving the university."[183] Frank was critical of the Edinburgh practice of rotating the clinical professors through the Infirmary's teaching ward every three months, claiming that students needed at least a year to fully understand the methods of one of their teachers. On December 14, 1795, Frank began his first course of lectures on special therapy and the pathology of internal diseases. Within three months, he managed to attract over 200 young local medical students and foreign physicians anxious to follow him on his rounds. On such occasions, the crowding around the beds was extreme, and the already vitiated air in the wards virtually suffocated patients and visitors alike.

To accommodate the new arrivals, Frank immediately added two wards but, given the structural characteristics of the building, they too were quite small. Since it was now virtually impossible for all visitors to witness the bedside proceedings, Frank went on once more to remodel the existing facilities, ending up with one 24-bed teaching unit divided into separate 12-bed sections for male and female patients. The dimly lit premises were better illuminated with large wax candles that improved physicians' inspection of their patients.[184] Frank usually made the morning rounds, assigning all incoming patients to the senior students, who took clinical histories and carried out physical examinations under the scrutiny of the professor and his entourage. All discussions among the medical personnel, as well as Frank's clinical lectures, were conducted in Latin.[185]

As described by contemporaries, Frank's morning rounds were quite instructive. His dignified and detached manner impressed those who accompanied him. A kind but somewhat distant man, he was concerned about the commotion created by the bedside teaching, especially insofar as it compromised patient comfort and caused further air pollution. He treated his patients with great respect, eliciting as much information as possible from them. His diagnostic acuity and wealth of medical knowledge kept his audiences engaged. Nothing pleased him more than hearing from his patients that their previous physician had bled them or provided a purgative. To the consternation of those around him, Frank declared that such therapeutic methods had only further debilitated the patient. Indeed, they had created an asthenic condition that, according to Brunonian concepts, required a strengthening regimen of wine, beef broth, and stimulating tonics. By contrast, the evening rounds with Cappellini were almost comical, as Frank's quite deferential assistant gallantly tried to imitate his master's erudition with extravagant statements delivered in a broken mixture of German and Latin.[186]

The educational value of Vienna's Allgemeines Krankenhaus was superior to that of the Edinburgh Infirmary. Based on the notions Frank had elaborated earlier at Pavia, the teaching regimen at the Allgemeines Krankenhaus involved both passive and active learning, since students were given opportunities to manage patients directly under professorial supervision. Although Vienna's potential patient pool was much greater than Edinburgh's, Frank, like Cullen before him, channeled only a select group through the narrow funnel of the Boerhaavian-sized teaching ward, leaving it up to students to take advantage of the broader spectrum of disease. Frank felt strongly that the presentation of too many teaching cases, with their sheer variety of complaints, would be detrimental to the process of medical education, overloading the student's memory and creating confusion. Frank also believed that, given the time constraints during rounds, it would be impossible for students, physicians, and professors to follow in detail the individual clinical progress of numerous patients. Instead, his goal was to allow students to focus in greater detail on a few typical cases, individualizing both diagnosis and management, a strategy consonant with the needs of a genteel medical profession preparing itself for private practice.

The Allgemeines Krankenhaus also played a greater role in medical research than the Edinburgh Infirmary. Frank's efforts to create a museum of pathological specimens brought pathological anatomy up to the level of medicine's junior partner, no longer completely subordinated to clinical knowledge. With the species-oriented disease classifications under attack from the Brunonian medical system, Frank sought to integrate significant anatomical data with his clinical observations. Moreover, aggressive experimentation with new drugs contributed to a better understanding of dosages and indications and eventually led to therapeutic skepticism.

Following Duschau's death, an autopsy was immediately scheduled. In Austria's state-sponsored institutions, the cumbersome permission procedures common in British voluntary infirmaries were not required for postmortem dissections. Since his arrival in Vienna, Frank had already gone beyond the Edinburgh model by allowing hospital practitioners together with senior medical students to perform dissections in the newly established death house. Here all pathological findings were to be carefully recorded and appended to the clinical chart. Frank's program suggested that he was convinced that a knowledge of the lesions discovered could not only illustrate the clinical evidence, but also act as a pedagogical corrective of the initial clinical impressions and thus provide a way to advance medical knowledge. Given similar differences in professional status between physicians and surgeons in the Austrian Empire, autopsies remained, as in Edinburgh and London, part of the surgical domain except for a handful of prestigious clinical teachers such as de Haen and Frank, who insisted on attending the procedures and seeking clinical correlations.

Convinced of the importance of pathological anatomy in understanding the nature of disease, Frank insisted on expanding the scope of postmortem dissections. The small, ill-ventilated autopsy room with its terrible stench had previously discouraged such examinations. Moreover, the hospital possessed only a few badly preserved pathological specimens to illustrate certain lesions, although before Frank's arrival in May 1795, a decision had been made to encourage senior physicians to provide additional preparations. Frank, in turn, issued a regulation in January 1796 establishing a pathological museum adjacent to the lecture hall. He hired Rudolf A. Vetter to be the prosector or pathologist for the hospital. New autopsy facilities were provided in a separate, well-ventilated house on the hospital's premises equipped with a kitchen. Vetter supervised the examinations—over 600 cadavers per year were provided for dissection—and prepared a number of pathological specimens for future demonstrations. He also lectured on pathological anatomy. Before the end of the century, the hospital possessed over 400 preparations to further the study of pathological anatomy.

The postmortem findings obtained from the body of Johann Duschau were not at all surprising. Although the bronchial tubes appeared to be clean, the chest was small, with the diaphragm pushed up by the liver and spleen. In addition to multiple pleural adhesions throughout the chest, the dissector discovered a major cavity full of pus in the lower lobe of the left lung. This apparent abscess had already perforated the diaphragm and invaded the spleen in two places, virtually destroying it. According to the surviving protocol, no other abnormalities were found. Frank's final diagnosis was typhus with pneumonia, although an underlying tubercular disease was probable. While Austrian physicians generally agreed that clinical observations could increase medical knowledge, bedside and pathological findings were employed to consolidate rather than to challenge contemporary theories and classifications of disease. Regardless of the extensive therapeutic experimentation, Frank's management of Johann Duschau's case suggests that, as in other contemporary European centers, medicine continued to support an eclectic but holistic view of the human body. Its functions in health and disease were explained with the help of vitalism and a number of neurophysiological as well as traditional humoral concepts.

Following an autopsy, all corpses were bundled up in sacks and loaded onto carts. With other deceased inmates, Johann Duschau's body may have been quickly conveyed to a nearby cemetery such as St. Mark's, outside the city gates, to avoid cadaveric contamination of soil and ground water.[187] Other patients were more fortunate. In an anonymous letter, one of them wrote: "Dear cousin: I was recently ill but now have returned from the hospital where everything went well. After laying there a few days, they took me through four courtyards to another room and my doctor could not find me. Days later, I was carried back again and so I kept playing hide and seek with the doctor. However, this movement apparently did me good and now I am healthy again except of some weakness in my limbs because of the [meager] hospital soup."[188]

NOTES

1. Royal Infirmary of Edinburgh, *Annual Report for the Year 1801*, Edinburgh, J. Hay, 1802, p. 1.

2. William Cullen, "Clinical cases and reports taken at the Royal Infirmary of Edinburgh from Dr. Cullen by Richard Hall, Edinburgh, 1772-3," MSS Collection, National Library of Medicine, Bethesda, MD.

3. Joseph Wilde, *The Hospital: A Poem in Three Books*, Norwich, United Kingdom, Stevenson, 1810, p. 8. For analysis see W. B. Howie, "Consumer reaction: A patient's view of hospitalized life in 1809," *Br Med J* 3 (1973): 534–36.

4. According to Infirmary records, only half as many people as usual applied for admission on Sunday. Most waited until Monday, the most popular day to enter. See Guenter B. Risse, *Hospital Life in Enlightenment Scotland: Care and Teaching at the Royal Infirmary of Edinburgh*, New York, Cambridge Univ. Press, 1986, p. 84.

5. Marjorie Plant, *The Domestic Life of Scotland in the Eighteenth Century*, Edinburgh, Edinburgh Univ. Press, 1952, pp. 161–62. More details can be found in Henry G. Graham, *The Social Life of Scotland in the Eighteenth Century*, 2nd ed., 2 vols., London, A. & C Black, 1900.

6. The statistics appeared regularly during the eighteenth century in the issues of *Scots Magazine*.

7. H. W. Hart, "Some notes on the sponsoring of patients for hospital treatment under the voluntary system," *Med Hist* 24 (1980): 447–60.

8. H. W. Hart, "The conveyance of patients to and from the hospital, 1720–1850," *Med Hist* 22 (1978): 397–407.

9. John Bellers, *Essay Towards the Improvement of Medicine*, London, Sowle, 1714, p. 6.

10. R. Mitchison, "Poor relief and health care in Scotland, 1575–1710," in *Health Care and Poor Relief in Protestant Europe 1500–1700*, ed. O. P. Grell and A. Cunningham, London, Routledge, 1997, pp. 220–33.

11. R. Mitchison, "North and south: The development of the gulf in Poor Law practice," in *Scottish Society 1500–1800*, ed. R. A. Houston and J. D. White, Cambridge, Cambridge Univ. Press, 1989, p. 219.

12. *Letters to the Patients in the Royal Infirmary of Edinburgh*, Edinburgh, J. Reid, 1772, p. 5. For England see R. Porter, "The gift relation: Philanthropy and provincial hospitals in eighteenth-century England," in *The Hospital in History*, ed. L. Granshaw and R. Porter, London, Routledge, 1989, pp. 149–78.

13. Risse, *Hospital Life*, pp. 105–06.

14. Ibid., pp. 98–101.

15. This declaration is dated January 31, 1771, and is available at the National Library of Scotland, Edinburgh.

16. For 1772 mortality statistics see *Scots Mag* 34 (1772): '28.

17. M. E. Fissell, "The disappearance of the patient's narrative and the invention of hospital medicine," in *British Medicine in an Age of Reform*, ed. R. French and A. Wear, London, Routledge, 1991, pp. 92–109.

18. William Cullen, Clinical lectures, Edinburgh, 177?–1773, MSS Collection, Royal College of Physicians, Edinburgh, p. 60.

19. A. J. Youngson, *The Making of Classical Edinburgh, 1750–1840*, Edinburgh, Edinburgh Univ. Press, 1966, p. 36.

20. For a biographical sketch see R. W. Johnstone, "William Cullen," *Med Hist* 3 (1959): 33–46; his consultation practice is analyzed in G. B. Risse, "'Doctor William Cullen, physi-

cian, Edinburgh': A consultation practice in the eighteenth century," *Bull Hist Med* 48 (1974): 338–51.

21. Cullen, Clinical lectures 1772–1773, p. 29.

22. More information on the admission routine can be found in Risse, *Hospital Life*, pp. 7–11.

23. L. J. Rather, "The six things 'non-natural,' " *Clio Med* 3 (1968): 337–47, and P. H. Niebyl, "The non-naturals," *Bull Hist Med* 45 (1971): 486–92.

24. W. Coleman, "Health and hygiene in the Encyclopédie: A medical doctrine for the bourgeoisie," *J Hist Med* 29 (1974): 399–421.

25. N. D. Jewson, "Medical knowledge and the patronage system in eighteenth-century England," *Sociology* 8 (1974): 369–85.

26. The concept of the *medicalization* of society was initially popularized in the writings of the *Annales* school of history in France, as well as by Michel Foucault. See, for example, Foucault's "The politics of health in the eighteenth century," in *Power/Knowledge: Selected Interviews and Other Writings, 1972–1977*, ed. C. Gordon, New York, Pantheon, 1972, pp. 166–82.

27. G. B. Risse, "Medicine in the age of Enlightenment," in *History of Medicine in Society*, ed. A. Wear, Cambridge, Cambridge Univ. Press, 1992, pp. 149–95. See also R. Porter, "The eighteenth century," in Porter et al., *The Western Medical Tradition, 800 BC to AD 1800*, Cambridge, Cambridge Univ. Press, 1995, pp. 371–475.

28. G. Rosen, "Medical care and social policy in seventeenth-century England," *Bull NY Acad Med* 29 (1953): 420–37, and J. H. Cassedy, "Medicine and the rise of statistics," in *Medicine in Seventeenth-Century England*, ed. A. G. Debus, Berkeley, Univ. of California Press, 1974, pp. 283–312.

29. I. Waddington, "The role of the hospital in the development of modern medicine: A sociological analysis," *Sociology* 9 (1973): 221–24.

30. See A. Wilson, "Conflict, consensus and charity: Politics and the provincial voluntary hospitals in the 18th century," *Engl Hist Rev* 111 (1996): 599–619. For details see John Aikin, *Thoughts on Hospitals*, London, J. Johnson, 1771, and John Woodward, *To Do the Sick No Harm: A Study of the British Voluntary Hospital System to 1875*, London, Routledge & Kegan Paul, 1974.

31. J. G. Humble and Peter Hansell, *Westminster Hospital, 1716–1966*, London, Pitman Med Pub., 1966, pp. 6–7. See also M. E. Fissell, "Charity universal? Institutions and moral reform in eighteenth-century Bristol," in *Stilling the Grumbling Hive: The Response to Social and Economic Problems in England, 1689–1750*, ed. L. Davison et al., New York, St. Martin's Press, 1992, pp. 121–44.

32. B. G. Gale, "The dissolution and revolution in London hospital facilities," *Med Hist* 11 (1967): 91–96, and G. W. O. Woodward, *The Dissolution of the Monasteries*, New York, Walter, 1966.

33. Petty expressed such ideas in a 1648 letter to Samuel Hartlib. See Harold J. Cook, *The Decline of the Old Regime in Stuart London*, Ithaca, Cornell Univ. Press, 1986, pp. 110–11.

34. For details see Lisa Rosner, *Medical Education in the Age of Improvement*, Edinburgh, Edinburgh Univ. Press, 1991.

35. Bellers, *Essay*, p. 14.

36. A. Borsay, " 'Persons of honour and reputation': The voluntary hospital in an age of corruption," *Med Hist* 35 (1991): 281–94.

37. For a useful overview see N. Phillipson, "The Scottish Enlightenment," in *The Enlightenment in National Context*, ed. R. Porter and M. Teich, Cambridge, Cambridge Univ.

Press, 1981, pp. 19–40. See also J. Clive, "The social background of the Scottish renaissance," in *Scotland in the Age of Improvement*, ed. N. T. Phillipson and R. Mitchison, Edinburgh, 1970, pp. 225–44.

38. The estimate for the year 1775 was 82,836, excluding the suburbs, according to William Creech. See *Letters addressed to Sir John Sinclair . . .* , Edinburgh, 1793, reprint, New York, AMS Press, 1982, pp. 24–25.

39. For more information see T. M. Devine, ed., *Improvement and Enlightenment*, Edinburgh, J. Donald Pub., 1989.

40. For an overview see Gordon Donaldson, *Scotland: Church and Nation Through Sixteen Centuries*, 2nd ed., Edinburgh, Scottish Academic Press, 1972, especially pp. 95–103.

41. Andrew M. Douglas, *Church and School in Scotland*, Edinburgh, St. Andrew Press, 1985, p. 49.

42. J. B. Morell, "The Edinburgh Town Council and its university, 1717–1766," in *The Early Years of the Edinburgh Medical School*, ed. R. G. W. Anderson and A. D. C. Simpson, Edinburgh, Royal Scottish Museum, 1976, pp. 46–65.

43. Edinburgh Infirmary, *An Account of the Rise and Establishment of the Infirmary or Hospital for the Sick Poor, Erected at Edinburgh*, Edinburgh, c. 1730, p. 2.

44. Ibid.

45. J. B. Morell, "The University of Edinburgh in the late eighteenth century: Its scientific eminence and academic structure," *Isis* 62 (1971): 158–72, and Anand C. Chitnis, *Scottish Enlightenment*, London, Croom Helm, 1976, pp. 124–94.

46. The role of Drummond is detailed in A. C. Chitnis, "Provost Drummond and the origins of Edinburgh medicine," in *The Origins and Nature of the Scottish Enlightenment*, ed. R. H. Campbell and A. S. Skinner, Edinburgh, J. Donald Pub., 1982, pp. 86–114.

47. Ninian Niving, *Jesus Christ in the Poor, or the Royal Infirmary of Edinburgh Recommended to the Charity of Well-Disposed Christians*, Edinburgh, Sands, Brymer, Murray & Cochran, 1739, p. 3.

48. A useful source is Edward Foster, *An Essay on Hospitals, or Succinct Directions for the Situation, Construction, and Administration of County Hospitals*, Dublin, W. G. Jones, 1768.

49. Hugh Arnot, *The History of Edinburgh*, Edinburgh, Longman & Cadell, 1779, p. 546.

50. Details are provided in Edwin F. Catford, *Edinburgh, the Story of a City*, London, Hutchinson, 1975, pp. 24–25.

51. See, for example, Edward Topham's letters from Edinburgh, written in 1774 and 1775, summarized in Michael Joyce, *Edinburgh: the Golden Age, 1769–1832*, New York, Longmans, Green, 1951, pp. 14–23.

52. William Creech, *Edinburgh Fugitive Pieces*, Edinburgh, G. Ramsay, 1815, p. 62.

53. A. J. Youngson, "The city of reason and nature," in *Edinburgh in the Age of Reason*, ed. D. Young et al., Edinburgh, Edinburgh Univ. Press, 1967, pp. 15–22.

54. Risse, *Hospital Life*, pp. 29–33. See also P. Mathias, "Swords and ploughshares: The armed forces, medicine, and public health in the late eighteenth century," in *War and Economic Development*, ed. J. M. Winter, Cambridge, Cambridge Univ. Press, 1975, pp. 73–90.

55. S. Selwyn, "Sir John Pringle: Hospital reformer, moral philosopher, and pioneer of antiseptics," *Med Hist* 10 (1966): 266–74.

56. For more details see John Aikin, *Thoughts on Hospitals*, London, J. Johnson, 1775, and William Blizard, *Suggestions for the Improvement of Hospitals and Other Charitable Institutions*, London, H. L. Galabin, 1796.

57. John Howard, *An Account of the Principal Lazarettos of Europe*, Warrington, United Kingdom, W. Eyres, 1789, p. 77.

58. G. B. Risse, "Cullen as clinician: Organization and strategies of an eighteenth-century medical practice," in *William Cullen and the Eighteenth-Century Medical World*, ed. A. Doig et al., Edinburgh, Edinburgh Univ. Press, 1993, pp. 133–51.

59. Robert Chambers, *Traditions of Edinburgh*, new ed., London, W. & R. Chambers, 1868, vol. 1, p. 105.

60. M. Nicolson, "Giovanni Battista Morgagni and eighteenth-century physical examination," in *Medical Theory, Surgical Practice*, ed. C. Lawrence, London, Routledge, 1992, pp. 107–08, and O. Keel, "Percussion et diagnostic physique en Grand Bretagne au 18e siècle: L'exemple d'Alexander Monro secundus," *Proc XXXI Int Congr Hist Med*, Bologna, Monduzzi Ed., 1988, pp. 869–75.

61. See George Martine, *Essays Medical and Philosophical*, London, A. Millar, 1740.

62. William Cullen, Clinical lectures delivered for John Gregory, Edinburgh, February–April 1772, MSS Collection, Royal College of Physicians, Edinburgh, p. 2. See also G. B. Risse, "Hysteria at the Edinburgh Infirmary: The Construction of a disease, 1770–1800," *Med Hist* 32 (1988): 1–22.

63. Wilde, *The Hospital*, p. 9.

64. George Fordyce, *A Dissertation on Simple Fever*, London, J. J. Johnson, 1794, p. 6.

65. William Cullen, *Nosology, or Systematic Arrangement of Diseases by Classes, Orders, Genera, and Species* (orig. ed. 1769), trans. from Latin, Edinburgh, W. Creech, 1800, p. 41. For details see W. F. Bynum, "Cullen and the study of fevers in Britain, 1760–1820," in *Theories of Fever From Antiquity to the Enlightenment*, ed. W. F. Bynum and V. Nutton, London, Wellcome Institute for the History of Medicine, 1981, pp. 135–47.

66. Cullen, *Nosology*, p. 37.

67. For details see G. B. Risse, "Typhus fever in eighteenth-century hospitals: New approaches to medical treatment," *Bull Hist Med* 59 (1985): 176–95.

68. Cullen, Clinical lectures, 1772–1773, pp. 129–30.

69. Ibid., p. 132.

70. Lester S. King, *The Medical World of the Eighteenth Century*, Chicago, Univ. of Chicago Press, 1958, pp. 193–226, and R. E. Kendell, "William Cullen's Synopsis Nosologiae Methodicae," in *William Cullen and the Eighteenth-Century Medical World*, pp. 216–33.

71. King, *Medical World*, pp. 123–55.

72. W. F. Bynum, "Cullen and the nervous system," in *William Cullen and the Eighteenth-Century Medical World*, pp. 152–62. For the cultural underpinnings of these ideas see C. Lawrence, "The nervous system and society in the Scottish Enlightenment," in *Natural Order: Historical Studies of Scientific Order*, ed. B. Barnes and S. Shapin, Beverly Hills, Sage, 1979, pp. 19–40.

73. King, *Medical World*, p. 141

74. Cullen, Clinical lectures, February–April 1772, p. 209. I am grateful to Michael Barfoot for sharing his unpublished manuscripts "Old Spasm: The medical theory and practice of William Cullen" and "Clinical medicine at the Edinburgh Royal Infirmary in the eighteenth century."

75. Cullen, "Therapeutics," in Institutes of Medicine, lecture notes, Edinburgh, 1772, MSS Collection, National Library of Medicine, Washington, vol. 7, p. 27.

76. Royal Infirmary of Edinburgh, *Report of a Committee on the State of the Hospital*, Edinburgh, 1818, p. 87.

77. W. B. Rabenn, "Hospital diets in eighteenth-century England," *J Am Dietetic Assoc* 30 (1964): 1216–21, and Samuel Davidson, *The History of Medicine*, Newcastle, S. Hodgson, 1791, pp. 103–50.

78. Royal Infirmary of Edinburgh, *Report of a Committee*, p. 68.

79. William Cullen, *First Lines of the Practice of Physic*, new ed., 4 vols, Edinburgh, C. Elliot, 1786, vol. 1, p. 194.

80. Risse, *Hospital Life*, pp. 177–239.

81. N. W. Kasting, "A rationale for centuries of therapeutic bleeding: Antipyretic therapy for febrile diseases," *Perspect Biol Med* 33 (1990): 509–16.

82. J. W. Estes, "Making therapeutic decisions with protopharmacological evidence," *Trans Stud Coll Phys Phil* 5 (1979): 116–37.

83. Benjamin Bell, *A System of Surgery*, 7th ed., Edinburgh, Bell, Bradfute & Dickson, 1801, vol. 3, p. 76.

84. Cullen, Clinical lectures, 1772–1773, p. 556. See R. B. Sullivan, "Sanguine practices: A historical and historiographic reconsideration of heroic therapy in the age of Rush," *Bull Hist Med* 68 (1994): 211–34.

85. Thomas Fowler, *Medical Reports on the Effects of Bloodletting, Sudorifics, and Blistering in the Care of the Acute and Chronic Rheumatism*, London, J. Johnson, 1795, p. 241.

86. For details see John Robertson, *A Practical Treatise on the Powers of Cantharides*, Edinburgh, Mundell, Doig & Stevenson, 1806.

87. Cullen, Clinical lectures, 1772–1773, p. 500.

88. Ibid., p. 51: "Let me tell you in general that you should never give the patient any hints with regards to the effects of medicines they are taking; the less medical knowledge they have, so much the better."

89. R. Passmore, "William Cullen and dietetics," in *William Cullen and the Eighteenth-Century Medical World*, pp. 167–85. See also J. W. Estes, "The medical properties of food in the eighteenth century," *J Hist Med* 51 (1996): 127–54.

90. See [John Stedman], *The History and Statutes of the Royal Infirmary of Edinburgh*, Edinburgh, Balfour & Smellie, 1778.

91. Wilde, *The Hospital*, p. 61.

92. Risse, *Hospital Life*, pp. 240–78; see also "Clinical teaching," Appendix C, pp. 340–50.

93. Hospital and university were not affiliated. See G. Ongaro, "L'insegnamento clinico di Giovanni Battista da Monte (1498–1551): Una revisione critica," *Physis Riv Int Stor Sci* 31 (1994): 357–69, and C. D. O'Malley, "Medical education during the Renaissance," in *The History of Medical Education*, ed. C. D. O'Malley, Berkeley, Univ. of California Press, 1970, pp. 89–102.

94. G. A. Lindeboom, "Medical education in the Netherlands, 1575–1750," in *History of Medical Education*, pp. 201–16, and E. C van Leersum, "Contribution to the history of the clinical instruction in the Netherlands," *Janus* 30 (1926): 133–51.

95. A. Cunningham, "Medicine to calm the mind: Boerhaave's medical system and why it was adopted in Edinburgh," in *The Medical Enlightenment of the Eighteenth Century*, ed. A. Cunningham and R. French, Cambridge, Cambridge Univ. Press, 1990, pp. 40–66.

96. Gerrit A. Lindeboom, *Herman Boerhaave: The Man and His Work*, London, Methuen, 1968, pp. 283–92. See also Lester S. King, *The Philosophy of Medicine: The Early Eighteenth Century*, Cambridge, Mass., Harvard Univ. Press, 1978.

97. See details in Thomas N. Bonner, *Becoming a Physician: Medical Education in Britain, France, Germany and the United States, 1750–1945*, New York, Oxford Univ. Press, 1995, especially pp. 103–41.

98. Michel Foucault, *The Birth of the Clinic*, trans. A. M. Sheridan Smith, New York, Vintage Books, 1975, pp. 54–63, and G. B. Risse, "Clinical instruction in hospitals: The Boerhaavian tradition in Leyden, Edinburgh, Vienna, and Pavia," *Clio Med* 21 (1987/88): 1–19.

99. Anonymous review of Home's *Clinical Experiments* in the *London Med J* I (1791): 1–2.

100. William Nolan, *An Essay on Humanity, or A View of Abuses in Hospitals*, London, J. Murray, 1786, p. 38.

101. Stedman, *History and Statutes*, pp. 74–75.

102. *The Dispensatory for the Use of the Royal Hospital in Edinburgh*, London, 1753, an English translation of the Latin version, *Pharmacopoeia Pauperum* (1748).

103. See also *Modern Practice of the London Hospitals*, 3rd ed., London, Crowder, 1770.

104. James Gregory, *Additional Memorial to the Managers of the Royal Infirmary*, Edinburgh, Murray & Cochrane, 1803, pp. 159–60.

105. Cullen, Clinical lectures, 1772–1773, p. 578. For an analysis see M. Barfoot, "Philosophy and method in Cullen's medical teaching," in *William Cullen and the Eighteenth-Century Medical World*, pp. 110–32.

106. Details are presented in Roy and Dorothy Porter, *Patient's Progress; Doctors and Doctoring in Eighteenth-Century England*, Stanford, CA, Stanford Univ. Press, 1989. See also Anne Digby, *Making a Medical Living: Doctors and Patients in the English Market for Medicine, 1720–1911*, Cambridge, Cambridge Univ. Press, 1994.

107. G. B. Risse, "The Brownian system of medicine: Its theoretical and practical implications," *Clio Med* 5 (1970): 45–51, and "John Brown," in *Klassiker der Medizin*, ed. D. von Engelhardt and F. Hartmann, Munich, C. H. Beck, vol. 2, pp. 24–36.

108. For a similar professional strategy in London see W. F. Bynum, "Physicians, hospitals and career structures in eighteenth-century London," in *William Hunter and the Eighteenth Century Medical World*, ed. W. F. Bynum and R. Porter, Cambridge, Cambridge Univ. Press, 1985, pp. 105–28. For more details see Susan C. Lawrence, *Charitable Knowledge: Hospital Pupils and Practitioners in Eighteenth-Century London*, New York, Cambridge Univ. Press, 1996.

109. This point is critical. Since the publication of Foucault's *The Birth of the Clinic*, historians have accepted his clear distinction between late-eighteenth-century French clinical instruction and the earlier "protoclinics" of Leyden, Edinburgh, and Vienna. See G. B. Risse, "Before the clinic was 'born': Methodological perspectives in hospital history," in *Institutions of Confinement: Hospitals, Asylums, and Prisons in Western Europe and North America, 1500–1950*, ed. N. Finzsch and R. Jütte, Cambridge, Cambridge Univ. Press, 1996, pp. 75–96.

110. Cullen, Clinical lectures, February–April 1772, p. 247.

111. Niving, *Jesus Christ in the Poor*, pp. 17–8.

112. Johann P. Frank, *Seine Selbstbiographie*, ed. E. Lesky, Bern, H. Huber, 1969, p. 95.

113. The observations were made by a German visitor in 1787. Max Neuburger, *Das alte medizinische Wien in zeitgenössischen Schilderungen*, Vienna, M. Perles, 1921, p. 111. For a more complete treatment of the daily life in Vienna during the eighteenth century consult Gerhard Tanzer, *Spectacle mussen seyn: Die Freizeit der Wiener im 18. Jahrhundert*, Vienna, Wien Bohlau, 1992.

114. Clinical case reproduced in Salomon Liboschitz, *Beyträge für die neuere Heilkunde*, Vienna, A. Doll, 1805, vol. 1, pp. 260–80.

115. Helmut Reinalter, *Am Hofe Joseph II*, Vienna, Ed. Leipzig, 1991, pp. 61–77.

116. Neuburger, *Wien*, pp. 110–11.

117. Ibid., p. 129.

118. For an overview see Hanns L. Mikoletzky, *Oesterreich, das grosse 18. Jahrhundert, von Leopold I bis Leopold II*, Vienna, Austria Ed., 1967, and Ernst Wangermann, *From Joseph II to the Jacobin Trials: Government Policy and Public Opinion in the Habsburg Dominions in the Period of the French Revolution*, 2nd ed, Oxford, Oxford Univ. Press, 1969.

119. Details about nutrition can be found in J. Komlos, *Nutrition and Economic Development in the Eighteenth Century Habsburg Monarchy: An Anthropometric History*,

Princeton, NJ, Princeton Univ. Press, 1989. A recent critique of this work is H. J. Voth, "Height, nutrition, and labor: Recasting the Austrian model," *J Interdis Hist* 25 (1995): 627–36.

120. For more information see Derek E. D. Beales, *Joseph II: In the Shadow of Maria Theresa, 1741–1780*, Cambridge, Cambridge Univ. Press, 1987, and David Good, *The Economic Rise of the Habsburg Empire, 1750–1914*, Berkeley, Univ. of California Press, 1984.

121. For a summary of Joseph II's reign see T. C. W. Blanning, *Joseph II and Enlightened Despotism*, New York, Harper & Row, 1970. The religious reforms are covered in Paul P. Bernard, *Jesuits and Jacobins, Enlightenment and Enlightened Despotism in Austria*, Urbana, Univ. of Illinois Press, 1971.

122. For biographical information see Paul P. Bernard, *Joseph II*, New York, Twayne, 1968, and more recently, Karl Gutkas, *Kaiser Joseph II, eine Biographie*, Vienna, P. Zsolnay, 1989.

123. Cited in Blanning, *Joseph II*, p. 3

124. For additional information see Erna Lesky, *Meilensteine der Wiener Medizin*, Vienna, W. Maudrich, 1981.

125. Bernhard Grois, *Das Allgemeine Krankenhaus in Wien und seine Geschichte*, Vienna, Maudrich Verlag, 1965, pp. 27–76.

126. K. Gutkas, "Kampf gegen die Armut: Sozialpolitik im Reformwerk Kaiser Joseph II," in *Was Blieb von Joseph II?*, International Symposium Melk 1980, Vienna, Niederoesterr Fonds, 1980, pp. 77–85.

127. Reinalter, *Am Hofe Joseph II*, pp. 61–77.

128. See critical essays in Leonard Bauer et al., *Von der Glückseligkeit des Staates: Staat, Wirtschaft und Gesellschaft in Oesterreich im Zeitalter des aufgeklärten Absolutismus*, Berlin, Duncker & Humbold, 1981.

129. G. Rosen, "Cameralism and the concept of medical police," *Bull Hist Med* 27 (1953): 21–42.

130. A valuable analysis is P. P. Bernard, "The limits of absolutism: Joseph II and the Allgemeines Krankenhaus," *Eighteenth-Cent Stud* 9 (1975): 193–215.

131. Details are provided in W. J. Callahan and D. Higgs, eds., *Church and Society in Catholic Europe of the Eighteenth Century*, Cambridge, Cambridge Univ. Press, 1979.

132. For details see Karl Weiss, *Geschichte der öffentlichen Anstalten, Fonde und Stiftungen für die Armenversorgung in Wien*, Vienna, R. Lechner, 1867.

133. See also Grois, *Das Allgemeine Krankenhaus*, pp. 11–26.

134. Details can be found in H. Wyklicky and M. Skopec, eds., *200 Jahre Allgemeines Krankenhaus in Wien*, Vienna, Vok, 1984.

135. See Johann P. X. Fauken, *Entwurf zu einem allgemeinen Krankenhause*, Vienna, 1784, and Johann Hunczovsky, *Medicinisch-chirurgische Beobachtungen auf seine Reisen durch England und Frankreich besonders über Spitäler*, Vienna, R. Graffer, 1783.

136. L. S. Greenbaum, "Health-care and hospital building in eighteenth-century France: Reform proposals of Du Pont de Nemours and Condorcet," in *Studies on Voltaire and the Eighteenth Century*, ed. T. Besterman, Oxford, Voltaire Foundation, 1976, pp. 895–930.

137. Dieter Jetter, *Wien von den Anfängen bis um 1900*, Wiesbaden, F. Steiner, 1982, pp. 48–52.

138. The information about hospital wards came from Wilhelm von Staffelt, a Danish writer who had visited Vienna in 1796. His account is reprinted in Neuburger, *Wien*, p. 160.

139. G. B. Risse, "Mozart and the Vienna world of medicine: Ideals and paradoxes," in *The Pleasures and Perils of Genius: Mostly Mozart*, ed. P. Ostwald and L. S. Zegans, Madison, CT, International Univ. Press, 1993, pp. 83–96.

140. Maximilian Stoll, *Über die Einrichtung der öffentlichen Krankenhäuser*, ed. G. A.

von Beeckhen, Vienna, C. F. Wappler, 1788, p. 38. Vienna's other hospitals engaged *Elisabetherinnen*, sisters belonging to the Order of St. Elizabeth, created by Pope Martin V in 1428.

141. From an anonymous tract, "Bemerkungen über das Civilspital" (1788), reprinted in Neuburger, *Wien*, pp. 101–02.

142. *Nachricht an das Publikum über die Einrichtung des Hauptspitals in Wien*, (1784), reprint, Vienna, Wiener Bibliophilen-Gesellschaft, 1960.

143. See E. Lesky, "Das Wiener Allgemeine Krankenhaus. Seine Gründung und Wirkung auf deutsche Hospitäler," *Clio Med* 2 (1967): 23–37.

144. For autobiographical details see Frank's *Selbstbiographie*. A biography based on primary sources is Hellmut Haubold, *Johann P. Frank, der Gesundheits-und Rassenpolitiker des 18. Jahrhunderts*, Munich, J. F. Lehrmanns Verlag, 1939.

145. Johann P. Frank, *System einer vollständigen medicinischen Polizey*, Vienna, C. Schaumburg & Co., 1786–1817. All quotations come from the selections in the English translation, *A System of Complete Medical Police*, ed. E. Lesky, Baltimore, Johns Hopkins Univ. Press, 1976. Wrote Frank: "The internal security of the state is the subject of general police science," adding that "a very considerable part of this science is to apply certain principles for the health care of people living in society," p. 12.

146. Frank links social conditions and disease in his "The people's misery: Mother of diseases," (1790), trans. H. E. Sigerist, *Bull Inst Hist Med* 9 (1941): 81–100. See also E. Lesky, "Johann Peter Frank and social medicine," *Ann Cisalpines d'Hist Soc* 4 (1973):137–44.

147. Johann P. Frank, *Ankündigung des klinischen Instituts zu Göttingen*, Göttingen, J. C. Dieterich, 1784, p. 4.

148. Frank, *Medical Police*, pp. 415 and 419.

149. Ibid., pp. 417–18.

150. Grois, *Das Allgemeine Krankenhaus*, pp. 77–84.

151. Excerpts from Frank's autobiography, published in 1802, reproduced in Neuburger, *Wien*, p. 138.

152. Frank, *Medical Police*, pp. 432–33.

153. Both Franks, father and son, were eventually forced to resign their positions and move to Russia, where they taught at the University of Vilnius. For details see Ramunas A. Kondratas, "Joseph Frank (1771–1842) and the Development of Clinical Medicine: a Study of the Transformation of Medical Thought and Practice at the End of the Eighteenth and Beginning of the Nineteenth Centuries," Ph.D. diss., Harvard Univ., 1977, and his article "The Brunonian influence on the medical thought and practice of Joseph Frank," in *Brunonianism in Britain and Europe*, ed. W. F. Bynum and R. Porter, London, Wellcome Institute for the History of Medicine, 1988, pp. 75–88.

154. Erna Lesky, *The Vienna Medical School of the 19th Century*, Baltimore, Johns Hopkins Univ. Press, 1976, pp. 8–12. For a contemporary defense of Frank's therapies see Thomas Cappellini, *Gesundheits-Taschenbuch für das Jahr 1802*, Vienna, 1802.

155. G. B. Risse, "Scottish medicine on the Continent: John Brown's medical system in Germany, 1796–1806," in *Proceedings of the XXIII Inter Congress Hist Med*, London, Wellcome Institute for the History of Medicine, 1974, vol. 1, pp. 682–87, and "The History of John Brown's Medical System in Germany during the Years 1790–1806," Ph.D. diss, University of Chicago, 1971.

156. Frank, *Medical Police*, pp. 410–11.

157. Ibid., p. 428.

158. Ibid., pp. 412–13.

159. Ibid., p. 428.

160. Neuburger, *Wien*, p. 110.

161. For details see Risse, "John Brown's System," especially pp. 199–210.

162. Frank, *Medical Police*, p. 428.

163. A similar therapeutic approach employed by Frank and his son Joseph was documented in the latter's *Ratio instituti clinici Ticinensis*, preface by Johann P Frank, Vienna, Camesina, 1797. German trans. by F. Schäffer: *Heilart in der klinischen Lehranstalt zu Pavia*, Vienna, Camesina, 1797. For an analysis see G. B. Risse, "Brunonian therapeutics: New wine in old bottles?" in *Brunonianism in Britain and Europe*, pp. 46–62.

164. For his clinical management see Anton de Haen, *Heilungsmethode in dem kaiserlichen Krankenhause zu Wien*, trans. E. Platner, Leipzig, Weygand, 1779.

165. His therapeutic preferences are documented in Maximilian Stoll, *Heilungsmethode in dem praktischen Krankenhause zu Wien*, 3rd ed., 7 vols., Breslau, 1783–1796.

166. For eighteenth-century remedies see J. Worth Estes, *Dictionary of Protopharmacology: Therapeutic Practices, 1700–1850*, Canton, MA, Science History Pub., 1990.

167. Frank, *Medical Police*, p. 429.

168. J. C. Kramer, "Opium rampant: Medical use, misuse, and abuse in Britain and the West in the 17th and 18th centuries," *Br J Addict* 74 (1979): 377–89.

169. Neuburger, *Wien*, p. 140.

170. L. Auenbrugger, "On percussion of the chest" (1824), trans. J. Forbes, *Bull Inst Hist Med* 4 (1936): 373–403.

171. See *Journal der Erfindungen* VI (1797): 4–40.

172. Joseph Frank, *Erläuterungen der Brownischen Arzneilehre*, Heilbronn, Class, 1797.

173. Frank, *Medical Police*, p. 410.

174. For an overview see E. Lesky, "The development of bedside teaching at the Vienna Medical School from scholastic times to special clinics," in *History of Medical Education*, pp. 217–134, and M. Nicholson, "Gerard van Swieten and the innovation of physical diagnosis," in *Medicine and Change: Historical and Sociological Studies of Medical Innovation*, ed. I. Löwy, Paris, INSERM, 1993, pp. 49–68.

175. J. Boersma, "Antonius de Haen, 1704–1776, life and work," *Janus* 50 (1961–62): 264–307.

176. Risse, "Clinical instruction in hospitals," 12–16.

177. See, for example, O. Keel, "La problematique institutionelle de la clinique en France et l'etranger de la fin du XVIIIe siecle a la periode de la Revolution," *Can Bull Hist Med* 2 (1985): 183–204.

178. C. Probst, "Aerztliche Forschung am Krankenbett im Zeitalter der Aufklärung," in *Festschrift für Hermann Heimpel*, ed. by colleagues of the Max Planck Institute. Göttingen, Vandenhoeck & Ruprecht, 1971, pp. 568–98.

179. Probst, "Forschung," pp. 591–97.

180. Johann G. Reyher, *Ueber die Einrichtung kleiner Hospitäler in mittlern und kleinern Städten*, Hamburg, 1784, p. 2.

181. For an overview see E. Lesky, "Klinische Arzneimittelforschung im 18. Jahrhundert," *Beitr Gesch Pharmazie* 29 (1977): 17–20. See also K. W. Schweppe and C. Probst, "Die Versuche zur medikamentösen Karzinomtherapie des Anton Störck (1731–1803)," *Wien Med Wochenschr* 5 (1982): 107–117, and see also K. W. Schweppe, "Anton Störck und seine Bedeutung für die ältere Wiener Schule," *Medizinhist J* 17 (1982): 342–56.

182. For a comparative analysis see O. Keel, "The politics of health and the institutionalization of clinical practices in Europe in the second half of the eighteenth century," in *William Hunter and the Eighteenth-Century Medical World*, pp. 207–56.

183. Frank, *Medical Police*, p. 341.

184. Neuburger, *Wien*, p. 138.

185. E. Lesky, "Johann P. Frank als Organisator des medizinischen Unterrichts," *Sudhoffs Arch* 39 (1955): 1–29.

186. Observations made by the German physician Karl Friedrich Burdach (1776–1847) during a visit to Vienna toward the end of the eighteenth century; reprinted in Neubauer, *Wien*, pp. 143–45.

187. Neuburger, *Wien*, p. 160. See also Risse, "Mozart."

188. The quote is from a letter written in 1794; reprinted in Neuburger, *Wien*, p. 134.

6

HUMAN BODIES
REVEALED

Hospitals of Post-
Revolutionary Paris

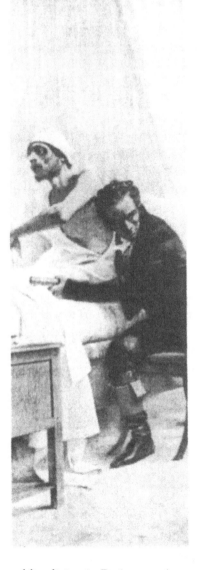

Hospitals are a measure of civilization: they are more appropriate to a nation's needs and better kept when the people are more united, more humane, and better educated.

Jacques Tenon, 1788[1]

The hospitals of Paris, designed originally as asylums for misfortune and suffering, have become the center of solid medical instruction. Clinical schools are formed under the auspices of the most celebrated men, from whose lessons a studious youth seeks instruction with ardor.

Félix S. Ratier, 1823[2]

A former soldier seeks rest

Around Christmas 1818, Jacques Dumesnil, a married 60-year-old shawl maker and retired soldier living in Paris, experienced intense back pains, for which he decided to consult a doctor. Formerly in good health, Jacques now felt his vitality ebbing. For almost two years now, he had been bothered by a nagging cough followed by expectoration of viscous, partly transparent phlegm. Although the cough was now almost continuous, Jacques had gradually gotten used to it, trying to perform his daily chores. Nothing is known about his family or friends, and he may have lived alone. In any event, getting older was not a good prospect. The physician Jacques consulted prescribed sulfur baths at the local Hôpital St. Louis, an institution specializing in skin diseases. A single deep soaking did not immediately lessen the pain, but over the next several days he felt much better. By early February 1819, however, Jacques' cough had intensified and his sputum became thick and dark. Alarmed by the symptoms and hoping to get a "rest," he applied for admission at a public hospital where former members of the military like Jacques were often welcome.[3] His destination: the Hôpital Necker, a charitable neighborhood institution for members of the parishes of St. Sulpice and du Gros Caillou.[4] It was a busy institution: during 1818, the hospital had admitted a total of 1,223 patients who remained there for an average of 30 days.[5]

Poor workers such as Jacques were increasingly viewed with some alarm and fear by the authorities. Restoration Paris had recently witnessed a steady increase in population. Each year, more than 10,000 new arrivals streamed into the capital from nearby regions. The 1817 census had disclosed a population of 714,500, mostly young, poor immigrants. They overran the central city, creating a maze of lodging houses, workshops, and small factories. While contributing decisively to the city's economic growth and early industrialization, Paris' working class also littered the narrow, winding streets with refuse that created a pestilential miasma still considered harmful to health.[6] Higher mortality and crime rates became the concern of hygienists and reformers, who often looked to hospitals for information documenting this seemingly progressive moral and physical degradation.[7] Epithets such as "barbarians" and "savages" were commonly used to describe the poor. These concerns sprang from the fact that, as in Edinburgh and Vienna, all social classes lived and mingled together, their status expressed by the vertical distinctions in housing that relegated the poorer folk to drafty attics.[8]

Occupation determined both social and economic status. Whether Jacques, the shawl maker, was a small artisan selling his own products or simply a wage earner in the clothier system is not known. The former retained their traditional artisanal structures and were better off than the latter, whose wages were slowly dropping while their working hours and conditions deteriorated. If Jacques was a worker, he could have been receiving some aid from his own parish. By a constitutional charter of June 1814, Catholicism had become France's state religion. Once more, gifts and donations to the ecclesiastical authorities were encouraged. A Society for Good Works formed part of the Paris Congregation, a new lay organization created by the pious upper classes.[9]

At the time of Jacques' arrival, admission policies at the Necker Hospital allowed free access only to sick poor parishioners from St. Sulpice and du Gros Caillou. Strangers were excluded to protect the parish's limited funds. Before the Revolution, when the institution was known as the Hospice de Charité, baptismal certificates and a confession had been traditional admission requirements. Given the time-honored reputation of hospitals as "gates to heaven," these preconditions made sense, since the institution only wanted to admit Catholics in good standing who needed to be prepared for salvation in the event of death. Wards were named after saints, and many featured individual altars where the visiting priest could say daily mass. In 1802, all Parisian establishments adopted triage procedures, seeking to slow the avalanche of potential patients. Many candidates were sent to a central admission office and examined by physicians who determined their suitability for inpatient care. Pregnant women and the mentally ill were systematically excluded from the Necker Hospital together with the "unclean" suffering from venereal or other obvious communicable diseases. Armed with a *billet d'entrée* listing name, condition, and time of admission, Dumesnil may still have sought out the parish priest to provide a recommendation or certificate attesting to his eligibility for free care.

The Necker Hospital—the name honored Suzanne Curchod Necker (1739–1794), who had sponsored and diligently administered the institution in its early pre-Revolutionary years—was located on the rue de Sevres toward the southwest, some distance from the center of Paris, an area surrounded by fields and gardens and thus potentially considered salubrious. The façade of its square, two-floor administrative building was unimposing, attached to a high wall surrounding an ample courtyard on one side and a large garden on the other. Upon entering the former, future patients encountered the side of a large chapel attached at right angles to the two main wards and the building housing the pharmacy, latrines, and laundry, as well as the living quarters and refectory for the religious personnel. The elongated wards located beyond the chapel could only be reached through a long, narrow corridor interrupted by an entrance to the kitchen. These wards were flanked by another larger courtyard reserved for convalescent males on one side and another enclosure employed for drying the laundry on the other. Although providing a fair amount of light and air, the entire tau-cross plan had been originally designed for a Benedictine monastery, and no amount of remodeling could successfully adapt the available space for its new functions.[10]

Like other hospitals, the Necker Hospital segregated male and female patients. Inmates were also separated according to four distinct medical categories: fever, malignant fever, surgical (injuries), and convalescents. Originally housing 120 patients before the Revolution, the hospital had somewhat expanded its capacity. It now counted 136 beds, 65 for males and 71 for females, with 80 beds reserved for individuals suffering from ordinary diseases, including fevers, 26 for those requiring surgery, and 30 for convalescents.[11] Together with a change of name—during the Revolution it was known as the Western Hospice—the Necker Hospital had acquired a new water supply and furnishings in 1802. Walls were painted and whitewashed. As in other contemporary European hospitals, the procedure was carried out using a lime solution meant to absorb carbon dioxide from the walls. For the first time since its founding in 1778, the hospital's main building had also been substantially remodeled. Removal of the first-floor ceiling provided the various wards with greater height and a larger volume of air. High windows were extended down to improve circulation. Female convalescents, no longer forced to perform institutional chores, were provided with an outside promenade on land shared with the Hôpital des Enfants Malades to speed up their recovery.

The staff consisted of 10 Sisters of Charity and a resident physician—originally a volunteer—aided by two surgeons, a *garçon chirurgien*, or resident, a visiting surgeon, and an apothecary. At the time of Jacques Dumesnil's admission in February 1819, René Théophile Laennec (1781–1826) was the resident physician of the hospital, appointed to the post in 1816, while Dr. Baffos was the surgeon. Originally from Brittany, Laennec had apprenticed with his uncle, a surgeon, before going to Paris.[12] He was a member of the Society for Good Works.[13] Like other small Parisian institutions, the Necker Hospital also had three *infirmiers* or male attendants available for caregiving, together with the religious personnel, a visiting chaplain, and a sacristan. A porter and gardener, together with a number of aides, *garçons* and *filles de service*, completed the hospital personnel.[14]

The Sisters were in charge of all departments, including the kitchen, laundry, and pharmacy. Called *soeurs grises*—gray sisters because of their habits—they were part of an order created by St. Vincent de Paul and Louise de Marillac in 1633 during the Counter-Reformation's religious revival. Based on their vows, these women had performed a wide combination of religious, administrative, and caregiving duties during the Ancien Régime. Following the revolutionary turmoil, five sisters presided once more over the wards, working under the direction of a veteran administrator, Sister Clavelot. For almost 20 years they had managed the institutional accounts, widely admired as models of clarity and exactness.[15] Indeed, Clavelot and the other Sisters were proud of their efficient stewardship and generous provisions of clothing for Necker's inmates. Following the Revolution, the Sisters of Charity had again been recognized as religious caregivers with the proviso that they no longer involve themselves in medical matters. Indeed, when Jacques came to the institution, the Sisters' functions were limited to religious and housekeeping activities, while physicians controlled both the hospital kitchens and pharmacies. The average cost per patient was 1 franc and 16 sous per day, among the lowest in the Parisian hospital system.[16] Frugality and efficiency, however, remained unrelated to institutional mortality. The official figures for 1818, the year before Jacques' admission, were reported to be 17.4%, a statistic virtually unchanged in more than three decades.[17]

In his own lifetime, the status and treatment of a patient like Jacques had changed significantly. Before the Revolution, he would have been seen as a pious recipient of traditional Christian charity, provided with rest, food, and simple care that ennobled both the patrons of the institution and its religious caregivers. In addition to caring for his basic physical needs, the religious personnel would have concentrated on his spiritual life through frequent prayers, masses, and reception of sacraments. Now, however, Monsieur Dumesnil had become a poor citizen-patient with a right to hospital care. In return, he was prepared to be an object of medical observation, diagnosis, and treatment. His diseased body would be subjected to carefully organized physical examinations designed to reveal the underlying pathological changes taking place in his various organs. Jacques's flesh was to become a teaching object, a valuable specimen in which to detect the relentless progression of a disease's natural evolution and ultimately the locus for discovering the suspected organ pathology through dissection on the autopsy table.[18]

Ancien Régime: Paris and its hospitals

On the eve of the Revolution, Paris already had a population of nearly 700,000. The eighteenth-century growth of the city had been impressive: by the year 1700 the metropolis held 500,000 people. The increase had been especially rapid in the 1770s and 1780s. Most new inhabitants came from France's provinces, constituting a rather mobile conglomerate fascinated by city life, excited about anonymity and freedom, and hopeful of employment. To care for the indigent among them, the city had more than 48 charitable institutions housing close to 20,000 inmates, many of them old, infirm, and orphaned.[19] As throughout Catholic Europe in the eighteenth century, most Parisian charitable institutions suffered from the traditional evils of financial corruption and inefficiency, while declining religious fervor had markedly diminished donations and bequests. To stimulate giving, ecclesiastical administrators continued the tradition of favoring the will of benefactors at the expense of inmates. Donors still expected to be rewarded for their charitable acts by grateful, praying residents. The residents themselves, many of whom came from the uprooted population of beggars and vagabonds inspiring fear on the streets of Paris, were subject to a new kind of social control and confinement, a *politique d'enfermement* in charitable institutions that increasingly combined the role of hospital and prison.

A century earlier, religious goals and the new security concerns of cities and towns had forged a compromise, fostering the creation of a single, uniform system composed of *Hôpitaux-générales* or general hospitals in France.[20] Responding to additional mercantilist considerations, idle inmates were put to work, as in Protestant workhouses, making textiles and other consumer goods. In sharp contrast with remaining smaller charitable establishments, these general hospitals possessed complex infrastructures and were staffed by religious caregivers, including the traditional Augustinian nuns, but also by two new groups that acquired a national profile: the Brothers of Charity of St. John of God, brought to France in 1601 by Marie de Medicis, and the previously mentioned Sisters of Charity inspired by St. Vincent de Paul.[21] Together these orders staffed hundreds of institutions, both large and small, equipped with their own pharmacies and dead houses, and assisted by a specialized staff of physicians and surgeons. Besides providing social order and economic productivity, the new hospices were organized to offer spiritual redemption and salvation.[22]

As the plague raged in Rome, the General Hospital of Paris was created in 1656 through the consolidation of several charitable houses.[23] Among them were the Bicêtre (males) and Salpêtrière (females), reserved for the disabled, the chronically ill, the aged, and presumed lunatics, together with vagrants, beggars, and prostitutes. Newborns went to the Foundlings Hospice, while the Pitié and St. Antoine orphanages admitted young children. The other traditional assistential institution in France was the Hôtel Dieu—"God's hostel." Located in larger French towns, especially in the north of the country God's hostels took in only the sick and abandoned poor. Many, like the Hôtel Dieu of Paris, were medieval foundations located in the center of the city. Placed under municipal control in 1505, the Parisian Hôtel Dieu reached a capacity of more than 1,000 beds. By the eighteenth century it was supported by a combination of private, municipal, and state funds and was supervised by a *bureau* of leading citizens together with a council of laymen that included magistrates, financiers, and wealthy bourgeois.

By the late eighteenth century, this traditional welfare network featured an estimated 1,961 so-called hospitals throughout France, products of unique historical circumstances and patronage. They remained scattered around the country but lacked geographic or structural unity. Most institutions were small establishments at the parish level with only a few beds. Their income came from a patchwork of sources that included rents, produce, or income from land, houses, and mines owned by the institution, supplemented with feudal dues, trusts, and legacies. Therefore, the entire system remained vulnerable to fluctuating economic conditions in France, particularly local crises, including agricultural failures and labor disputes. Faced with high food costs (50% of all expenditures) and high labor costs (another 25%), administratively inefficient institutions faced financial difficulties and needed further private donations or municipal subsidies. A gradual decrease in the former forced the secularization of the traditional hospital system and transformed charity from a religious obligation to a social duty.[24]

In France, as elsewhere in Catholic Europe, this process demanded some form of standardized administration, first unsuccessfully attempted by the crown. Protests that donors should not control endowments from beyond the grave continued to fall on deaf ears, although royal efforts to limit further private donations had some effect. Thus, the French hospital network remained a collection of markedly different institutions with distinctive administrations, sources of income, and patient populations. In theory, larger units were to be run by a *bureau* or administration composed of Church officials, the king, the nobility, and representatives from the community. The last served somewhat reluctantly, supervising daily affairs. In theory at least, a *bureau*'s activities could be reviewed by a general assembly and royal inspectors, but the system's inherent complexity both before and after the Revolution proved impervious to reform, since elected officials usually failed to carry out their unwelcome duties.

After the mid-eighteenth century, this essentially dual system of hospices and

Hôtel-Dieu hospitals came under increased scrutiny and criticism as Enlightenment ideals of physical health painted an optimistic picture of the possibilities of prevention and recovery. Views such as Montesquieu's, suggesting that the state owed its members "a way of life not injurious to health and a place in the public hospital in case of illness,"[25] were echoed by others, although the common perception of hospitalization remained linked with last resort and death. New expectations about the usefulness of medical intervention facilitated the establishment of a vigorous marketplace where consumers representing all social classes searched for health care options.[26] Given the rather unfavorable popular view of contemporary medical professionals, calls were issued for the licensing and state control of physicians and drugs. At the same time, the hospital's welfare function was increasingly judged as wasteful, and general hospitals were accused of promoting idleness and actually increasing the number of dangerous vagrants. Hospitals and hospices no longer functioned as agents of moral rehabilitation.[27]

A precipitating event in the growing debate about the role of hospitals was the week-long fire in December 1772 that severely damaged the gargantuan Hôtel Dieu of Paris. The original medieval building, located on both sides of the Seine, had become a sprawling complex with 112 low-ceilinged *salles* or wards reached through narrow corridors. More than 3,500 patients were crowded into 1,200 beds, with the heels of one inmate to the shoulder of another.[28] As the editor of the famous *Encyclopédie,* Denis Diderot (1713–1784), described it, the institution was "the biggest, roomiest, richest and most terrifying of all our hospitals. . . . Imagine every kind of patient, sometimes packed three, four, five, or six into a bed, the living alongside the dead and dying, the air polluted by this mass of sick bodies, passing the pestilential germs of their affections from one to the other, and the spectacle of suffering and agony on every hand."[29]

Impressed by the miserable conditions, Louis XV ordered the demolition of the Hôtel Dieu in 1773, but his death and the ascension of Louis XVI to the throne delayed execution of this order. But what would become of the hospital's thousands of inmates who could not be accommodated in any of the existing facilities? Thus the monarch was persuaded to accept an alternate plan calling for the reconstruction of the remaining parts of the Hôtel Dieu, a scheme that was submitted to the Academy of Sciences for further study. The Academy, a semiofficial body composed of *savants*, many of them prestigious scientists, was already engaged in articulating reforms in several areas of society. Its purpose was to fashion rational recommendations for French society and thus influence public opinion and perhaps, ultimately, royal decisions.

Between 1775 and 1785, the initial debate about the future of the Hôtel Dieu spilled over into general discussions about reform of the entire Ancien Regime's hospital system. Reacting to the squalor and overcrowding observed in larger city hospitals, experts suggested better accommodations for the sick poor closer to their homes, facilitating visits by family and friends. Two important leaders in this movement were Louis XVI's finance minister, A. Robert J. Turgot (1727–1781), and his successor, Jacques Necker (1732–1804), a Swiss Protestant, whose dismissal by the King in 1789 ignited the storming of the Bastille. In 1780, Louis XVI appointed a physician, Jean Colombier (1736–1789), as inspector of hospitals and prisons. Colombier, in turn, was instrumental in further medicalizing the Bicêtre and Salpêtrière hospices belonging to the Hôpital Général of Paris. In 1781, Colombier created separate infirmaries on the premises of these almshouses, staffed by a physician in chief, surgeon, apothecary, and nurses, based on contemporary military models. Through Necker's influence, the king also supported the creation of a new institution, the Hospice de Charité, a smaller 120-bed facility, the future destination of Jacques Dumesnil.[30]

To make such a neighborhood hospital a reality, the minister's wife, Suzanne, writer and mother of Germaine, the famous Madame de Staël, was placed in charge of the project. Madame Necker was a popular figure in Paris, and her prominent salon was frequented by French and foreign literati. Bypassing the archbishop of Paris, she quickly acquired an old monastery vacated by the Benedictines of Notre Dame de Liesse and remodeled it into a hospital for the sick and poor parishioners of St. Sulpice and du Gros Caillou. Although its architectural features were out of step with the newer tenets of hospital ventilation and hygiene, the institution soon became a model for would-be hospital reformers.[31]

Acting as a self-appointed administrator, Madame Necker admitted her first patients in September 1778 after converting the monastic dormitories into wards. To staff this hospital, she had contracted with a dozen Sisters of Charity, who together with the Augustinian nuns were the traditional custodians of French hospital life. Before the Revolution, the Sisters had nearly 4,000 members serving in hundreds of charitable establishments throughout France. After several months of probation in provincial institutions, the recruits came to the mother house in Paris to be trained for their activities, which included home visits to the poor, teaching in parish schools, and caring for the sick poor in hospitals and hospices. Once they had taken the vow—an annual, not a perpetual, pledge—the Sisters waited for the mother house to place them.

Wherever they were assigned, the Sisters were viewed as agents of piety in a hospital environment repeatedly portrayed as corrupting, especially to children. The Sisters' contracts with a charitable institution such as the Hospice de Charité at St. Sulpice detailed all conditions of hospital service. Among the most important were the Sisters' demands for day-to-day management, including the hiring and firing of lay servants, running the institutional pharmacy, and performing most caregiving functions, including spiritual assistance. Indeed, the Sisters were frequently in charge of the inmates' nutrition and performed procedures such as bloodletting and wound dressing, activities that increasingly brought them into conflict with attending physicians and surgeons.[32]

In 1784, the Hospice de Charité hosted a commission from the Royal Academy of Sciences composed of future Paris Mayor Jean S. Bailly (1736–1793), chemists Antoine L. Lavoisier (1743–1794) and Jean Darcet (1725–1801), the mathematician Pierre S. de Laplace (1749–1827), and the physicist Charles A. Coulomb (1736–1806), as well as the surgeon Jacques Tenon (1724–1816). This visit stood in marked contrast to the opposition encountered by those same commissioners at the Hôtel Dieu, where wary trustees and nuns refused the Academicians access to the hospital's registers. Madame Necker, however, was proud of her model institution and encouraged favorable publicity for her charity. Four years before the commission's inspection, she had published a small pamphlet detailing her rationale for establishing the institution, stressing the importance of hygiene, especially clean, odorless air, although her hospital continued to be criticized for its lack of proper ventilation.[33] In fact, after its first year of operation, the Hospice de Charité reported in 1780 an overall mortality of 17.4%. Madame Necker tried to blame the unfavorable statistics on the influx of consumptive individuals and the elderly in advanced stages of malnutrition, who preferred to die in the hospital rather than alone.

In fact, the Hospice's high institutional mortality continued the following year—it was now over 21%—prompting its savvy administrator to halve the number of reported deaths by simply not counting those inmates who were considered incurables. More than personal pride was at stake. High mortality at the Parisian Hôtel Dieu—virtually 25%—had already sparked an intense debate concerning the ideal size of hospitals. Reformers such as the Neckers and Academy members advocated smaller, more efficient, and more hygienic institutions. In truth, the Hospice de Charité was an experiment explicitly designed to provide its patrons with empirical proof of its superiority, crucial for the development of future institutions. By 1785, François Doublet (1751–1795), the first salaried resident physician at the Hospice, and Colombier had carried out their own inspection tour of various establishments that resulted in important publications proposing the conversion of existing welfare institutions into medical installations for anatomical, physiological, and clinical studies.

Among the foreign visitors who included the Hospice de Charité on their tour of French hospitals was the British hospital reformer John Howard, who briefly inspected the premises in January 1786. Howard was sufficiently impressed to pronounce the hospital a "noble example of private charity," but his recommendation to wash the men's wards apparently went unheeded.[34] Using pertinent information supplied to him by Sister Cassegrain, head of the original Sisters of Charity working in the Hospice de Charité, Academy commissioner Jacques Tenon eventually featured the institution in his second report on hospitals in 1786. His major criticism was the high mortality rate—men 14%, women 20%—second only to that of the Hôtel Dieu. Although no clear explanation concerning these differences emerged, it was argued that women—less expendable as homemakers—delayed admission until they were quite sick.[35]

Doublet, for his part, published an article in 1788 extolling the Hospice de Charité's showcase quality and inherent capacity to reduce mortality. Since it served St. Sulpice, the largest parish of Paris, Doublet argued that the exemplary hospital was well positioned to generate statistics that would accurately reflect the prevailing epidemiology of the city. On the basis of such data, future hospital admissions could become more selective, with the Sisters of Charity accepting only those applicants who could be restored to health.[36] For its part, the commission from the Academy of Sciences continued to count all institutional deaths. In his final 1788 report, Tenon blamed the high mortality at the Hospice on "the gravity of the ailments being treated there" plus the "limited amount of air the patients have to breathe."[37] Necker's remodeling of the religious facilities had not provided the necessary ventilation, especially in the women's ordinary fever ward, with its low ceilings and high windows. However, Tenon praised the well-maintained toilets located away from the wards, between two gardens, as contributing to institutional hygiene.

Tenon's final report counted 6,236 acutely ill hospitalized patients in Paris. With the addition of 15,000 foundlings and 14,000 ailing and poor adults in custodial care, the total burden of the Parisian hospitals and hospices reached over 35,000 inmates, nearly 5% of the city's total population. The "medical" beds for sick inmates comprised about 38% of the total, the rest being occupied by the chronically ill and aged. With regard to the Hôtel Dieu, the report confirmed and expanded the earlier critiques of the crowded and dreadful conditions, the waste and inefficiency, the lack of hygiene and organization, and, above all, the squalor and degradation created by a system that officially operated as a charity. Tenon's recommendations—he had toured British hospitals in 1787—aimed at making the institution "an instrument for recovery" in the tradition that went back to Renaissance hospitals like the Florentine Santa Maria Nuova and was later stressed again by various Enlightenment thinkers.[38] For this purpose, patients needed to have individual beds, sufficient air, and smaller wards not exceeding 40 beds. Trained nursing personnel and regular medical supervision were absolutely necessary.

While the Academy of Sciences debated the issue, the burned-down wing of the Hôtel Dieu had already been reconstructed; the recommendation to replace the deadly institution with four smaller hospitals administered and supplied by a "community center" with emergency service was academic. Nevertheless, Colombier, who had supervised the restoration, established a comprehensive code for regulating the hospital's medical services after July 1787. His ambitious goal was the transformation of "God's hostel" into a medical and surgical establishment devoted to the care of acutely and chronically ill patients. A year later, the hospital minutes reflected the physicians' new influence in the administrative decision-making process. Tasks such as the movement of patients (admissions and discharges), dietary prescriptions, and the use of drugs—all previously carried out by the Augustinian nuns, who had done so since the mid-seventeenth century—had been transferred to medical professionals.

Day-to-day operations, however, continued to be entrusted to the religious orders, whose spiritual agendas increasingly clashed with the medical goals. The cloistered Augustinian nuns, under the rule of Prioress Sister de la Croix, had vowed to devote their lives consciously to reenacting the life and works of Christ, including his good works of ministering to the sick. In their view, "God's hostel" was still a charitable Christian shelter open to all without restrictions. Hospital routines such as admission, washing of hands and feet, confession, prayers, and the sacraments, as well as feeding and clothing, continued to be viewed as religious rituals to be performed in an atmosphere of respect and piety. The nursing nuns were shocked by the behavior of medical professionals, who were noisy and disrespectful and who operated on patients publicly in their beds. Moreover, doctors mocked religion and clergy, dismembered those who died in the institution, and summarily discharged presumed convalescents. A report presented to the archbishop of Paris and the royal government in 1789 dramatically presented these complaints, characterizing the medical actions as "tyrannical despotism," immoral, and highly detrimental to the patients.[39]

With religious goals continuing to play key roles in French institutional management, the battle lines between religious nurses and medical professionals were clearly drawn by the eve of the Revolution. The ensuing power struggle was over the administrative control of these institutions devoted to the sick. Physicians blamed overcrowding on open admission and lengthy stays, which resulted in three or more needy persons occupying each bed. They also denounced high mortality rates and blamed them on the lack of institutional hygiene, as well as deficient dietary programs.

Although increasingly conscious of the deficiencies of its traditional network of hospices and hospitals, the Ancien Régime was unable to overcome the formidable organizational and financial barriers to comprehensive reform.[40] Enlightenment views concerning health and the physiocratic tenets about the economic impact of disease on populations generated a number of proposals to improve hospital management and caregiving. Many of the blueprints for new establishments were presented during the last two decades before the Revolution, and became the basis for further discussions and recommendations presented during the Revolutionary years.[41] Indeed, many of the Ancien Régime's advocates for reform, including Tenon of the Academy of Sciences and the anatomist Felix Vicq d'Azyr (1748–1794) of the Royal Society of Medicine, reemerged as prominent and influential members of Revolutionary committees and commissions. These men provided the necessary continuity and information to spark a new round of debates on the role of hospitals that was to change forever the character of these institutions.

Hospital reform: The fate of France's "curing machines"

After 1789, the subject of hospital reform consumed the time and effort of numerous legislators, government officials, and commissions as they pondered the possibility of transforming French hospitals into what Tenon called "machines" or instruments for the *art de guerir* or healing art. The obstacles were formidable, since most institutions performed both confinement and restorative functions within a set of archaic administrative and financial structures. During the Ancien Régime, two major issues had already been highlighted and debated: the failure of hospices and hospitals to function as agents of moral rehabilitation and their resistance to shifting from religious to medical objectives. The results were institutions of delinquency and terror, as well as breeding grounds for cross-infection and death. But how could charitable relief be provided and hospitals fulfill a primarily medical role? During more than a decade of fact-finding missions, discussions, and legislation, these two somewhat overlapping questions continued to be handled separately.

At the end of the Empire, the torturous evolution of the post-Revolutionary French hospices and hospitals had the paradoxical result of returning them to their Ancien Régime status as charitable institutions. However, gone were the traditional sources of financial support, a combination of endowment income derived from feudal trusts and rents of property, as successive revolutionary governments seized and then sold most of the hospital property providing such funds. The result was a drastic cut in services as well as a spate of institutional mergers and closures. With new bequests lagging, funding had come first from central government loans, followed by emergency bailouts from regional and local authorities, until the whole financial mess was eventually turned over to local hospital commissions composed of private persons, often donors, who operated the hospitals on a basis of service contracts by the early 19th century.

Fueled by such financial exigencies, hospitals were forced to streamline their operations and reduce the cost of care per patient. The vigorous attack on religious caregivers, including the breakup of their congregations and demand for an oath to the Revolution, forced many to leave the institutions, weakening their administrative hold on most hospitals. Return of the nursing orders under Napoleon, however, reflected their peerless qualities as caregivers and willingness to work for low wages. The medicalized character of the institutions they returned to was obvious. If anything, the French medical profession had won the war over the institutional control of hospitals. Overcrowding, the nemesis causing internal chaos and high death rates, was, in time, drastically reduced, in part, through a decrease in patient admissions because of screening and triage, as well as because of faster turnover achieved by the earlier discharge of convalescents. Many indigents were referred to welfare bureaus, and the ambulatory sick were treated at home. By the early 1810s, those who were allowed to enter hospitals found cleaner and better ventilated premises and a bed for each.

During the period of the National Constituent Assembly (May 1789 to October 1791), one momentous change took place that crippled the financial power of the French hospital system. On November 2, 1789, the Assembly ordered the seizure of all Church property, including that of the religious orders, a 400-million-livre asset, while abolishing all feudal dues and other privileges that represented nearly 60% of all charitable income. As noted, this single measure severely eroded all hospitals' financial base and impaired services offered by the Church and the hospitals.[42] In addition to their loss of income from the seizure of their endowments, all institutions were affected by the prevailing inflation and the increase in hospital expenses. This fact, coupled with the proliferation of indigents, led the Constituent Assembly to hastily provide loans and back down on the sale of hospital properties, ordering hospitals to continue administering their own holdings on a provisional basis.

Another Committee on Mendicity composed of philanthropists, clerics, and physicians addressed the urgent needs of the poor in 1790. Among its tasks was to investigate the nature and magnitude of the administrative, financial, and sanitary problems of existing hospitals through questionnaires, surveys, and personal visits. The inquiry focused on 20 establishments identified by Tenon in his 1788 report, including those located in Paris and its surroundings. In a series of reports issued between 1790 and 1791, the Committee struggled with the perennial questions: using what method, who could define the good or worthy poor as opposed to the able-bodied beggar who did not deserve aid and who could become a criminal threat? As always, the distinction was critical, since Ancien Régime proposals had already pointed out that French hospices were undesirable social welfare institutions because they promoted idleness and corruption instead of restoring spirituality. The Committee's final blueprint, read to the Assembly on January 31, 1791, suggested that local governments should decide who was entitled to public assistance. To protect worthy people from corruption, it was necessary to separate them from existing hospices and provide them with home-based relief, including visits by physicians and distribution of medicines by dispensaries, a scheme common in Protestant countries. Family members would act as natural nurses.[43]

However, the Committee also realized that there were other good poor persons without family support for whom the hospital remained a necessary destination during illness. For such individuals, hospital care was to be a right. Communities with more than 4,000 people would therefore need to retain a number of small hospices and hospitals, each of them with a capacity of 150 patients. Larger metropolitan areas required an additional central institution for complicated surgical cases, treatment of venereal problems, and isolation of contagious patients. A medical triage procedure would sift from the masses of apparently ailing indigents those persons who were really sick and deserved to be admitted for treatment. They would be assigned to the various hospitals according to their ailments.

Dual management, at home and in the hospital, would improve patients' morale through contact with friends and family while preventing idleness and moral decay. This scheme, it was believed, would primarily benefit young children and the elderly. To implement these recommendations, the Committee on Mendicity suggested the centralization of all relief functions by the state since, in their view, only the government had a chance to deal with the serious problem of poverty in France. Such a measure also made sense financially since it would streamline aid and manage it more efficiently. By restricting assistance to the truly needy, deinstitutionalization would also save money and curtail waste in the hospitals themselves. Equally important, this plan would prevent overcrowding and thus improve institutional hygiene. Better ventilation and fewer hospital-induced fevers could be achieved through architectural changes such as additional windows and smaller wards.

With regard to the Hospice de Charité, the Committee requested hospital accounts in April 1791 as it began surveying all Parisian charitable institutions. This time the information was provided by Sister Braujon, the mother superior, who had succeeded Sister Cassegrain. Together with the parish priest of St. Sulpice, Monsignor Marnaud, and with support from the Duchess of Duras, another friend of the Neckers, Sister Braujon now administered the institution. All religious personnel had taken an oath of loyalty to the Revolution. Madame Necker had given up the direction of the Hospice in 1788 and two years later accompanied her husband into exile to his native Lausanne.

François La Rochefoucauld-Liancourt (1747–1827), an Ancien Régime aristocrat, and chairman of the Committee was apparently impressed by the efficient operation of the Hospice de Charité but concerned about its excessive institutional mortality rate, which contrasted with the apparent "good care that patients receive in this hospital." According to information supplied to the authorities, the Hospice had reduced the cost per patient to an economical 17 sous per day, while the Committee had calculated the expense for a medical welfare patient at 18 sous per day. Here the size of the Hospice, with its small staff and bureaucracy, was obviously responsible for such favorable statistics, and these low expenditures were henceforth frequently cited in other national reports.[44]

To deal specifically with medical questions, the Constitutional Assembly created in September 1790 a separate Committee on Salubrity or Health that included all Assembly physicians. Concerned about the scope of the Committee on Mendicity's jurisdiction, the members of this new committee, led by Joseph I. Guillotin (1738–1814), then professor of the Paris Medical School, quickly established their own jurisdiction by including all aspects of public health, medical education, and hospital medicine. Committee members worried about their public image and low esteem among all sectors of the population, and they were reluctant to become ensnared in new welfare schemes being propounded by the rival Committee that would reduce physicians to civil servants. A plan to reform French medicine prepared by Vicq d'Azyr was presented to the Committee on Health in an attempt to shore up the role of medical professionals. It proposed the union of medicine and surgery and suggested a new curriculum stressing clinical skills and employing large hospitals in the training of French medical students. In fact, each of the four proposed medical schools was to be closely affiliated with teaching hospitals. Departmental chairmen at the university would simultaneously hold leading positions at the various hospital services. This plan also had the support of Pierre J. G. Cabanis (1757–1808), an important physician and reformer, who articulated his ideas in *Observations sur les hôpitaux*, written in the same year. To improve quality, Cabanis even favored unfettered competition among medical practitioners in the marketplace, with educational excellence instead of licensing as the path to success.[45]

Like Vicq d'Azyr, Cabanis favored steps to medicalize the hospitals further and transform them into laboratories for the study of disease. Before placing these institutions within the medical system, however, efforts were needed to change them from "magazines of corrupted air" contaminating the inmates into cleaner, better-organized establishments. Thus the author preferred smaller 100- to 150-bed hospitals such as Madame Necker's Hospice de Charité. Here physicians would have more time to observe and study fewer patients, thus reaching better diagnoses as well as prescribing adequate treatments. Put in charge of most forms of patient care, including diet and drugs, medical professionals visiting the patients several times a day would learn their trade and manage the patients more effectively. Based on such ideas, the Committee on Health presented its final report in September 1791 before being disbanded, along with the Committee on Mendicity, as the work of the Constitutional Assembly came to an end. Since no action was taken, these recommendations simply became guidelines for future discussions and legislative proposals.

During the life of the Legislative Assembly (October 1791 to September 1792), the former Committee on Mendicity was replaced by a new Committee on Public Assistance under the chairmanship of Tenon. The veteran reformer wasted no time in requesting further aid for the financially ailing hospitals. Although the Assembly responded favorably and voted some funds, further aid was refused until all institutions had presented their reports of past expenditures. Unfortunately, the war against Austria in the spring of 1792 shifted the attention of the lawmakers to military questions, especially the creation of a powerful army. Perhaps even Jacques was drafted. During that year, 1,400 physicians and surgeons joined the military medical corps. In spite of urgent civilian needs, welfare reform became a low priority.[46]

Undaunted, the new Committee submitted its welfare reform proposals in June 1792 based on recommendations of the previous committee. During the summer, confusion over the control of Paris' hospitals led the municipality to resume its authority and create its own hospital commission. Financial problems were becoming more acute, and previous loans to the institutions could not be repaid. To make matters worse, the Legislative Assembly issued a decree in August 1792 ordering the breakup of all religious congregations and the sale of their houses. This move devastated the internal economy of the hospitals since many religious caregivers were forced to leave. In a further escalation of anti-Catholicism, hospital chapels were closed, priests dismissed, and religious services such as confession, communion, and last rites suspended. When lay replacements were hired in the hospitals, the balance of power within most institutions finally shifted toward the physicians. The effect was a drastic reduction in patient admissions because of medical screening; the Hôtel Dieu in Paris reduced its inmate population from 2,500 to 1,500.

Early during the Convention before Thermidor (September 1792 to July 1794), more attacks were leveled against the existing hospices and hospitals, which were characterized as symbols of Ancien Régime decadence and corruption. In a further escalation of the rhetoric, they were now categorized as "tombs of the human race" and *maisons de repression* (houses of repression) contributing to the problem of mendicity.[47] Indeed, since these institutions were perceived as embarrassing royal leftovers, calls were issued to eliminate them altogether. In the meantime, a change of name was proposed for the hospitals devoted to the sick. Henceforth they were to be known as *maisons de santé* (houses of health), which, although cosmetic, was reflective of the current sentiment. Meanwhile, hospital income continued to plummet, reduced to about 20% of the endowment earnings available during the Ancien Régime. To make matters worse, institutions were now required to pay taxes by January 1793. A month later, however, the Convention was forced to provide further money to the minister of the interior for hospital aid, a practice periodically repeated to make ends meet. Most of the funds, however, went toward the aid of civilian hospitals treating sick and wounded soldiers. In the meantime, France's rapid mobilization continued: in 1793, the nation had 650,000 under arms; by February 1794, 1,200,000.[48]

A new Committee on Public Assistance created by the Convention seemed committed to the work of its predecessor, presenting in March 1793 a plan for national assistance. Once again, home care was depicted as less destructive to the moral fiber of the poor and considered less costly than institutional care. Moreover, hospital utilization was to be restricted to individuals who had no home or relatives, as well as those afflicted with chronic conditions. Therefore, the French assistential system needed to be divided into hospices for the young and aged and the *maisons de santé*. This time, the reformers were more successful in persuading the legislature to adopt some of their proposals. In June 1793, a law created a system of public assistance for infants and the aged. Each *arrondissement* (city district) was to have a shelter for the aged and maternity care together with a limited number of city hospices. However, the Convention, primarily involved in military matters, stopped short of creating an administrative system for managing these institutions, thus foiling the implementation of the public assistance legislation.

Conditions in Paris before Thermidor deteriorated further because of the large number of sick and needy paupers—one estimate counted 60,000 of them—together with wounded soldiers who literally were overrunning the hospitals still under communal control. A new commission emerged in March 1793 to supervise assistance to the needy until a comprehensive welfare system could be created. An architect was hired to improve the buildings of existing hospitals and make them more sanitary. Higher patient turnover led to less overcrowding and lower mortality rates. Two measures by the Convention in October and December 1793 put further pressure on the former religious personnel still working in hospitals to take their oaths of loyalty to the Revolution on penalty of being fired and considered traitors. Their diminished presence led to the gradual abolition of the Sisters' apothecary, replaced by professional male pharmacists.

Like other institutions devoted to the care of sick paupers during the Convention, Jacques' Hospice de Charité also suffered a name change in 1792: it was henceforth known as the Hospice de l'Ouest or Western Hospice. In line with the earlier secularization efforts that had abolished all religious ceremonies, even the hospital's chapel had been converted into a storage facility. The order of the Sisters of Charity was disbanded and their Parisian mother house closed. However, many of the Sisters took the required loyalty oath and were allowed to continue their caregiving functions as lay volunteers. Younger and more worldly than their Augustinian counterparts at the Hôtel Dieu, they managed to survive the turmoil of the Terror. In truth, their caregiving remained vastly superior to the services being rendered by salaried servants.[49]

Finally, at the peak of Jacobin radicalism, the Convention passed its famous decree of 23 Messidor (July 11, 1794) ordering the immediate confiscation by the state of all hospital property, a move that effectively nationalized the hospitals since they lost all their remaining income. In return, the government promised to meet hospital expenses and assume responsibility for their debts. Given the financial constraints resulting from the war, this measure spelled disaster for the existing hospitals. It ensured further closures, mergers, and cuts in services. Moreover, the new constraints signaled the virtual end of the hospital as a welfare institution, opening the way for the medical profession to consolidate its power and pursue the goals of treatment, teaching, and research.

After the fall of Robespierre and during the Thermidorean Convention from July 1794 to October 1795, the earlier principles proclaimed by the Committee on Mendicity continued to be supported as part of the Revolutionary rhetoric, but the approach to hospital reform was quickly abandoned. The Committee on Public Assistance's earlier plan for a national scheme to control and finance welfare as well as hospitals was scrapped. Such designs were now completely unrealistic because of the bankruptcy of the French hospital system. Anticipating its forthcoming demise, the Committee, in a new report to the Convention dated January 1795, suggested that private charity would once more be the solution for France's indigent problem.

Unfortunately, the sale of hospital properties had proceeded at a rapid pace— more than half were quickly disposed of—and funds from the government to replace the lost income were sporadic and slow in coming. Efforts to counter the devastating effects of the 23 Messidor decree finally emerged in August 1795 as the Convention postponed any further sales. The only solution for hospitals was once more to reduce expenses through greater efficiency, a difficult task given the current inflation in food prices. As the welfare role of the French hospital vanished, government leaders became increasingly enthusiastic about its function within a reformed system of medical education. This transformation was to proceed along the lines previously set out by Guillotin and Vicq d'Azyr in their report of 1791. Indeed, creation of the new *écoles de santé* (schools of health) in late 1794 designated teaching hospitals as the primary institutions for training health professionals.[50]

Because of the administrative confusion and financial crisis afflicting the French hospital system, serious consideration was given during the Directory (1795–1799) to abandoning centralized control and returning welfare to local parishes. In the end, the authorities decided to retain control and supervision of the system by placing it under the newly created Ministry of the Interior. Financially, however, the law of October 7, 1796, put all hospitals under the jurisdiction of local municipal governments and regional departments or prefectures. Each community was to appoint a five-member commission to run the daily operations of its own hospitals, while towns with more than 100,000 inhabitants would have a board chosen by the departmental government. Since no further state funding was forthcoming, all remaining income from local hospital property would be pooled by a municipality and redistributed to each institution according to need. To facilitate such financing, the 1794 legislation selling hospital property was repealed and further nationalization of properties postponed. In spite of such measures, the government was forced to provide emergency funds to keep some institutions from folding, but it failed to prevent the closure of a number of hospices in small communities.

Legislation in 1798 confirmed previous decrees regarding local support for hospitals, while the national government, in a burst of bureaucratic zeal, continued to monitor and regulate all expenditures. In Paris, expenses were now about six times higher than income, forcing drastic service reductions in institutions— 20 were left—through consolidation. With the Department of the Seine in arrears on hospital salaries, many hospital employees failed to be paid for 15 months. Instead, they were compensated with hospital supplies at the expense of patient care, leading to bread shortages, meatless soups, few drugs, and no bed linens. Not surprisingly, previous problems of institutional overcrowding ceased, and expenses decreased as the needy stayed away. The crisis prompted a partial reintroduction of funding methods employed during the Ancien Régime in the form of town taxes such as the *octois* or tolls on food supplies entering cities, while charitable donations were again eagerly sought. At this point, the visions of early hospital reformers appeared to have ended in total failure, while piety and charity had sunk to dangerously low levels.[51]

At the end of 1798, new legislation attempted to correct previous deficiencies, establishing clearer lines of authority and finally abandoning the centralized financing scheme. Instead, hospital management was placed in the hands of private contractors with the goal of improving conditions. The new system consisted of five different companies, each responsible for one aspect of the assistential complex that included children, the aged, the poor and incurables, hospices and the sick, and the Salpêtrière. The decision, reached by François de Neufchateau, Minister of the Interior, was predicated on the assumption that fixed sums of money, stipulated in these service contracts, would produce substantial savings to the municipalities. Within this entrepreneurial framework, low-paid caregiving nuns returned to many of the institutions, since the previous oath of allegiance was no longer required. Able inmates were also given employment and remuneration according to their abilities. Although daily food rations were severely curtailed, and new linen and clothing supplies remained virtually nonexistent, the Western Hospice, now led by Sister Clavelot, survived.[52]

During the Consulate (1799–1804), French hospitals remained in critical condition. After being stripped of their income in 1789 by the Constituent Assembly, most of them failed to recover in spite of the laws passed by the Directory. Food and other supplies were scarce, and previous promises of humanitarian aid were not fulfilled. Local hospital commissions now became permanent powerful bodies. They reported to the prefect of their department, who, in turn, accounted to the minister of the Interior. New fiscal directives clashed with the traditional mission to take in all the needy. In 1802, a new triage system was created as more prospective inmates requested admission. Those previously accepted to institutions of the *hôpital général* were no longer automatically accepted unless they were elderly, without families or resources. In addition, convalescent stays were shortened to three days and indigents were referred to welfare bureaus.

In Paris, a new 11-member Conseil General d'Administration des Hôpitaux de la Seine emerged. Among the Council members were the hospital reformer Cabanis; Antoine A. Parmentier (1737–1813), who had amended the existing pharmacopoeia; and Michel A. Thouret (1748–1810), dean of the local École de la Santé. Among their early accomplishments were attempts to regularize hospital finances through a number of cost-cutting measures, including further personnel reductions and liquidation of debts incurred during the Revolutionary years.[53] Unlike the Sisters of Charity, their Augustinian sisters at the Hôtel Dieu were rapidly dwindling in spite of efforts to recall those who had been expelled earlier. In difficult financial times, just finding enough food for their charges was a great accomplishment for these tireless workers.

During the Empire, previous reformers had insisted that it was more rational and economical to deal with the poor on a home-centered basis than in hospitals, but the time had long passed for bold experiments. While retaining central control, the 1806 law merely addressed a number of organizational issues regarding hospitals. The General Council developed new disciplinary regulations with a series of penalties for rules violations. Again, strict criteria of need were stressed for all hospital admissions, and the appointment of hospital physicians now had to follow a competitive process of nomination. On the financial front, further institutional mergers occurred as the authorities again utterly failed to grasp the realities of hospital management. Hospitals once more welcomed private charity, channeled through the Ministry of the Interior. As during most of the eighteenth century, donors were given rights of admission and the privilege to sit on hospital governing boards. At stake was the need to secure additional funds since tax money could not cover the costs of managing the civil establishments.

Institutional staffing continued to be a problem, with the public still supporting the presence of religious sisters in hospitals. Poor pay forced the rapid turnover of ancillary lay personnel. In truth, Catholic nurses were virtually irreplaceable on hospital wards, although they now had to obey regulations set by the administrative commissions and were prevented from reorganizing into powerful orders. In fact, representatives of all nursing orders were called to meet with Napoleon in December 1807 to discuss the current needs of nursing and hospital care.[54] With sisters again playing prominent caregiving roles, hospital life in some respects returned to pre-Revolutionary routines, as priests were again allowed to conduct mass and dispense the sacraments.

On the positive side, there were attempts to improve patient comfort within a more hygienic environment. Hospital authorities now only allowed the installation of single three-foot-wide beds, allowing greater space between them to facilitate air circulation, nursing, and medical rounds. Not only did the wards become less crowded through patient transfers and the assignment of one patient per bed, but floors and walls were periodically whitewashed to prevent miasma. Administrators also promised to place more stoves in the wards during cold winters and make bathing a regular component of the therapeutic program. In turn, patients were to wear distinctive hospital clothing—cotton in summer, wool in winter—and comply with regulations. One reformer even suggested that patients of similar age and occupation should be grouped together in the wards for mutual support and encouragement.[55]

Bedside and autopsy table: New approaches to disease

The most prominent outcome of the post-Revolutionary era for French hospitals was the dominant presence of the medical profession and the execution of its pedagogical and research agendas in the wards. Particular styles of scientific thought are never generated in a vacuum. They emerge within specific cultural and institutional contexts that define and restrict the range of observations and discoveries.[56] New ideas, exemplified by the works of Cabanis, Philippe Pinel (1745–1826), Marie-François Xavier Bichat (1771–1802), and Laennec, created a further impetus toward empirical approaches to knowledge and the systematic collection of a body of medical and surgical information wherein internal diseases could also be conceived in localized, anatomical terms. These new structural and physiological conceptions were expressed in a renewed interest in pathological anatomy and the development of techniques of physical examination within hospital settings.[57]

Cabanis and Pinel had already been part of a pre-Revolutionary group of French physicians convinced that sense impressions were the basic building blocks of all ideas and knowledge. This popular ideology had its roots in the work of philosophers such as Locke and Condillac, who had concluded that sensations were the only true psychological events for the construction of perception, understanding, judgment, and memory. Cabanis and Pinel frequently visited the salon of Mme. Helvetius at her suburban villa in Auteuil, a meeting place of Enlightenment philosophes and social reformers who espoused this philosophy. In time, both physicians came to be known as medical ideologues for their belief that observation would expose the existence of analogies and differences among the various diseases through the discovery of certain constant relations and differential criteria.[58] The result would be a superior construction and precise classification of human disease, leading to greater diagnostic and therapeutic certainty. Previous medical systems stressing rationality—including those of the Scotsmen William Cullen and John Brown—were suspect to Pinel and Cabanis, too narrowly drawn to encompass the manifold panorama of human infirmity displayed in hospital settings.[59]

Together with such radical empiricism came a profound skepticism regarding causality. Besides tacitly believing that nature was regular and constant in its operations, Cabanis was reluctant to speculate about the ultimate causes of health and disease, as well as the nature and essence of the vital principle believed to be operating within human bodies. For Cabanis, most causes remained mysteriously concealed, and nature displayed an inherent and inexplicable variability. Instead of building successive medical systems that placed nature into temporary straitjackets, Cabanis preferred to channel the physicians' efforts toward direct observation and description of bedside events. He himself had used this method before coming to Paris.[60] For Cabanis, as for Cullen and Frank before him, the *clinic*—meaning bedside contacts between physician and patient—was to be the locus of medical research and education.

Following the Revolution, medical men had achieved total power over the management of their hospital patients and the dissection of their corpses. As one contemporary Salpêtrière physician indicated, the poor who entered the public hospitals made a contract with the state, in effect transferring ownership of their bodies.[61] Dissections, although feared by many inmates and an incitement to occasional escapes from the wards, were seen by physicians as the patient's final contribution to society. At the same time, however, the procedure was viewed as a sort of sacrilege, especially by religious caregivers who supported the notion of bodily integrity for the afterlife.[62] As more anatomical findings were correlated with clinical phenomena, physicians doubled their efforts to detect internal lesions and abnormalities in the living patient. Jean N. Corvisart's (1755–1821) "meditations on death"—meaning the study of dissected bodies—were not to be a "vain curiosity," but simply the vehicle for "distinguishing diseases by certain signs and constant symptoms."[63]

Parisian hospitals were true museums of pathology. As hospital physicians systematically dissected all those who perished within the institution, virtually every patient revealed a variety of lesions, many of them unsuspected by either patients or their caregivers. At first, the mandatory and rather frequent postmortem examination were superficial and incomplete. Confusion and error were still common since many cadaveric changes were not fully understood. Moreover, autopsies seldom shed light on any causes of disease, proximate or remote, and often failed to disclose the immediate reason for death. Nevertheless, gross pathological findings were now considered the principal, not supplementary, criteria for diagnosis and classification of diseases. As Bichat had remarked in 1800, nosologists such as Cullen had erred in their classifications because of their indifference to postmortem examinations and the pathological knowledge they yielded. During the early 1800s, this more integrated anatomoclinical approach to disease gradually became the norm as surgeons and physicians tried to merge their respective frames of reference.

While Cabanis, Pinel, and Corvisart pursued their efforts to expand the knowledge of clinical medicine, another reformer, Bichat, had arrived in Paris in June 1794 and began his research under the direction of Pierre J. Desault (1738–1795), chief of surgery at the Hôtel Dieu. Bichat pursued surgical subjects conducive to his projected military career, including the anatomy, physiology, and pathology of bones and joints. At the Hôtel Dieu, autopsies had been performed routinely on all surgical patients since the seventeenth century. In fact, since the 1710s, courses based on anatomical demonstrations and dissections were held there routinely. Working in such a milieu, Bichat turned his attention away from whole organs, focusing instead on their constituent parts. Not surprisingly, he soon concluded that "ignorance of organic affections, resulting from a total neglect of postmortem examination, is the cause that has misled the ancient practitioners on most diseases."[64] Although he worked without a microscope, Bichat carried out numerous experiments in which tissues were subjected to desiccation, putrefaction, and chemical actions.[65]

Six months after Bichat's arrival, plans earlier formulated by the Health Committee for three new *écoles de santé* to be located in Paris, Montpellier, and Strasbourg were implemented. Among the goals of the Revolutionary government were the unification of medicine and surgery. As one member, Anton F. Fourcroy (1755–1809) indicated, legislators wished to "eradicate that ancient separation between two estates that has caused so much trouble. Medicine and surgery are two branches of the same science."[66] In spite of this claim, however, Fourcroy's elaborate blueprint for the organization of instruction at the new school envisioned separate courses for internal and external pathology. While placed under one academic roof, both medical and surgical collectives continued to defend the integrity of their own disciplines. Soon, François Chopart (1743–1795) and Pierre F. Percy (1754–1825) developed the surgical pathology course tailored to the needs of future army surgeons. It was mostly nontheoretical and focused strictly on discrete, localized lesions. Concentrating on trauma, the course divided diseases topographically according to soft and hard parts. In 1795, François Doublet and Joseph F. Bourdier planned the medical pathology course. Medicine followed its traditional approach of presenting diseases within their natural historical evolution and as components of an interlocking classification schema. Pathology remained holistic and subservient to bedside findings, explained by a deliberately vague and speculative pathogenesis based on vitalistic principles. Thus, both the surgical and medical groups continued their own separate approaches to the phenomena cf disease.[67]

In addition to the designated wards in both the Hôtel Dieu—for *maladies externes* (surgery)—and the Hôpital de la Charité—for *maladies internes* (medicine), an ever-expanding body of teachers and students now descended on the hapless inmates of other institutions within the extensive Parisian hospital system. Pinel, who by 1794 had become chief physician at the Salpêtrière, was put in charge of a 200-bed infirmary, where he used a 30-bed ward to make detailed observations employing his much vaunted "analysis." While Pinel still tried to fit the protean manifestations of disease observed in the hospital wards into diagnostic categories that were in harmony with his 1798 nosology, however, new postmortem findings continually undermined the existing clinical classifications.

In September 1798, a plan for curricular reforms of the École de Santé in Paris affirmed that "the art of healing is one and indivisible and that as a consequence there is only one pathology." Suggestions were made to integrate the two courses of pathology—"the way a trunk is followed by its branches"—into a new synthetic view of pathology.[68] A year later, Bichat published a pair of reports on bone and joint pathology that attempted to bring medicine and surgery together. The articles disclosed a new physiology and pathology of the synovial system, with Bichat pointing out the reactivity of the serous fluids in the joint space. As he attempted an intellectual convergence of medical and surgical ideas, Bichat stressed that organs were complex entities, with their component tissues distributed into a number of anatomical categories, such as the cellular, arterial, venous, muscular, mucous, serous, synovial, and glandular types. Bichat's ideas were consonant with sensualist views held by French scientists and physicians. Transcending the static surgical approach, however, Bichat was interested in establishing a relationship between altered tissues and functions. According to his scheme, tissue lesions determined the appearance of clinical symptoms, a radical reversal that placed pathological anatomy in a dominant position with regard to clinical medicine.[69]

Bichat's *Traité des membranes en général et diverses membranes en particulier* appeared in 1800. The book claimed to represent a new science of anatomy and pathology based on a simple classification of bodily linings, their distribution in several organs, and particular susceptibility to disease. During a course taught in 1801–1802 at the Hôtel Dieu, Bichat expounded on his new membrane theory by locating the seats of disease in all of his 21 subtypes of solid tissue. As autopsy reports demonstrated, Bichat's dissections at the Hôtel Dieu involved numerous victims of so-called dropsical diseases, including anasarca, pleurisy, pericarditis, and peritonitis. Although his premature death precluded further studies, Bichat's tissue theory was quickly assimilated into the pathological works of influential physicians such as Gabriel Andral (1797–1876), Gaspard L. Bayle (1774–1816), Laennec, Jean Cruveilhier (1791–1874), and Pierre A. Piorry (1794–1879).[70]

In 1803, Bichat's unfinished five-volume *Traité d'anatomie descriptive* appeared posthumously, completed by colleagues. Bichat's introduction summarized his fundamental approach: "dissect in anatomy, experiment in physiology; follow the disease and make a postmortem examination in medicine; this is the three-fold path without which there can be no anatomist, no physiologist, no physician." In less than two years, he had established new links between physiology and pathological anatomy. What made Bichat's approach unique was his willingness to transcend the traditional surgical approach of studying particular local lesions in isolation. Instead, Bichat sought to cross anatomical boundaries by searching for systemic pathological actions affecting the whole body, including inflammation. This goal was achieved by employing the medical doctrines of sensibility and irritability. Bichat's holistic explanations were expected to make sense of the pathological variety encountered at the autopsy table. Moreover, some abnormal pathological configurations could possibly be detected clinically before death. In combining the surgical and medical approaches, Bichat's greatest legacy was the creation of a new pathophysiology capable of guiding clinical medicine. His publications established the essential basis for a systematic program of anatomical-clinical synthesis.[71]

Further efforts to correlate clinical and autopsy findings were made by Laennec, Necker Hospital's resident physician at the time of Jacques Dumesnil's admission. The less-focused internal vision of pathology had been closely associated with traditional medical agendas espoused by hospital practitioners in Edinburgh and Vienna. The attending physician witnessed the dissection of his former patient, identified morbid appearances in certain organs, and thus supplemented the clinical knowledge of the diseases he had managed with the pathological findings. Moreover, lesions were often correlated with age, sex, and the seasons to establish "anatomical constitutions" or susceptibilities consonant with other medical and epidemic factors. Finally, whenever possible, pathological anatomy furnished physiologists and clinicians with glimpses of reciprocal influences between the diseases and the states of entire organ systems. At first, this traditional auxiliary role to the clinic continued to dominate the Paris faculty and found expression in the teachings of Pinel and the courses of internal pathology at the *École*.[72]

Shortly after arriving in Paris in April 1801, Laennec registered at the local *École* and started to follow Corvisart's course at the Hôpital de la Charité. He also took a private anatomy course from the surgeon Guillaume Dupuytren (1777–1835), already *chef de travaux anatomiques* at the *École pratique de dissection* linked to the medical school. As a result of these experiences, Laennec published articles on peritoneal inflammation and other bodily membranes in Corvisart's *Journal de Mèdecine*, setting off a dispute with Dupuytren over the classification of anatomical lesions. Employing a strictly utilitarian approach, Dupuytren's emphasis was concentrated on localized pathology, since surgery required an intimate knowledge of particular organs, vessels, and nerves, as well as specific anatomical relationships. Such a practical approach represented the traditional surgical thought collective and it obviously also fulfilled the pedagogical needs of future surgeons taught at the school.[73]

For Laennec, however, there was another way of mapping out the body and interpreting its morbid appearances, which differed from the traditional descriptive approach employed by the anatomists. Their exposition of organic lesions followed the actual order of dissection, with diseases classed according to their seats, not their nature. The alternative strategy championed by Bichat, and now Laennec, was both anatomical and clinical, a path that would force a total reorganization of contemporary nosology.

While Laennec's elevation of pathological anatomy was perceived as nothing less than revolutionary by his followers, many of the issues raised in establishing clinical-pathological correlations were still in dispute at the time of Jacques' admission. Among the most difficult was the question of etiology; could pathological anatomy, through its study of lesions, point to the true causes of a disease? Some of Laennec's colleagues speculated that the lesion itself was the cause rather than an effect, questioning whether or not morbid appearances actually determined the evolution of physiopathological processes. While conscious of the limitations inherent in the anatomical approach, Laennec nevertheless tried to establish criteria by which practitioners could link lesions, functions, and causes. He agreed that pathological anatomy was becoming the science of all visible changes produced by disease, the new basis for nosology and most certain guide to medical diagnosis.[74] However, his opposition to any dogmatic formulations prompted him to reject a strict organicism—the concept that all disease was localized in organs—while continuing to promote the importance of a dynamic physiological view regarding pathological phenomena. In Laennec's opinion, the new pathology had to provide facts applicable to clinical medicine. "Without [pathology] diagnosis is always either impossible or prone to uncertainty," he declared in 1809.[75] Medicine needed to become more anatomical and surgery more medical.

Physical diagnosis: Laennec and the stethoscope

If medical diagnosis was to be based on the structural and functional abnormalities of the various organ systems, post-Revolutionary French physicians needed to probe the bodies of their patients closely before death for necessary clues. Becoming an excellent diagnostician was to become a coveted goal of medical practitioners.[76] As one French author asserted, to possess such skills would provide physicians with a measure of confidence and aplomb bound to inspire confidence and even admiration in patients.[77] In fact, in time, diagnostic accuracy and prognostication easily displaced therapeutics as the criterion on which to judge medical efficacy. Even if the sickness turned out to be severe or incurable, such a diagnosis was deemed quite useful. Patients' uncertainty vanished and anxiety lessened; palliative measures could be instituted. Relatives could be summoned, affairs settled, confession heard, and last rites administered.[78]

As articulated in France during the early nineteenth century, the science of semeiotics or interpretation of symptoms was based on the twin interpretations of the sick persons' complaints and the language of their organs. The former, elicited through careful history taking, was believed to be always fraught with error. In the view of many French physicians, most hospital patients tended to exaggerate their complaints, while others either tried to invent or carefully hide them, especially if they were stigmatizing, as in the case of venereal diseases. François Merat, a student of Corvisart, warned hospital physicians about the ignorance of the lower classes, who, in their coarse language, were either incapable of adequately expressing their complaints or, having read some popular medical tracts, tried to frame their suffering using what physicians perceived to be a ridiculous, if not humorous, pseudomedical terminology. To facilitate communication, Merat recommended that physicians avoid employing technical terms such as *dyspnea*—a hallmark of inexperienced young practitioners—using instead common language and asking a set of "yes" or "no" questions.[79]

A superior strategy was to interpret organic functions through careful, frequent observation of the sick, coupled with systematic exploration of the nervous, digestive, respiratory, circulatory, and genitourinary organ systems.[80] To obtain a more complete clinical picture, Corvisart, like his colleagues in Edinburgh and Vienna, went beyond history taking to actively examining his patients.[81] The inventory of symptoms was joined by bodily inspection and palpation. In 1806, Corvisart announced the reintroduction of Leopold Auenbrugger's method of percussion in his own work *Essay on Diseases of the Heart*. The procedure consisted of striking parts of the body, notably the chest, with the palm of the hand, thus eliciting a series of sounds and tactile sensations. Percussion was especially important in lung diseases, as the normal resonance of these air-filled organs could change, revealing areas of dullness that suggested the presence of fluid or inflammatory deposits. Two years later, in 1808, Corvisart published a French translation of the Austrian physician's *Inventum Novum*, thereby providing a critical impetus for the integration of pathological anatomy and physical diagnosis. Another academic, Pierre Piorry, developed an indirect method of percussion that employed a small hammer and an ivory plate called the *pleximeter* to detect similar changes. His prize-winning presentation of 1826 signaled the advent of another valuable technique for improving physical diagnosis.[82]

Another diagnostic scheme, developed in the early 1800s by François Chaussier (1746–1828), the first professor of anatomy and physiology at the Paris Medical School, recommended a five-step procedure to check vital functions—respiration, circulation, voluntary motion, sensibility, temperature, and sleep. He then tested sensory activities such as vision, smell, hearing, taste, and touch, followed by mental ones, including perception, memory, and judgment. These examinations continued with an assessment of nutritional status, digestion, secretions, excretions, and genital functions. A brief interrogation of the patient, disclosing individual circumstances such as age, gender, constitution, lifestyle, occupation, previous health, onset of symptoms, and prior treatment preceded or followed this functional review.[83]

French physicians believed that mastering diagnosis was part of an expanding and specialized clinical knowledge that would pay off in the form of prestigious hospital posts and lucrative private practices. This belief stood in sharp contrast to the uncertainty and ignorance displayed by healers whom the medical profession labeled "dangerous empirics."[84] Within that same context, Pinel's earlier nosological efforts had been advertised as removing "the emphatic promises of charlatanism which pretends to cure all diseases and does not see in the violence and order of their symptoms anything but a sort of harmony and gathering of preservative efforts."[85] Early-nineteenth-century practitioners thus strained to achieve precise diagnoses and to issue equally accurate prognoses of their carefully constructed disease entities. The new level of medical certainty rooted in anatomical–clinical correlations was part of a strategy of professional and social rehabilitation for men who had witnessed the low public opinion of their activities before and after the Revolution. The catch phrase "medicine of observation" became emblematic of efforts that also stressed scientific respectability.[86] However, while the rhetoric was impressive, public opinion remained skeptical. "Society repeats the trite accusation that medicine is a conjectural art," complained Corvisart as he enumerated the "obstacles and snares" responsible for the uncertainty that was popularly attributed to medicine. To deflect such criticisms, Corvisart suggested that humanity stop demanding "health from the healing art" and abandon hopes for greater longevity.[87]

After accepting the post of resident physician at the Necker Hospital in 1816, nearly two years before Jacques Dumesnil's admission, Laennec continued to employ another physical examination technique: direct auscultation. This procedure, of Hippocratic origins, consisted in listening with the ear directly applied to the patient's chest for respiratory and cardiac sounds. Direct auscultation, however, like direct percussion, was limited because physicians often failed to discern the expected sounds while making their suffering patients even more uncomfortable. In addition, this technique raised concerns about professional rights of access to the bodies of the sick, particularly in the case of paying patients. In hospitals, the privacy of patients was less of a concern to caregivers, but the practice was made somewhat repugnant by the sometimes unwashed, foul-smelling inmates.

Shortly after assuming his post at the Necker Hospital, Laennec claimed to have discovered that heart and lung sounds could be amplified and transmitted through a rolled-up notebook. In the introduction to his treatise, Laennec insisted that he had made this discovery around October 1816 after being called to the bedside of a private patient, a plump young woman suffering from heart disease. Faced with the awkward and potentially embarrassing prospect of pressing his ear to her chest, Laennec rolled a sheaf of paper—probably one of his hospital notebooks—into a cylinder to listen for chest sounds at a distance. To his utter surprise, the improvised tube transmitted the sounds quite clearly.[88] Eventually, Laennec reproduced the acoustics of the improvised, fragile instrument using a one-foot-long wooden cylinder one and one-half inches in diameter, equipped with a funnel-shaped cavity at the end to further enhance the sound. The cylinder could be disassembled into two parts for easier carrying. It was called a *stethoscope*— from the Greek *stethos*, meaning "breast" or "chest," and *skopein*, meaning "to explore."[89] Moreover, this instrument could be employed through light clothing.

Armed with this device, Laennec would develop a systematic examination technique and organize his acoustic findings. The first such examination in the hospital, on March 8, 1817, involved a 40-year-old woman with bilateral pneumonia ("respiration explored with help of the cylinder"). As a novel form of physical diagnosis, indirect, stethoscope-mediated auscultation was not a sudden discovery but part of a process. Already familiar with sounds obtained from placing their ears directly on the patient's chest, physicians such as Laennec faced the task of correlating a host of newly obtained tones with the familiar pathology derived from dissections. This meant working with a large number of carefully selected patients and cadavers. Using the (often tubercular) patients in a ward reserved for acute fevers, Laennec came to link a number of chest sounds with the underlying changes in the lungs. He apparently combined the skills of a good listener with those of a consummate dissector.

Laennec's findings were first published in a two-volume text, *De l'auscultation médiate, ou traité du diagnostic des maladies des poumons et du coeur*, published in 1819. The book illustrated his ideas of how to achieve an anatomical–clinical synthesis. It not only extended techniques of physical diagnosis as important adjuncts of the new pathological anatomy, but also established the legitimacy of an approach that melded medical and surgical perspectives.[90] Indeed, Laennec sought to emphasize the superiority of what he called the "anatomical" instead of the clinical or "symptomatic" description of diseases. Moreover, "morbid anatomy must, I think, be considered as the surest guide of the physician, as well to the diagnosis as to the cure of diseases," he wrote.[91] Laennec's diagnostic successes depended on the sick poor who died in the Necker Hospital. Among the largest group of his patients were textile and fashion workers, including Jacques.

Auscultation provided a dynamic picture of the lesions within the natural evolution of the disease under study.[92] Although the purpose of extensive pathological knowledge was primarily diagnostic, Laennec also insisted that this information would influence therapeutics. In a final word of caution, he spoke of pathological anatomy's "obscure points," including the frequent inability to distinguish among slight macroscopic changes, the confusion between causes and effects, and postmortem artifacts. While conscious of the limitations inherent in the anatomical approach, Laennec nevertheless tried to establish criteria by which practitioners could equate lesions, functions, and causes. As the case of Monsieur Dumesnil demonstrates, he kept extensive records of many of his public hospital cases, although the actual writing of clinical histories and autopsy reports was assigned to his students. Such documentation was included in his 1819 book. An expanded second edition followed in 1826, presenting more clinico–pathological correlations based on chest sounds.

Life at the Necker Hospital

Laennec, together with his interns and students at the Necker Hospital, carefully interviewed and examined prospective patients such as Jacques Dumesnil. By this time, a small room had been outfitted at the hospital to screen new arrivals medically, since the Sisters of Charity no longer functioned as institutional gatekeepers. Perhaps Laennec had some preference for cases that would provide opportunities for practicing auscultation. Patients accepted by the institution were assigned to different wards according to their presumptive diseases. Jacques' destination was the Salle St. Joseph, a 28-bed ward reserved for male fever patients, where he occupied bed 28 (labels placed in front of the beds contained numbers for reference purposes). By this time, difficult-to-clean wooden beds had been replaced by single iron-framed ones prudently spaced three feet apart to allow proper circulation of air, caregivers, and students.[93] These beds, with their blue cotton covers, were surrounded by white curtains in the summer, blue ones during the winter.

As elsewhere, rituals at the Necker Hospital included at least two daily medical visits, one in the morning by the chief physician and pharmacist, one in the afternoon by an assistant, in each case accompanied by interns and students. Laennec described his average day as extremely busy. He got up before 7.30–8.00 AM, providing some consultations even while dressing. Rules specified that he had to visit all patients twice a day and more often if they were quite sick. Morning rounds were made at 8 AM in the company of two Sisters of Charity, the apothecary, the nurse in charge of the ward, and students. Laennec checked the *cahier de visite* or ledger containing medical orders written the previous night, listened to a verbal progress report from the Sister in charge, and allowed the surgeon to perform minor procedures such as bloodletting and bandaging. New prescriptions were dictated in Latin at the bedside. After rounds, Laennec was supposed to supervise the preparation of the remedies ordered earlier.[94] All these activities were repeated during late afternoons and evenings, with a one-hour break for supper. Finally, Laennec devoted the last hour before bedtime at 11 PM to his correspondence.[95]

Visits to individual patients during rounds were at the center of well-choreographed rituals that patients awaited with great anticipation. Before Laennec's arrival, all cleaning chores had to be completed, with bedpans and spittoons collected for possible inspection by the caregivers. Physicians and students were periodically reminded of the psychological impact of these visits, with suggestions that the *chef de service* always act in a consoling and reassuring manner even when recovery was not expected. In the opinion of shrewd clinicians, such an attitude was more efficacious than all the available remedies. Frequent testimony of interest from physicians was deemed important, and the round makers were encouraged to question patients occasionally about matters "extraneous to the visit" that, in the view of one author, "more than once contribute to a better night, [and] decreased anxiety, as well as deaden[ing] the pain through the magic influence of calm, care, and security."[96] After all, the progress of a patient's bodily ills was closely linked in the medical mind of the time to the emotional reactions to sickness.

Jacques' chest was carefully examined on February 13, 1819, the day after his admission. Physical examinations now assumed greater importance than ever before. They were preferably carried out during the day to allow for better light. Presumably Jacques was febrile, but neither temperature nor pulse readings are available. Instead, we are left with selected information including detailed descriptions of physical signs of disease elicited by the physicians. According to Laennec, an echo could be heard—upon percussion—while the patient's respiration remained strong. The *pectoriloquy* (pectus, breast, and loqui—"to speak") consisted of an exaggerated sound of words or fremitus heard through the chest wall, a new sign of disease discovered by Laennec with the help of the stethoscope. For the resident physician, this finding usually suggested a cavity or consolidation of lung tissue immediately below the placement of his cylinder. As the examination proceeded, the echo continued to be evident under Jacques' right armpit and toward the top of the lung just next to the joint between the clavicle and the humerus. For the experienced Laennec there probably was little doubt: Jacques suffered from a cavity at the top of the right lung.[97] The diagnosis was *phthisis* (tuberculosis), the most common and most lethal disease in contemporary Paris.[98]

But what to do? Dietary orders were now a central component of a cautious medical regimen that largely followed the natural history of the disease in question. As Pinel declared, "dietetics offers endless resources if it is skillfully used and strictly delimits medication.[99] Unlike the Latin drug prescriptions, these recommendations were deliberately issued in a loud, intelligible voice and in French to inform the patient and thus avoid future misunderstandings and bickering with the nurses when meals were served.[100] A key food was the vegetarian or meat *bouillon*, a traditional French soup, with half a bowl first served with the medications upon rising at 6.30 AM. Other servings were distributed at three-hour intervals throughout the day. Wine was de rigeur: it retained its traditional religious and cultural value and therefore was liberally provided to both adults and children together with the prescribed medical diet.

At the Necker Hospital, the midmorning bouillon was followed by a 2.30 PM collation with baked potatoes and bread with jam. Supper was at 5 PM, with bread and meat and more bouillon served at the discretion of the caregivers. In the case of tuberculosis, a milk-based diet—cow or goat's—with potato or cassava starch, and rice or barley, was traditional. Rest was important, although several physicians advised early ambulation and the use of chairs for convalescents still too weak to spend much time wandering through common halls. Here "the pleasure of company or conversation might speed convalescence, and so might innocuous diversions," including a pool table, swings, bowling games, short walks, and gardening.[101] Friends and relatives were always encouraged to visit. At the Necker Hospital the wards were ventilated as well as possible through the enlarged windows, and some institutions also burned aromatic leaves to neutralize the pervasive stench.

Regarding Jacques' treatment, Laennec probably followed a palliative approach since he seemed to share the general opinion that phthisis could not be cured: "the tubercular affection, like cancer, is absolutely incurable, inasmuch as nature's efforts towards effecting a cure are injurious and those of art are useless."[102] Like others, Laennec admitted that this disease had been subjected, with little success, to a great variety of often opposing and contradictory treatments. A few patients were subjected to bloodletting or had leeches applied on chest areas considered to be affected. The intent was merely to diminish the inflammatory process in the underlying lung tissues. There was no hope of preventing the development of tubercles.

Although medical practitioners throughout Europe had since the 1770s become more skeptical about prevailing treatments, the new pathological anatomy failed to provide any new guidelines for action. At the turn of the century, French therapeutics remained purely empirical, deprived of all causal or theoretical underpinnings traditionally employed to justify the use of drugs. In fact, the ubiquitous and extensive nature of the organic lesions prevalent in patients created the impression that the vaunted healing power of nature was inadequate to stem the force of disease. Perhaps nature actually contributed to the formation of lesions. This had led Corvisart, for example, to question one of the central features of ancient Greek medicine: the essentially harmonious character of an individual's constitution, the idiosyncratic humoral blend sustained by the body's internal forces. In Corvisart's less optimistic perception, constitutional variations contributed to the formation of multiple diseases as organ systems were subjected to the destructive influences of particular lifestyles and occupations. Unfortunately, local lesions could seldom be reversed by generalized treatments. The best therapy, based on the presence of lesions exposed by pathological anatomy, was surgery. Once established, the lesions seemed irreversible and the long-term prognosis fatal. Since neither the external symptoms of a patient's illness nor the art of medicine were able to detect these internal bodily events in their early stages, most therapeutic efforts were merely palliative. The new ontology of disease based on such lesions converted hospital physicians into spectators who helplessly witnessed the relentless natural progression of these diseases without being able to arrest them or address the physical and psychological needs of patients.[103]

Yet, as Laennec's experience with private patients showed, there was always hope of a spontaneous cure for phthisis. Laennec accepted the possibility that once emptied of pathological material, lung cavities could actually heal by producing a cartilaginous cover. Collapse and scarring were also possible outcomes observed in several autopsies. To dissolve and soften existing lesions and promote the evacuation of tubercular material, patients were given alkaline products, including lime water, salt of ammonia, carbonate of soda and ammonia, and aromatic oils, including camphor.[104] In Laennec's somewhat optimistic vision, the body occasionally made efforts to mature and evacuate the tuberculous matter, so that the perceived pectoriloquy could also be interpreted as a positive sign of possible recovery. To prevent excessive coughing, patients such as Jacques received small doses of an extract of belladonna mixed with syrup and a mucilaginous tisane or tea prepared with gum Arabic powder to facilitate expectoration. At the Necker Hospital, physicians also dispensed pills or a syrup containing a mixture of narcotics to reduce coughing and facilitate sleep. These remedies contained opium, seeds of black henbane—hyoscyamus—and root of hound's tongue—cynoglossus—prepared with saffron and myrrh.[105]

At this time, periodic revisions of existing pharmacopoeias and the wholesale elimination of ineffective drugs were in full swing. French hospital physicians usually had been allowed to prescribe freely from among an array of medications stocked in an institution's pharmacy. But, after 1803, doctors began following the *Pharmacopée à l'usage des hospices civils* prepared by Parmentier, a dispensatory sponsored by the Conseil General d'Administration des Hôpitaux, of which Parmentier was a member. Like their colleagues in other European countries, French practitioners became skeptical of the therapeutic powers of numerous traditional compounds, preferring instead to employ a few simple drugs, including purgatives, emetics, tonics, and painkillers and, as Pinel declared, "assist the healing powers of nature and provide a solid base for the art of medicine."[106] A veritable foe of polypharmacy, Pinel strongly suggested that "the physician's medication should be simple and scientific. It should comprise only uncomplicated substances such as alkalis of soda and potash, ammonia, mineral acids, a few neutral salts, oxides of antimony, iron, mercury, etc. prepared with the greatest precision."[107]

In general, Laennec and other French physicians rejected bloodletting, blisters, stimulants, and the inhalation of various gases in the treatment of phthisis. However, impressed by the therapeutic qualities of the mild climate near the sea, Laennec advocated the creation of an "artificial marine atmosphere" in a hospital ward with the help of fresh seaweed spread around the premises.[108] He also followed the ancient practice of cauterizing the patient's chest—documented in Hippocratic writings and experienced by Theodoros Prodromos in Byzantium. The procedure consisted in the application of an incandescent copper or iron rod below the clavicles and scapulas creating up to 12–15 burns, an ordeal to which few patients dared to submit. Instead, eighteenth-century physicians now produced isolated blisters with potassium hydroxide, a popular caustic, placed on the patient's inner thigh to limit the inflammatory force of the disease and thus prevent the secondary miliary eruption of tubercles throughout the body.

For the next two months, Jacques apparently had no additional symptoms. During this time, however, the pectoriloquy was repeatedly verified by Laennec and his students. As mentioned in his notes on the case, if the stethoscope was placed under Jacques' right clavicle, one could obtain a sound suggesting that he was actually breathing directly through the wooden cylinder itself. Examiners also noticed that to obtain a more obvious pectoriloquy, it was necessary to press the cylinder lightly on the patient's body. If they pressed harder, the sound became quite muffled. Laennec surmised that the presumed tubercular lesion was located very close to the surface of the lung; if the cylinder was pressed harder, the pectoriloquy became softer and consequently less evident. These examinations, often performed for the benefit of students, raised the issue of patient comfort. However, the stethoscope was easy to apply and did not noticeably disturb patients such as Jacques, since the sounds could be obtained through the bed clothing. Since available case notes were designed to bolster the stethoscopic findings, no mention was made of other diagnostic studies such as the examination of the patient's sputum, a common routine. In Jacques' case, the expectorated matter must have had the appearance of dull white granules, believed to originate in the softened tubercles and caverns of the lung. Another expert of this disease, Bayle, compared them with well-boiled rice, whereas the Hippocratic writings had referred to them as grains of hail. When physicians placed the secretions in a jar filled with water, the somewhat cheesy matter rapidly fell to the bottom, dividing into small lumps and giving the water a milky tint.[109]

At the Necker Hospital, Jacques was cared for by a small nursing staff of Sisters of Charity and their lay assistants. The Sisters had successfully guided the institution through the turmoil of the Revolutionary period. Now, during the Bourbon Restoration, nursing had definitely taken a back seat to medicine. At the center of previous controversies between Sisters and attending physicians had been matters of diet. In most cases, hospital doctors had strongly opposed as detrimental to patient recovery all the snacks, soups, and cookies provided as charitable gestures. In the eyes of the religious caregivers, the issue of feeding continued to be inextricably linked to notions of humanitarian care seldom stressed by the new graduates of the Parisian medical school. The hard-working Sisters continued to pride themselves on their provision of compassionate care, talking with the patients, calming their fears, and consoling them in their hours of greatest suffering.

Because of their administrative and clinical experience, the nuns nonetheless remained powerful competitors, particularly to inexperienced young students prowling around the wards. As with their pre-Revolutionary predecessors, their religious identification also insulated them from images of seduction and promiscuity traditionally attached to those nursing functions involving intimacy and physical contact. The rivalry between the physicians and the Sisters was variously expressed in a series of conflicting discourses mixing images of female compassion and male callousness with recalcitrant religious authority, dangerous quackery, and scientific enlightenment.[110]

But could the average physician maintain a sympathetic and caring attitude in hospitals? Laennec, like Corvisart, seems to have been aware of the psychological status of his poor patients. In an experiment conducted among wounded soldiers from Brittany hospitalized at the Salpêtrière in 1814, Laennec placed them together in a single ward and assigned to the unit some Breton physicians who spoke their dialect. The patients' emotional and physical improvement confirmed Laennec's impression that these new opportunities for socialization and mutual support between patients and caregivers had important healing qualities.[111] The same effect could be achieved through a liberal visiting policy, allowing patients easier access to relatives and friends.

On April 17, Jacques complained of a light pain in his abdomen. At this point his lower legs became slightly swollen; pressing the skin around the ankle retained an impression of the finger. His genitals were also mildly infiltrated with fluid. Laennec examined the patient's chest with his stethoscope. Respirations were weak, tending to be heard more toward the back right area of the chest cavity, and now were accompanied by crackling sounds suggesting the presence of fluid. These sounds were also heard on the left side of the chest. From that time on, the patient's condition gradually deteriorated until May 15. His abdomen swelled considerably and offered an obscure fluctuation to the feeling hand, while his legs grew in size. His penis and scrotum were enormously distended. The patient now experienced a light but constant pain in his abdomen, but otherwise, he felt rather well. He urinated infrequently, but without any pain. Jacques' thirst was moderate; his appetite was small, but his overall strength was not noticeably diminished.[112]

Subjected to repeated stethoscopic examinations by Laennec and his entourage, Jacques' chest echoed a bit less on the right side than on the left. His respirations were faint and accompanied by an intermittent gurgle, always in the upper right portion of his chest. The rales were not apparent in the lower thoracic cavity but were replaced there by a slightly mucous sound. Pectoriloquy was faint under the right armpit and collarbone. An ominous note was added to the diagnostic sheet: pulmonary edema of the right lung. The patient's heartbeat became extremely feeble. Like most of his contemporaries, Laennec probably refused to share the gloomy news with his patient, afraid that the truth would snuff out Jacques' persistently upbeat attitude concerning his prognosis.

During the next few days, Jacques seemed to feel better. His breathing was a bit stronger and less uncomfortable. The swelling in his abdomen, thighs, and genitals subsided. He even coughed and spat much less than he had since his admission. Spring was in the air, and a tenuous optimism began to grip him; he thought that he was getting better. But the hoped-for improvement was temporary. Soon the edema in Jacques' legs reappeared and his abdomen swelled considerably, now displaying an obvious fluctuation. As the last days of May passed, the patient continued rapidly to waste away and weaken. New strong pains toward the left iliac area of his lower abdomen created significant discomfort, and he could sleep only on his back. His breathing became very labored. As Laennec remarked on May 29, one could barely hear it without the help of the cylinder, and on the right side of the chest the breath sounds were replaced by a partially sibilant mucous sound. Conscious to the end, Jacques Dumesnil finally died on June 5, 1819, and a routine autopsy was scheduled to begin 15 hours later. He had been hospitalized for 114 days.[113]

Since the Revolution, the availability of cadavers for dissection obtained from Parisian hospitals was quite impressive. At this time, the large Hôtel Dieu furnished close to 5,000 bodies per year. Hospital dissections, however, carried a significant additional risk of infection for those who carried them out. In the early nineteenth century, over 60% of the dissecting students in Paris were said to have been affected by what was then euphemistically called *hospital fever*, at times highly lethal.[114] Laennec probably was anxious to dissect his former patient, hoping to confirm his stethoscopic findings at a time when the new findings with this instrument were still tentative and subject to further refinement for his forthcoming book. Jacques' body was characterized by a purple face, swollen abdomen, and swollen legs, with thin, spindly arms. The right side of his chest contained almost half a pint of a limpid, yellowish secretion that flowed out of the chest as the sternum was lifted, even though the body was on its back. Laennec and his colleagues noted that the secretion was contained between the sternum, mediastinum, and lung. The fluid was forced back toward the superior, posterior, and exterior part of the thoracic cavity, and it adhered lightly to the pleura near the ribs. This adherence took place in the middle of a yellow, opaque, membranous lining that was very firm, appearing almost cartilaginous near the top of the lung. Did this represent early natural healing? On other areas of the pleura, dissectors discovered a scattering of small, white, opaque tubercles as big as millet grains.[115]

According to the report, these tubercles were lifted easily by scraping the pleura with the blade of a scalpel. All three lobes of the lung were fused together with scar tissue. Many tubercles had developed on the internal surface of these cellular cysts. In the upper lobe the tissue was flaccid, almost dry, with no traces of blood oozing out even after some venules were cut; the color of the tissue was extremely dark gray-blue. At the very top of the lung, Laennec noticed two dilated bronchial tubes that seemed to turn into a dead end in a section of lung tissue as big as a nut that was extremely firm and difficult to cut. The left lung was a bit larger than the right. Attached to the pleura by two or three thin, white, rather firm membranes, the lung was immersed in almost four ounces of a thin, watery fluid. The tissue was also crepitant, reddish, and infiltrated with a sputum-like secretion but without a trace of tubercles. The abdominal cavity contained at least four pints of liquid. A large number of dark yellow tubercles riddled the entire liver. On the entire interior surface of the peritoneum Laennec and his students discovered a soft, opaque secretion presenting as a very thin line with colors ranging from pale yellow to reddish to black. This membranous secretion featured an enormous number of white, opaque tubercles similar to those found on the right pleura but larger, about the size of a hemp seed.

Since the case was titled by Laennec as "coexistence of pectoriloquy and egophony in a subject attacked by partial hydrothorax sometime after the recovery from a tuberculous excavation," it certainly is possible that our resident physician had remained somewhat optimistic about Jacques' chances of recovery until the middle of May, when generalized swelling and wasting away signaled a downhill course. Laennec was also interested in linking tuberculosis with certain occupations and working conditions.[116] No doubt, along with others, this case played an important role in further shaping the opinions Laennec expressed about the disease in his 1819 treatise. Again the body of a working-class hospital patient had exposed its mysteries, contributing to the growth of medical knowledge and the prestige of physicians such as Laennec.

Parisian hospitals: Teaching and research

The pre-Revolutionary Paris Medical School did not officially include clinical training in its curriculum, although it had supported an elaborate system of surgical apprenticeship since the 1740s. Working without pay in exchange for training, 50–70 *externes*—a two-year stint for young surgeons—trained with a dozen *commissionaires* who received meals there together with another dozen *compagnons* or *internes* in charge. Interns lived in the hospital and worked under a chief resident student, the *gagnant-maitrise*. He, in turn, reported to a chief hospital surgeon.[117] Since surgeons significantly outnumbered physicians, they regularly took care of both surgical and medical patients admitted to the hospital. Before the Revolution, the Hôtel Dieu's status as a surgical training institution—contested earlier by the College of Surgery—received a decisive boost with the appointment of Pierre J. Desault (1738–1795) as *chef de service* in 1785. Desault converted the rather informal training experience into an elaborate educational program that combined hands-on bedside teaching with lectures and surgical demonstrations. Both were delivered in a new amphitheater, while the postmortem dissections took place in the morgue. After 1787, Desault oversaw the reforms implemented by Colombier, then the inspector of hospitals and prisons, to achieve a measure of medical control over the internal management of the institution. This generated the previously discussed series of bitter confrontations with the Augustinian nuns.[118] At the same time, Colombier and others issued calls for the unification of medicine with surgery and the creation of clinical training in which students would play a hands-on role.

Another important institution for pre- and post-Revolutionary clinical instruction in Paris was the Hôpital de la Charité—not to be confused with Jacques' hospice—a 230-bed hospital devoted exclusively to male patients. Here Louis Desbois de Rochefort (1750–1786) had initiated a private course of bedside instruction in 1780, largely based on Stoll's contemporary Viennese model. In 1788, Rochefort was succeeded by his able assistant, Corvisart, who also made daily morning rounds with students, examining and prescribing for his own 40-bed ward patients. Like Cullen in Edinburgh and Stoll in Vienna, Corvisart was particularly interested in using the patient's symptoms and physical signs to improve the diagnostic skills of his students. To obtain a more complete clinical picture, Corvisart employed palpation and Auenbrugger's direct percussion. As in Frank's Vienna, his mandatory autopsies attempted to link clinical and pathological manifestations of disease.[119]

As Pinel declared in the 1790s, the best medical teachers were patients. Following his appointment in 1791 as chief physician at Bicêtre, Pinel began teaching at the institution's infirmary. Convinced of the value of bedside observations, Pinel suggested that both physicians and students walking the wards regularly take detailed notes on the various manifestations and stages of disease. Since many individuals suffered from several ailments simultaneously, their symptoms were quite variable and confusing. Pinel therefore advocated an observational strategy, his so-called analysis, designed to break down difficult and often baffling manifestations of disease. Methodically, Pinel tried to separate and assemble them into distinct symptom sequences that could be related to specific disease descriptions available in his nosology.[120]

By the fall of 1792, the war had already killed many army physicians; civilian and military hospitals suffered severe shortages of qualified surgeons and physicians. Although Vicq d'Azyr had provided a blueprint for a unified medical-surgical school a year earlier through the Committee on Health of the Constitutional Assembly, no legislative action had followed. To make matters worse, the Legislative Assembly in August 1792 abolished all "privileged associations," including universities, scientific societies, and professional guilds. Educating replacements for the medical military corps came to be a makeshift effort loosely based on anatomical dissections, apprenticeships, and hospital experience. Then, in August 1793, new legislation virtually doubled the size of the French army. All remaining physicians, surgeons, pharmacists, and even medical students between the ages of 18 and 40 became eligible for the draft. Reforming France's educational system became urgent as the shortage of trained military surgeons worsened. Finally, Antoine F. Fourcroy (1755–1809), a former member of the Ancien Régime's Academy of Sciences, was charged with preparing a new education plan modeled after formal surgical apprenticeships. Pinel's 1793 essay on the "clinical training of physicians" provided further suggestions for medical reform, including once more the union of medicine and surgery and the prominent use of hospitals for clinical education.[121]

Prompted by France's chronic shortage of qualified medical personnel and the abbreviated path of medical studies, the number of students soared. Although access to the wards was restricted, instructors soon witnessed their clinical rounds degenerate into disorderly spectacles compromising both bedside teaching and patient welfare. In 1796, for example, one foreign observer at the Hôtel Dieu described in vivid detail the surgical rounds conducted by Philippe J. Pelletan, Desault's successor. As the professor went from bed to bed, he was pushed around by a crowd of noisy students, five deep, who pushed from behind onto the patient's bed. Others, unable to witness the proceedings, climbed on stools and nearby bed frames to catch a glimpse. Broken furniture and constant shoving and shouting between master and students were routine.[122]

During the Directory, France still urgently needed more practitioners to support its imperial ambitions. The official enrollment in 1798 was 900 medical students but a year later it rose to 1,200, creating serious difficulties for both in-structors and students because of a lack of resources. To accommodate the ever-growing number of students and foreign observers, instructors such as Corvisart and Pinel soon found it necessary to create programs of self-study. On May 29, 1801, Corvisart founded the Society for Medical Instruction at the Charité Hos-pital, a mutual teaching association designed especially for fourth-year students under the supervision of experienced teachers. Directed by gifted clinicians such as Bayle and Jean J. Leroux des Tillets (1749–1832), the Society sought to pro-vide its students—who included Jacques' attending physician, Laennec, and the experimentalist François Magendie—with a somewhat structured clinical educa-tion that imitated pre-Revolutionary models of private apprenticeships. Clinical research and instruction thus rapidly became a shared enterprise between teach-ers and students, allowing the latter a more active role.[123] A certain methodolog-ical rigor guided these efforts. An admission chronicle, daily progress notes, and a final discharge summary together with frequent autopsy reports constituted the clinical case record. Later these data were increasingly subjected to statistical analysis.

With consensus about a new program of medical teaching and investigation in sight, French physicians and students were optimistic that traditional medical notions could be challenged and even replaced with new knowledge obtained at the bedside and in the autopsy room of a hospital. Students examined patients, wrote clinical notes, and assisted in the performance of postmortem examinations. This makeshift partnership of teachers and students, originally promoted by a shortage of medical personnel, ultimately became the decisive innovation in French medical education. It eliminated the still largely passive type of instruction where-by students followed their professors on rounds as spectators. Later, the associa-tion between professors and students became critical when new techniques such as Laennec's auscultation method emerged. Learning such listening skills de-manded not only collaboration and a closer relationship between teacher and stu-dent, but also an independent hands-on approach by the students themselves try-ing to interpret the sounds detected by the famous cylinder.[124]

During the Consulate, on February 23, 1802, a new *Réglement Général pour le Service de Santé des Hôpitaux et Hospices Civils de Paris* appeared, creating a system of house officers based in part on pre-Revolutionary surgical models. The *élèves internes* in medicine and the *compagnons* in surgery resided in the hospital, while others, the *élèves externes*, just regularly visited the wards. The former served for four years, the latter for three; both had a chance to advance to resident physi-cian and ultimately to *chef de service*. The positions were assigned to those who passed a public examination. They rotated for one year through the main teach-ing hospitals—Hôtel Dieu, Charité, Hôpital des Veneriennes. In 1802 the gov-ernment authorized 24 *internes* positions, with the number slowly expanding to 30 by 1830. Its ostensible pedagogical purpose was to create a medical elite, but economic goals loomed larger: ensuring the regularity of hospital services and providing chiefs of service with competent young physicians on call who could troubleshoot and take care of all routines and emergencies in their absence.[125]

Interns usually spent a busy day on the wards. In the morning, they had to be on hand when the chief of the service made his rounds—usually between 8 and 9 AM—although surgeons such as Dupuytren made their visits much earlier, at 5 AM. In the afternoon, the interns made rounds again from 4 to 7 PM, registering their visits in journals called *cahiers de visite*. They usually remained on call for 24 hours and received free meals and lodging in the hospital. By requiring long hours on call and providing few opportunities to leave the institution, the system completely isolated young physicians from friends and family, as well as society at large. The hospital became not only their home, but also their entire universe. Most interns hailed from the provinces and, separated from their families, they constituted a lonely group in search of companionship.[126] When not making rounds on the wards, they usually gravitated toward the *salle de garde*—literally, the room for watchmen—a form of emergency and admission room at the heart of the hospital provided with living quarters for the house staff on call. Here not only were critical cases managed, but the overworked interns could relax, eat meals, organize boisterous parties, and bond. Their total immersion in patient management, especially constant monitoring of disease manifestations, was congruent with the original objective of the French medical leaders: to reconstruct the natural evolution of individual diseases. To achieve this goal, continuous observation of the unfolding symptoms and physical signs of a limited number of select patients was required, followed by systematic pathological confirmation and thus legitimation at the autopsy table. To transcend individual variations and achieve a degree of certainty in their disease constructions, multiple observations had to be carried out on a large population of patients. For this purpose, the Parisian hospital network provided a setting unparalleled anywhere else in the world.

Whether this intense scientific scrutiny of hospital patients—now reduced to the sum of their diseased organs—favored further depersonalization and even callousness toward suffering remains unclear. There was always a potential conflict between the professional aspirations of physicians and the needs of patients, but much depended on individual personalities in this new paternalistic relationship.[127] Patients were often terrified of hospitalization, sad and anxious after admission to the wards, but some came to respect the diagnostic skills of their physicians and remained hopeful of recovery. French practitioners, in turn, became proud of their diagnostic prowess but remained pessimistic about cures, although keen to provide their charges with all the necessary aids to bolster their natural healing forces. This involved providing proper rest and food but also improving the emotional state of the patients. Following the return of religious personnel to hospitals, the sacraments were routinely administered only at admission, since at any later time they could suggest an impending fatal outcome and thus dash the patient's hopes of recovery.[128] In Pinel's view, the psychological aspects of illness should never be neglected. Depression was common. Comforting words, whether uttered by physicians or nurses, could provide welcome reassurance.[129]

Such humanitarian exhortations suggest that students and house staff may have displayed indifference toward the plight of their patients, partly explained as a social class phenomenon but perhaps also as a function of the vast panorama of misery and suffering experienced on the crowded wards. Detachment and toughness were defensive adjustments learned within the rarefied atmosphere of these hot-houses of pathology. Because of military demands during the Revolution, the educational machinery to train scores of medical professionals had been cranked up under emergency conditions and kept in high gear during the Directory and Napoleon's reign. Still in high gear during the Bourbon Restoration, it now created by the 1820s a progressive glut of French medical graduates, with foreign students—many from America—increasingly joining them for rounds and lectures.[130]

The patient's body:
Centerpiece of medical learning

After publishing the first edition of his treatise, Laennec retired to his ancestral home in Brittany for two years on account of his own chronic ailment, which he considered "nervous." True to his own views, he lived near the seashore in the hope that the milder climate would bring about his recovery from a condition he attributed to stress and malnutrition. Upon returning to Paris in late 1821, Laennec resumed his post at the Necker Hospital until March 1823, when he received an appointment at the Charité Hospital. Among other honors, he was nominated to the chair of medicine at the College de France. Although he also continued to see an increasing number of private patients, Laennec devoted most of his energy to hospital practice and writing. The second edition of his book was published only weeks before his death on August 13, 1826. At the age of 45, Laennec died from tuberculosis, the disease he had so carefully studied.[131] In his final years, at both the Necker and Charité hospitals, Laennec was surrounded by physicians and students, many of them foreign visitors—including a contingent from Edinburgh—who were anxious to learn about the artful cylinder that could detect the presence of several diseased organs. In time, Laennec's stethoscope and its multiple varieties would become the symbol of medical professional identity. In Jacques' time, however, this instrument merely epitomized the newly negotiated access to the human body and the epistemological shift resulting from physical examinations of the sick.

Although the so-called medicalization of the hospital had its early roots in

Byzantium and was further advanced during the Renaissance in Italy, the Enlightenment fostered ideal conditions for a central medical presence in institutions devoted to the care of the sick.[132] In France this process was quite remarkable, linked to particular political, economic, and cultural contexts before and after the Revolution. During the Ancien Régime, many hospitals had remained discredited welfare institutions with primary custodial functions. Their transformation into medical organizations occurred during the tumultuous Revolutionary years and under successive governments, including the Consulate and the Empire. However, the hospital system could not have survived without the enduring presence of the religious nurses, who may have seemed like an anachronism to their medical brethren, but who not only kept these establishments functioning in the face of overwhelming budget cuts, but also provided personal care to ease the sufferings of those who were admitted.

What was truly unique about the French hospital experience? First of all, the size and number of institutions comprising the Parisian hospital system devoted to sick care was greater than that of any urban area of the world.[133] Moreover, traditional French welfare schemes and class differences accentuated the depersonalization and loss of autonomy of the hospitalized poor, contributing to greater bureaucratic control and a new physician–patient relationship.[134] With institutional cross-infections and persistent high mortality, these hospitals provided the necessary human tools for advances in clinical medicine and pathological anatomy. In the controlled ward environments, substantial numbers of inmates, alive and dead, were selected for systematic study, classification, and dissection.

Most remarkable were the implications of accurately mapping the sick body with the new techniques of physical examination. As another strategy to achieve greater diagnostic certainty and improve professional identity, these investigations came to rest on the discomfort of poor hospital inmates whose privacy could be violated in the quest for new knowledge. Although both the pleximeter—the thin ivory plate placed on the skin to be struck by a small hammer in indirect percussion—and the stethoscope were ostensibly developed to ameliorate patient discomfort, they were also designed to distance the examiner from his lower-class patients and thus prevent contagion. The new world of sounds and tactile sensations became the exclusive patrimony of professionals, displacing the role of patients' as providers of information about their illnesses previously deemed essential. This shift had significant implications for the healing relationship. Paradoxically, these new diagnostic rituals came to reinforce the importance of physicians' own sense perceptions and their capacity to individualize the art of medicine. In time, intimate explorations employing the stethoscope created new opportunities for personal relationships with those being examined, including performance of the healing touch. Although threatened by newer methods of bodily scanning and now employed by other health professionals, the successors of Laennec's cylinder remain the most visible and powerful symbols of Western physicians.

Another important French development was the creation of a comprehensive program of medical education and research centered on clinical studies in hospitals. This system was highly competitive, hierarchical, and predicated on the continuous presence and teaming up of physicians, interns, and students, whose narrow goal was to acquire diagnostic skills and advance the medical knowledge of particular diseases. In the ensuing decades, the Paris Medical School and its teaching hospitals became the most famous medical-educational institutions in the world, a Mecca for thousands of foreign students anxious to make ward rounds with some of the most distinguished French clinicians and surgeons.[135] To this day, this method of bedside teaching at hospitals—previously noted in Edinburgh and Vienna—has remained one of the central aspects of medical education. New in Paris, however, was the strategy of total immersion in hospital life—reflected in management routines with long and exhausting hours of work—that similarly survive as a rite of passage for professional and later specialty certification. Both aspects of Western medical training endure, based on the original premise that frequent bedside vigils are indispensable for obtaining the necessary clinical understanding and experience.

Although events in Edinburgh and Vienna hinted at a modest role for the hospital in medical research, Parisian institutions went considerably further. They became the central space for the creation of new medical knowledge, the source of medical certainty and professional authority. Suffering patients became clinical research material. Faced with a bewildering array of patient complaints and symptoms, French physicians gradually demoted the often unreliable patient histories. Pathological findings obtained under more controlled circumstances at the autopsy table became central. In a complete turnabout—a veritable epistemological break[136]—pathology came to rule clinical medicine, narrowing medicine's attention to those acute complaints that could be rapidly correlated with significant internal lesions otherwise undetectable by the eye. The human body ceased to be a mysterious black box and was reduced instead to a collection of organ systems and tissues in constant flux. In the end, the collective effort of a generation of practitioners and students working in Parisian hospital wards and dissection rooms provided the foundations for an approach that sought the answers to human illness in an anatomical–clinical synthesis soon to become both the hallmark and the shortcoming of modern medicine.[137]

NOTES

1. Jacques Tenon, *Memoirs on Paris Hospitals* (1788), ed. with intro. by D. B. Weiner, Canton, MA, Science History Pub., 1996, p. 43. For a summary of Tenon's ideas see L. S. Greenbaum, " 'Measure of Civilization': The hospital thought of Jacques Tenon on the eve of the French Revolution," *Bull Hist Med* 49 (1975): 43–56.

2. Félix S. Ratier, *A Practical Formulary of the Parisian Hospitals* (1823), trans. from French, Edinburgh, R. Buchanan, 1830, p. 7.

3. S. Barsa and C. R. Michel, *La Vie Quotidienne des Hôpitaux en France au XIXe Siècle*, Paris, Hachette, 1985, especially pp. 30–40.

4. This case summary, titled in Laennec's hand "Coexistence of pectoriloquy and egophony in a subject attacked by hydrothorax (partial) some time after the recovery from tuberculous excavation" (my trans.), was written up by one of his students. Musée Laennec, Bibliothèque Universitaire de Nantes, MS Classeur I, lot b, feuilles 183–88. This case is also listed in L. Boulle et al., eds., *Laennec, Catalogue des Manuscripts Scientifiques*, Paris, Masson, 1982, p. 28. I am grateful to Dr. Jacalyn Duffin for allowing me to study a copy of this manuscript and to David Barnes and Deirdre O'Reilly for helping me decipher and translate the document.

5. Lydie Boulle, "Hôpitaux Parisiens: Malades et maladies à l'heure des Revolutions," Ph.D. diss, École Practique des Hautes Études, Paris, 1986. The pioneering publication in this field remains Erwin H. Ackerknecht, *Medicine at the Paris Hospital, 1794–1848*, Baltimore, Johns Hopkins Univ. Press, 1967.

6. For details see Louis Chevalier, *La Formation de la Population Parisienne au XIXe Siècle*, Paris, Presses Univ. de France, 1950.

7. Louis Chevalier, *Labouring Classes and Dangerous Classes*, trans. F. Jellinek, New York, H. Fertig, 1973.

8. See Guillaume de Bertier de Sauvigny, *The Bourbon Restoration*, trans. L. M. Case, Philadelphia, Univ. of Pennsylvania Press, 1966, especially pp. 236–67 and pp. 257–64.

9. Ibid., pp. 300–27.

10. For a detailed floor plan see Conseil General d'Administration des Hospices (Seine, France), *Plans des hôpitaux et hospices civils de la ville de Paris*, Paris, 1820. The Necker Hospital—a former monastery—had only three sides, with the chapel forming one of the axes, and retained the traditional interior courtyard.

11. A temporary expansion to 140 beds occurred on January 1, 1814, to house victims of a typhus fever epidemic.

12. For details see Jacalyn Duffin, *To See with a Better Eye: A Life of R. T. H. Laennec*, Princeton, Princeton Univ. Press, 1998.

13. For an overview of the French institutional context consult G. Weisz, "The medical elite in France in the early nineteenth century," *Minerva* 251 (1987): 150–70, and his *The Medical Mandarins, the French Academy of Medicine in the Nineteenth and Early Twentieth Centuries*, New York, Oxford Univ. Press, 1995.

14. See extract from Conseil General d'Administration des Hospices (Seine, France), *Rapport fait au conseil general des hospices* (1816), in Raymond Gervais, *Histoire de l'Hôpital Necker (1778–1885)*, Paris, A. Parent, 1885, pp. 136–37.

15. Ibid.

16. See the chart in Michael Friedländer, *Entwurf einer Geschichte der Armen und Armenanstalten nebst einer Nachricht von dem jetzigen Zustande der Pariser Armenanstalten und Hospitäler insbesondere in November 1803*, Leipzig, Göschen, 1804.

17. Gervais, *Histoire*, p. 73.

18. In providing us Jacques' name, Laennec may have violated a law of medical confidentiality passed in 1810, but this medical case was probably intended to remain unpublished, recorded as part of his early stethoscopic findings. See Boulle, "Hôpitaux Parisiens," pp. 54–55. See also R. Villey, *Historie du Secret Médical*, Paris, Seghers, 1986.

19. See Daniel Roche, *The People of Paris*, trans. M. Evans and G. Lewis, New York, Berg, 1987, especially pp. 9–98, and his "A pauper capital: Some reflections on the Parisian poor in the seventeenth and eighteenth centuries," *French Hist* 1 (1987): 182–209.

20. For a summary of French charitable institutions in the early eighteenth century see M. Joerger, "The structure of the hospital system in France in the Ancien Régime," in *Medicine and Society in France*, ed. R. Forster and O. Ranum, trans. E. Forster and P. Ranum, Baltimore, Johns Hopkins Univ. Press, 1980, pp. 104–36. More details are provided in Laurence Brockliss and Colin Jones, *The Medical World of Early Modern France*, Oxford, Clarendon Press, 1997.

21. M. C. Dinet-Lecomte, "Les soeurs hospitalieres au service des pauvres malades aux XVIIe et XVIIIe siècles," *Ann Demogr Hist* (1994): 277–92.

22. For a sketch of these issues see C. Hannaway, "Medicine and religion in pre-Revolutionary France: Introduction," *Social Hist Med* (1989): 315–19. For more information see John McManners, *The French Revolution and the Church*, New York, Harper & Row, 1969.

23. For details consult Olwen H. Hufton, *The Poor of Eighteenth-Century France, 1750–1789*, Oxford, Clarendon Press, 1974, and Richard F. Elmore, "The Origins of the Hôpital General of Paris," Ph.D. diss., Univ. of Notre Dame, 1975.

24. An important source is Jean Imbert, *Le Droit Hospitalier de l'Ancien Régime*, Paris, Presses Univ. de France, 1993. See also Daniel Hickey, *Local Hospitals in Ancien Regime France: Rationalization, Resistance, Renewal*, Montreal, McGill-Queens Univ. Press, 1997.

25. Montesquieu, *The Spirit of the Laws*, Book 33, chap. 29, p. 25.

26. C. Jones, "The great chain of buying: Medical advertisement, the bourgeois public sphere, and the origins of the French Revolution," *Am Hist Rev* 101 (1996): 13–40.

27. For details see Matthew Ramsey, "The popularization of medicine in France, 1650–1900," in *The Popularization of Medicine, 1650–1850*, ed. R. Porter, London, Routledge, 1992, pp. 97–133, and his earlier book, *Professional and Popular Medicine in France, 1770–1830*, New York, Cambridge Univ. Press, 1988.

28. P. A. Richmond, "The Hôtel-Dieu of Paris on the eve of the Revolution," *J. Hist Med* 16 (1961): 335–53.

29. L. Perol, "Diderot, Mme Necker et la reforme des hôpitaux," *Stud Voltaire 18th Cent* 311 (1993): 219–32, and R. Mortier, "Diderot et l'assistance publique, où la source et les variations de l'article 'Hôpital' de l'Encyclopédie," in *Enlightenment Studies in Honor of Lester G. Crocker*, ed. A. J. Bingham and V. W. Topazio, Oxford, Voltaire Foundation, 1979, pp. 175–85.

30. Besides the small showcase hospice in the parish of St. Sulpice, other projects completed at this time were a 22-bed hospital for the Paris College of Surgery (1774), the Vaugirard Hospital (1780) for newborns affected with venereal disease, and the 40-bed Cochin Hospital (1782).

31. Gervais, *Histoire*, pp. 7–18. See also L. W. B. Brockliss, "Medical reforms, the Enlightenment, and physician-power in late eighteenth-century France," in *Medicine in the Enlightenment*, ed R. Porter, Amsterdam, Rodopi, 1995, pp. 64–112.

32. See C. Jones, "Sisters of Charity and the ailing poor," *Soc Hist Med* 1 (1989): 339–48.

33. For excerpts of this document see Gervais, *Histoire*, pp. 18–21. On the Neckers see L. S. Greenbaum, "Jacques Necker and the reform of the Paris hospitals on the eve of the French revolution," *Clio Med* 19 (1984): 216–30.

34. John Howard, *An Account of Lazarettos of Europe*, Warrington, U.K.: W. Eyres, 1789. See also J. Lough, "John Howard's account of French prisons and hospitals, 1775–1786," *Stud Voltaire 18th Cent* 284 (1991): 385–99.

35. For details see Lindsay B. Wilson, *Women and Medicine in the French Enlightenment: The Debate over "Maladies des Femmes,"* Baltimore, Johns Hopkins Univ. Press, 1993.

36. Francois Doublet, "Hospice de Charité, an 1788," *Journal de med* 82 (1790): 193–234, also cited in H. Mitchell, "Politics in the service of knowledge: The debate over

the administration of medicine and welfare in late eighteenth-century France," *Social Hist* 6 (1981): 190.

37. Tenon, *Memoirs,* pp. 39–43.

38. L. S. Greenbaum, " 'The commercial treaty of humanity': La tournée des hôpitaux anglais par Jacques Tenon en 1787," *Rev d'Hist Sciences* 24 (1971): 317–50.

39. L. S. Greenbaum, "Nurses and doctors in conflict: Piety and medicine in the Paris Hôtel Dieu on the eve of the French revolution," *Clio Med* 13 (1978): 247–67.

40. L. S. Greenbaum, "Scientists and politicians: Hospital reform in Paris on the eve of the French revolution," *Proc Consort Revolut Eur* (1973): 163–91.

41. For this point see G. Rosen, "Hospitals, medical care, and social policy in the French Revolution," *Bull Hist Med* 30 (1956): 124–49. For details of some of the plans see L. S. Greenbaum, "Jean Sylvain Bailly, the Baron of Breteuil, and the four new hospitals of Paris," *Clio Med* 8 (1973): 261–84.

42. A useful overview of the revolutionary changes is provided by Mary C. Gillett, "Hospital Reform in the French Revolution," Ph.D. diss., American University, 1978, and John E. Frangos, *From Housing the Poor to Healing the Sick: The Changing Institution of Paris Hospitals under the Old Regime and Revolution,* Madison, NJ, Fairleigh Dickinson Univ. Press, 1997.

43. See Dora B. Weiner, *The Citizen-Patient in Revolutionary and Imperial Paris,* Baltimore, Johns Hopkins Univ. Press, 1993, pp. 84–87 and 321–27.

44. This report of the Committee on Mendicity (Poverty Committee) is quoted in Weiner, *The Citizen-Patient,* p. 39. See also I. Woloch, "From charity to welfare in revolutionary Paris," *J Mod Hist* 58 (1986): 779–812, and, for more details, see Alan Forrest, *The French Revolution and the Poor,* New York, St. Martin's Press, 1981.

45. P. J. G. Cabanis, "Sur les hôpitaux," in *Ouevres Complètes de Cabanis,* Paris, F. Didot, 1823, vol. 2, pp. 315–62. For a biography of Cabanis see Martin S. Staum, *Cabanis: Enlightenment and Medical Philosophy in the French Revolution,* Princeton, Princeton Univ. Press, 1980.

46. D. B. Weiner, "French doctors face war, 1792–1815," in *From the Ancien Regime to the Popular Front: Essays in the History of Modern France in Honor of Shepard B. Clough,* ed. C. K. Warner, New York, Columbia Univ. Press, 1969, p. 59.

47. See Gillett, "Hospital Reform," p. 104. The speaker was Barère de VievZac, a member of the Committee on Mendicity of the Constituent Assembly.

48. Weiner, "French doctors face war," p. 60.

49. Colin Jones, "The Daughters of Charity in Hospitals from Louis XIII to Louis Philippe," in *The Charitable Imperative,* ed. C. Jones, London, Routledge, 1989, p. 197. Following the decrees of July 27 and September 2, 1792, the entire hospital property of the former Hospice de Charité was apparently confiscated by the government since it was considered to be owned by *émigrés.*

50. Gillett, "Hospital Reform," pp. 132–56. See also L. E. Sabin, "The French Revolution: The forgotten era of nursing history," *Nurs Forum* 20 (1981): 225–43.

51. Forrest, *The French Revolution,* pp. 55–71.

52. Gillett, "Hospital Reform," pp. 157–90.

53. Weiner, *Citizen-Patient,* pp. 139–46.

54. D. Weiner, "The French Revolution, Napoleon, and the nursing profession," *Bull Hist Med* 46 (1972): 274–305.

55. J. F. Couzin, *Essai sur l'Hygiene des Hôpitaux,* Paris, Bechet, 1813, pp. 40–41.

56. This approach was articulated by Ludwig Fleck, "On the question of the foundations of medical knowledge," trans. T. J. Tren, *J Med Philos* 6 (1981): 237–56. For a more

extensive treatment see Fleck's *Genesis and Development of a Scientific Fact*, ed. T. J. Tren and R. K. Merton, Chicago, Univ. of Chicago Press, 1979.

57. Toby Gelfand, *Professionalizing Modern Medicine,* Westport, CT, Greenwood Press, 1980, especially pp. 58–79.

58. G. Rosen, "The philosophy of ideology and the emergence of modern medicine in France," *Bull Hist Med* 20 (1946): 328–39.

59. G. B. Risse, "The quest for certainty in medicine: John Brown's system of medicine in France," *Bull Hist Med* 43 (1971): 1–12.

60. See Staum, *Cabanis,* p. 95, and L. J. Jordanova, "Reflections on medical reform: Cabanis' Coup d'Oeuil," in *Medicine in the Enlightenment*, pp. 166–80.

61. The physician in question was Nicholas Chambon de Mantaux (1748–1826). For details see T. Gelfand, "A clinical ideal: Paris 1789," *Bull Hist Med* 51 (1977): 397–411.

62. C. Jones and M. Sonenscher, "The social functions of the hospital in eighteenth-century France: The case of the Hôtel Dieu of Nîmes," *French Hist Stud* 13 (1983): 172–214.

63. Jean N. Corvisart, *An Essay on the Organic Diseases and Lesions of the Heart and Great Vessels*, trans. J. Gates (1812), facsimile, New York, Hafner, 1962, p. 16.

64. See Russell C. Maulitz, *Morbid Appearances: The Anatomy of Pathology in the Early Nineteenth Century*, New York, Cambridge Univ. Press, 1987, pp. 19–31.

65. For a full treatment of this subject see John E. Lesch, *Science and Medicine in France: the Emergence of Experimental Physiology, 1790–1855*, Cambridge, MA, Harvard Univ. Press, 1984.

66. Fourcroy quoted in Maulitz, *Morbid Appearances*, p. 39.

67. Ibid., pp. 36–59.

68. Ibid., pp. 60–105.

69. John Pickstone, "Bureaucracy, liberalism, and the body in post-revolutionary France: Bichat's physiology and the Paris school of medicine," *Hist Sci* 19 (1981): 115–42.

70. J. Duffin, "Gaspard-Laurent Bayle et son legs scientifique: Au delà de l'anatomie pathologique," *Can Bull Med Hist* 3 (1986): 167–84.

71. L. S. King, *The Medical World of the Eighteenth Century*, Chicago, Univ. of Chicago Press, 1958, pp. 290–96. For more details see Elizabeth Haigh, *Xavier Bichat and the Medical Theory of the Eighteenth Century,* London, Wellcome Institute, 1984.

72. G. B. Risse, "La synthèse entre l'anatomie et la clinique," in *Histoire de la Pensée Médicale en Occident*, ed. M. D. Grmek, Paris, Ed. du Seuil, 1997, vol. 2, pp. 177–97.

73. Maulitz, *Morbid Appearances*, pp. 73–78.

74. R. T. H. Laennec, *A Treatise on Diseases of the Chest*, trans J. Forbes (1821), facsimile, New York, Hafner, 1962, pp. xix–xxv.

75. Maulitz, *Morbid Appearances*, pp. 83–103.

76. For a comparative view see G. B. Risse, "A shift in medical epistemology: Clinical diagnosis, 1770–1828," in *History of Diagnostics*, ed. Y. Kawakita, Osaka, Tanaguchi Foundation, 1987, pp. 115–47.

77. L. J. Renauldin, "Diagnostic," in *Dictionnaire des Sciences Médicales*, Paris, Panckoucke, 1814, vol. 9, pp. 163–69.

78. F. Merat, "Interrogation," *Dictionnaire des Sciences Médicales* 1818, vol. 25, p. 527.

79. Ibid., pp. 525–26.

80. P. Jolly, "Semeiotics," in *Encyclopedie Méthodique*, Paris, Agasse, 1830, vol. 13, p. 1.

81. See R. Porter, "The rise of physical examination," in *Medicine and the Five Senses*, ed. W. F. Bynum and R. Porter, Cambridge, Cambridge Univ. Press, 1993, pp. 179–97. For a comparative analysis of the various European teaching centers see O. Keel, "La prob-

lematique institutionelle de la clinique en France" (in two parts), *Can Bull Med Hist* 2 (1985): 183–204 and 3 (1986): 1–30.

82. G. B. Risse, "Pierre A. Piorry (1794–1879), the French master of percussion," *Chest* 60 (1971): 484–88.

83. Renauldin, "Diagnostic," 167–69.

84. Ibid., pp. 163–64.

85. Philippe Pinel, *La Médecine Clinique*, 2nd ed., Paris, Brosson, 1804, p. xxvii. The epistemology of both Pinel and Bichat was derived from Condillac but mediated in important ways by the example of Lavoisier's chemistry. See William R. Albury, "The Logic of Condillac and the Structure of French Chemical and Biological Theory, 1780–1801," Ph.D. diss., Johns Hopkins Univ., 1972, pp. 187–254.

86. T. D. Murphy, "The French medical profession's perception of its social function between 1776 and 1830," *Med Hist* 23 (1979): 259–78. This plan of professional advancement was also reflected in Corvisart's publications. See W. R. Albury, "Heart of darkness: J. N. Corvisart and the medicalization of life," *Hist Reflection* 9 (1982): 17–31. Also consult Ramsey, *Professional and Popular Medicine*.

87. Corvisart, *Essay on Organic Diseases*, p. 21.

88. For a new analysis of the events see M. D. Grmek, "L'invention de l'auscultation médiate, retouches à un cliché historique," *Rev Palais de la Découverte* 22 (1981): 107–16.

89. On the title page of his book, Laennec quoted a passage from Hippocrates—Epidemics III: "Pouvoir explorer est, a mon avis, une grande partie de l'art." See the original edition of *De l'auscultation médiate, ou traité du diagnostic des maladies des pou, ons et du coeur* , 2 vols., Paris, Brosson & Chaude, 1819.

90. In the introduction to his famous work, Laennec acknowledged that "morbid anatomy, since the commencement of the present century, throughout Europe, and more especially in Paris, has been productive of many improvements and discoveries." See Laennec, *Diseases of the Chest*, p. xxx.

91. Ibid., p. xxxiii.

92. See J. Duffin, "Vitalism and organicism in the philosophy of R.T. H. Laennec," *Bull Hist Med* 62 (1988): 525–45.

93. Gervais, *Histoire*, p. 50.

94. Ibid., p. 23.

95. This information, conveyed in a letter dated April 22, 1817, by Laennec to a friend, Courbon-Perusel, was included in a biography written by Alfred Rouxeau. Private communication from Jacalyn Duffin.

96. J. F. C. Coste, "Hôpital," *Dictionnaire des Sciences Médicales*, 1817, vol. 21, p. 460.

97. According to several authors, the term *tuberculosis* seems to have been coined in 1839 by the German physician Johann L. Schönlein. For details concerning Laennec's views of this disease see J. Duffin, "Unity, duality, passion, and cure: Laennec's conceptualization of tuberculosis," in *Maladie et Malades, Historie et Conceptualisation, Mélanges en l'honneur de Mirko Grmek*, ed. D. Gourevitch, Geneva, Libraire Droz, 1982, pp. 333–46.

98. V. P. Comiti, "Incidence et prévalence de la pathologie pulmonaire au temps de Laennec," *Rev Palais Dec* 22 (1981): 124–29. For a general history of the disease consult René and J. Dubos, *The White Plague: Tuberculosis, Man, and Society* (1952) reprint, New Brunswick, Rutgers Univ. Press, 1987, and R. Y. Keers, *Pulmonary Tuberculosis: A Journey Down the Centuries*, London, Baillière Tindall, 1978.

99. Philippe Pinel, *The Clinical Training of Doctors, An Essay of 1793*, ed. D. Weiner, Baltimore: Johns Hopkins Univ. Press, 1980, p. 78.

100. Coste, "Hôpital," p. 465.

101. Ibid., p. 84.

102. Laennec, "Phthisis pulmonalis," in *Diseases of the Chest*, p. 17.

103. For an overview see E. H. Ackerknecht, "Die Therapie der Pariser Kliniker zwischen 1795 und 1840," *Gesnerus* 15 (1958): 151–63. I am indebted to an unpublished paper by Randall Albury, "Corvisart and Broussais: Human individuality and medical dominance," given at the conference "History of Scientific Medicine in Paris, 1790–1850: A Reinterpretation," College of Physicians of Philadelphia, 1992.

104. René T. Laennec, *Traité de l'Auscultation Mediate,* 2nd ed. (reprint), Paris, Masson Ed., 1927, vol. 1, pp. 703–13.

105. See Isidore Bricheteau, *Medical Clinics of the Hospital Necker*, trans. from French, Philadelphia, A. Waldie, 1837, pp. 26–27. Other details about the contemporary treatment of phthisis can be obtained from the article by the anatomist Jacques P. Maygrier, "Phthisie," in *Dictionare de Sciences Médicales*, 1820, vol. 42, pp. 105–54.

106. Pinel, *Clinical training*, p. 78.

107. Ibid., p. 82.

108. Laennec, *Traité de l'Auscultation*, vol. 1, p. 717.

109. G. Andral, *The Clinique Médicale, or Reports of Medical Cases,* condensed and trans. by D. Spillan, London, H. Renshaw, 1836, p. 462.

110. Jones, "Sisters of Charity," 345–48.

111. J. Duffin, "Private practice and public research: The patients of R. T. H. Laennec," in *French Medical Culture in the 19th Century*, ed. A. La Berge and M. Feingold, Amsterdam, Rodopi, 1994, pp. 118–48.

112. See MSS Musée Laennec.

113. Ibid.

114. The information was provided by Pierre F. Percy (1754–1825), a military surgeon. See his article "Dissection" in the *Dictionnaire des Sciences Médicales*, 1814, vol. 9, p. 649.

115. Autopsy findings are reprinted in MSS Musée Laennec. See also Duffin, "Unity, duality, passion and cure," p. 341.

116. Duffin, "Private practice and public research," pp. 16–18. Using the occupations of 646 of Laennec's hospital patients, the author discovered that textile and fashion workers made up 23.5% of the total.

117. T. Gelfand, "Gestation of the clinic," *Med Hist* 25 (1981): 169–80. See also his *Professionalizing Modern Medicine*, pp. 98–115.

118. Gelfand, *Professionalizing Modern Medicine*, pp. 116–25.

119. Laurence Brockliss has tried to dispel the notion that pre-Revolutionary medical education was highly inadequate and therefore ripe for a sweeping reform. See L. W. Brockliss, "L'enseignement médical et la Révolution: essai de réévaluation," *Hist de l'Education* 42 (1989): 79–110, and an English version, "Practical medical training in eighteenth-century France," in *History of Scientific Medicine in Paris, 1790–1850, A Reinterpretation*, forthcoming.

120. Pinel, *La Médecine Clinique*, pp. v–xxvi.

121. "The healing art should be taught only in hospitals: this assertion needs no proof. Only in the hospital can one follow the evolution and progress of several illnesses at the same time and study variations of the same disease in a number of patients," Pinel, *Clinical Training*, p. 67.

122. The witness was a German surgeon from Göttingen, Georg Wardenburg. See O. Marx, "The practice of precepts: An episode of bedside teaching from the past," *Surgery* 59 (1966): 469–71.

123. M. J. Imbault-Huart, "Concepts and realities of the beginning of clinical teaching in the late eighteenth and early nineteenth centuries," *Clio Med* 21 (1987–88): 60.

124. Although 10 years later, the experiences of Laennec's successor, Chomel, offer in-

teresting points of comparison. See L. S. Jacyna, "Au lit des malades: A. F. Chomel's clinic at the Charité, 1828–9," *Med Hist* 33 (1989): 420–49.

125. For more information consult Raymond Durand-Fardel, *L'Internat en Médecine et en Chirurgie des Hôpitaux et Hospices Civiles de Paris*, Paris, G. Steinheil, 1904. Another important source of information in English is Leonard Groopman, "The *Internat des Hôpitaux de Paris*: The shaping and transformation of the French medical elite, 1802–1914," Ph.D. diss, Harvard Univ., 1986.

126. Sauvigny, *Bourbon Restoration,* pp. 257–58.

127. Some of these issues are aptly stressed in A. B. Astrow, "The French Revolution and the dilemma of medical training," *Persp Biol Med* 33 (1990): 444–56. See also Mireille Wiriot, *L'Enseignement Clinique dans les Hôpitaux de Paris entre 1794 et 1848*, Paris, Chaumes, 1970.

128. F. E. Fodere, "Malade," *Dictionnaire des Sciences Médicales* 30 (1818): 168.

129. Pinel, *Clinical Training*, p. 84

130. J. H. Warner, "The selective transport of medical knowledge: Antebellum American physicians and Parisian medical therapeutics," *Bull Hist Med* 59 (1985): 213–31, and by the same author, "Remembering Paris: Memory and the American disciples of French medicine in the nineteenth century," *Bull Hist Med* 55 (1991): 301–25.

131. For details see J. Duffin, "Sick doctors: Bayle and Laennec on their own phthisis," *J Hist Med* 43 (1988): 165–82.

132. A. Thalamy, "La médicalisation de l'hôpital," in *Les Machines à Guerir*, ed. M. Foucault et al., Paris, Institute de l'Environment, 1976, pp. 43–53.

133. Most of the clinical teaching in French hospitals, as in their counterparts in other European countries, was carried out on a limited number of patients, usually about 30, which was the size of a regular ward. To observe and examine in detail hundreds or perhaps thousands of inmates would have been hopelessly confusing and almost impossible within the time frame of daily rounds. The French advantage consisted in drawing the best teaching cases from a vast institutional population.

134. Foucault has stressed the role of the hospital as an institution of power and control that subjected individual patients to a new medical and administrative discipline. See his *The Birth of the Clinic*, trans. A. M. Sheridan Smith, New York, Vintage Books, 1975. The best interpretation of his approach is the introduction to *Reassessing Foucault*, ed. C. Jones and R. Porter, London, Routledge, 1994, pp. 1–16, written by the editors.

135. For details see John H. Warner, *Against the Spirit of System: The French Impulse in Nineteenth-Century American Medicine*, Princeton, Princeton Univ Press, 1998.

136. The concept of a *rupture epistemologique* was employed by various French philosophers of science, including Gaston Bachelard and Georges Canguilhem. See Canguilhem, *Ideology and Rationality in the History of the Life Sciences*, trans. A. Goldhammer, Cambridge, MIT Press, 1988, pp. 10–11. The thesis espoused by Michel Foucault is that these changes were not merely cumulative but also significant enough to alter the entire structure and organization of medical knowledge.

137. For an excellent synthesis see William F. Bynum, *Science and the Practice of Medicine in the Nineteenth Century*, Cambridge, Cambridge Univ. Press, 1994.

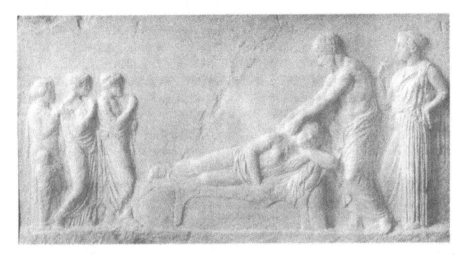

Incubation. Asclepius touches a sick person. ca. 400 BC. Votive bas relief from the
Asclepian temple at Piraeus, Athens Museum. (Wellcome Library, London)

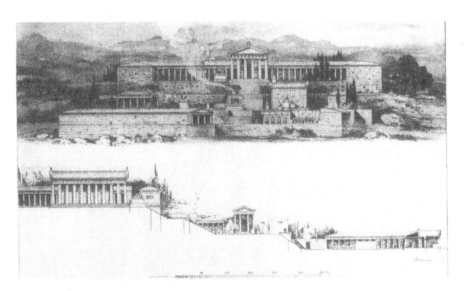

Asclepieion on the island of Cos in Hellenistic times, second century BC. Reconstruction by
P. Schatzmann, 1932 (Wellcome Library, London).

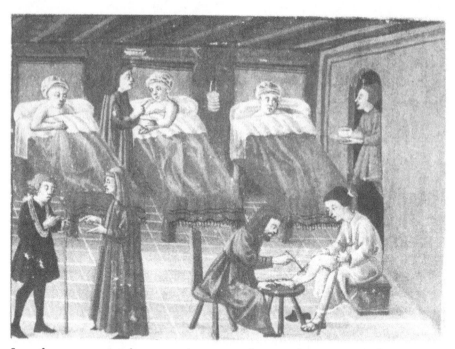

Scene from a monastic infirmary ward ca. 1400; infirmarer takes the pulse; attendant brings food; consulting barber surgeon attends to a leg ulcer; ambulatory patient with arm in sling gets advice. MSS Gaddiano 24 (Biblioteca Medicea Laurenziana, Florence, Italy).

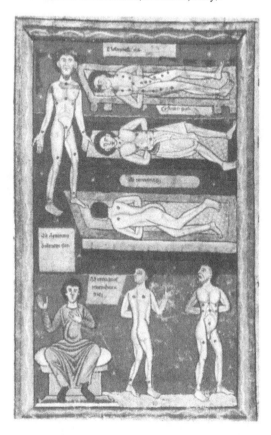

Late 12th Century maps of the human body displaying sites to be cauterized in the treatment of disease (MSS, Bodleian Library, Oxford).

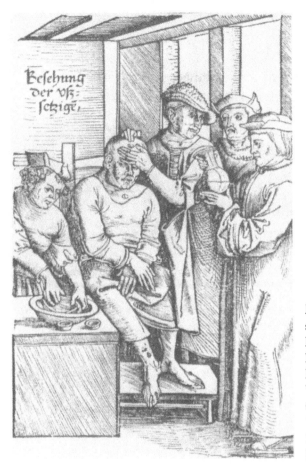

Medical examination of a person suspected of suffering from leprosy in the early 1500s. Physicians examine facial lesions, urine, and blood. Woodcut from Hans von Gersdorff's book *Feldbuch der Wundarztney,* published in 1540 (National Library of Medicine, Bethesda).

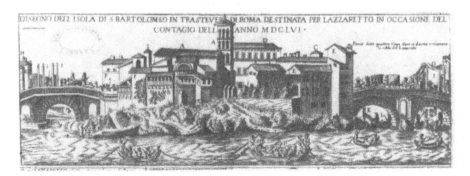

Sketch of the dwellings on the island of St. Bartolomeo on the Tiber River in Rome, converted into a makeshift lazzaretto during the 1656 plague epidemic. The engraving depicts the transport of suspected victims across the bridges, and the disposal of the dead in boats for burial downstream (NLM).

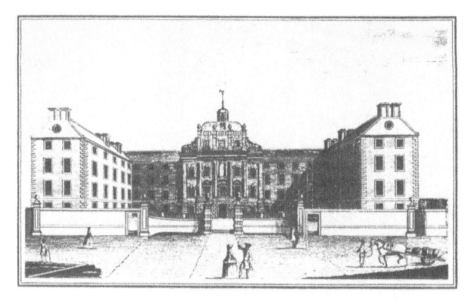

View of the Royal Infirmary of Edinburgh, the Palladian mansion designed by William Adam, ca. 1780s (Lothian Health Board, Edinburgh, UK).

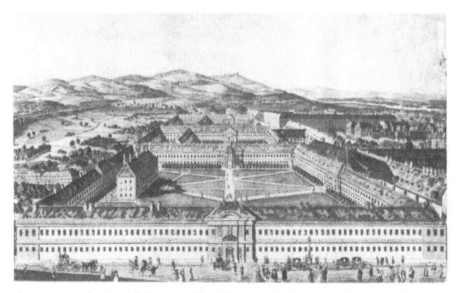

A panoramic drawing of the remodeled Viennese almshouse—with its multiple courtyards—that opened as the Allgemeines Krankenhaus in 1784. The contemporary copper engraving was created by Joseph and Peter Schaffer (Institute for the History of Medicine, Vienna, Austria).

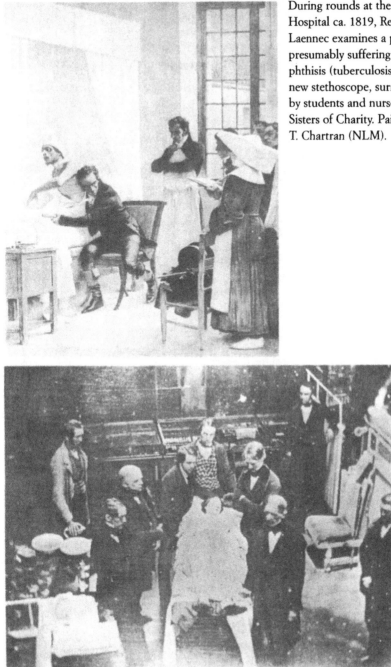

During rounds at the Necker Hospital ca. 1819, René T. H. Laennec examines a patient presumably suffering from phthisis (tuberculosis) with his new stethoscope, surrounded by students and nurses, the Sisters of Charity. Painting by T. Chartran (NLM).

Daguerrotype of one of the earliest operations under ether anesthesia on a female patient, performed at the Massachusetts General Hospital in 1846, formerly in the possession of Dr. William Morton, who stands at the head of the table dressed in a checkered vest. Dr. John C. Warren is at the right, near the bottom of the operating table (Courtesy of the Countway Library and S. Borack, Boston).

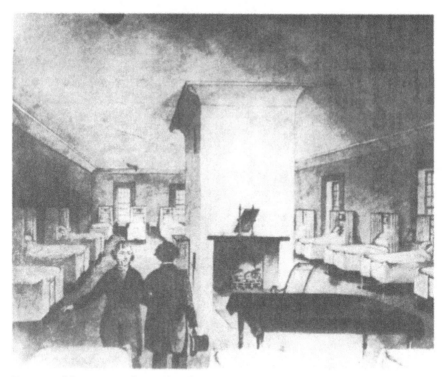

Drawing of the interior of a ward at the Massachusetts General Hospital, ca. 1845, depicting patients and two visiting physicians (Courtesy of Public Affairs, MGH, Boston).

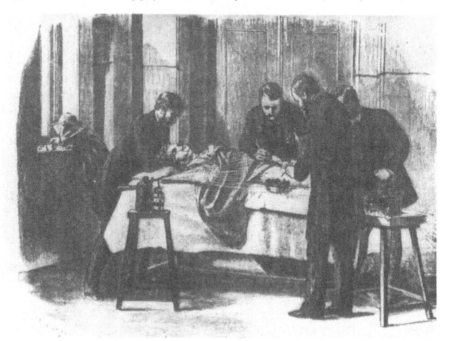

Use of a portable carbolic acid spray during a surgical operation performed by adherents of Lister's antiseptic methods in the late 1870s, perhaps including Lister's assistant, William Watson Cheyne. Wood engraving from his book *Antiseptic Surgery* (1882) (NLM).

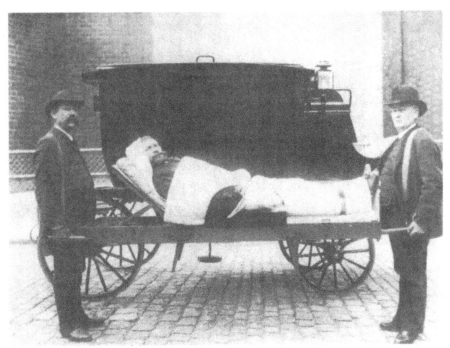

Cholera epidemic of 1892. Sanitary workers of the city of Hamburg transport patients suspected of harboring the disease to the local hospitals (Photo, courtesy of Hamburg's Staatsarchiv).

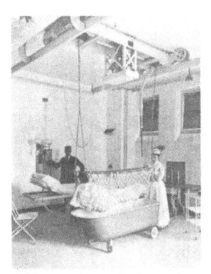

Cold water treatments for fever patients in the 1890s. Photograph from the New York Hospital's "House of Relief" branch depicting a patient and nurse with an operator working the electric lift to submerge the patient in a tub. (Hodson, *How to Become a Trained Nurse,* 1898.)

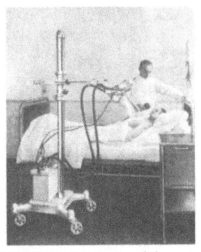

Mobile high voltage Nanos radiology unit for bedside use reflects the new advances being made in X-ray engineering around 1930 (*Brit J Radiol* 5 (1932):256)

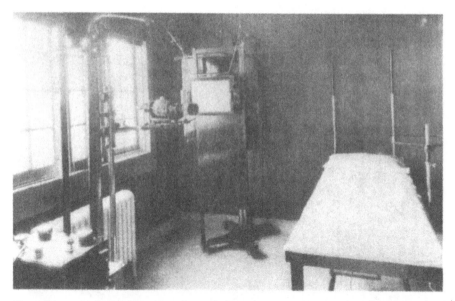

New diagnostic facilities: a room for radiological examinations with a fluoroscope and X-ray machine, Madison General Hospital, 1930 (Photo, courtesy of MGH Archives, madison, Wisconsin).

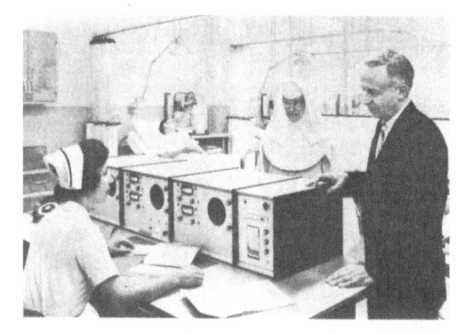

Cardiac Care Unit, Mercy Hospital, late 1960s. Nurse-coordinator Gottstine confers with cardiologist O'Brien and hospital director Sister Mary Sacred Heart (Mercy Hospital, *75 Years of Caring,* Buffalo, 1979).

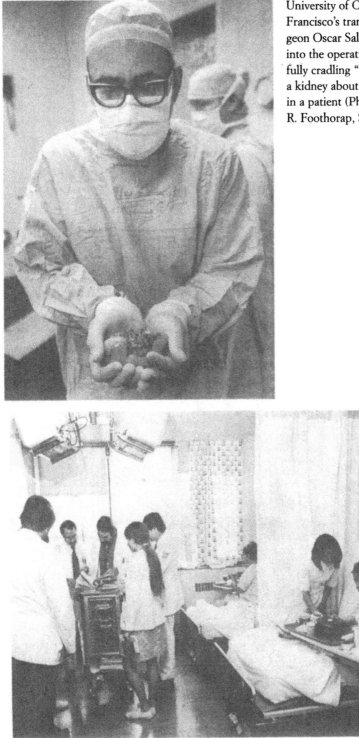

University of California, San Francisco's transplantation surgeon Oscar Salvatierra walks into the operating room, carefully cradling "the gift of life," a kidney about to be implanted in a patient (Photo courtesy of R. Foothorap, San Francisco).

UCSF's Moffitt Hospital ca. mid 1970s. Four-bed ward similar to that available for transplant patients in the early 1980s (UCSF Archives).

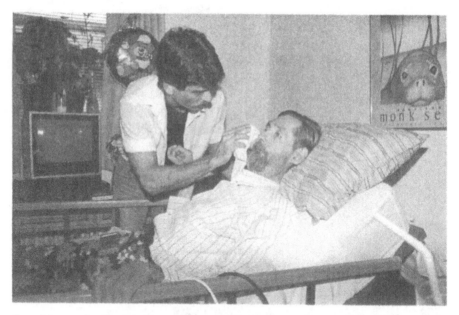

Caregiving at the Coming Home Hospice, San Francisco (Courtesy of G. P. Ray, Santa Cruz).

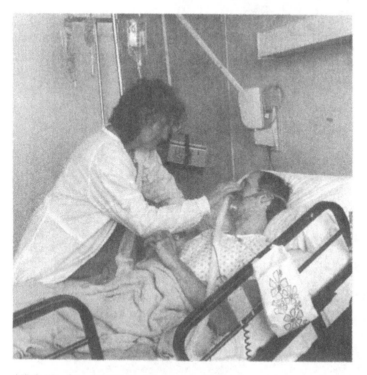

AIDS Ward at SFGH in 1986: nurse Diane J. comforts Fred H., one of the patients (Courtesy of G.P. Ray, Santa Cruz).

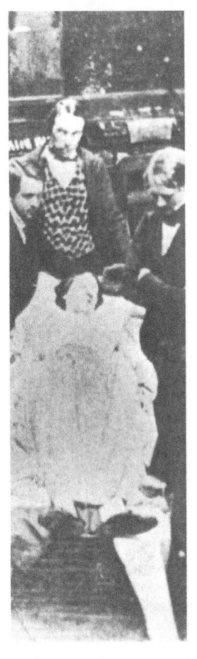

7

MODERN SURGERY
IN HOSPITALS

Development of Anesthesia
and Antisepsis

AMERICA: WARREN AND
ANESTHESIA

In this very hour while I am speaking, how many human creatures are cheated of pangs which seemed inevitable as the common doom of mortality, and lulled by the strange magic of the enchanted goblet, held for a moment to their lips, [go] into a repose which has something of ecstasy in its dreamy slumbers . . . the fierce extremity of suffering has been steeped in the waters of forgetfulness and the deepest furrow in the knotted brow of agony has been smoothed forever.
Oliver Wendell Holmes, 1847[1]

Life in a voluntary
American hospital

On the afternoon of March 7, 1845, an 18-year-old "domestic from Ireland," Alice Mohan, limped into the Massachusetts General Hospital (MGH) in Boston with a swollen right knee. She told the admitting house surgeon, possibly Charles F. Heywood, that the problem had started two months earlier, in the middle of the winter, after she had slipped on the ice and struck her knee. Considerable swelling, acute pain, and bruises followed, with persistent tenderness and discomfort, especially when the leg was in motion.[2] Perhaps the accident was God's punishment for her sins. At this time, most Irish immigrants were denied admission; instead the hospital referred them to the local almshouse. By contemporary standards, the Irish were considered members of a steadily growing population of foreigners who

failed to conform to the prevailing models of industry and self-help. Alice's occupation, however, qualified her as deserving of care at the MGH if the sickness
was not trivial. Indeed, the original proposal for establishing the hospital had accepted the premise that "servants generally undergo great inconveniences, at least
when afflicted with sickness," and that their private care in the families they were
serving was difficult since the mistress of the house was usually otherwise engaged.
In an institution such as the MGH, young servant girls "would find an alleviation of their sufferings which must gladden the heart of the most frigid to contemplate."[3]

In 1845, MGH was a small 60-bed establishment almost half occupied by paying patients, a radical departure from the Edinburgh model restricted to the sick
poor. In early March three physicians, two clergymen, and four naval officers occupied private rooms. They even preferred to bring their wives or servants to attend them. The bulk of the other paying patients were wives, domestics, mechanics,
laborers, mariners, farmers, and traders. Vigilance and fiscal monitoring were periodic responsibilities of the hospital's trustees, who made their weekly visits at all
hours of the day and night, inspecting the food, checking household arrangements,
and talking individually with the patients.[4] More than a third of all qualified applicants for admission could be accommodated. No one suffering from contagious
or venereal diseases or incurable conditions could enter. Alice's admission could
have been arranged by a subscriber, perhaps her employer, or even an officer of
the corporation, who had a right to one of the "free" beds. As in Europe, it was
not uncommon for masters to rid themselves of sick or injured help by sending
them to the hospital.[5] Sixty-two female domestics got free beds in 1845, making
up more than half of all female admissions and close to 75% of those hospitalized in this category.[6]

In the mid-1840s, Boston had a population of about 140,000. As the financial
center of New England, the city supplied the capital for an industrial hinterland
that included Lowell's textile centers and Salem's shoe manufacturing. Boston had
retained its own small-scale industries, with their craftsmen, artisans, and traders,
a culturally homogeneous community without large slums or a stigmatized workforce. Bostonians formed a confident, self-contained community, proud and firm
in their belief that progress could be achieved through self-reliance, willpower,
and hard work.[7] However, since the early 1840s, poor Irish immigrants such as
Alice had been arriving by the thousands, driven by a combination of political and
economic factors that accelerated after 1845 because of the great potato blight.
Unskilled, penniless, and mostly unemployed, the starving Irish clustered in old
Boston, transforming many areas into overcrowded slums. Poverty and degradation quickly stigmatized this ethnic group, its members linked to alcoholism, crime,
and prostitution. In their quest to join the city's labor force, many Irish women
were welcomed as domestics; New England had a shortage of servants because
natives usually found more lucrative, less demeaning jobs. Soon, women like Al-

ice found employment in middle-class households, who valued their joviality, their loyalty, and especially their low wage demands. By 1845, Irish domestic workers in Boston numbered around 2,000.[8]

On admission, Alice's knee was considerably swollen, especially around the patella, with some tenderness on deep pressure and a distinct fluctuation suggesting the presence of fluid. For comparative purposes, both knee joints were measured; the right one was one inch larger in circumference. The patient was ordered to rest in bed. Two daily douches with cold water were ordered for the affected joint, to be followed by alcohol washings. Since the bathing only caused further pain, the attending surgeon changed the order the following day, recommending instead that a full pitcher of cold water be dashed daily on the troublesome joint. Thus, Alice began life in the hospital, a stay punctuated by a series of conventional attempts—some reaching back to antiquity—to cure her swollen knee. John Collins Warren (1778–1856), chief of surgery and professor of anatomy and surgery at the Massachusetts Medical College (Harvard), directed her care. He visited the hospital on Tuesdays and Thursdays and operated on Saturday mornings in the amphitheater. Given the high proportion of paying patients, hygiene and good nursing seemed to be institutional priorities, but the original female caregiving staff—four head nurses and five assistants—was poorly paid and drawn from the local servant population. The institution had also hired a chambermaid and two waiters to attend to their needs. When an epidemic of erysipelas broke out in the institution that spring, Warren, ever aware of the potentially dangerous contamination of postoperative wounds, blamed the infection on deficient nursing and the "retention of foul matters" in the beds.[9] Bedridden patients were sponged daily with soap and water and their bed clothes ventilated. Ambulatory inmates took showers and a warm bath every second or third day.

Late in March, both a tobacco poultice and placement of leeches failed to reduce Alice's swelling. A blister was applied below the patella in May, followed by warm water and alcohol applications and more leeches. By June the skin around the knee peeled off, and the joint was bandaged after rubbings with palm oil. So far, Alice's suffering had been considered part of the therapeutic regimen, but persistent pain during motion and no improvement in September prompted the surgeons to prescribe some fomentations with an opium extract. Later, Alice was given hypodermic morphine injections to block the burning pain caused by the caustic. Because the wound only yielded some thin, whitish fluid, the resulting ulceration was packed with peas to stimulate further draining, but lack of progress forced the use of an iron cautery. Could the purifying fire cleanse the rotting flesh? Finally, in November, the surgical staff gave up their efforts at counterirritation, simply prescribing a house diet and morphine for pain.

At this point, Alice's stay had already far exceeded the average hospitalization for free-bed holders, which was reported to be about five to seven weeks.[10] Why was she kept so long in the hospital? Conventional medical stereotypes suggested that, as a young Irish woman, Alice probably possessed a scrofulous bodily constitution, little physical endurance, and higher sensitivity to pain. Such individuals often suffered from "white" swellings in their joints, especially in the knees and ankles.[11] "White" joint infections were indeed quite common among the sick poor, reflecting the widespread presence of this disease among Boston's young Irish immigrants. The condition—an ulceration of the synovial membrane with formation of multiple abscesses—was linked to tubercles in the lungs. Limited to one joint, and frequently triggered by trauma, the "scrofulous disease" was deemed incurable. Palliation, especially pain control, seemed the only option.

Within this framework, Alice's conservative management, doggedly pursued for many months, was obviously succeeding. Indeed, the repeated scarifications and caustic burns had created a stubborn, draining ulcer at the knee that prevented purulent matter from poisoning the interior of the body.[12] In any event, the goal of her individualized regimen was to restore bodily energies through rest, regular food, and localized draining designed to assist nature in the elimination of unwanted humors. At a time when professional identity was closely linked to therapeutic prowess and moral integrity, both physicians and surgeons tried to maintain a clinical posture of moderation and trust in the healing powers of nature.[13] The conservative behavior of the hospital's surgeons mirrored, in part, that of its leading physicians, including James Jackson (1777–1867), the chief of the medical department, Walter Channing (1786–1876), and John Ware (1795–1864). To be sure, surgery exhibited some differences from medical intervention, since its technical procedures were based on universal anatomical landmarks and physiological processes. However, given the paucity of actual interventions, most surgical activities also followed the principle of specificity. Individualized approaches were tailored to the characteristics of particular patients and their constitutional, ethnic, social, moral, and physical condition.

The new year found Alice still on the ward, somewhat more comfortable but the target of further palliative practices. On January 13, 1846, the attending surgeons created an "issue," another small scarification kept open again by the use of a pea or another foreign body attached to a string for quick removal. As before, the intent was to drain harmful fluid stubbornly remaining in the joint that was blamed for the pain and restricted motion. New scarifications were made in March, May, and June 1846, alternating with other applications of the caustic potassium solution. By July, these various procedures were battling an expanding abscess that now reached deep inside the knee joint. A fistula needed to be drained by poultices, cold water dressings, and 12 leeches. Moreover, progress notes reveal that the patient was now almost constantly constipated, requiring frequent enemas, no doubt the result of inactivity and morphine injections.

Because of the degree of Alice's disability, a return to her employer seemed out of the question. Caregivers, for their part, must have been under considerable pressure to discharge a patient whose social dependency was being encouraged by a lengthy hospital stay. It also undermined institutional statistics, published annually for subscribers. Moreover, the chronic nature of the case was contrary to the hospital's aims as an institution for acute medical interventions. But just then, the hospital authorities were inaugurating an expansion of the original Bulfinch building in July 1846, increasing the institution's capacity by about 60 beds, to be devoted mostly to poor patients and thus lessening the pressure to vacate available beds.[14] Thus, Alice remained. By now she was a familiar face in the institution, a veteran inmate cheered on daily by a staff of hard-working nurses who mainly engaged in housekeeping chores. Most of these low-skilled caregivers were about Alice's age and probably were also of Irish ancestry. To cope with prolonged suffering, one could imagine her drawing strength from relationships with nurses and other patients.

What were Alice's relations with the surgeons? Ostensibly, they periodically hurt and burned her knee, draining the tuberculous abscesses and ulcers and then providing narcotics to lessen the pain. By early September, the use of ipecac, an emetic to clear her stomach, increased her nausea and vomiting, forcing attending physicians to apply a blister to her stomach. More morphine and brandy were given for pain. The right knee was still being attended to with cold water washings, followed by the application of a flannel cloth, but the pain and distress persisted. For two more weeks, Alice was quite uncomfortable. She continued to suffer from nausea, vomiting, and considerable weight loss that could be attributed to the suspected consumption. By October, the painkillers had become less effective (was she becoming addicted?) and the whole right limb was covered with lint four inches above and below the knee joint, exposed to an irritating mustard poultice.[15]

A month later, Alice's general condition had deteriorated significantly and she now was bedridden.[16] Constant pain required increasingly high, daily doses—four to eight grains—of morphine. What were her chances of preserving an infected limb that stubbornly refused to respond to local treatments and a therapeutic approach consisting solely of rest, a nourishing diet, and pain control?[17] Once a trivial traumatic swelling, Alice's knee had evolved into a chronic, life-threatening condition. Why were the surgeons continuing to treat her lesion conservatively? What about a more radical approach, most likely an amputation of the leg above the knee joint? Indeed, crippling surgery seemed the only way to save Alice's life. Ironically, this solution was not considered wise for "persons belonging to the lower classes of society who have to support themselves by their bodily labor."[18] There were also fears that an amputation might trigger the tuberculous disease in other portions of the body.

MGH surgeons emphasized their conservatism in an age when surgical procedures were limited by pain and the risks of postoperative infection. Earlier that same year, a visiting hospital surgeon, Henry J. Bigelow (1818–1890), had admonished his Harvard students not to "identify surgery with the knife, with blood and dashing elegance. Distrust surgical intrepidity and boldness," he had added. The purpose of surgery was "to save and not to destroy, and an operation is an avowal of its own inadequacy."[19] Such a stance seemed to produce more favorable results. According to published statistics, John C. Warren had performed a total of 40 leg amputations at MGH, with a 25% mortality rate. Warren's private clientele fared even significantly better: 5.5%. Another visiting surgeon, George Hayward (1791–1863), had reported in 1840 an overall mortality of 21% for all amputations performed in the institution, with an even higher rate for those carried out on the thigh: 26%. This rate compared favorably with those of famous European hospitals, such as the Edinburgh Infirmary, which reported a 27.5% death rate at the time.[20]

But surgery was about to change in Boston. Rumors were flying around the hospital about a new fluid that caused patients to sleep and not feel pain while they were being cut. If Alice Mohan had heard about the events of October 16 and 17 in the hospital's amphitheater, she probably also knew that Warren had decided against employing the "letheon" again. Its discoverer apparently refused to divulge the nature of the agent he employed, ostensibly to gain time and secure a patent for the magic vapor. A routine operation scheduled for October 27 on a 14-year-old girl named Sarah Everett, who suffered from a bony tumor on her right upper arm, was carried out by Warren without anesthesia. Fortified by 100 drops of laudanum—an alcoholic extract of opium—the patient had been placed in the operating chair. Sarah endured a four-inch incision over the swelling, described as the size of a walnut, followed by the application of bone pliers to crush and remove the excessive bone. Like most such procedures, there was a fair amount of bleeding and pain. In time, Sarah would mend.[21] Was Alice next?

Philanthropy in Boston: The Massachusetts General Hospital

When Dr. E. D. Fenner, one of the editors of the *New Orleans Medical and Surgical Journal*, came briefly to Boston—the "Athens of America"—in May 1846, he was impressed by the social prestige and wealth of its medical elite. After visiting the MGH, he wrote: "This is a most perfect and beautiful hospital, whose only fault consists in its being unnecessarily fine in its equipment." Fenner described the new physical facilities, observing that the beds "appear to be fully as neat and comfortable as those of the Tremont or Astor Hotels. In short, everything about this establishment is in more magnificent style than I ever expected to see about a hospital" and concluding that "it is by no means exclusively a charity hospital, but is designed also as a resort for all such as are either absent from their homes, or who cannot be well attended to at home."[22]

A backward glance at the origins of this voluntary hospital begins on March 10, 1810, with a meeting of prominent, powerful Bostonians. The city was then

enjoying a commercial boom. Called by the Rev. John Bartlett, chaplain of the local almshouse, the group planned to discuss the fate of the physically and mentally ill residing there. Bartlett had already visited the new republic's two existing
general hospitals: the Pennsylvania Hospital in Philadelphia, opened in 1756, and
the New York Hospital, operating since 1791. He had also heard about the new
ideas for the management of the insane in Europe following the French Revolution.[23] Attending the meeting in Boston were Jackson and Warren, who were persuaded to take the initiative in seeking broad financial support for the establishment of a hospital.[24] On August 20, 1811, the two men issued a circular letter
inviting subscriptions "for a hospital for the reception of lunatics and other sick
persons." In their appeal, both physicians—who had trained at the Edinburgh Infirmary and its London counterparts—pointed out that "hospitals and infirmaries
are found in all the Christian cities of the Old World," as well as in American
cities such as New York and Philadelphia. Jackson and Warren were also keenly
aware of the educational value of such institutions.[25]

The circular elicited quick, enthusiastic responses. On February 25, 1811, the
Massachusetts legislature chartered a corporation composed of 56 distinguished
figures of the Commonwealth headed by James Bowdoin.[26] This group heading
the new hospital, named the Massachusetts General Hospital, held its first organizational meeting in April 1811. A board of trustees composed of 12 persons,
chosen annually, was required to lay before the entire corporation at its annual
meeting the treasurer's institutional accounts. To help with the finances, the corporation received an estate from the legislature as an endowment, provided that
the trustees could raise an additional $100,000 within five years through match-
ing donations and private subscriptions. The hospital charter extended the "advantages of this institution" to all worthy persons, regardless of citizenship, station in life, or economic means. Indeed, MGH was to be conceived as an
establishment available to the Commonwealth's general working population, rich
and poor. Planners in Boston especially targeted "mechanics, journeymen, and apprentices, laborers, and domestic servants, mere sojourners in the city with no connections near at hand ready to pour oil and wine into their wounds when they are
in need of relief."[27] These people were the deserving poor, whose lack of caregiving family members exposed them to the dangers of prolonged illness and des-
titution.

By an act of the state legislature, the hospital corporation was authorized in
1814 to grant annuities on lives. This activity led in that same year to the formation of a separate Massachusetts Hospital Life Insurance Company.[28] Although
founded primarily as a fund-raising institution, this company soon extended its
activities to investment and banking and had a powerful influence on the industrialization of New England. One-third of its net profits became payable to the
hospital and thus remained a key source of income. In December 1816, a public
fund-raising campaign was launched, although priority was assigned to the open-

ing of an insane asylum. State support was based on political affinities between the governing Federalist party and the hospital's leading supporters. As in Europe a few decades earlier, the driving ideology was mercantilist, with the Federalists viewing the state as a sailing vessel on which both the captain and his officers had a duty to protect the welfare of their crew. By March 1817, the drive had already obtained over $100,000 to meet the conditions of the legislative grant. Donations were received from citizens in all walks of life. Two of the more bizarre gifts were a 273-pound sow and an Egyptian mummy from Thebes.[29]

After examining several sites for a general hospital, a committee recommended the purchase of the Allen Street Estate, a four-acre tract on the banks of the Charles River with excellent exposure to fresh summer breezes, always a primary consideration when planning a well-ventilated hospital. The land was bought for $20,000, and Charles Bulfinch (1763–1844), designer of the State House and leading architect of the period, was selected to visit similar institutions in New York and Philadelphia and report his findings.[30] The legislature, in turn, authorized the provision of granite blocks for the hospital's construction, to be prepared and fitted by convicts from the nearby state prison. Although competing bids were received by the board of trustees, Bulfinch's plan for the hospital was selected on January 25, 1818. The imposing and ornate three-story building was designed in the classical Greek revival style, with an elegant portico and gables topped by a dome. The rectangular structure consisted of a central core surrounded on each side by a wing. Its interior design owed much to Adam's Royal Infirmary of Edinburgh, with its emphasis on segregating the patients and facilitating their institutional control. All floors were linked through central stairways. Service areas, including the kitchen, laundry, wood bins, and morgue, together with a sickroom for dying patients, were shifted to the basement. Both upper floors contained administrative and staff rooms in the center, surrounded by wards and smaller rooms for paying patients on the wings. Supported by the portico, the domed amphitheater, with its large skylight, towered over the building. It was designed for lectures and surgical operations. In a departure from previous models, Bulfinch created separate rooms for the resident nursing and medical personnel adjacent to the facilities housing patients. Another innovation featured central heating and ventilation, as well as interior plumbing and toilets with water closets.[31]

The hospital's cornerstone was laid on July 4, 1818, but construction proceeded slowly during the next three years. At last, Jackson and Warren were notified early in 1821 that the block-type hospital would be ready for patients on September 1. To prepare for its occupancy, a retired ship's master was appointed superintendent and his wife the matron on April 1. The first patient, a 30-year-old sailor, was admitted on September 3. Boston had acquired not only another imposing landmark on the banks of the Charles River, but also a state-of-the-art medical facility. As soon as the hospital opened, students from Harvard College's medical school followed their professors from the Boston Almshouse to the new premises, where the first surgical operation—for an anal prolapse—was performed on September 21. In 1823 the building was finally completed, with a capacity of 73 beds. After both the medical school and the hospital were in operation, Jackson and Warren issued a pamphlet in 1824 in which they reemphasized the link between the caring and educational roles of the MGH.[32] Moreover, like its Parisian counterparts, the institution also promoted clinical research, best exemplified by Jackson's studies on typhoid fever. To place the hospital's finances on a more stable basis, the trustees approved a new subscription method in 1825 whereby anyone who donated $100 per year would have a free bed at his disposal in the hospital.

While prayer, meditation, and perhaps Bible readings may have been allowed, Sunday worship was prohibited since it was felt that it could produce "an unfavorable excitement in patients." However, the hospital had been clearly conceived and was run as an interdenominational charitable institution, although most of the sponsors and trustees were Unitarians. Later, in 1842, John C. Warren donated the sum of $1,000 to create a fund for the purchase of religious and moral books as part of an institutional library and a reflection of the hospital's spiritual agenda. "It must be obvious to every reflecting mind," declared the trustees, "that seasons of bodily infirmity and sickness present peculiarly favorable opportunities for making useful impressions upon the character and for affording Christian comfort and consolation."[33]

By 1830, the establishment on Allen Street and the Harvard Medical School had become the dominant medical institutions in New England. By necessity, the number of patients remained small, and surgical operations were seldom scheduled, in spite of Warren's publications and professional eminence. Bostonians, however, including hospital trustees, truly believed that the quality of care given to patients at the MGH was at least comparable to that provided at the Pennsylvania or New York hospitals. Teaching and clinical research continued, and accounts of the management of selected surgical cases was now routinely published in the *Boston Medical and Surgical Journal.*

More and more, the institution reflected the major orientation of its medical staff, which was concerned with practicing a therapeutically less aggressive medicine compared to that of other prominent American institutions on the Eastern seaboard. From the beginning, Jackson's medical treatments had been relatively conservative, deemphasizing the aggressive "heroic" approaches of the day, including excessive purging and bloodletting. Jackson also attacked Brunonianism, the Scottish alternative medical system based on the use of stimulants, notably wine and opium.[34] Another example of this approach was Jacob Bigelow's 1835 publication, *A Discourse on Self-Limited Diseases.*

In 1836, the hospital's admission process was entrusted to an assistant house physician but was still subject to regulations and final approval by the trustees, who had controlled admissions before. This change was apparently prompted by the trustees' inability or unwillingness to make the necessary personal inquiries—as stipulated by the rules—into the financial status of poor applicants to determine their "deserving" status. On the practical level, the new regulations simplified MGH's admitting procedures, thus also attracting more paying patients, who during that year made up more than half of the hospital population. Their preferential admission forced the rejection of numerous poor people, especially "persons of color," while favoring the entry of merchants and clergymen who paid for their care.

Discussions about an expansion of the facilities were held as applications for admission increased in the late 1830s.[35] After almost two decades, the trustees of the hospital acknowledged that a higher level of charitable giving had become necessary if the institution was to fulfill its earlier assistential goals.[36] Following the retirement of Jackson, a number of young physicians who had studied medicine in Parisian hospitals took over. They included Jacob Bowditch's son, Henry I. Bowditch (1808–1892), who promoted the use of Laennec's stethoscope; Oliver Wendell Holmes (1809–1894), the famous physician and man of letters; and John C. Warren's son, the surgeon Jonathan Mason Warren (1811–1867).[37] To promote more business, new surgical equipment had been acquired by John C. Warren during a visit to Europe in 1838. This decision was made in spite of the fact that the institution was now running a worrisome deficit and had been forced to curtail by two-thirds the number of free beds previously offered to the poor. It was expected that the excellent surgical reputation of the institution, still resting on that of Warren, would attract more paying inmates and lead to more surgeries.

With the appointment in 1839 of a new superintendent, Charles Sumner, a former sea captain (not to be confused with the famous anti-slavery senator), the trustees continued to emphasize the special status of the MGH as a place of first rather than last resort. "The design of this hospital is different from that of many others, inasmuch as it is intended as a retreat in sickness for those who can and do pay their own board as well as those whom sickness or accidents may have deprived of the means of doing so," the annual report declared. The institution had successfully transcended the early stigma of being another "poor-house under a new name," and the trustees insisted that "a large part of the community now understands that if from any cause they cannot be taken care of in the bosoms of their own families, there is no other situation where they can more respectably, comfortably and economically place themselves than in your hospital."[38]

The early 1840s witnessed further hospital expansions. Sumner ran a tight ship. He increased efficiency and reduced expenses, but the number of poor patients being turned away increased to the point where Bowditch, then an assistant physician, made generous contributions to the free-bed fund, thereby almost doubling the admissions of those without resources.[39] Since MGH's sister charity, the McLean Asylum for the insane, was running a surplus in its operation, the trustees pledged to shift this money to MGH in the hope of expanding its services in the face of growing local needs. The visiting medical and surgical staff, composed of three physicians and three surgeons, was now in firm control of admissions and proceeded to improve the hospital's clinical record keeping. A new superintendent, John M. Goodwin, replaced Sumner in 1841, and for the first time in years, administrative savings allowed an increase in the number of those admitted to free beds—climbing to more than half of the total number of patients accepted by the institution. Part of this change was due to the more rapid turnover of paying inmates, mostly males (the gender ratio was 3:1). The poor occupying free beds, however, stayed on average three times longer, leading to charges that they had selected the hospital as their "comfortable home."[40]

By 1845, calls for more hospital accommodations were common in Boston. In the opinion of some medical leaders, another charitable facility was needed, especially in East Boston, which was quickly becoming the manufacturing center of the city. The perception that MGH had "grown into a colossal institution" but could not admit all applicants was widely shared in the city. "By the very nature of its organization, there are many free beds, so-called, actually purchased by wealthy gentlemen, who have given large sums of money to the hospital—and they have the privilege of sending their friends, and indeed, any person they may choose, to occupy them—and while there, they receive every possible attention, without cost to themselves or additional expense to their kind patrons." By contrast, the number of persons paying by the week was insufficient, a reason for the recent successful subscription to enlarge the building. The goal was to create more room for additional paying inmates, part of the "constant rush of strangers to the city, now the great commercial center of the north," while also continuing to admit a class of respectable sufferers—locally employed poor like Alice—who could not afford to pay their hospital fees.[41]

Management of pain: A professional goal

Pain remains a complex human problem. While pain can be framed as physiological phenomenon or a mental state, thresholds for its perception and meaning are constructed and modulated by culture. Awareness and expression of pain—there is a very rich vocabulary in all languages dealing with types of pain—and its relief have always engaged humankind. Faced with the reality of pain, healers have traditionally assumed that it is a natural event associated with vitality, an important and useful alarm signal—in classical antiquity, the bark of a guardian dog—necessary for triggering internal recovery. Moreover, if pain could be constructed as a positive manifestation of the body's ability to defend itself and drive out disease, painful counterirritation procedures in vogue until the nineteenth century such as blistering, cupping, moxa (burning a small cone of herbs placed on particular areas of skin), and cauterization, experienced by patients from Aristides and Prodromos to Janet Williamson and Alice Mohan, would only enhance the healing effects. By contrast, lack of pain—like that experienced by leprosy sufferers—was associated early on with skin damage and infection.[42]

If ancient healers often considered pain in a positive physiological light, Christianity likewise stressed its moral qualities. Suffering was thus viewed as both punishment (Old Testament) and redemption (New Testament). Its redemptive quality was closely linked to the suffering Christ. "Pain is the chastisement of a Father or, at least, that it is in some way or another ordained for, or instrumental to good. Otherwise evil and pain would be in their effects on sufferers, long-lived."[43] Uncoupled from such religious meanings, pain came to be associated with disease and disorders in the Cartesian human machine to be avoided or conquered. During the Enlightenment, this secularization and a new view of human physiology as directed by the nervous system radically changed the cultural meaning of pain.[44] As noted earlier, nervous sensibility and excitability came to be seen as critical for the maintenance of a healthy balance. Within this world of nerves, physical pain became for some an excessive, harmful stimulus, capable of derailing internal harmony and sustaining imbalances of the body's vitality.[45] Other sufferers and medical practitioners, however, continued to view pain as a positive manifestation closely linked to vitality and individual physical and moral strength, a clinical warning system that also monitored recovery. This ambivalence had survived to our own day.[46]

Pain suppression through the use of alcoholic beverages, mandrake extracts, hemp vapor, and opium extracts can be traced back to early civilized life in the Middle East and Europe. By the Middle Ages, medicated sponges soaked in solutions of opium, hemlock, leaves of mandragora, henbane, and wild ivy were employed for surgical interventions. In 1540, Paracelsus advocated the use of "sweet vitriol" (ether) for similar circumstances, and the surgeon Ambroise Pare achieved local anesthesia through the compression of nerves. In the eighteenth century, vigorous debates ensued about the wisdom of using anodynes or painkillers, especially the traditional opium preparations employed since antiquity. Here the debates between adherents of William Cullen and John Brown over the characterization of opium as either a sedative or a stimulant merely reflected the growing utilization of this drug for lessening pain, either as an item of the official materia medica or as an ingredient in patent medicines dispensed by quacks. With the discovery of nitrous oxide by Joseph Priestley in 1772 and Beddoes' use of gases, including ether inhalations, in the treatment of tuberculosis, the stage was set for further experimentation. In 1800, Humphry Davy expounded on ether's possible anesthetic qualities. Practitioners, however, hesitated to employ these gases, aware of their capacity to depress vitality and even cause death, effects attributed to the poisonous nature of these compounds.[47]

Among the leading factors responsible for the events of October 1846 at MGH, when ether anesthesia was first introduced to render patients temporarily uncon-

scious for surgery, was the evolution of American dentistry. Originating as a domestic and folk practice performed by itinerant blacksmiths and tooth drawers,
dentistry had hitherto been mainly restricted to the extraction of infected teeth,
a procedure also performed by physicians and surgeons. However, by the late
eighteenth century, a new marketplace for a broader range of dental services, especially among the wealthy and middle-class urban populations, favored greater
professionalization. Not only were extractions still common, but dentists now offered a wide variety of fillings and replacements, the latter in the form of bridges
and dentures. The coming of age of American dentistry is best exemplified by the
1793 appointment of one surgeon-dentist, R. C. Skinner, to the staff of the New
York Dispensary, as well as the New York Hospital and Almshouse.[48] In 1801
Skinner published his influential book, *A Treatise on the Human Teeth.*

In Boston, the dental tradition went back to silversmith Paul Revere in the
1760s, followed by the surgeon-dentist Josiah Flagg, who, after a brief itinerant
practice, had settled in Boston in 1795. Flagg—the "Boston dentist" par excellence—had also devised the first dental chair with an adjustable headrest. Aided
by the influx of competently trained surgeon-dentists from Europe, especially
France, professional dentistry in America became popular, especially in the growing commercial centers along the eastern seaboard. Most dentists offered the traditional procedures associated with their craft, especially tooth extractions. However, following Flagg, they also began to stress oral hygiene and the importance
of tooth retention. Given its narrow anatomical focus, non-life-threatening character, and technical developments in restorative procedures and prosthetic devices
using porcelain, dentistry was increasingly in demand during the 1820s and 1830s.
A small professional elite sought to achieve legitimacy and standing in a field
crowded by inferior, untrained "dental bunglers." The existence of "an almost
standing army of dentists in the United States" and public complacency concerning
their professional qualifications remained a serious problem in the absence of state
licensing or regulations.[49]

In spite of such efforts, the medical profession continued to hold dentistry in
lower social and professional esteem since its members, devoted to a manual craft
and locked into an overt commercial competition, failed to satisfy the ideals of
professional gentility. Physicians in New England were alarmed by the rate of increase of their dental brethren. In 1844, the fear in Boston was that dentists would
soon outnumber physicians, since there seemed to be an ever greater demand for
them—in their eyes, caused by the bad work of half of the profession. Tooth decay was viewed as a universal evil and was blamed on poor diet. Physicians de-
riding the lack of science and the "mechanical" character of dentistry were transparent in their professional jealousy. Dentists commanded high fees, often higher
than medical ones, and the public seemed to be willing to pay.[50] For dentists, the
road to cultural recognition was manual education and the achievement of dexterity: "Hands should be educated as well as the head" read one editorial, espe-

cially that most delicate sense of touch that, "if not so necessary for the success of the operation, is all important for the feelings and welfare of the patient."[51] Moreover, in another demonstration of the value of competition, dentists designed their own instruments, making them increasingly small and light.

Because of the accompanying pain, surgery at this time had to be performed at incredible speed to prevent death from shock and blood loss. Although spiritual fortitude and manual dexterity were critical, the best operators had to be fast, a fact that severely limited the range of elective procedures to be performed. Because of secondary infections, interventions involving cavities such as the chest and abdomen were not attempted. Each operation was a brutal ordeal, especially for the patient. By the 1840s, moderating voices were heard within the profession preaching restraint in the popular practice of amputations, even though this injunction diminished a surgeon's income. An 1845 editorial commented that "in regard to amputations, the greatest modern impression is the frequency with which they are abstained from. When surgeons first got into the way of operating, limbs were removed without scruple and frequently without just cause. They would appear sometimes to have been lopped off as if to prove how well the body could maintain its existence without them."[52] Commenting on the expansive nature of surgery as reflected in Jacob Bigelow's 1845 *Manual of Orthopedic Surgery*, another Boston reviewer remarked that "the free manner of cutting up the cordage of the living human body which is now practiced here and there and everywhere, is well calculated to astonish those who have been lubricating tendons all their professional days to no purpose."[53]

While Alice Mohan's knee was being subjected to daily sinapisms—mustard plasters—Gilbert Abbott, a 20-year-old printer with a congenital tumor on the left side of his face and neck, awaited surgery in a nearby ward. Always weak and sickly, he had been admitted to the men's surgical ward on September 25, 1846. On examination, the mostly soft tumor could be made to disappear by compression. It consisted of tortuous, indurated veins extending from the surface deep below the tongue. But what to do? This problem seemed more cosmetic than life-threatening. Finally, John C. Warren decided to expose the swollen veins by dissection for the purpose of placing a ligature around them, although the prospect of knives in his face must have been simply terrifying to Gilbert. Confined to MGH's surgical ward for almost three weeks, he must have been anxious. Outside, the unusually warm Indian summer throughout New England had produced a second crop of wild raspberries for picking until a "Nor'easter" blew through the city, causing damage to ships.[54]

Warren sent a note on October 14 to Dr. William Morton, requesting his presence for the purpose of administering ether to the patient. Morton, who was engaged in private dental practice, had already successfully administered the anesthetic two weeks earlier to one of his patients. Before him, another dentist, Horace Wells, from Hartford, Connecticut, had administered nitrous oxide successfully during tooth extractions. Allowed by Warren to demonstrate its anesthetic qualities before his medical school class in 1844, Wells attempted to extract a student's tooth, but the experiment had failed to produce complete insensibility and the dentist was laughed out of Boston.[55] Now, two years later, Morton had obtained Warren's consent to administer his "letheon" to a surgical patient. Since no patients in private practice were available in the next few days, Warren selected Abbott for this fateful experiment and scheduled the operation for Friday, October 16, 1846.[56] The selection of a Friday was unusual; to maximize the presence of physicians and medical students, all operations were performed on Saturday mornings in the hospital's amphitheater. However, given Wells' previous failure with nitrous oxide, Warren perhaps wanted to avoid another possible embarrassment by deliberately operating in front of a small group of staff members.[57]

At the appointed time, Gilbert was led into the theater and seated in an operating chair. Warren and a number of colleagues gathered around the sufferer. Breaking the oppressive silence, Warren announced to his incredulous audience that "a test of some preparation was to be made for which the astonishing claim had been made that it would render the person operated upon free from pain." Unfortunately, Dr. Morton failed to appear, and after waiting for 15–30 minutes, a frustrated Warren is said to have commented somewhat sarcastically that "I presume he [Morton] is otherwise engaged," a pronouncement that elicited a "derisive laugh" from those attending. However, as Warren brandished a knife to begin his surgery, Morton entered the operating room from a side door. Apologizing for his delay, he informed Warren that "he had been occupied in preparing his apparatus which consisted of a tube connected with a glass globe." Warren turned to him, saying, "well, sir, your patient is ready." Morton applied the tube to Abbott's nostrils, telling him to inhale the ether, and after four to five minutes, Abbott appeared to be asleep. Now it was Morton's turn to tell Warren that "your patient is ready, sir."[58]

Warren now made a two and one-half inch incision over the center of the external tumor, just beneath the edge of the jaw, extending through the skin and subcutaneous tissue. To his great surprise and that of his retinue, the patient "did not shrink nor cry out." A layer of fascia was dissected off, disclosing a network of large veins and small arteries, but hemorrhaging was slight and no vessel required ligature. During the dissection, however, the patient began to move his limbs and cry out, uttering "extraordinary expressions, and these movements seemed to indicate the existence of pain." Warren quickly passed a curved needle with a ligature under the tumor, compressed it, and tied the mass, filling the wound with a small compress and lint. The extremely brief and limited operation was over, the experiment with the anesthetic agent seemingly a partial success.[59]

After Abbott recovered his faculties and before being returned to the ward, he told his surgeons what they wanted to hear: he had not experienced any pain but simply an unpleasant scraping sensation. After the dressings were removed

the next day, the wound was filled with potash—potassium carbonate—but venous bleeding occurred for several hours, checked with sponges, ice packs, lint,
and compression. Emboldened by this favorable turn of events, Warren enlisted
George Hayward the following day to remove a large, fatty subcutaneous tumor
from the right shoulder of a woman who had entered the hospital as an outpatient. The unnamed individual volunteered to be placed under the effects of
letheon and again, after a few minutes, was completely insensitive, allowing Hayward to incise the skin and extirpate the growth.[60] By Sunday, Gilbert Abbott
was resting comfortably and displayed a good appetite, receiving some broth with
soaked toast. A week later, following the use of poultices, the slough of the wound
was removed, uncovering a healthy granulating surface sprinkled with potash and
then dressed with lint soaked in warm water. While the tumor retained its previous size, no blood vessels could be detected in it, and the incision began to heal.
Although no further complications ensued, Gilbert remained in the hospital for
another month as a convalescent and was finally discharged on December 7.

First amputation under ether anesthesia, 1846

With Abbott slowly recovering from his surgery, a decision to amputate Alice Mohan's leg must have been reached in early November, following Hayward's replacement of Warren as chief of the hospital's surgical service. After checking with
his former superior, Hayward agreed to continue the moratorium on further ether
inhalations until Morton changed his mind about sharing the nature of letheon
with the hospital's surgical staff and exempting MGH from patent rights to its
use. On November 6, Morton visited Hayward at the suggestion of Henry Bigelow,
offering to employ his letheon in a "capital" operation to truly demonstrate its
anesthetic qualities. Alice's amputation had already been scheduled for the following day. Hayward again conferred with Warren. He demanded that, in exchange for providing another experimental subject, Morton would have to reveal
in a letter the true nature of his compound, as well as grant the hospital's surgical staff permission to employ it in future operations. Perhaps reluctantly, Morton agreed, and, after further consultations between Hayward and other visiting
surgeons, Alice's amputation under letheon anesthesia was scheduled for the following day. This information was transmitted to the Harvard medical students
and was also widely circulated among members of Boston's surgical fraternity.

On Saturday morning, November 7, 1846, a pale, emaciated Alice Mohan was
carried to the surgical amphitheater on a stretcher by two male attendants. They
were accompanied by the house surgeons, Heywood and Lambert. Just then, the
tall clock on the hospital's stairway rang 11 times. An hour earlier, Alice had ingested 100 drops of laudanum. Clad in a white sheet covering her entire body,
she faced the operators and a curious, standing-room-only audience assembled to

witness what promised to be an extraordinary event. Surrounding Hayward were other visiting surgeons, including John C. Warren, Henry Bigelow, Samuel Parkman, Samuel D. Townsend, and J. Mason Warren, the last chosen to assist in the surgery. Warren Senior had already addressed the audience, reading Morton's permission letter. The operating table, located at the center of the domed room, was covered with white linen next to another table featuring surgical instruments and ligatures also covered by clean cloth. Lifted by the attendants, Alice was placed on the operating table on her back, with the lower extremities projecting beyond its edge but "duly" supported, presumably by some temporary contraption.

Hayward now came forward, announcing that he and the other surgeons had agreed to let Dr. Morton administer his preparation to the patient. This was the cue for the dentist to make his appearance on the stage, stylishly dressed in a blue frock coat with brass buttons and carrying the mysterious glass globe containing the magic potion. With all preliminary arrangements completed, Morton took a central position behind the patient and ordered her to begin breathing the mixture. Alice, however, confronted with the pungency of the vapor, refused at first to inhale it. At last, with Morton adjusting the mouthpiece to fit her, she began breathing and seemed unconscious—"completely under its influence" within three minutes. With Hayward in charge and Warren Junior assisting, the femoral artery was compressed at the groin and the right thigh transfixed at its middle. After cutting in rapid succession two skin and muscle flaps and retracting them, Hayward had another assistant compress the artery while Mason sawed off the bone. A slight sprinkling of blood was stopped with bone pliers, and the chief vessels were secured with ligatures.[61]

According to eyewitnesses, the audience remained quiet and tense, with only occasional murmurs as the surgery proceeded with lightning speed. As the last ligature was placed about two minutes later, Alice began to groan and cry a little, but the procedure was essentially over. Once the amputated leg had been taken away, a single dressing dipped in cold water and secured around the stump was applied to compress the wound. Alice, quickly returning to consciousness, seemed surprised that the amputation had already taken place.[62] According to the operative notes, the blood loss was small. "With regard to the influence of the preparation inhaled, the patient asserts that she was entirely insensible until the last artery was being secured" read the clinical chart. Bigelow later stated that Alice failed to answer several questions put to her throughout the few minutes of the operation, a sign that she was "evidently completely insensitive to pain or other external influences." However, she was said to have uttered a mild cry when the sciatic nerve was divided.[63]

Alice's immediate postoperative period was quite routine. She displayed a very feeble pulse and cold, sweaty skin. She also began moaning because of phantom pain in the amputated limb and received another 50 drops of laudanum. By 2 PM, however, Alice had sufficiently recovered to talk "very pleasantly" with her caregivers and ask for a cup of tea. An hour later, Hayward removed the compresses and some remaining blood clots, then carefully checked the ligatures, brought the flaps together to cover the bone, and secured them with six separate sutures. Finally, the entire stump was carefully dressed and covered with bandages moistened in cold water. Perhaps this was the turning point in Alice's illness. The peccant humors had been carried away together with her infected leg. More than a year of suffering was about to end.

Alice was not the only one operated on that morning using an anesthetic. Barely half an hour later, John C. Warren stepped into the amphitheater to face Betsy Magrun, a 53-year-old widow from Duxbury with a tumor the size of a pigeon attached to the left side of her jaw. Betsy had also been premedicated with laudanum at 10 AM and, placed in an operating chair, was ordered to inhale Morton's preparation for about three minutes before falling asleep. Warren then proceeded to remove an entire fragment of the "carcinomatous affection," ligating three major arteries and cutting across the submaxillary gland. The patient remained insensible until the bone was being sawed into, then "suffered" while a cold compress was applied. The wound continued to bleed freely in spite of efforts to compress it with numerous sponges. Finally, after Betsy had been returned to her bed in the ward, another ligature was placed around the incision by J. Mason Warren, who was assisting his father, and both Hayward and Bigelow also inspected it. In spite of these circumstances, the patient's wound, but perhaps not her disease, was healed, and she was discharged November 30.[64] Three weeks of clinical trials at the MGH to determine the effects of letheon—sulfuric ether—in surgery were over.

In marked contrast to Alice Mohan and Betsy Magrun, Theophilus Petier, a 35-year-old Canadian farmer, was subjected to an emergency amputation of his left lower leg without an anesthetic just a week later. Petier had been brought into the hospital at 5 PM following an accident on November 16 at the Boston and Lowell Railroad yard. In an intoxicated state, he had attempted to get on a moving car, missed his foothold, fell on the rails, and had the leg crushed by one of the car wheels. After his arrival, the patient was brought into a bathroom for cleansing, laid on a table, and had the amputation at 7 PM under the direction of Hayward without uttering a complaint. Two hours later, somewhat sober, he realized the nature of the surgery and had to be restrained with the use of a straitjacket.[65]

Alice Mohan, meanwhile, had a gradual recovery punctuated by a series of temporary setbacks. Because of her severe muscular spasms on the operated thigh, a nurse was ordered to sit constantly next to her, compressing the stump with her hand to avoid any break in the ligatures. With laudanum administered freely to decrease pain and facilitate sleep, Alice became more comfortable (her manner was even described as "vivacious") on November 9, barely two days after the surgery. All stitches were removed on the 13th, with the lips of the stump now brought together by a single plaster. However, a week later, the patient experienced sudden pain and a gush of blood in the stump, which was immediately treated with arterial compression in the right groin and a tourniquet "for the sake of perfect security." Half an hour later, with the compression procedures suspended, no further bleeding ensued. From that point on, Alice recovered rapidly. With an improved appetite, she started to gain weight and became ambulatory, walking through the ward on crutches by early December.

When Abbott's minor surgery had been concluded, Warren is said to have turned to those present and exclaimed: "Gentlemen, this is no humbug, the conquest of pain has been achieved." The pointed reference to "humbug" was made in the context of contemporary professional struggles in America, and referred to the growing popularity of hypnotism and other mesmeric practices in surgery. Even the editors of the *Boston Medical and Surgical Journal* felt compelled to write in the November 18, 1846 issue that "an impression exists in Boston that a remarkable discovery has been made. Unlike the farce and trickery of mesmerism, this is based on scientific principles and is solely in the hands of gentlemen of high professional attainments who make no secret of the matter or manner."[66]

Two days after Alice Mohan's surgery, Henry Bigelow presented a paper on the employment of inhalation anesthesia to members of Boston's Society of Medical Improvement, having provided earlier an abstract to be read before a session of the American Academy of Arts and Sciences on November 3.[67] Bigelow shared with his audience a chronological account of the events, mentioning Warren's and Hayward's first interventions in October, followed by a series of human experiments conducted by Bigelow himself with sulfuric ether. Bigelow stressed that "medicated inhalation," including the use of ether, had been tried before for pain control, as well as for respiratory and gastrointestinal conditions. The results had been uncertain, in part because of the idiosyncratic responses of the subjects. Some became excited and uncontrollable after a few breaths, while others were notably sedated, even paralyzed. Such differences, Bigelow suggested, were partly dosage related, stemming from differences in the amount of ether inhaled, a problem to be corrected through the employment of a standardized inhaler, a two-necked glass globe that allowed the entrance of air through one opening and the exit of vapor through a mouthpiece on the other. The patient's expired air, in turn, was diverted from the globe through a valve designed to avoid dilution of the vapor. To enlarge the evaporating surface, the globe was filled with sponges soaked in the ether.

Bigelow went on to describe a number of successful cases from Dr. Morton's dental practice that he had personally observed. Pulse readings and the state of pupillary dilation were included. Most states of unconsciousness were achieved within about three minutes, at which point the apparatus was immediately withdrawn and the surgical extractions performed in the next minute or two, just before most patients awoke. In some cases, nausea and vomiting followed. The transfer of this procedure from dentistry to surgery obviously presented new challenges. The level of unconsciousness to be achieved had to be somewhat deeper and more sustained, without creating excessive excitement or a semicomatose condition that would make surgery impossible. Previously, surgeons employing ether had run into trouble, as their patients remained drowsy or nearly comatose for extended periods. "The process," concluded Bigelow, "is obviously adapted to operations which are brief in their duration, whatever be their severity."[68] Dental extractions, amputations, and the alleviation of functional pains such as muscular spasms seemed the ideal indications.

Having placed ether inhalation within the context of previous therapeutic efforts, Bigelow was now keen to stress the novelty of this approach to surgical procedures, citing "ignorance of an universal application and immense practical utility that prevented such isolated facts from being generalized." Consequently, he now awarded the "invention" to Charles T. Jackson and William Morton, defending their right to take out a patent since they were the rightful "proprietors." Here Bigelow conceded that scientific discoveries had traditionally been rewarded not by patent and profit, but by fame, honor, and academic positions, especially in the medical field, which was more philanthropic than most. "Many will assent with reluctance to the propriety of restricting by letters patent the use of an agent capable of mitigating human suffering," Bigelow admitted, but peculiar circumstances made the employment of letheon an exception. Among them was its potential for abuse, and the need for restricted access since its action was still unknown. Above all, however, Bigelow argued, patents were common in the otherwise secretive and competitive "mechanical art of dentistry," adding, however, that the generous proprietors had already ceded their rights to MGH and could be persuaded to do likewise for other members of the medical profession "as soon as necessary arrangements can be made for publicity of the process."[69]

In 1793 the U.S. Congress had enacted a law granting patents to inventors of products or processes that "promote the progress of science and useful arts." Then, in 1836, a new Patent Office began to award patents—usually for a term of 17 years—within a framework that sought to encourage creativity and reward inventors. Dentists immediately took advantage of such legislation, protecting their new processes for making false teeth. In medicine, however, most patents had been sought by greedy manufacturers of nostrums containing secret ingredients, conferring a certain aura of unscrupulousness on the entire process.[70]

While linking the patent issue with the needs of an entrepreneurial and less professionalized dental community, Bigelow was really trying to seize control of the etherization method as a way to advance Boston's surgical community. His own flashy professional demeanor and self-advertisement had already generated widespread criticism among his more traditional peers. The argument employed by Bigelow and his colleagues was that the use of letheon had to be restricted to a small group of responsible practitioners "to prevent it from being abused and falling into the power of low, evil-minded, irresponsible persons."[71] There was still a fair amount of stigma attached to ether as a recreational drug. So-called ether frolics were widely popular in New England among the upper classes, and with its inebriating influence, ether was closely associated with another problematic substance: alcohol. To move sulfuric ether from recreational to professional use linked with science demanded a cautious approach. Much was at stake if surgery was to benefit from inhalation anesthesia, and the range of experiences needed to be restricted lest dangerous side effects and even accidental deaths mar or stop once more a most encouraging development.[72]

The following day, the *Boston Daily Advertiser* reprinted Bigelow's article without including the controversial passages about the patenting issue. Then Bigelow's father, Jacob, wrote a letter on November 28 to a friend in London, Francis Boot, enclosing the newspaper article. After a quick transatlantic crossing, the information was published in an issue of the *London Medical Gazette* on December 18. Informed of Bigelow's paper that same day, the prominent London surgeon Robert Liston immediately went out to obtain sulfuric ether, spending the weekend perfecting a proper inhaler. By Monday, December 21, Liston was ready and went on to perform an amputation of the thigh—an operation similar to that carried out on Alice Mohan—using ether anesthesia, the first such procedure outside of the United States.[73]

The significance of ether anesthesia

Exactly five weeks after Alice's operation, John C. Warren teamed up once more with Morton. The patient was Mary Muldrave, a 50-year-old Irish widow, who had been admitted 10 days earlier with a fungous tumor the size of a walnut attached to her left canine tooth. Sitting in the operating chair and taking a few breaths of ether, the patient fell asleep, and Warren was able to make an incision under the upper lip, crush the tumor with his special pliers, place two ligatures, and apply the cautery to prevent any bleeding before the patient awoke. According to the clinical chart, Mrs. Muldrave was discharged "well" on December 24.[74] At the instigation of Morton's attorney, R. H. Eddy (also the U.S. patent officer in Boston),[75] Warren Senior, meanwhile, felt pressured to issue an official statement on November 30 about the new discovery. His account of the events that had transpired at the MGH during the past six weeks was communicated to the *Boston Medical and Surgical Journal.*

Warren described the known sequence of events, from Morton's initial request and Abbott's partially successful surgery to his own subsequent meeting with the chemist Jackson, who claimed to have suggested the use of ether.[76] Warren also explained the decision not to perform further etherization until the patent matter had been resolved. With Morton's letter granting the hospital free use of the

method, surgeries under ether resumed with Mohan and Magrun, followed by two
tumor removals by Warren Junior on November 12 and November 21. Warren's
conclusion was that all the cases proved "a decided mitigation of pain" but that
the etherization method needed to be employed with great caution because of its
stimulation of both the heart and the respiration rate. This meant that it should
"never be employed except under the inspection of a judicious and competent
person."[77]

After her nearly two-year ordeal, a reborn Alice Mohan was discharged "well"
from the MGH on Tuesday, December 22, 1846, just before the Christmas holiday. The hospital's trustees had voted to provide her with a $25 wooden leg pros-
thesis,[78] but she undoubtedly faced an uncertain future.[79] Alice was the first patient ever to tolerate a significant surgical procedure under anesthesia. As Bigelow
and others had pointed out, pain control had been an important professional issue since the 1750s, although the dangers of iatrogenic harm and drug addiction,
especially with opium, had caused surgeons repeatedly to avoid employing the
substances already available. In addition, ether inhalation, although not designed
to prolong the speedy interventions, provided surgeons with a more pliable patient—at least after an initial unpredictable period of excitement—thus increasing the ease and safety of a particular surgical procedure. According to Hayward,
the insensibility "disarms the operative part of our calling of the terror with which
it is uniformly regarded by patients" and in more protracted cases would prevent
possible shock.[80] Still, uncertainties about the preparation and action of sulfuric
ether remained, and the patient's need for a vital supply of oxygen during anesthesia had already become clear.

Because of the hazards linked to their administration, the use of anesthetics
increased professional control and patient dependence. Although opportunities
for a widespread technological solution to the problem of surgical pain was at
hand, surgeons found themselves returning to the principle of therapeutic specificity, which remained a hallmark of professional identity and status. A veritable
"calculus" of suffering ensued whereby surgeons made only selective use of anesthesia after assessing the individual characteristics of the patient they were planning to operate on.[81] Among the criteria employed in making such a determination were important cultural, social, and religious considerations.[82]

Finally, the "discovery" of ether anesthesia in Boston must be placed firmly
within the context of contemporary Boston medicine and surgery, especially its
local struggles for professional and cultural identity in an atmosphere of sectari-
anism that included the spread of mesmerism. Lacking licensing or any other legal standard, the profession's only stronghold was the local Boston Medical Society. A year later, this state of affairs led to the establishment of the American
Medical Association in an effort to provide national legitimacy and identity. At
MGH, ether anesthesia decisively enhanced the institution's reputation as an international medical teaching and research center. The new eastern wing expan-

sion was nearing completion, and together with the western addition already in use, the hospital's capacity nearly doubled, allowing the admission of more private patients, as well as sick and destitute Irish immigrants. A plaque in the old amphitheater, now known as the Ether Dome, still proclaims it the site of the first public use of ether. Although the qualifier was meant to acknowledge the earlier use of ether on private patients by Crawford W. Long of Georgia, the public nature of the demonstration and the presence of witnesses were absolutely critical for the subsequent success of the procedure. Linking the origins of surgical anesthesia with Boston hospital medicine became a matter of intense local professional pride. Boston's reputation as one of America's foremost medical centers, even rivaling the traditional front-runner, Philadelphia, was to grow. More than 20 years later, one author asked: "was it not in Boston that the pain-annulling property of sulfuric ether was discovered, the stupendous boon of anesthesia being thus, under Providence, given to mankind?"[83]

SCOTLAND: LISTER AND ANTISEPSIS

To be shut up with strangers inside huge walls and folding gates, tho' its so far prison like, still it is not that, it is a hospital and tho bleak and dreary looking, I was there under the wise dispensation of God.

Margaret Mathewson, 1877[84]

From the Shetlands to Victorian Edinburgh

Explaining that she was going to seek advice regarding her arm, Margaret Mathewson traveled to Edinburgh in early 1877 to consult surgeons at the Royal Infirmary. Living in Mid Yell on the Shetland Islands, this 29-year-old unmarried daughter of a poor parish teacher was experiencing swelling, pain, and dysfunction of her upper left arm near the shoulder, a complication of a three-year respiratory ailment. When the shoulder got worse after an accident while performing harvest chores, Margaret had consulted the local parish minister, who made an incision over what appeared to be an abscess and provided her with some ointment to periodically dress the draining wound. The cut failed to close, leaving behind a fistula that eventually prompted Margaret to decide on another course of action. Over the objections of her parents, who were "prejudiced against the Infirmary," she decided to travel to Edinburgh.

For more than a century, hospitals had been considered dangerous places that spread infection and caused death. This so-called hospitalism had become a major dread, jeopardizing the hospital's role as a house of recovery. Margaret, however, had no such dread of hospitals, and she informed her brother Arthur that she had known other "girls who had gone there just to take a rest from service for a few weeks,"[85] much as Janet Williamson had at the same Infirmary nearly a century earlier. Armed with a letter of recommendation from her minister, she journeyed south by sea to Leith in the company of a neighbor bound for Australia. After reaching her boarding house in Edinburgh, Margaret contacted her cousin Martha, living in the city, only to be confronted by some bad news: another smallpox epidemic threatened the Scottish capital.[86]

Also troubling the city's medical community at the time was the perceived collapse of the Edinburgh Medical School. This had been predicted in an article on February 12 in London's *Daily Telegraph* on the occasion of the death of Sir William Fergusson (1808–1877), the famous Scottish surgeon and former assistant to Robert Knox. The English newspaper suggested that "the Great Northern Lights"—meaning the great masters of the healing art who had made Edinburgh famous during the first half of the century—were rapidly vanishing and that the Medical School was sinking "into the dark shadow of eclipse." Categorizing the allegation as an example of "patronizing Cockney superiority," a leading Edinburgh newspaper cited the presence in the city of thousands of students from throughout Britain and many other nations as sufficient testimony that Edinburgh remained one of the world's great medical centers.[87]

For two days, Margaret rested after her voyage before walking with her cousin to the Royal Infirmary on Friday, February 23, 1877. All prospective surgical patients went to the old High School located east of the original Adam building erected in 1741.[88] Upon reaching the higher plateau, both women were impressed by the majesty of the buildings. The Infirmary's neighboring High Street quarter now had a population of over 30,000 but few sanitary facilities. Without plumbing facilities in many older buildings, the traditional emptying of individual bedpails into streets and gutters continued unabated. Although frigid sea breezes from the northeast periodically swept away the "diabolical combinations" of odors, the sewage frustrated all efforts at domestic cleanliness. As ever, black smoke billowed from hundreds of city chimneys. No wonder Edinburgh had a higher mortality rate than any British city except Glasgow.[89]

Earlier in the century, the original Infirmary had become excessively overcrowded, and surgery was performed on Sundays at a church across the street. In 1829, the managers—fearing that air circulation around the Infirmary would be impaired by new construction—purchased the two-story school building erected in 1777 along the nearby yards. To convert the facilities into a surgical hospital, internal partitions were removed, and new walls stopped short of the roof to facilitate ventilation. The remodeling included a new surgical amphitheater that accommodated 100 students. On each floor, a long corridor separated eight- or nine-bed wards. When the surgical unit opened in 1832, the total capacity was 72 beds, but it was soon increased to 80 and for a time housed 103 patients.

Earlier needs for space and air circulation had prompted in 1833 the purchase of the old Surgeons' Hall constructed in 1697. Other buildings on what was known as Surgeons' Square followed. The new facilities offered opportunities for reallocating surgical beds, which was important to James Syme (1799–1870), holder of the university's chair of clinical surgery.[90] In the days before anesthesia, Edinburgh was well known for its surgical training and featured renowned figures such as Charles Bell (1774–1842), Robert Liston (1794–1847), and Fergusson. As in other European and American centers, the range of major surgical operations remained limited, featuring primarily amputations, removal of bladder stones, ligation of aneurysms, mastectomies, and trepanations. All interventions required special dexterity and great speed, with postoperative shock and septic complications killing nearly half of the patients. In spite of such conditions, the surgical facilities became overcrowded in the early 1840s.

Syme had been placed in charge of three smaller wards with about 30 beds. Unlike London, with its multiple hospital facilities, bedside teaching in Edinburgh was concentrated in one institution, and the large number of students enrolled at the university severely limited direct patient contact. To fulfill his academic duties, Syme lectured in the amphitheater, regularly using patients under his care for the demonstrations. Following the first administration of chloroform by the professor of obstetrics, James Y. Simpson (1811–1870), at the Infirmary in November 1847, surgical interventions rapidly multiplied. In response to Syme's concerns about insufficient space, the Infirmary managers planned and built a three-story New Surgical Hospital connected to the old High School. Officially opened in April 1853, the new facilities provided 128 additional beds, prompting a rearrangement of the Infirmary's whole surgical department. Syme was now given 72 beds—62 in the old building and the rest in the new one—but complaints about their salubrity and ventilation persisted.

At the hospital's gate, meanwhile, Margaret and her cousin were met by the porter. They asked him the name of the best professor of surgery. The unhesitating reply: Dr. Lister. Of Quaker heritage, Joseph Lister (1827–1912) was one of Britain's most successful (albeit controversial) surgeons. Born near London, he had pursued a college and medical career at the nonsectarian University College in the capital. There he had been present when Liston performed his first major surgical operation under ether anesthesia in December 1846, nearly six weeks after Alice Mohan's leg amputation in Boston. The success of such operations promised a new phase in the development of clinical surgery, and Lister took steps to broaden his experience after graduating in 1852. His first destination had been Edinburgh, where Syme was already considered one of the most prominent surgeons of the day. First appointed supernumerary house surgeon at the Infirmary, Lister quickly consolidated his friendship with Syme, married his daughter, and obtained positions at the hospital. He became resident house physician in 1854 and assistant surgeon two years later, a significant achievement given the clannishness of his Scottish colleagues. In 1860, he obtained the Regius Professorship of Surgery at the University of Glasgow, taking charge of the surgical wards of the Royal Infirmary there a year later.[91]

Concerned about postsurgical wound sepsis, Lister by 1865 had begun to develop a method of antisepsis based on the employment of carbolic acid to cleanse wounds. Although controversial, this approach attracted numerous visitors from all over the world to Glasgow's Infirmary. In 1869, following Syme's stroke and subsequent resignation, Lister assumed Edinburgh's chair of clinical surgery on the condition that the hospital authorities provide him "with the means of giving my lectures in connection with the Infirmary."[92] In many respects, his choice as an attending surgeon placed the Royal Infirmary at the center of British surgery. His classes were the largest in the land, numbering each year more than 350 students. Not surprisingly, Lister's fame was also partly responsible for attracting a steady stream of patients to the Infirmary.

Unknown to the women standing at the gate, however, were the rumors flying around the infirmary that Lister was now negotiating with King's College, London, concerning the chair in surgery left vacant by Fergusson's death. As reported in the newspapers two days before Margaret's trip to the Infirmary, Lister had been presented with a memorial at the end of his afternoon lecture. The document, signed by more than 700 current and former students, expressed deep regret at the prospect of his leaving Edinburgh. Confronted in the crowded classroom, Lister was said to have insisted that he had not the remotest intention of accepting the appointment and that his local position was much better than any in London or elsewhere. In fact, aware of the current doubts about the quality of instruction at the Edinburgh Medical School, Lister told his adoring students that clinical surgery in London was a "sham."[93]

As Margaret and her cousin headed for Surgeons' Hall, their hearts must have sunk. In contrast to the classical features of its façade, the interior appeared gloomy and dingy, the corridors badly lighted, and the wards overcrowded, with beds everywhere. A sense of inferiority and dread gripped the women, with Margaret commenting that "a strange smell pervaded the building of distant carbolic acid, stale tobacco smoke and ancient boiled beef."[94] Directed to the Infirmary's upper waiting room, the two women ascended a long flight of stairs flanked by an iron railing, where they encountered one of Lister's house surgeons, William Watson Cheyne (1852–1932). To her utmost surprise, Margaret recognized him as a former neighbor and minister's son from the island of Fetlar. Cheyne, formerly a demonstrator in anatomy at the University, had just returned from a visit to Vienna and Strasbourg to monitor Lister's antiseptic system on the Continent.[95]

After a few questions, Cheyne briefly examined Margaret's shoulder in an adjacent room, reassuring her that the joint was not luxated. Instead, she was told that there was still an abscess in the shoulder joint, with a smaller one near the collarbone. Margaret was then ordered to wait with other patients for Lister in the lobby next to the stairway. Sitting patiently on a bench, the two women witnessed around noon the entrance of a dignified "elderly looking gentleman," followed by Cheyne and about 20 students, who went into a big room located next to the first landing below them. Unwittingly, Margaret and Martha also observed the outcome of an amputation. After they heard piercing screams inside—the door was left ajar—eight students came out of the room carrying an unconscious man in a long basket outfitted with pillows and sheets. Another student followed, carrying the patient's lower leg rolled in silk paper and dripping blood. As her cousin began to faint, Margaret had to admit that this was indeed an ominous beginning for her odyssey.[96]

Soon thereafter, the professor stepped out of the operating room with his entourage. Cheyne motioned Margaret into an examination room, where he introduced her to Lister. "The professor seemed to be a kind and good man," she later remembered.[97] After questioning her in detail in his soft, low voice, Lister examined the lesion with a four-inch-long silver probe to ascertain the existence of dead bone fragments. He was also curious about the numerous bruises over her chest left by the repeated use of plasters to treat her stubborn cough. Lister promised to listen "some day" to her chest with a stethoscope—he carried none with him—and, speaking to his assembled audience, concluded that Margaret indeed had a consumptive disease that, in his view, had providentially turned from the lungs to the shoulder joint, a seemingly hopeful development.[98] Lister's decision: admit her to the hospital.

Margaret was already prepared for admission, having brought along her own nightdress and some money. After saying goodbye to her cousin and entrusting her with her purse, she was directed to an eight-bed ward in the Infirmary's Old High School building, where the head nurse assigned her to the last remaining bed in one of the rooms. Several of Lister's other surgical wards were presently filled with no fewer than 15 patients. Some larger beds held up to three occupants—mostly children—a consequence of the professor's rather liberal admission policy, which caused severe, chronic overcrowding. In the smaller wards, extra mattresses were placed on the floors at night for ambulatory patients.[99] The remodeled building had never been designed as a hospital, and its only virtue remained the prominent location that promised some ventilation.

While Infirmary practitioners had certain discretionary powers to accept patients, admissions were still closely monitored by the managers. Any excess numbers, as well as long-term hospitalizations—over 40 days—prompted requests to the surgeons controlling such beds to write letters explaining the reasons for their actions. In certain cases, the surgeons' assistants also made personal presentations to the managers on behalf of their masters. Lister was not immune to such controls and was required periodically to justify the extended stays.[100] By 1877, the combined Old and New Surgical Hospitals had 190 beds distributed among five surgeons: three ordinary surgeons and the two professors, Lister and Syme. Lister believed that accommodating as many as 70 individuals by means of extra beds and "shake downs" in his wards would not jeopardize these patients since his antiseptic method was capable of preventing hospitalism. He even went so far, in the mid-1870s, as to suspend the annual cleaning of the wards because of the great demand. The six wards contained approximately 10 beds each, supplemented by six 2-bed rooms for pre- and postoperative patients, an arrangement not ideal for nursing functions. At the time of Margaret's admission, construction of a new Infirmary at Lauriston Place, southwest of the present site, was well underway. To improve hygiene, the new establishment was to be composed of smaller separate units or pavilions—a plan debated by the French Academy of Sciences before the Revolution nearly a century earlier—according to criteria elaborated by the new reformer of nursing, Florence Nightingale (1823–1910) and others.[101]

Hospitalism and the "new" nursing

Concerns about the salubrity of hospitals and the threat of "hospital distempers" had been voiced during the eighteenth century, as exemplified by the writings of John Pringle, John Howard, Johann P. Frank, and Jacques R. Tenon. Institutionally acquired fevers—mostly of the typhus variety—became more common as the number of hospitalized patients soared, overwhelming the existing facilities. Contemporary opinion favored the notion that the origin and propagation of hospital fevers was due to general environmental miasma, the traditional malodorous vapors emanating from the sick and their infected wounds. Ventilation and cleanliness were widely advocated to cope with the situation. Since the 1750s there had been frequent recommendations to empty particular wards and "whitewash" them with chemical solutions. In Edinburgh, proper air circulation around the Infirmary plateau continued to be a high priority. This concern was largely responsible for the managers' worry that further construction in the vicinity would impair free movement of air.[102]

By the nineteenth century, complaints concerning the salubrity of hospitals multiplied, voiced by the increasingly active surgeons, who observed a growing incidence of postoperative wound infections leading to pus formation, abscesses, and fatal sepsis. At the Edinburgh Infirmary, Syme had complained in 1827 about the lack of primary wound closures and their increased suppuration following surgery.[103] But miasma emanating from sick patients could not explain the frequency of puerperal fever in lying-in institutions, and the latter suggested that hospital-acquired disease might come from the presence of putrefaction, perhaps carried by surgeons themselves. By the 1840s, the changing of clothes, a ban on the performance of autopsies, and even a moratorium on medical practice after a case of fever were measures recommended in many European hospitals to control this scourge.[104] In Edinburgh, professor of obstetrics James Simpson, who wrote a series of articles and reports on hospitalism, concluded in 1848 that current hospitals were "crowded palaces" creating unhygienic conditions that could be avoided only by evacuating patients to smaller buildings or cottages with private rooms.[105]

In 1869, Simpson once more proposed that existing large hospital structures be exchanged for smaller buildings made of wood or iron to avoid what he defined as hospitalism, a high institutional mortality based on the proliferation of septic conditions among inmates. "The man laid on an operating table in one of our surgical hospitals is exposed to more chances of death than the English soldier on the field of Waterloo," Simpson argued.[106] With the help of statistics comparing the mortality of patients with major limb amputations in selected voluntary hospitals (41%) and provincial private practice (10.7%), he complained about the "pitiless and deliberate sacrifice of human life," urging a reform of the existing hospital system.[107] The question was quickly taken up that same year at the next meeting of the British Medical Association in Leeds. Here various authors challenged the accuracy of Simpson's statistics, suggesting that private and Infirmary surgeons encountered vastly different populations affected by industrial trauma and disease, employing therefore different criteria for selecting a procedure such as amputation. Moreover, the habits and poverty level of the patients all materially affected the results of surgical intervention. In the end, British medical professionals agreed that hospitals were necessary evils, perhaps dangerously unhygienic shelters, but good for the working poor, medical instruction, and scientific observation.[108]

Simpson and his critics recognized that hospitalism had a structural component. Increased mortality seemed linked to the size of an institution, suggesting a revolution in hospital construction that would favor smaller and independent units in the form of temporary pavilions or cottages.[109] Experiences during recent conflicts in the Crimea and the American Civil War seemed to confirm these observations. Because of a lack of additional space, this rearrangement was impossible in crowded metropolitan areas unless existing hospitals were to be disbanded to distant suburbs and rebuilt as veritable hamlets with a large number of temporary sheds or pavilions. To avoid the free passage of polluted air from one unit to another, Simpson's final proposal was to remodel existing wards and create separate exits for each of them, as well as for the stairways and corridors connecting them.[110] Only through such a system of individual ventilation and self-purification could hospitalism be controlled.[111] As part of the architectural proposals, one surgeon even suggested an octagonal central hall, with the medical and surgical wards extending out from the center, with totally detached facilities for fever patients.[112]

Following Simpson's death, the debate was joined in 1874 by John E. Erichsen (1818–1896), one of Britain's foremost surgeons and clinical professor at University College, London. His four lectures on hospitalism closely followed the Franco-German War, in which medical experiences in the field suggested that septic complications of wound management were lowest for soldiers attended in

temporary, drafty canvas tents. Hospitalism was said to be caused by a septic influence, a morbid condition of the atmosphere capable of infecting wounds and
then spreading to the rest of the body. Under such circumstances, hospital overcrowding per se was only a relative factor. It was the nature of the hospital environment more than the number of cases that generated this pestilential atmosphere. But what to do about it? Erichsen identified factors involved in the problem,
including the patient's health, social status, and occupation, surgical skills, and
postoperative wound-healing techniques currently available.[113]

Finally, Erichsen focused on the effects of the hospital environment on patients. He agreed that older hospitals were simply big houses, three or four stories high, constructed in such a way that the air flowed freely through staircases
and corridors from the basement to the upper floors. Once contaminated at its
source, however—namely, in basements housing kitchens, cellars, washing facilities, and the dead house—or at first-floor outpatient departments, this septic and
contagious atmosphere inevitably diffused throughout the rest of the building regardless of other ventilation in the wards. The solution, therefore, was to remove
all such ancillary facilities to separate buildings, as well as to establish an independent isolation ward for patients suffering from erysipelas and suppurating
wounds. Moreover, all unnecessary furnishings were to be removed, with the surgical wards closed once a month for disinfection, and caregiving personnel and
patients were required to wear easily washable clothing.[114] For many medical leaders, sanitary governance of a hospital was now considered of equal priority with
medical care.[115] Erichsen was quite impressed with the quality of newly constructed hospitals in the United States. He especially liked the plans prepared by
a former Union Army officer, John S. Billings (1838–1912), for a hospital near
Washington, D.C., with its individual pavilions and elaborate ventilation system.
For Erichsen, antiseptics were unnecessary since hospital hygiene could be
achieved through better architectural planning and internal management.[116]

Erichsen's ideas influenced thought about hospital management throughout
Britain, including Edinburgh. Since wholesale demolition of existing hospital facilities in the country was not feasible, how could such institutional hygiene be
achieved, and who would be responsible for achieving and monitoring it? Apparently not the nursing staff. Despite occasional calls for improvement, nursing
at the Edinburgh Infirmary had remained virtually unchanged since the eighteenth
century.[117] Poor working conditions, low pay, and lack of training were the three
most notable deficiencies. Those willing to work were selected from the ranks of
local domestic servants and needy widows, often dysfunctional individuals. Lacking the most elementary skills, many of these women were subjected to long hours
of hard labor, performing domestic chores such as scrubbing floors, carrying
corpses to the morgue, and feeding and attending the sick. Exhausted and overwhelmed, many drowned their sorrows in whisky and laudanum, easily available
but quickly addictive restoratives.[118]

As the Edinburgh Infirmary expanded its physical facilities and the scope of its medical and surgical care, the older system of an exclusively matron-dominated hospital staff had ended with the appointment of a house governor in 1837, followed by a treasurer-superintendent in 1844. While building maintenance and hospital provisions improved, the nurses continued to be a lowly support group, technically working under the matron and totally separated from the medical staff. Without direct supervision, hospital nursing remained primarily a housekeeping activity, coupled with disorganized efforts at patient assistance. Nurses were expected to clean wards, make beds, attend patients, and carry medicines to and from the apothecary shop. Day nurses worked 7 AM to 11 PM shifts and received meager food allowances. Patients requiring special attention needed temporary supernumerary nurses since the night nurses were mostly old charwomen and scrubbers working from 11 PM until 5 PM the next afternoon. Night watching was a farce since the women, tired and poorly fed, got little rest during the day and were usually fast asleep at night. Time off from duties occurred only every two weeks.

A 1859 report on Infirmary nursing by Joseph Bell, one of Syme's house surgeons, was not very encouraging, although Florence Nightingale had paid a visit to the Infirmary two years earlier. Syme's 72 patients were cared for by 9 women under the direction of a Mrs. Lambert and a Mrs. Porter, each responsible for 36 beds and praised for their "strong Scottish sense and capacity."[119] The remaining seven functioned as night nurses, with major responsibilities for scrubbing and cleaning the wards and corridors. Because of the risk of postoperative complications, student dressers took four-hour watches for postoperative patients. The matron or governess still hired the cooks, chambermaids, and ordinary nurses. The last were often characterized as "old and useless drudges, ignorant and not always sober." One observer spoke of their "filthy ways and reeky gowns," a comment that could also, however, have been applied to the surgeons.[120]

Increasingly, these conditions called for radical change if hospitals wanted to expand the range as well as improve the success of medical and surgical interventions. In 1860, Nightingale's Training School for Nurses was inaugurated at St. Thomas' Hospital in London to supply a cadre of young, competent nurses.[121] Florence Nightingale's school stressed the vocational aspects of nursing and trust in God's mystical providence.[122] This philosophy had been shaped by earlier visits to Paris, where Nightingale studied with the Catholic Sisters of Charity, and Germany, where she observed the activities of the Protestant Deaconess Institute in Kaiserswerth.[123] Ritual, discipline, and loyalty followed a military model—based on her experiences during the Crimean War—that also extolled the virtues of character and sacrifice.[124] Another influential nursing model in Britain was the Anglican sisterhood of Saint John's House, which eventually took over the care at University College Hospital in 1862.[125]

Nightingale's training program also fostered attempts to improve nursing at the Edinburgh Infirmary in 1860. A specially appointed committee suggested improved wages and conditions to attract a better class of women while providing greater supervision and probationary training. In Presbyterian Edinburgh, sisterhoods were out of the question. From early 1863 to 1864, a trial period for training a group of probationers under the direction of a Mrs. Taylor was successful, but disputes arose concerning the cost of providing the nurses with mandatory beer allowances. Qualitative improvements in the workforce were modest. In 1866, an independent supervisor, Anne Sidey, was appointed to formally distinguish nursing duties from the housekeeper's domestic responsibilities. This decision established a so-called mixed system in which the entire nursing staff was to be supervised by a female superintendent and probationers accepted for in-house training. Sidey remained in charge until 1871, finally resigning for health reasons.

Confronted with this vacancy, the Infirmary's new superintendent, Charles H. Fasson, went on to create a more complex nursing hierarchy. In October 1872, the first Lady Superintendent of Nurses at the hospital, Elizabeth Barclay, was appointed. Barclay had been trained at St. Thomas' Hospital under the auspices of the Nightingale Fund and had experience in German war hospitals during the Franco-Prussian conflict of 1870–1871.[126] She was allowed to bring with her a small group of trained nurses quickly known as "the Nightingales," who assumed the newly created posts of day and night assistant superintendents, plus day and night staff nurses, assistant nurses, and probationers-in-training.

By contemporary standards, the Nightingales received better pay and worked shorter hours: days from 7 AM to 8.30 PM and nights from 8.30 PM to 9 AM. Problems remained with the reduced off-duty hours: two and a half hours for meals, one hour of rest, and one and a half days off duty for every two weeks of work. Not surprisingly, reports in 1873 indicated that some nurses had been found sleeping on vacant beds or wrapped in blankets on chairs. However, the Nightingales no longer performed heavy cleaning chores. These duties had been transferred to ward assistants. To provide the new nurses with the comforts of home, a house on the grounds of the Infirmary was converted into a Nurses' Home.[127] At this time, night nursing came to be considered critical in saving lives, but ironically, it remained the most neglected aspect of the reforms.[128] In contrast to a report on night nursing in London hospitals,[129] Edinburgh in 1873 still had some night nurses burdened with scrubbing duties. They made their rounds with candlestick in hand, towel over the arm, and were frequently caught sleeping on duty.[130] Some local women of rough appearance and surly manners were described by their middle-class supervisors as "slovenly young ones of the lowest class." Efforts were undertaken to reclassify some of these women as scrubbers, but this led to conflicts since they often owed their positions to personal recommendations from medical staff members.

As elsewhere, changes in nursing care at the Infirmary were gradual. To the chagrin of the Nightingales, wards remained noisy and patients could hardly rest, as both lower-class patients and nurses created a "perfect riot of laughing and talking" vividly described by Margaret Mathewson.[131] In spite of the Nightingale leadership, properly trained personnel remained scarce. By 1874, the public in Britain had become aware of the importance of skilled nursing in hospitals, and the presence of Nightingale trainees boosted people's expectations of recovery. Although supervisory personnel were trained in the new nursing, staff nurses were still from the old school, paying less attention to patient cleanliness and diet. Many could not adapt to the new circumstances, but their loyalty and experience were still considered assets. Some older women left, and others were pensioned off. Former night nurses were retained as scrubbers and ward maids.

As the old guard passed from the scene, the issue of selective recruitment of new probationers became very important. While the emphasis was on youth and formal training, traditionally older but experienced women displayed that "motherliness of nature" still considered the most precious attribute.[132] At the same time, the Nightingales sought to adopt a new asexual identity—shunning earlier stereotypes of promiscuity—with authority to exercise power over male patients.[133] In addition to personal qualities, the new nurses needed to acquire a broad range of necessary skills. Among them were increasingly the preservation of institutional and patient hygiene, both domestic duties now upgraded and provided with a medical rationale. Other critical Victorian attributes were the Nightingales' presumed moral qualities and character. These were seen as essential in preserving the hospital's traditional spiritual care function, now increasingly displaced by newer medical agendas.

Nursing reform was largely predicated on the acquisition of specific skills. It therefore demanded a program of systematic instruction financed in Edinburgh by a Nursing and Training Fund. Training took place on the wards under the direction of head nurses, who taught the essential practical duties in patient care as defined by medical practitioners. Between visits and rounds, nurses were told to watch symptoms, recognize emergencies, and write reports about the events. Additional classes were given by the nurse superintendent. Infirmary practitioners were also recruited to assist in this teaching and training. Joseph Bell, for example, lectured on surgical nursing and appliances, anatomy, obstetrics and gynecology, as well as physiology, since nurses needed to have elementary knowledge of medicine to be valuable helpers.

The transition to a regimented, hierarchical nursing system was stressful. Given the paucity of trained personnel, there was considerable institutional turnover, since trained nurses and probationers were in great demand at other institutions and in private nursing. Because nurses were social equals with medical and surgical personnel, friction among them increased. Some nurses tended to advise and prescribe, and others almost ignored the existence of resident physicians and surgeons.[134] The long hours on duty caused battle fatigue and called for stimulants. Not surprisingly, perhaps, Barclay had a breakdown due to alcohol and opium addiction. Pressured by Nightingale—who as "Mother-Chief" continued to correspond with many of her former students—Barclay resigned in 1874. Her replacement was the assistant superintendent, Angelique L. Pringle (1846–1920), a favorite pupil of Nightingale, nicknamed "Pearl," and a graduate of the St. Thomas' Hospital Training School. Small, modest, and self-effacing, Pringle was an expert nurse and manager, although she disliked being in charge.[135]

In Britain, medical and surgical staffs were quickly won over by the new nursing model. In fact, they defined and shaped it as an adjunct to their own work. At Edinburgh, however, Lister's relations with the new nurses remained ambiguous. Because of his faith in antisepsis, Lister perhaps undervalued the importance of the nurses' sanitary work and spiritual assistance. In fact, as competition between dressers—who were medical students—and nurses ensued in the application of surgical bandages, Lister chose to perform his own bandaging or delegated it solely to his closest assistants. Although staff vacancies were filled with newly trained probationers such as Mary Logan, who later befriended Margaret, the old guard remained in charge. The crusty but kindly Janet Porter, who had served under Syme—she was already in her seventies—continued as Lister's staff nurse from 1869 to 1877. Porter apparently ruled her flock with an iron hand, and tensions may have existed between her and the Nightingales assigned to the professor's surgical wards concerning the scope and priority of their duties. Because the nurses were good soldiers, their perceived loyalty was to the institution, and they studiously avoided interfering with the medical functions.[136]

By the time of Margaret's arrival, the Edinburgh Infirmary had made steady advances in training nurses and probationers. Some were hired as matrons or head nurses in other institutions around the country.[137] Managers agreed that progress had occurred, admitting that "efficient and careful nursing is a most important feature in an hospital."[138] During Lister's last year in Edinburgh, the Infirmary boasted that its nursing staff was widely recognized for its efficiency and the excellent training furnished with the cooperation of the medical and surgical staffs. Awards were also given to nurses specially employed in training new probationers. In all, since Barclay's 1871 appointment, the quality and number of personnel had increased, including a complement of ward assistants.[139] The expense was not trivial, but the usually cost-conscious hospital managers seemed determined to shoulder this additional financial burden.[140] In fact, from 1872 to 1874, expenditures for nurses' salaries rose nearly 50%, and in 1877, Lister's last year in Edinburgh, they had almost doubled since Barclay's appointment.[141]

In that year, Margaret Mathewson provided vivid glimpses of the new ward conditions created by the Nightingale nursing system. In recounting some of the daily routines, she mentioned the Saturday evening washing of the patients' feet with the assistance of ambulatory patients, a procedure reminiscent of medieval religious rituals. Equipped with soap and towels, nurses and volunteers went along the beds, taking special care of the children, who were also bathed twice a week. Although everyone was allowed to wear his or her own clothes, bed linens and bed clothing were laundered twice a week.[142] Finally, following Lister's departure, the Infirmary's head nurses were judged competent enough by the surgeons to administer hypodermic injections. This could be done based on medical instructions, with the surgeons measuring out the dosages. Unusually powerful dosages were still given by resident physicians and surgeons.[143]

By the late 1870s, contemporary nursing was perceived as an honorable profession but was deemed subservient to medical and surgical needs. The Nightingales exemplified a new spirit of self-respect and group identity, generating a "salutary influence on the whole tone of ward life."[144] This vote of confidence in their abilities dovetailed with contemporary perceptions that efficient nursing lowered the hospital's death rate and increased the comfort of patients. Declared an anonymous Infirmary nurse: "Much may be said about antiseptic and septic wards, modes of dressing, modes of operating, as modifying mortality in the surgical house. Really good devoted nursing has its own power and is a most appreciable though often utterly forgotten factor in the sum."[145]

Lister and the antiseptic system of surgery

Following Lister's return from Glasgow to Edinburgh in October 1869, he was embroiled in a controversy with former colleagues and managers in Glasgow. Stressing the salutary effects of his system of treatment, the professor had admitted that the hospital wards in that city had been among the most unhealthy in the kingdom. Lister went on to paint a gruesome picture of the Glasgow Royal Infirmary, especially the new surgical hospital, where he had first developed the tenets and methods of his antisepsis. Remnants of a shallow burial pit containing the corpses of cholera victims from the 1849 epidemic were exposed near the lower male accident wards, and another part of the building ended at the old cathedral churchyard, its ground holding nearly 5,000 decomposing bodies.

Betraying his old-fashioned miasmic views, Lister insisted that the surgical wards were vitiated, functioning under conditions "utterly inconsistent with health in the patients." Further deterioration was due to overcrowding, a condition for which Lister also blamed the hospital authorities. Anxious to provide access to Glasgow's deserving poor, the managers had added a number of extra beds. Lister portrayed himself as "engaged in a perpetual contest with the managing body," his "firmness" preventing further evils, although he "sometimes felt it a questionable privilege to be connected with the institution."[146] Citing the lack of cases of pyemia and hospital gangrene after strict employment of his methods, Lister boasted that hospitalism could be easily conquered inside hospital walls without tearing them down or building smaller cottages.

Lister developed the foundations of his antiseptic system during his Glasgow years. Publication of the first papers on antiseptic surgery occurred in 1867 following a presentation at the British Medical Association meeting in Dublin. According to Lister, there were two forms of inflammation. The direct one was necessary for healing by first "intention"—meaning that the parts of a wound would unite directly, without the formation of scar or granulation tissue—while the indirect type, subject to putrefaction, was a reaction to the presence of dead tissue in wounds, including decomposed blood and lymph. Referring to Pasteur's recent discoveries, Lister declared that airborne living germs caused this fermentation. Therefore, he reasoned, if surgeons could find a substance capable of killing these germs or preventing their access to the dead tissues in the wound, such putrefaction could be avoided.[147]

By 1868, Lister had constructed a rather flexible theory of putrefaction based on "zymotic" fermentation widely shared by Victorian surgeons, physicians, and public health officials. But how could such decomposition be prevented? Most surgeons attempted to heal surgical wounds by first intention, carefully cleansing and closing them, keeping them dry, and sometimes exposing them to air. Lister was pessimistic—perhaps in response to conditions in the Glasgow Infirmary—and was resigned to healing wounds by a clot and granulation. To protect wounds from airborne ferments, they were covered with dressings soaked in disinfectants such as carbolic acid—which was widely available—to prevent putrefactive odors. This approach was hardly original and could easily be traced back to French surgeons of the early 1860s.[148] Since gaping wounds were filled with blood clots and serum, dressings needed to be covered by carbolic plaster or cloth to prevent discharges from reaching the air and initiating the feared decomposition. Even surgical incisions were not sutured. Glasgow surgeons spoke derisively of such practices as "carbolic acid mania" and explained Lister's system as a theory based on false premises bolstered by practical coincidences.[149] During the next decade, Lister recast these explanations and adopted Pasteur's language of germs without abandoning reliance on carbolic acid as the antiseptic of choice.[150]

After his arrival in Edinburgh, Lister addressed the 1871 British Medical Association meeting in Plymouth, where his emphasis was again on the germ theory of putrefaction. He extensively discussed Pasteur's latest work and Tyndall's air experiments with floating dust.[151] "I do not ask you to believe that the septic particles are organisms," explained Lister, nor did he wish to question the issue of spontaneous generation. He simply wanted his audience to believe that these particles, whatever their nature, had a chemical energy and a power of self-propagation responsible for the putrefaction found in unprotected wounds. Without such a concept, no true antiseptic rationale could be constructed. His lengthy paper then went on to discuss in detail an updated method of antisepsis involving the use of carbolated cotton wool, oiled silk dressings, and the introduction of a spray.

Carbolic acid in low dilutions had caused an unusual flow of serum during the first day following surgery, and a special exit had to be provided in the form of

drainage tubes. In fact, the danger of tension created by retained fluids could itself cause inflammation and suppuration. In Lister's opinion, employing smaller
quantities of a more diluted (1:100) carbolic acid solution and dispersing it in a
fine mist would allow the droplets to cleanse the atmosphere immediately surrounding a wound of all agents of putrefaction, thus avoiding fateful contamination and subsequent sepsis. For this purpose, a large, hand-activated spray machine nicknamed the "donkey engine" was created. This manual pump, introduced
without prior testing or experimental proof of efficacy, was to be operated during surgery by a relay team of perspiring assistants, supplemented by the periodic
dressing of wounds.[152] Another practical innovation was Lister's employment of
antiseptic catgut for arterial ligatures. He also announced that since his arrival
in Edinburgh nearly two years earlier, his surgical wards at the local Infirmary
had not experienced a single case of pyemia, hospital gangrene, or erysipelas,
even though the beds were placed much closer to each other than in other institutions.[153]

Some further changes in Lister's method were reported by an observer in 1873.
The carbolic acid solution had been strengthened again to 1:40, and a new spray
machine with a foot-activated bellows was introduced.[154] Late that year, a Birm-
ingham surgeon, Sampson Gamgee, a former student of Lister's, visited Lister's
Infirmary wards and produced a critique of the antiseptic method. Gamgee tried
to separate the theoretical underpinnings from the antiseptic practice. In spite of
Pasteur's work, the airborne theory of germs remained controversial, since it
seemed incapable of accounting for all the phenomena involved in wound healing or putrefaction. This prompted Gamgee to concentrate on the practical aspects of Lister's method, which he found too focused on the employment of carbolic acid; no serious experimental effort had been made to ascertain the efficacy
of other compounds and approaches to wound healing.[155]

In 1875, Lister returned once more to an issue closely linked to his antiseptic
system. "The word hospitalism which some years ago found its way from Edinburgh to the Continent, no longer terrifies us," he announced. After citing the
success of his treatments in the prevention of wound infection abroad, especially
in Germany, Lister again focused on the Edinburgh Infirmary. He was proud of
his work during the past six years, accomplished under adverse conditions. Yes,
the wards assigned to him were small and overcrowded, and an isolation ward for
erysipelas cases had been converted into a regular unit because of a shortage of
beds. Most of the time, there were more patients than beds in these wards, forcing inmates to share them. Under these conditions, Lister had even suspended in
1872 the annual ward cleanings, since they would have required the removal of a
large patient population. "My wards are more severely tried, I believe, than those
of any other surgeon in the kingdom," he commented. In spite of such extreme
conditions, Lister reported only one case of pyemia and none of gangrene. The
pyemia had probably resulted from dressings left unchanged for over a week. Lis-

ter insisted that the antiseptic method prevented putrefaction and dangerous secretions, the true local causes of hospitalism. Paradoxically, "if we take cleanliness in any other sense than antiseptic cleanliness, my patients have the dirtiest
wounds and sores of the world," affirmed Lister. None of his arguments was buttressed by statistics; they were meant to be simply taken on faith.[156]

At Edinburgh, Lister lectured twice a week to a class of several hundred students. The amphitheater, also employed for surgical operations, was a square room
with a large window facing north. It featured a blackboard and sink but no basins
for hand washing, which was considered unimportant. The worn floor was blood-
stained, sprinkled with sawdust. At the center stood an ordinary kitchen table surrounded by a semicircle of upholstered chairs reserved for foreign visitors. After
the students had taken their seats, Lister would walk in, accompanied by his entourage of assistants and house surgeons. He took his place on an old worn horse-
hair-covered chair. If surgery was contemplated, an instrument clerk came with
two others carrying the carbolic acid spray and chloroform bottle, towel, and
tongue forceps. Patients for these demonstrations were chosen from among Lister's hospital patients. Clad in ordinary garments or towels, they were brought
into the theater by dressers. Some seemed to appreciate the attention, but the
mood was solemn, almost eerie. Order and quiet prevailed.[157]

The surgical ritual began with Lister greeting his patients. He was characterized as courteous, modest, and gentle. His kindness to children often prompted
their parents to donate money to the Infirmary.[158] Lister seemed comfortable in
Scotland, tolerant of the melancholic, almost phlegmatic character of its people,
except for their evangelical zeal, which he tried to ignore. In fact, after attending
Sunday morning services in an Episcopal church, Lister often came to the Infirmary to dress the serious surgical patients, thereby breaking Scotland's revered
Sabbath, a visit welcomed by patients but unpopular with the staff.[159] He always
kept his distance, addressing colleagues and assistants by their last names. While
his self-confidence grew, his disciples remained insecure and fearful of committing errors that would expose the antiseptic system to criticism. Thus, no spirit of
camaraderie and friendship blossomed. In the theater, Lister—who was not a
graceful speaker—tried to explain his cases strictly within the context of his surgical principles.

Lister insisted on using cumbersome bandaging techniques. He was a fastidi-
ous and compulsive surgeon, unwilling to delegate; he performed most dressing
changes himself or supervised selected dressers. As a result, Lister spent a great
deal of time and energy on the wards.[160] While in Edinburgh, he changed
from plaster to oiled silk as a protective barrier. Eight layers of carbolic acid-im-
pregnated gauze overlapped the silk and were expected to absorb wound secretions. For additional protection from germs, the occlusive muslin gauze was first
dipped in a mixture of resin, paraffin, and carbolic acid. Other antiseptics, in-

cluding boric acid and zinc, were also employed. In November 1875, Lister had the opportunity to demonstrate his antiseptic method personally for members of the British Medical Association meeting in Edinburgh.[161] A desire for portability and fewer operating personnel led Lister to adopt a steam-generated sprayer. It produced a suffocating mist of highly irritating chemical vapor in the operating theater and wards. In fact, the caustic spray resulted in great discomfort for the operating team and patients inhaling it.[162]

Not everyone in Edinburgh was in favor of the antiseptic method. Just after Lister's arrival, between November 1869 and June 1870, James D. Gillespie's various surgical patients were treated only with clean water dressings and dry lint; the senior acting surgeon claimed to have a mortality rate of less than 4%. His report stressed that "great attention was paid to the proper nourishment of the patient and carefully regulated hygiene."[163] In his 1873 introductory address to the new medical students, one professor and ordinary physician to the Infirmary, George W. Balfour, suggested that Lister's belief in Pasteur's vital theory of fermentation and the method of antiseptic surgery based on it increased Infirmary expenditures, when it was evident that "under almost any other theory similar results might be attained for a merely nominal sum."[164] The lack of comparative clinical trials necessary for claiming the validity of the new method continued to hamper its acceptance, especially in the surgical circles of London.

James Spence (1812–1882), appointed to the Edinburgh chair of systematic surgery in 1864 and author of a surgical textbook, objected to the label *antiseptic* as meaning Listerian. For Spence, the term was not to be restricted to any special method of wound management since every surgeon employed treatments designed to avoid septic complications, including the open-air method. He preferred non-volatile agents such as solutions of chloride of zinc that could be easily applied and required no dressings.[165] Spence tried to keep an open mind about Lister's procedures, and some of his house surgeons certainly employed them. Like other surgeons in Britain, he complained about Lister's reluctance to compile statistics and divulge surgical mortality. Lister was a perfectionist obsessed with failure, and he therefore revised his techniques constantly. Failures were always attributed to minute breakdowns in execution or to nursing problems, prompting questions about the practicality of a treatment rendered ineffective by the slightest error. Lister's statement that practitioners of his method had to believe in the germ theory to carry out his procedures properly created resistance and produced few disciples. Since he never published a book, Lister's lack of a systematic exposition of his theory and his therapeutic rationale hampered the diffusion of his system.[166] Finally, Lister's repeated theoretical shifts, based on the new understandings in bacteriology, further confused his followers.

Patrick H. Watson, an ordinary acting surgeon at the Infirmary, was another of Lister's critics. Watson argued that carbolic acid was an irritating and powerful poison, destroying skin around the wound, stimulating secretions, preventing local granulation, and causing deep cysts that required drainage. Having absorbed the compound through their wounds, some patients exhaled carbolic acid, excreted an olive-colored urine—sometimes tinged with blood—and experienced dizziness. In fact, many wounds needed to be protected from carbolic acid to prevent such absorption. Alexander G. Miller, an assistant surgeon at the time of Lister's 1877 departure to London, found carbolic spray equally troublesome. In his experience, it made surgeons perspire, their septic sweat dripping on the patients' wounds, and those wearing glasses were virtually blinded by the mist. Standing in such a carbolic atmosphere for more than an hour was bad for the health of surgeons. They retained a bad taste in their mouths, could not enjoy dinner, and worried about their scanty, highly colored urine.[167] Joseph Bell, another Infirmary colleague, followed Spence in advocating natural healing by leaving wounds alone and avoiding tension. For Bell, Lister's method was labor intensive and disturbed the patients with frequent wound redressing. Finally, for Thomas Keith, "extra surgeon for ovarian disease" at the Infirmary and member of the "natural school," the accent was also on simplicity, hygiene, atmospheric purity, and cleanliness. Keith employed soap and distilled water and boiled his sponges, determined to achieve first intention healing by paying attention to environmental factors. Dry, infrequent dressings, coupled with uniform gentle pressure and absolute rest were part of his routine.

Not surprisingly, Lister's antiseptic method was expensive as well as complicated. After his arrival in Edinburgh, the Infirmary's managers reported for the year 1870–1871 a 1,200 pound increase in general expenditures due to the increased number of surgical inpatients and their extended stay.[168] The following year witnessed a 30% increase in the cost of dressings, especially carbolic acid plasters.[169] By 1875, the expenditures for antiseptic dressings had jumped another 40% and managers became concerned, trying to increase the number of annual subscriptions to avoid further deficits. Two years later, as Lister headed south to assume his new post at King's College, London, complaints about the increased costs were still heard, but efforts to economize now finally bore fruit, allowing the Infirmary to show a modest surplus. Anxious managers, however, reassured their subscribers that the cuts had not affected patient comfort or recovery.[170]

After Lister's departure, Spence's successor, John Chiene (1843–1923), proposed in November 1877 to reduce the increased expenditures and simplify antiseptic techniques. Their cost to the Infirmary had grown during Lister's tenure from about £200 to nearly £1,000 per year. Chiene proposed replacing the gauze with cheaper paper and saving on thick gauze dressings by employing small sponges that retained carbolic lotion and absorbed wound discharges. This method avoided full dressing changes and prevented the use of irritating spray for superficial wounds, especially ulcers, thus facilitating scabbing and producing no increase in mortality.[171]

Infirmary life: An eyewitness account

Margaret shared the usual aversion to hospitals and fear of infection, but on entering the ward she was pleasantly surprised to find a bed with white covers, clean sheets and pillows, in a room "so tidy and neat enlivened by a nice fire."[172] Furnished with three large windows, the walls of Margaret's ward in Surgeon's Hall were 16 feet high, and the roof had four air holes to promote ventilation. Above the fireplace was a bookcase containing a number of tomes—mostly religious in nature—for the use of patients, together with a copy of the house rules. Framed pictures adorned the walls. A long table with "lots of lotions, bottles and dressing stuffs" stood near the door. Between the beds were high-legged tables for the placement of meals, and under the windows were drawers for storing the patients' belongings. Margaret's initial impression was that "all the patients seemed quite at home and not suffering very much," as they acknowledged in silence the new arrival.[173]

The nurse in charge of the Women's Surgical Ward, Mary Logan, appeared, asking the patient to make herself comfortable and take off her boots. Logan was one of the "Nightingales" described by an earlier patient as having a bright face and blue eyes. Kind and calm, Logan seemed someone who could talk about Beethoven and Balzac and use proper Latin medical terminology.[174] A card with Margaret's name, birthplace and residence, employment, and sponsorship was filled out and placed over her bed. Margaret's midday arrival coincided with dinnertime, and another nurse wearing a print dress, white apron, and cap came in with a tray of food: soup, bread, potatoes, and beef. Shortly thereafter, at 3.30 PM, mail was distributed, followed an hour later by another ringing of the bell. It announced afternoon tea with bread and butter and the arrival of visitors, who were allowed to stay for two hours. At 7.30 PM, supper was served with bread and milk. Before bedtime at 8 PM, Logan read a chapter from the Bible and said a prayer. Ambulatory patients were told to get back into their beds and the gas was turned down in the fireplace. At 8.30 PM, the 12-hour day shift ended and the lights were out.

On her first day in the hospital, Margaret was awakened at 5.30 AM by another ward nurse, who ordered her to get up and make herself "generally useful," assisting with caregiving chores. By 9 AM, breakfast was served, including bowls of porridge and fresh milk, coffee, and bread before the next nursing shift started half an hour later. Logan appeared at 10 AM with 40 yards of gauze that needed to be cut into strips 3 inches wide and 20 feet long by patients "who had the use of their hands." With this task completed, the ward patients began looking for Lister as early as 10.30 AM. An hour later, there was a great commotion as students started filing arm in arm into the Infirmary from the nearby university and carriages stopped at the gates, discharging the surgery professors, Spence and Lister, who conducted the noon-hour rituals.

Finally, at 12.45 PM, Lister, with Cheyne and about 40 students in tow, came downstairs to Margaret's ward.[175] In addition to examining a few other patients, Lister came to see Margaret and kindly ordered her to disrobe, something she very reluctantly did in public. Lister once more went over the particulars of the case and then allowed Cheyne to cover her wound with carbolic acid dressings before the rounds ended at 1 PM. Just before the dinner hour, students came through the wards as dressers. Their activities, including the lancing of infected wounds and abscesses, spoiled some patients' appetites. A strange and intriguing attraction—Margaret even drew a sketch of it in her diary—was Lister's machine, popularly known as the "puffing Billy,"[176] with steam hissing from its safety valve and a warm carbolic spray issuing from a nozzle onto the surgical dressings. The sharp, intoxicating clouds filled the air and choked both the patients and operators, causing quite a stir but apparently "keeping down the pain of dressing."[177]

Following her admission, Margaret spent several days in an eight-bed ward before being transferred to a two-bed waiting room in anticipation of her planned surgery. Meanwhile, her wound continued to be covered daily with carbolic acid lotion. These solemn dressing sessions under Lister's direction were complex affairs. Lister greeted his patients, usually with a smile. In an almost choreographed fashion, clerks and dressers, removed clothing and cut old bandages with pointed scissors. No nurses were in attendance. Before proceeding, Lister and his assistants dipped their own hands in large tin basins of carbolic acid lotion. At Lister's stern command "spray please," a clerk carrying the metal container approached the bed and aimed its fine mist at the naked wound while also soaking numerous layers of gauze in carbolic acid. After they ascertained that there was no pus—confirmed by the lack of a putrefactive odor on the old dressings—the wound was drenched with a borax lotion and covered with another strip of oiled silk. The carbolized bandage was generously spread around the wound and often had to be fastened with safety pins.[178]

On March 10, Margaret was called upstairs by a German physician—Lister always had a number of foreign visitors—for a more formal presentation to surgeons and students in the teaching and operating hall simply known as the "theater." With other patients similarly slated for the teaching session, she patiently waited for hours in an adjacent vestibule ominously named the "dark room" before being dismissed and allowed to return to her ward. "I was truly glad as I was shaking with fear and cold beside,"[179] confessed Margaret. A similar summons the next day was more successful. Lister himself presented her case before an audience of about 40 gentlemen. Speaking in clear, deliberate English, Lister once more went through the essentials of Margaret's clinical history and presented the previous diagnosis, namely, that she suffered from a "singular case of consumption of the lungs," together with an abscess in the shoulder joint and another near the collarbone. As Lister ordered her to turn around for the audience to observe the back of her shoulder, patting her reassuringly on the arm, Margaret spotted a diagram of her swollen arm chalked on a blackboard, with special marks indicating the place and extent of the planned surgical procedure. Since sepsis had seemingly been abolished by antiseptic means, Lister now was involved in extending the frontiers of bone and joint surgery, including nontraumatic lesions such as Margaret's.

Lister shared the contemporary view that scrofulous joint disease was primarily an expression of heredity and constitutional weakness that could also give rise to tubercular lung disease.[180] Defined as a chronic inflammation affecting structures of lower vitality like joints and bones, the disease attacked the periosteal and synovial structures, especially those in the knee, elbow, and ankle, creating a jelly-like deposition followed by ulceration and abscess formation. Lister's colleague, Spence, believed that in the early stages of the disease, rest, a nutritious diet, fresh air, and local bandaging or the application of a plaster appeared to stop the process among upper-class individuals who seemed otherwise healthy. Children also frequently recovered. However, among the poor who came to hospitals for treatment—such as Alice Mohan in Boston—the symptoms usually progressed until amputation became necessary.[181]

The issue facing Lister was whether to amputate the entire arm at the shoulder socket or remove portions of the joint cavity together with the head of the humerus, a procedure pioneered by Liston and Syme in the 1830s. Amputation placed the patient at greater risk of shock and infection, although this procedure had caused only 28% mortality in Glasgow during Lister's tenure there.[182] If performed early, before the muscles were completely atrophied, excision provided a chance to eliminate the lesion altogether while preserving a partially functional limb. If the patient was in tolerable health, this more complex but less drastic operation produced only about 20% mortality.[183] The resulting scar tissue linking bone and the surrounding fibrous tissue allowed some movement. Surgeons also hoped that such an extraction would arrest or at least palliate the coexisting lung disease.

Upset by the extent of the planned surgery—she had hoped that it would not be so serious an operation—Margaret nearly fainted. She had to be helped out of the room and taken downstairs to her bed, with orders for a nurse to remain at her bedside and keep her company.[184] Later, after Margaret had settled down, she was allowed to take a walk outside. Upon her return to the ward, she was informed that surgery had been scheduled for the following day and that she could not have anything to eat beforehand, since the chloroform anesthesia frequently caused severe vomiting. On March 12 a worried Margaret, undressed but wrapped in a blanket, was called upstairs for her surgery. Sitting next to the fireplace in the waiting room, she remained there for nearly three hours before Cheyne stopped by to inform her that surgery had been postponed. Apparently, word had gotten around that Lister intended to leave Edinburgh for London, and many patients now crowded his operating schedule. Holding one of their weekly meetings that same day, the Infirmary's managers sternly demanded that the excess number of patients currently in the surgical wards be eliminated. In fact, the governors gave the Infirmary surgeons only two weeks to discharge them, threatening to halt all further admissions except for emergency injuries.[185] Margaret, meanwhile, returned to her bed, welcomed by the shouts of her ward mates. However, she had missed her dinner and had to content herself with tea and a light supper.

For the next two weeks, Margaret was summoned daily to the amphitheater for possible surgery, only to be informed that her turn was yet to come. Emergency procedures obviously had priority over a nonlethal, slowly draining joint. The mood in the ward was upbeat, and rather than wearing her down, the emotional roller coaster of her impending surgery seemed to help Margaret get used to her surroundings. Teasing from her roommates never seemed to end. She actually came to believe that nothing was going to happen: "fear had given way to confidence."[186] The downside was that without her daily midday dinner, Margaret was losing considerable weight. On March 23, Cheyne unexpectedly showed up in the ward after breakfast to inquire about the size of Margaret's recently ingested meal. She immediately began to suspect that surgery was imminent. Indeed, at about 10:30 AM, one of the nurses told her to undress, and at 1 PM Cheyne personally accompanied her upstairs to the amphitheater where Lister was already waiting and the gallery was filling up with students. Smiling and bowing toward the patient, Lister greeted Margaret, asked her to step up to a chair set at the side of the central table provided with a blanket and two pillows, and then ordered her to lie down. In addition to the usual crowd in the gallery, four gentlemen— presumably dressers in blue check aprons—were sitting around an old kitchen table. Cheyne then laid a folded towel saturated with chloroform over the patient's face and ordered her to breathe while Lister gently put his hand on her left arm, trying to reassure her. "I did feel encouraged to hope for the best," Margaret recalled.[187] Gradually, she felt herself perspiring and growing weak, but she was conscious enough to say a brief prayer, fearful that she would never wake up but prepared to enter "the dark valley of the shadow of death."[188]

After Margaret became unconscious, Lister cut into the shoulder joint and removed it. This decision, however, had not been communicated to the patient. When she finally woke up, Margaret found herself in a two-bed ward with a six-week-old baby operated on the same day for a harelip. She thought first of her arm: was it off or not? Still groggy from the anesthetic, she sat up to feel for it but could not find it because a bulky, heavy bandage covered her left side from the waist to the neck. Sadly, she concluded that amputation had indeed taken place. Then, after somewhat loosening the bandages, she discovered to her delight that the left arm was still attached, thanks to God, but closely bandaged to her waist. Grateful for this divine act of mercy, Margaret started to cry, thus alerting one of the nurses, who suggested that she continue resting. Later, she awoke quite nauseated and received a brief visit from her brother Arthur, who was immediately ushered out because of her frequent vomiting. On the orders of Nurse Logan, a "No Visitors" sign was posted on the door.

Logan was concerned about the condition of both patients who had just undergone surgery. She and Cheyne checked Margaret's pulse every half hour and entered the measurements on a card. The patient was somewhat febrile and was given ice to chew, together with a glass of laudanum for her increasing pain.[189] As expected, Margaret had a difficult postoperative recovery. Early the next day, she remained feverish and nauseated because of the chloroform taste in her mouth. Quite thirsty, she demanded sips of lemonade and was fed teaspoonfuls of ice by the nurses. Fortunately, the pain in the shoulder seemed to be decreasing. As usual, Lister made his noon visit to the surgical wards with the students. Local newspapers were now reporting that negotiations between King's College and Lister had progressed to the point where it was virtually certain that the professor would leave for London.[190]

Lister asked Margaret whether she was experiencing pain and then ordered her to sit up so that he could personally dress the wound. Margaret meekly indicated that the wound was quite sore, but she tried to hide the true intensity of her pain from the assembled crowd of medical students. Lister immediately became angry when he discovered that the patient had already loosened the original bandages. To avoid further embarrassment, Cheyne quickly interceded, attributing Margaret's action to the side effects of chloroform. Lister relented but admonished the patient to check with Nurse Logan whenever the dressing became uncomfortable. Then he went on with the dressing, exposing the gauze to his carbolic acid spray and then covering it with chloride of zinc ointment. Worried about joint and muscular stiffness and retraction after surgery, Lister also carried out a full range of passive movements of the limb after each dressing. He now seized Margaret's left arm to move it away from the body, triggering a sudden and excruciating pain that caused the patient to almost scream and nearly faint. With a corner of the bed sheet firmly between her teeth to muffle any sounds, Margaret tried to survive the ordeal. Aware of her suffering, Lister stopped, praising the stoicism of the Scottish people. Addressing his entourage on March 25, he also observed that "I have great fear of putrefaction setting in here and you all know its outcome. Thus, I will look anxiously for the second day or third day between hope and fear. I hope this chloride of zinc will preserve it but it is only an experiment."[191]

Lister's casual remarks to the students had a devastating impact on Margaret. "This set me to meditate seriously as I plainly saw there was little or no hope of my recovery," she wrote later, adding that she thought, "now it will be best to review my religious hope for eternity." Unfortunately, her brother was turned away at the door, and Margaret wondered whether she would ever see him again. Nurse Logan, meanwhile, continued to check her pulse every 15 minutes, encouraging the sipping of ice and telling Margaret that her survival depended on it. The nurse admitted that if she had been in that situation, Lister's remarks would have disturbed her too. In fact, under the circumstances, she admired Margaret's poise and faith in God. Febrile and with a high pulse rate, the patient apparently fell into a delirious slumber, dreaming and murmuring about Jesus taking her to the gate of heaven but stopping in front of it, only to remark that she had to return to earth for a while longer and "tell more sinners the way of salvation."[192]

Cheyne, who had periodically monitored her pulse during the crisis, also indicated that Margaret had successfully negotiated the "turning point either for life or death." With both her fever and her pulse rate declining, the surgeon now believed that the patient was over the worst. For her part, she felt reborn, "returned from the grasp of death and the spirit world." Surgery had been the catalyst for this spiritual revival. Next morning, Lister made an unexpected appearance in the ward just to see Margaret. Smiling and holding out his hand to greet her, the professor complimented her on her apparent recovery and promised to come back later for a scheduled redressing of the surgical wound. He then did something quite unexpected. Lister folded his hands, closed his eyes, and stood for a few minutes in silent prayer before walking out of the room.[193]

Encouraged by Lister's prayer, Margaret's spirits soared. The power of Jesus was healing her. At noontime, as her arm was readied for another dressing, the famous surgeon again prayed with closed eyes for a few minutes before telling his audience that the wound was neither inflamed nor putrid.[194] Somewhat surprisingly, this favorable outcome was credited to the zinc chloride, not the carbolic acid. Lister also expounded on the postoperative complications related to chloroform, revealing that he had been forced to administer several ounces of the anesthetic to keep Margaret down during the lengthy operation and stating that it took more than an hour to revive her. After waking up, she had been given a teaspoon of brandy and a drink of lemonade. Two days later, Margaret seemed on the mend, now able to drink and retain some fluids.

Lister left for London in early April to finalize his new appointment.[195] Ordered to remain on her back in bed for the next two weeks, Margaret was provided with a daily jug of fresh milk and some solid food. Logan encouraged her to eat, grow strong, "and give the house a good name." Cheyne had remained behind and carried out the wound dressings. Another consumptive and new roommate, Lindsay Mathie, was operated on in the same small room by rolling her bed next to the window. Although bed sheets obstructed Margaret's view, the entire episode, from chloroform administration and the flash of instruments to the final wakening slap on her face and chest with a cold towel, brought back bad memories. Unfortunately, by the end of April, Lindsay began to suffer from severe headaches and became wildly irrational. For those patients who were now ambulatory like Margaret, her eventual death and wake at the Infirmary's mortuary was a "solemn call." "I wonder who will be next from this ward?" asked Margaret.[196]

A week after Lindsay's death, Robert Roxburgh, who had succeeded Cheyne as resident surgeon on May 21, appointed another dresser. His clumsy wound care routines elicited significant bleeding and "dreadful" pain for Margaret. Moreover, the bandages were too tight, and she had trouble sleeping at night. To complicate matters, she had returned to one of the ordinary wards and was forced to share a bed with another inmate because of overcrowding. Lister's Edinburgh tenure was coming to an end. In June and July, weekly Infirmary statistics revealed that there were close to 300 surgical patients in the house. Tired and weary, Margaret tried to shield her sore, bandaged shoulder each time she climbed into an already occupied bed. By mid-July she had even lost her place on a shared cot, telling her brother in a letter that "I had to lie just in any bed who would let me in."[197]

Lister, who had returned in August and came to dress Margaret's wound, removed three drainage tubes and expressed his satisfaction that she understood the importance of exercise to prevent future joint problems. Lister insisted that Margaret's case had been an experiment, that he had first meant to amputate her arm but felt sorry to cause such a loss to a young working woman. Providentially, concluded Lister, the surgery had been a perfect success. Although she had suffered a great deal, it appeared that Margaret's wound might eventually close and she would have a satisfactory range of motion. Besides performing the traditional chores, Margaret made herself useful throughout her long stay by playing with hospitalized children and visiting with other patients, especially on Sundays, when ambulatory patients were allowed to attend church services in a makeshift chapel and volunteers flooded the wards, bringing baskets of flowers and fruits and singing hymns with inmates.[198] Everyone seemed to admire her spiritual strength and kindness to others. Margaret remembered Logan saying that "this is just the way here and it always helps to keep us cheery, as that's the best half of our medicine."[199] By late August, it was decided to send Margaret to the Infirmary's convalescent home. Surgical beds were at a premium, and recovering patients—especially those who lived far from Edinburgh—needed more time to regain their strength. Sadly, Margaret bade farewell to her roommates and the nurses: "I do like to think on many happy hours and days spent in and about the Infirmary," she later admitted.

Providing aseptic surgery: A new role for hospitals

On July 30, Lister had appeared in person before the Infirmary managers and officially resigned his position. He was, however, asked to remain in charge until the appointment of his successor.[200] In late September, he finally left for London with four men who were to form the nucleus of his staff there: W. Watson Cheyne as house surgeon, John Stewart as clerk, and two students. With missionary zeal they headed south to promote the "antiseptic system" among surgery's unconverted. The voluntary British hospital movement, however, was in turmoil. Although hounded for decades by the specter of hospitalism, the London establishments affiliated with medical schools were being flooded with patients, attracted by the successes of medicine and surgery in both diagnosis and treatment. Institutional reforms continued to be advocated, especially the provision of separate infectious disease hospitals and isolation wards for the reception of patients suffering from erysipelas and gangrene.[201]

In Edinburgh, meanwhile, Margaret went to a convalescent home located two miles west of the city in the village of Corstorphine. Capable of accommodating about 50 patients, this compound had opened 10 years earlier on a five-acre site with tree-lined gravel paths, flower beds, and lush lawns protected from the northern winds. The house featured a housekeeper, nurse, chaplain, and gardener, and the food was wholesome and plentiful.[202] Residents participated in weekly concerts, singing, reciting poems, and acting in plays. Margaret established a good relationship with Nurse Skeene, a probationer under Lister, who insisted on educating her patients in dressing their own wounds and dealing with elementary first aid. This was particularly important to people who lived in rural areas without physicians. Patient education could save lives and prevent unnecessary readmissions.[203]

Margaret remained for three weeks in Corstorphine before being sent back to the Infirmary in late September for a checkup. Given the shortage of beds, she stayed in the hospital for only a week. Back at the convalescent facility, Margaret was informed a few days later that Lister would pay his last visit to Edinburgh. Obtaining a pass from the housekeeper, she returned to the Infirmary, although it was not her dressing day. Lister was apparently delighted to see Margaret and insisted on dressing her arm for the last time. Talking to his students, he admitted that "I have a great pleasure in seeing this case today and there is a marked progression here since I saw it last. What a useful experiment this is. It was really as singular a case as I have had for some years."[204] Margaret was officially discharged from the Infirmary as cured on October 23, 1877. She told Nurse Logan that "I like you best as I have been longest and feel more at home. I was treated with kindness and civility."[205]

After a period of rest at Campbelltown, where her brother Walter was the lighthouse keeper, she sailed back to the Shetlands. A month later, in January 1878, her wound began to discharge again. Following a written consultation with Chiene—who adhered to Lister's antiseptic method—she obtained a rubber tube for the purpose of inserting it into the still draining wound. By the summer, Margaret was able to consult Watson Cheyne on his visit to Fetlar during a holiday. In August the wound finally healed, and when she wrote about her hospital experiences in the summer of 1879, Margaret was able to perform all her indoor work chores. Her account was originally meant to be a personal memento of her journey into the world of Victorian surgery, but soon she distributed a few copies to friends in the belief that her narrative would encourage other sufferers on the island to seek similar relief.[206] Unfortunately, her reexposure to the harsh climate on Mid Yell and the discomforts and hardships of her rural domestic life precipitated a decline in Margaret's general health over the next two years. She died of consumption of the lungs on September 28, 1880.

Margaret Mathewson's death came amid vigorous debates about the future role of British voluntary hospitals. As her case demonstrated, their traditional charitable character was rapidly being replaced by the notion that such institutions could provide what was perceived as a scientifically based level of surgical care unmatched even by that given to the upper classes in their homes. "A patient is a natural specimen of disease upon whom all the resources of medical art and science are to be lavished," commented one editorialist, adding that "a hospital is now not merely a place in which the sufferings are relieved, but a place in which they receive benefits open to scarcely any other class in the community." Such benefits could also be bestowed on middle- and upper-class paying patients in separate facilities with private rooms.[207]

Based on his wound treatment, Lister credited himself with the decline in hospital fevers and improved surgical outcomes. Under presumed heroic circumstances, his chemical fix had prevailed over those who wanted to tear down old teaching hospitals and replace them with disposable cottages. Many of his contemporaries, however, insisted that the increasing success of surgical management was due to general sanitary, dietary, nursing, and architectural reforms, not the application of caustic antiseptics.[208] In the final analysis, Lister's surgical "revolution" did not derive from a single, sudden innovation engineered by the professor and his followers. More realistically, it was accomplished by a convergence of several trends within the surgical, medical, nursing, hospital, and public health fields, each of them increasingly applying the tenets of a new hygiene gradually based on bacteriology. "The advantages of hospitals to a great extent consist in the thoroughly organized appliances for the treatment of all the forms and complications of disease, in the trained nursing, and perhaps even more in the general order and complete adaptation of everything to the relief and cure of suffering."[209] Surgery, encouraged by anesthesia and antisepsis, could promise recoveries and cures. Thus, by the 1880s, the medicalized hospital, previously threatened with extinction as the house of decay and death, emerged cleansed and better organized, ready to meet the needs of a growing number of middle-class patients.

NOTES

1. Introductory lecture given by Wendell Holmes at the Harvard Medical School on November 3, 1847, as quoted by John C. Warren in *The Influence of Anesthesia in the Surgery of the Nineteenth Century*, Boston, privately printed, 1906, p. 31.

2. Alice Mohan's clinical evolution was documented in the surviving surgical casebook for the year 1845–1846 of the Massachusetts General Hospital, MSS Collection, F. A. Countway Library of Medicine, Boston. I am grateful to Richard J. Wolfe, Curator of the Rare Book Collection, for his assistance.

3. See Nathaniel I. Bowditch, *A History of the Massachusetts General Hospital*, Boston, J. Wilson & Son, 1851, p. 6.

4. *Annual Report to the Board of Trustees of the Massachusetts General Hospital for the Year 1843*, Boston, J. Loring, 1844, p. 8.

5. See Margaret Gerteis, "The Massachusetts General Hospital, 1810–1865: An Essay on the Political Construction of Social Responsibility During New England's Early Industrialization," Ph.D. diss, Tufts University, 1985, pp. 120–21.

6. *MGH Annual Report* (1845), pp. 8–9.

7. For an overview see Oscar Handlin, *Boston's Immigrants*, Cambridge, MA, Harvard Univ. Press, Belknap Press, 1959, especially pp. 1–24. See also Peter R. Knights, *The Plain People of Boston, 1830–1860: A Study in City Growth*, New York, Oxford Univ. Press, 1971.

8. Handlin, *Boston's Immigrants*, pp. 61–62. See also P. Goodman, "Ethics and enterprise: The values of the Boston elite," *Am Q* 18 (1966): 437–51.

9. *Boston Med Surg J* 33 (Aug. 13, 1845): 38–39. See also Gerteis, "The MGH, 1810–1865," pp. 76–78.

10. *MGH Annual Report* (1846), p. 11.

11. William Nisbet, *The Clinical Guide*, 2nd ed., Edinburgh, J. Watson, 1800, pp. 156–58.

12. Benjamin C. Brodie, *Pathological and Surgical Observations of Diseases of the Joints*, London, Longman, Hurst Rees, Orme & Brown, 1818, especially, pp. 209–58.

13. See John H. Warner, *The Therapeutic Perspective: Medical Practice, Knowledge, and Identity in America, 1820–1885*, Cambridge, MA, Harvard Univ. Press, 1986, especially pp. 11–80.

14. *Boston Med Surg J* 35 (October 7, 1846): 205. See also the pamphlet *The Trustees of the Massachusetts General Hospital to the Public*, Boston, Eastburn's Press, 1844, p. 11.

15. W. O. Baldwin, "Mustard poultices applied extensively to the surface," *Boston Med Surg J* 32 (Mar. 5, 1845): 95–97.

16. One of her surgeons, George Hayward, later commented in a paper read before the Boston Society for Medical Improvement on April 12, 1847, that Alice would "have sunk from the combined influence of her previous debility and the shock of the operation." *Some Account of the First Use of Sulphuric Ether by Inhalation in Surgical Practice*, Boston, 1847, p. 6.

17. See Robert Liston, *Elements of Surgery*, 2nd ed., London, Longman, Orme, Brown, Green, 1840, pp. 86–87, and Samuel Cooper, *The First Lines of the Theory and Practice of Surgery*, 7th ed., London, Longman, Orme & Co., 1840, pp. 318–19.

18. Brodie, *Pathological and Surgical Observations*, p. 247.

19. *Boston Med Surg J* 33 (Jan. 21, 1846): 502. Because of the expected opening of new wings, the hospital in February 1846 doubled the number of its visiting professionals.

20. See George Hayward, *Statistics of the Amputations of Large Limbs that Have been Performed at the Massachusetts General Hospital*, Boston, D. Clapp, 1850, and P. F. Fee, "Remarks on the statistics of amputation," *Boston Med Surg J* 35 (Aug. 26, 1846): 72–73.

21. Extracted from MGH surgical case book, year 1845–1846, MSS Collection, Countway Library, Boston.

22. "Dr. Fenner's letter from Boston," *Boston Med Surg J* 35 (Sept. 23, 1846): 152–53.

23. Bowditch, *A History of the MGH*, pp. 3–9.

24. Both had extensively studied medicine in Europe, with Jackson serving nine months as a surgical dresser at London's Guy's and St. Thomas' hospitals, and Warren spending a year at Guy's and then another in Edinburgh, with bedside instruction at the Royal Infirmary. A third year had been spent in Paris, studying in the hospitals there with Corvisart and Dupuytren.

25. "The means of medical education in New England are at present very limited and totally inadequate to so important a purpose. . . . A hospital is an institution absolutely essential to a medical school, and one which would afford relief and comfort to thousands of the sick and miserable. On what other objects can the superfluities of the rich be so well bestowed?" Quoted in Bowditch, *A History of the MGH*, p. 8.

26. The charter asserted that "the hospital, thus established, is intended to be the receptacle for patients from all parts of the Commonwealth, afflicted with diseases of a peculiar nature, requiring the most skilful treatment and presenting cases for instruction in the study and practice of surgery and physic. Persons of every age and sex, whether permanent residents of the town, or occasional residents therein, citizens of every part of the Commonwealth, as well as strangers, from other states and countries, those in indigent circumstances, who, while in health, can gain by their labour a subsistence for themselves and their families." From Act of Incorporation, in State of Massachusetts, *Acts and Resolves* (1811), chap. 94, Massachusetts State Archives, Boston. Copy in Countway Library, Boston.

27. Ibid. See Gerteis, "The MGH, 1810–1865," pp. 17–54

28. See *Proposals of the Massachusetts Hospital Life Insurance Company, August 18, 1823*, Boston, J. Loring, 1823. For details see Gerald T. White, *A History of the Massachusetts Hospital Life Insurance Company*, Cambridge, MA, Harvard Univ. Press, 1955.

29. For a summary see Leonard K. Eaton, *New England Hospitals, 1790–1833*, Ann Arbor, Univ. of Michigan Press, 1957, pp. 29–55.

30. L. K. Eaton, "Charles Bulfinch and the Massachusetts General Hospital," *Isis* 41 (1950): 8–11.

31. For more details and floor plans see Eaton, *New England Hospitals*, pp. 81–99.

32. "The administration of public infirmaries very properly embraces a two-fold object: the relief of the sick and the instruction of medical students. With a view to the promotion of both these ends, the Massachusetts Hospital, while it gives accommodation to the full extent of its means to the sick poor, gives also admission, which was at first conditional but is now free, to the students of the medical class attending the lectures of the physicians and surgeons. . . . Students are admitted to the patients to enable them to become practically conversant with the symptoms of disease and the operation and influence of medicinal agents." J. Jackson and J. C. Warren, pamphlet, MSS Collection, Countway Library, Boston.

33. *MGH Annual Report* (1842), p. 9

34. See James J. Putnam, *A Memoir of Dr. James Jackson*, Boston, Houghton, Mifflin & Co., 1905, pp. 257–62. See also Eaton, *New England Hospitals*, pp. 169–79.

35. *MGH Annual Report* (1836), pp. 3–4

36. *MGH Annual Report* (1838), pp. 5–9.

37. *MGH Annual Report* (1837), pp. 3–4.

38. *MGH Annual Report* (1839), pp. 4–5.

39. *MGH Annual Report* (1840), p. 4.

40. *MGH Annual Report* (1841), pp. 3–5.

41. "A new hospital in Boston," *Boston Med Surg J* 32 (Apr. 2, 1845): 184–85. MGH and McLean Asylum were receiving almost a third of all charitable donations in Boston since the 1830s. S. A. Eliot, "Public and private charities in Boston," *North Am Rev* 128 (July 1845): 135–59.

42. For an overview see D. de Moulin, "A historical-phenomenological study of bodily pain in Western man," *Bull Hist Med* 48 (1974): 540–70. For details see Roselyne Rey, *History of Pain*, trans. L. E. Wallace, J. A. Cadden, and S. W. Cadden, Paris, Ed. La Dècouverte, 1993.

43. Harriet Martineau , *Life in the Sick-Room*, 2nd American ed., Boston, Crosby, 1845, p. 30.

44. D. Caton, "The secularization of pain," *Anesthesiology* 62 (1985): 493–501.

45. See also E. M. Papper, "The influence of romantic literature on the medical understanding of pain and suffering: The stimulus to the discovery of anesthesia," *Perspect Biol Med* 35 (1992): 401–15, and his *Romance, Poetry, and Surgical Sleep: Literature Influences Medicine*, Westport, CT, Greenwood Press, 1995.

46. For a synthesis see K. M. Dallenbach, "Pain: History and present status," *Am J Psychol* 52 (1939): 331–47, and details in David B. Morris, *The Culture of Pain*, Berkeley, Univ. of California Press, 1991.

47. N. A. Bergman, "Humphry Davy's contribution to the introduction of anesthesia: A new perspective," *Perspect Biol Med* 34 (1991): 534–41.

48. Malvin E. Ring, *Dentistry, an Illustrated History*, New York, A. N. Abrams, 1985, pp. 183–228. See also P. Benes, "Itinerant physicians, healers, and surgeon dentists in New England and New York, 1720–1825," in *Medicine and Healing*, ed. P. Benes, Boston, Boston Univ. Press, 1992, pp. 95–112.

49. A brief account of the Society and its annual conventions can be obtained in C. O. Cone, "Report on practical dentistry," *Am J Dent Sci* 9 (October 1848): 3–22.

50. "Multiplication of dentists," *Boston Med Surg J* 31 (Nov. 6, 1844): 285. See also R. B. Gunderman, "Dr. Horace Wells and the conquest of surgical pain: A Promethean tale," *Perspect Biol Med* 35 (1992): 531–48.

51. "Mechanical skill necessary for the dentist," *Boston Med Surg J* 31 (Oct. 16, 1844): 227.

52. *Boston Med Surg J* 32 (Feb. 19, 1845): 69.

53. *Boston Med Surg J* 32 (June 4, 1845): 366.

54. *The Boston Post*, Oct. 8, 1846, and Oct. 13, 1846.

55. The accepted chronology of events is presented in S. Stallings and M. Montagne, "A chronicle of anesthesia discovery in New England," *Pharm Hist* 35 (1993): 77–80. Wells' priority claims were presented in J. Wales, *Discovery of the late Dr. Horace Wells of the applicability of nitrous oxide gas, sulphuric ether and other vapors in surgical operations*, Hartford, E. Gear, 1852. Excerpts of Wells' account can be found in J. J. Herschfeld, "Horace Wells, pioneer in anesthesia and his defence of his discovery," *Bull Hist Dent* 33 (October 1985): 124–30.

56. J. C. Warren, "Inhalation of ethereal vapor for the prevention of pain in surgical operations," *Boston Med Surg J* 35 (Dec. 9, 1846) 375–79.

57. Abbott's operation was, of course, the first and landmark surgery ushering in a new era. It was thus widely celebrated and memorialized, including the commissioning of a painting by Robert C. Hinckley. For a fascinating glimpse of the circumstances surrounding the actual event and the painting, see L. D. Vandam, "Robert Hinckley's The First Operation with Ether," *Anesthesiology* 52 (1980): 62–70, and more recently Richard J. Wolfe, *Robert C. Hinckley and the Recreation of the First Operation Under Ether*, Boston, Boston Medical Library, 1993.

58. This exchange was provided by another eyewitness, Washington Ayer, "First public demonstration under ether, the account of an eye witness," *Boston Med Surg J* 135 (1896): 397, reprinted in the *Occidental Med Times* 10 (March 1896): 121–29.

59. Notes of Abbott's operation are in MGH's surgical casebook for the year 1845–1846, MSS Collection, Countway Library, Boston.

60. This case is barely mentioned in the numerous contemporary accounts. See, for example, H. J. Bigelow, "Etherization—a compendium of its history, surgical use, dangers, and discovery," *Boston Med Surg J* 38 (Apr. 19, 1848): 232.

61. D. D. Slade, "Historic moments: The first capital operation under the influence of ether," *Scribner's Monthly* (1892): 518–24.

62. The information has been brought together from the surgical report attached to Alice Mohan's clinical case; the account communicated by her surgeon, George Hayward, in his 1847 paper; Bigelow's recollections; and the published description by the medical student Daniel Slade, all cited above.

63. H. J. Bigelow, "Insensibility during surgical operations produced by inhalation," *Boston Med Surg J* 35 (Nov. 18, 1846): 314–15.

64. Case of Betsy Magrun, MGH surgical casebook for the year 1845–1846, MSS Collection, Countway Library, Boston.

65. Case of Theophilus Petier, MGH surgical casebook, 1845–1846.

66. Editorial, *Boston Med Surg J* 35 (Nov. 18, 1846): 324.

67. Bigelow, "Insensibility," 309–17.

68. Ibid., 316.

69. Ibid., 317.

70. J. Harvey Young, *The Toadstool Millionaires*, Princeton, Princeton Univ. Press, 1961, pp. 40–41. For more information on patents see Bruce W. Bugbee, *Genesis of American Patent and Copyright Law*, Washington, DC, Public Affairs Press, 1967.

71. Editorial, *Boston Med Surg J* 35 (Nov. 18, 1846): 324.

72. I have greatly benefited from the work of Alison Winter, who attempted to debunk the hagiographic historiography linked to the "discovery" of anesthesia; see her "Ethereal epidemic: Mesmerism and the introduction of inhalation anesthesia to early Victorian London," *Soc Hist Med* 4 (1991): 1–27.

73. For details see J. F. Fulton, "The reception in England of Henry Jacob Bigelow's original paper on surgical anesthesia," *N Engl J Med* 235 (1943): 745–46, and R. H. Ellis, "The introduction of ether anaesthesia to Great Britain," *Anaesthesia* 31 (1976): 766–77. After some initial hesitation, French surgeons also began to employ it in early 1847.

74. Case of Mary Muldrave, MGH surgical casebook for the year 1845–1846, MSS Collection, Countway Library, Boston.

75. *The Boston Post*, Oct. 11, 1846.

76. Further disputes about the priority of discovery broke out between Morton and Jackson. See, for example, Joseph L. Lord, *Memorial addressed to the trustees of the Massachusetts General Hospital in behalf of Charles T. Jackson, M.D. in relation to the discovery of etherization*, Boston, Thurston, 1849. Jackson's priority claims were rebutted by N. I. Bowditch, who continued to support Morton's claims. See his *The Ether Controversy*, Boston, J. Wilson, 1848.

77. Warren, "Inhalation of ethereal vapor," 375–79. Warren erroneously gave the date of October 17 for the operation on Gilbert Abbott, presumably because most elective surgical procedures were scheduled for Saturdays. An account of the developments from Morton's point of view was negotiated with Nathan P. Rice, who wrote under contract *Trials of a Public Benefactor*, New York, Pudney & Russell, 1859. See H. R. Viets, "Nathan P. Rice M.D. and his trials of a public benefactor," New York, 1859," *Bull Hist Med* 20 (1946): 232–41.

78. I am indebted to Richard A. Wolfe for this information, obtained from the minutes

of the hospital's Trustee Records not currently housed at the Countway Library and thus unavailable for study.

79. The Boston city directory for the year 1848 only lists a Philip Mohan, laborer, living in Jackson Court, but it is unclear whether he was related to Alice.

80. Hayward, *Some Account*, p. 6.

81. Martin S. Pernick, *A Calculus of Suffering: Pain, Professionalism and Anesthesia in Nineteenth-Century America*, New York, Columbia Univ. Press, 1985, especially pp. 148–67. A useful summary of the author's arguments can also be found in "The calculus of suffering in nineteenth-century surgery," *The Hastings Center Report* (April 1983): 26–36. According to Pernick's statistics, between 1853 and 1862, 32% of the major limb amputations following fractures at the Pennsylvania Hospital were carried out without anesthetics.

82. T. M. Johnson, "Contradictions in the cultural construction of pain in America," in *Advances in Pain Research and Therapy*, ed. C. S. Hill, Jr., and W. S. Fields, New York, Raven Press, 1989, pp. 27–37.

83. Editorial, *Boston Med Surg J* 81 (1869): 118. Boston's claim to priority was not without controversy: Bigelow described his version of the events in H. J. Bigelow, "A history of the discovery of modern anesthesia," in *A Century of American Medicine, 1776–1876*, Philadelphia, Lea, 1876, pp. 75–112. See also W. J. Friedlander, "The Bigelow-Simpson controversy: Still another early argument over the discovery of anesthesia," *Bull Hist Med* 66 (1992): 613–25.

84. Margaret Mathewson, "A Sketch of Eight Months as Patient in the Royal Infirmary of Edinburgh," 1877, p. 26. A copy of this manuscript is available at the Medical Archive Centre, Edinburgh University Library. The author stated that the account had been written entirely from memory for her own use. Later, Mathewson said that she complied quite reluctantly with requests from her friends in making this document public, and was keen in declaring that the story was not written to expose or censure the managers, officials, and physicians of the Royal Infirmary.

85. Letter to brother Arthur, Jan. 31, 1877, quoted in Martin Goldman, *Lister Ward*, Bristol, A. Hilger, 1987, p. 20.

86. *Edinburgh Evening News*, Feb. 14, 1877, p. 2.

87. Ibid., Feb. 13, 1877. For an overview of conditions in Scotland see Michael Lynch, *Scotland: A New History*, London, Century, 1991, pp. 397–421.

88. A contemporary medical visitor described it as "a grim, formal stone building of bastard classical design." See John R. Leeson, *Lister as I Knew Him*, New York, Wood & Co., 1927, p. 16.

89. Conditions were compared to those in Aleppo or Damascus. See "Sanitary state of Edinburgh," *Br Med J* II (July 1861): 108, and "Sanitary condition of Edinburgh," *Lancet* 1 (Feb. 19, 1870): 278. See also A. J. Youngson, *The Making of Classical Edinburgh, 1750–1840*, Edinburgh, Edinburgh Univ. Press, 1966, p. 36.

90. Edinburgh traditionally had two surgical professorships. For brief biographical information on Syme, consult his obituary: "James Syme," *Edinb Med J* 16 (1870–1871): 180–92.

91. For a brief biographical sketch see C. E. Dolman, "Joseph Lister," in *Dictionary of Scientific Biography*, New York, Scribner's, 1973, vol. 8, pp. 399–413. The standard biography is Rickman J. Godlee, *Lord Lister*, rev. 3rd ed., Oxford, Clarendon Press, 1924, and more recently, Richard B. Fisher, *Joseph Lister, 1827–1912*, London, Macdonald & Jane's, 1977.

92. A. Logan Turner, *Story of a Great Hospital: The Royal Infirmary of Edinburgh, 1729–1929*, Edinburgh, Oliver & Boyd, 1937, p. 239.

93. *Edinburgh Evening News*, Feb. 22, 1877, as reported by the *Lancet* 1 (Mar. 10, 1877): 361. The remark was deemed "foolish and offensive" by some of his London colleagues. Lister defended his remarks in "Clinical surgery in London and Edinburgh," *Lancet* 1 (Mar. 31, 1877): 475–77.

94. Mathewson, "Sketch," p. 7.

95. Wm. Watson Cheyne, *Lister and His Achievement*, London, Longmans, Green, & Co., 1925, p. 30.

96. Mathewson, "Sketch," p. 6. Mathewson's narrative was also presented in W. B. Howie and S. A. B. Black, "Sidelights on Lister: A patient's account of Lister's care," *J Hist Med* 32 (1977): 239–51.

97. Mathewson, "Sketch," p. 7.

98. Lister was said to be somewhat ambiguous about the relationship between tuberculosis—a pulmonary disease—and what were widely known as scrofulous joint infections. The latter were treated as ordinary wounds with irrigations employing carbolic acid lotion. See Lister's Lectures on Surgery taken by Richard T. Jones, October 1868–April 1869, lect. 46.

99. Mathewson, "Sketch," p. 43. Such overcrowding was ironic, since Lister had blamed his unfavorable working conditions on the managers of the Glasgow Infirmary for providing an excessive hospital population while he was working there.

100. For example, Royal Infirmary of Edinburgh, Minutes of the Meeting of Managers, 26 Mar. and 2 Apr. 1877.

101. For details of this protracted process see "Medical News," *Edinb Med J* 16 (1870–1871): 478–80, and Turner, *Story of a Great Hospital*, pp. 224–38.

102. See, for example, S. Selwyn, "Sir John Pringle: hospital reformer, moral philosopher, and pioneer of antiseptics," *Med Hist* 10 (1960): 266–74.

103. James Syme, *Contributions to the Pathology and Practice of Surgery*, Edinburgh, Sutherland & Knox, 1848, pp. 72–73, as quoted in E. D. Churchill, "The pandemic of wound infection in hospitals: Studies in the history of wound healing," *J Hist Med* 20 (1965): 390–404.

104. See Oliver Wendell Holmes, *The Contagiousness of Puerperal Fever*, Baltimore, Williams & Wilkins, 1936.

105. The nineteenth-century overcrowding of provincial English hospitals has been documented by S. Cherry, "The hospitals and population growth: Part 1, the voluntary general hospitals, mortality and local populations in the English provinces in the eighteenth and nineteenth centuries," *Pop Stud* 34 (1980): 59–75.

106. J. Y. Simpson, "Our existing system of hospitalism and its effects," *Edinb Med J* 14 (March 1869): 818. A similar argument is made by Simpson in "Hospitalism: Its influence upon limb amputations in the London hospitals," *Br Med J* I (June 12, 1869): 533–35.

107. J. Y. Simpson, "System of hospitalism," *Edinb Med J* 14 (June 1869): 1084–1115.

108. P. Leslie, "Admission of patients into hospitals," *Br Med J* II (Sept. 4, 1869): 282. The issue of poor patient nutrition as a key factor in the postoperative complications has been documented for Glasgows's Royal Infirmary. See D. Hamilton, "The nineteenth-century surgical revolution—antisepsis or better nutrition?" *Bull Hist Med* 56 (1982): 30–40.

109. A contemporary example was the new pavilion-style St. Thomas' Hospital in London. See G. Goldin, "Building a hospital of air: the Victorian pavilions of St. Thomas' Hospital, London," *Bull Hist Med* 49 (1975): 512–35. For further information see Lindsay P. Granshaw, "St. Thomas' Hospital, London, 1850–1900," Ph.D. diss., Bryn Mawr, 1981.

110. T. Holmes, "On 'hospitalism,'" *Lancet* 2 (Aug. 7, 1869): 194–96, and (Aug. 14, 1869): 229–30; also see the editorial in *Lancet* 2 (Aug. 7, 1869): 201–02, with responses from Simpson in "Some propositions on hospitalism," *Lancet* 2 (Aug. 28, 1869): 295–97;

(Sept. 4, 1869): 332–35; (Sept. 26, 1869): 431–33; (Oct. 2, 1869): 475–78; (Oct. 16, 1869): 535–38; and (Nov. 20, 1869): 698–700.

111. See also the editorials "Hospitalism and statistics," *Lancet* 2 (Aug. 26, 1871): 297–98, and "Hospitalism," *Lancet* 2 (Sept. 16, 1871): 403–04.

112. F. P. Atkinson, "A few remarks on the construction and internal management of hospitals with a view to the lessening of pyemia and the spread of contagious diseases," *Edinb Med J* 16 (1870–1871): 37–39.

113. J. E. Erichsen, "Lectures on hospitalism," *Lancet* 1 (Jan. 17, 1874): 84–86, and (Jan. 24, 1874): 122–26.

114. Ibid., *Lancet* 1 (Jan. 31, 1874): 151–54; (Feb. 14, 1874): 221–24. Old habits died slowly. One observer remembered that surgeons still wore their bloodstained surgical coats spotted with pus, failed to wash their hands following dissections, and had their ligatures dangling from their coats. See Leeson, *Lister*, p. 3.

115. Editorial, "The sanitary aspects of English hospitals," *Lancet* 1 (May 29, 1875): 764–65.

116. "Under the present system we begin at the wrong end. Instead of preventing the possibility of atmospheric contamination by perfect hospital hygiene, we allow the septic poison to be engendered and then, before it can be implanted on the wound, seek to destroy it by the employment of chemical agents." J. E. Erichsen, "Impressions of American surgery," *Lancet* 2 (Nov. 21, 1874): 719. For an overview of the Listerian influence in the United States see G. H. Brieger, "American surgery and the germ theory of disease," *Bull Hist Med* 40 (1966): 135–45.

117. G. B. Risse, *Hospital Life in Enlightenment Scotland*, New York, Cambridge Univ. Press, 1986, pp. 75–78.

118. R. F. Lumsden, "On nursing in Scotland," in *Hospitals, Dispensaries, and Nursing*, ed. J. S. Billings and H. M. Hurd, Baltimore, Johns Hopkins Univ. Press, 1894, pp. 487–93. For details see K. Williams, "From Sarah Gamp to Florence Nightingale: A critical study of hospital nursing systems from 1840 to 1897," in *Rewriting Nursing History*, ed. C. Davis, Totowa, NJ, Barnes & Noble, 1980, pp. 41–75.

119. The information from Bell's report is quoted in Turner, *Story of a Great Hospital*, p. 208.

120. Leeson, *Lister*, p. 3.

121. Details are presented in Monica E. Baly, *Florence Nightingale and the Nursing Legacy*, London, Croom Helm, 1986, pp. 20–40 and 171–86, and in L. A. Monteiro, "Response in anger: Florence Nightingale on the importance of training for nurses," *J Nurs Hist* 1 (1985): 11–18.

122. Florence Nightingale, *Notes on Nursing*, New York, D. Appleton & Co., 1860. For a recent and critical biography of Nightingale see F. B. Smith, *Florence Nightingale: Reputation and Power*, London, Croom Helm, 1982, especially pp. 155–82. Nightingale's beliefs are reviewed in J. G. Widerquist, "The spirituality of Florence Nightingale," *Nurs Res* 41 (1992): 49–55.

123. Florence Nightingale, *The Institution of Kaiserswerth on the Rhine*, London, London Ragged Colonial Training School, 1851. For details see Irene Schuessler Poplin, "A Study of the Kaiserswerth Deaconess Institute's Nurse Training School in 1850–1851: Purposes and Curriculum," Ph.D. diss., Univ. of Texas, May 1988.

124. C. L. Cordery, "Military influences on Nightingale's reforms of modern nursing: The dominance of ritual and tradition," in *History, Heritage and Health*, ed. J. Covacevich et al., Brisbane, Australia Society of Historical Medicine, 1996, pp. 193–96.

125. C. Helmstadter, "Robert Bentley Todd, Saint John's House, and the origins of the modern trained nurse," *Bull Hist Med* 67 (1993): 282–319, and P. Williams, "Religion, re-

spectability and the origins of the modern nurse," in *British Medicine in an Age of Reform*, ed. R. French and A. Wear, London, Routledge, 1991, pp. 231–55. In the late 1860s, questions were raised about the slow progress made by the Nightingale Fund in training the new nurses. See the editorials "Hospital nurses," *Lancet* 2 (October 1869): 622, and "Nursing in hospitals," *Lancet* 2 (December 1869): 817–18. For details see C. Helmstadter, "Old nurses and new: Nursing in the London teaching hospitals before and after the mid-nineteenth-century reforms," *Nurs Hist Rev* 1 (1993): 43–70, and "Doctors and nurses in the London teaching hospitals: Class, gender, religion and professional expertise," *Nurs Hist Rev* 5 (1997): 161–97.

126. Barclay's appointment included the statement that she "has devoted herself to hospital work from philanthropic motives which sought their realisation in a regular pursuit connected with the sick." Royal Infirmary of Edinburgh (hereafter RIE), Report of the Managers, 1 Oct. 1871–1 Oct. 1872, p. 12.

127. M. Barfoot, "To catch a Nightingale: Nursing reforms at the Royal Infirmary of Edinburgh, 1872–1900," in *New Countries and Old Medicine*, ed. L. Bryder and D. A. Dow, Auckland, Pyramid Press, 1995, pp. 256–62. For further discussion see M. E. Baly, "The Nightingale nurses: The myth and the reality," in *Nursing History: The State of the Art*, ed. C. Maggs, London, Croom Helm, ca. 1987, pp. 33–59.

128. See anon. letter, "Hospital nursing," *Lancet* 1 (February 1872): 204.

129. Editorial, "Hospital night-nursing," *Lancet* 1 (January 1872): 84. See C. Helmstadter, "The passing of the night watch: Night nursing reform in the London teaching hospitals, 1856–90," *Bull Can Hist Med* 11 (1994): 23–69.

130. Turner, *Story of a Great Hospital*, p. 214.

131. Entries from a diary kept by Nurse Pringle provide a vivid glimpse of conditions in the Infirmary's wards. Some of the entries are reproduced in Goldman, *Lister Ward*, pp. 39–44.

132. Anon., "Nurses and doctors," *Edinb Med J* 25 (1880): 1049. A plea by the more mature and now maligned nurses is contained in Anon., "Old time nurses. A plea for the middle-aged," *The Hospital* 15 (Feb. 17, 1894), nursing suppl.: cxcvii.

133. For details see Catherine A. Judd, "Hygienic Aesthetics: Sick Nursing and Social Reform in the Victorian Novel, 1845–1880," Ph.D. diss., Univ. of California, Berkeley, 1992.

134. Editorial, "Hospital nursing," *Lancet* 1 (February 1874): 205.

135. RIE, Report of Managers, 1 Oct. 1873–1 Oct. 1874, p. 13. In spite of Barclay's resignation, the managers expressed great satisfaction about the new nursing system, attributing to it a drop in institutional mortality from 8% to 6.6% for patients hospitalized more than 48 hours. For a biographical sketch of Pringle see Zachary Cope, "Angelique Lucille Pringle," in *Six Disciples of Florence Nightingale*, London, Pitman Med. Pub., 1961, pp. 35–46.

136. The issue was discussed in a review of the publication *Hints for Hospital Nurses*, written by Rachel Williams, a former Nightingale at the Infirmary. See *Edinb Med J* 22 (1877): 1006.

137. RIE, Report of the Managers, 1 Oct. 1874–1 Oct. 1875, p. 7.

138. Ibid., 1 Oct. 1875–1 Oct. 1876, p. 5. One casualty of the new institutional sanitation was the ward assistant's dining room, destroyed by fire in late April 1877. RIE, Minutes, 30 Apr. 1877.

139. RIE, Report of the Managers, 1 Oct. 1876–1 Oct. 1877, pp. 6–7.

140. In England, one letter signed "Economy" complained that half of the expenditures devoted to the care of patients were now directed to the nursing staff, their housing, and their laundry expenses. See "New systems of nursing," *Lancet* 1 (June 1876): 839.

141. RIE, Report of the Managers, 1 Oct. 1873–1 Oct. 1874, p. 27, and 1 Oct. 1876–1 Oct. 1877, p. 35.

142. Although some clothing was permanently stained or destroyed by both wound discharges and silver nitrate, Margaret was indignant about the greed of her fellow patients in requesting replacements from the institution. See Mathewson, "Sketch," p. 32.

143. RIE, Minutes, 24 Dec. 1877.

144. Anon., "Nursing in the Edinburgh Infirmary," *Edinb Med J* 21 (1876): 929–33.

145. Anon., "Edinburgh Infirmary nursing, by one of the staff," *Edinb Med J* 25 (1880): 1051. For an analysis of Nightingale's views see C. E. Rosenberg, "Florence Nightingale on contagion: The hospital as moral universe," in *Healing and History*, ed. C. E. Rosenberg, New York, Science Hist. Pub., 1979, pp. 116–36.

146. J. Lister, "On the effects of the antiseptic system of treatment upon the salubrity of a surgical hospital," *Lancet* 1 (Jan. 1, 1870): 4. The managers angrily responded in a letter published in the journal two weeks later, blaming Lister for the overcrowding since he kept his patients longer than the other surgeons. Lister's rejoinder, published February 5, defended his accomplishments and the credit his system had brought to the Glasgow Infirmary.

147. J. Lister, "On the antiseptic principle in the practice of surgery," *Br Med J* II (Sept. 21, 1867): 246–48. See also "On a new method of treating compound fracture, abscess, etc.," *Lancet* 1 (July 27, 1867): 95–96, followed by "On the antiseptic principle in the practice of surgery," *Lancet* 2 (Sept. 21, 1867): 353–56, and "Illustrations of the antiseptic system of treatment in surgery," *Lancet* 2 (Nov. 30, 1867): 668–69. Lister's papers can also be found in Joseph Lister, *The Collected Papers of Joseph Baron Lister*, 2 vols., Oxford, Clarendon Press, 1909.

148. See J. Wood, "Address in surgery," *Lancet* 2 (Aug. 9, 1872): 183.

149. "Medical men cannot be too cautious in mounting hobbies or in being led away by the seductive influence of discovery. There is nothing more calculated to shake the faith of the public in our art." D. C. Black, *Br Med J* II (Sept. 4, 1869): 281.

150. For an excellent analysis of Lister's shifting ideas see C. Lawrence and R. Dixey, "Practising on principle: Joseph Lister and the germ theories of disease," in *Medical Theory, Surgical Practice*, ed. C. Lawrence, London, Routledge, 1992, pp. 153–215.

151. For a summary of contemporary ideas see Arthur E. Sansom, *The Antiseptic System*, Philadelphia, Lippincott, 1871. Regarding Tyndall's work see P. D. Olch, "The contributions of John Tyndall to wound infections and putrefaction," *Surg Gynecol Obstet* 116 (1963): 249–54.

152. J. Lister, "Address in surgery," *Br Med J* II (Aug. 26, 1871): 225–33.

153. Ibid. For a summary of Lister's views by a contemporary resident surgeon at the Royal Infirmary see J. Cumming, "On antiseptic surgery," *Edinb Med J* 17 (1871–1872): 985–1011.

154. R. J. Godlee, "On the antiseptic system as seen in professor Lister's wards at Edinburgh," *Lancet* 1 (May 17, 1873): 694–95 and (May 24, 1873): 769–71.

155. S. Gamgee, "The treatment of wounds on the antiseptic method," *Lancet* 1 (Jan. 3, 1874): 9–10 and (Jan. 10, 1874): 50–52. For Lister's science and method see N. J. Fox, "Scientific theory and social structure: The case of Joseph Lister's antisepsis, humoral theory and asepsis," *Hist Sci* 26 (1988): 367–97.

156. J. Lister, "An address on the effect of the antiseptic treatment upon the general salubrity of surgical hospitals," *Br Med J* II (Dec. 25, 1875): 769–71.

157. Leeson, *Lister*, p. 78.

158. Hector C. Cameron, *Reminiscences of Lister*, Glasgow, Jackson, Wylie & Co., 1927, p. 43.

159. Leeson, *Lister*, pp. 69–73.

160. Cameron, *Reminiscences*, p. 85.

161. J. Lister, "Demonstrations of antiseptic surgery before members of the BMA in the operating theater of the Royal Infirmary, 4th and 5th August, 1875," *Edinb Med J* 21 (1875): 193–205 and 480–87. For an account of his earlier improvements see J. Lister, "On recent improvements in the details of antiseptic surgery," *Lancet* 1 (Mar. 13, 1875): 365–67, (Mar. 20, 1875): 401–02, (Mar. 27, 1875): 434–36, (Apr. 3, 1875): 468–70, (May 1, 1875): 603–05, (May 22, 1875): 717–19, and (June 5, 1875): 787–89.

162. Cameron, *Reminiscences*, p. 88.

163. A. Bennett, "Notes with observations on cases treated in the surgical wards VIII, IX, X, XI, and XII, Royal Infirmary, Edinburgh, under the care of Dr. Gillespie," *Edinb Med J* 16 (1870–1871): 676–87.

164. G. W. Balfour, "Introductory address delivered at the opening of the Edinburgh Medical School on 3d November 1873," *Edinb Med J* 19 (1873–1874): 486.

165. C. Roberts, "The action and use of antiseptics in surgical practice," *Lancet* 1 (Apr. 27, 1872): 570–71.

166. Cheyne, *Lister and His Achievement*, pp. 29–30. Indeed, Cheyne himself later published such a text: *Antiseptic Surgery*, London, Smith, Elder & Co., 1882.

167. J. Chiene, "The antiseptic dressing of wounds," *Edinb Med J* 23 (1877): 550–54.

168. RIE, Report of the Managers, 1 Oct. 1870–1 Oct. 1871, pp. 3–4.

169. "An improved mode of surgical treatment, although it may increase the expense, is a matter entirely for the decision of the medical officers." See RIE, Report of the Managers, 1 Oct. 1871–1 Oct. 1872, p. 17.

170. RIE, Minutes, 14 May 1877, and RIE, Report of the Managers, 1 Oct. 1876–1 Oct. 1877, p. 20.

171. Chiene, "The antiseptic dressing of wounds," 509–12.

172. Mathewson, "Sketch," p. 11.

173. Ibid., p. 12.

174. See William E. Henley, "Staff-nurse, new style," a poem originally published in *Cornhill Magazine* in 1875, reproduced in Goldman, *Lister Ward*, pp. 44–45.

175. A near-contemporary sketch described physicians as "men of buckram and infallibility" who gravely shook their heads and looked beyond their patients with sphinx-like eyes as if they searched for the mysteries of an unknown world within their bodies. *The Hospital* II (May 28, 1887): 3.

176. The term appears in Arthur Conan Doyle, *Round the Red Lamp*, New York, Appleton & Co., 1894, pp. 9–19, and is reprinted in Goldman, *Lister Ward*, pp. 71–76.

177. Mathewson, "Sketch," p. 18.

178. Leeson, *Lister*, p. 18.

179. Mathewson, "Sketch," pp. 40–41.

180. John E. Erichsen, "Scrofula and tubercle," in *The Science and Art of Surgery*, 7th rev. ed., London, Longmans, Green & Co., 1877, vol. 1, pp. 320–30.

181. James Spense, *Lectures on Surgery*, 2nd ed., Edinburgh, Adam and Charles Black, 1875, especially pp. 266–77.

182. The statistics presented by J. Y. Simpson, however, were meaningless, since the Glasgow Infirmary reported only seven arm amputations for disease from 1861 to 1868. In the Royal Infirmary of Edinburgh for the same period there were only six such cases, with a 33% mortality rate. See his "Our existing system of hospitalism and its effects," *Edinb Med J* 14 (Mar. 1869): 1106–08.

183. Erichsen, "Excision of joints," in *The Science and Art of Surgery*, vol. 2, pp. 241–52.

184. Mathewson, "Sketch," p. 42.

185. RIE, Minutes, 12 Mar. 1877.

186. Mathewson, "Sketch," p. 62.

187. Ibid., p. 66. This method of chloroform administration by dripping the fluid on a towel either folded in layers or shaped into a cone and placed over the patient's face, required smaller quantities of the anesthetic and was therefore less dangerous.

188. Mathewson, "Sketch," p. 66.

189. Ibid., p. 68.

190. *Edinburgh Evening News*, Mar. 24, 1877.

191. Mathewson, *Sketch*, p. 74.

192. Ibid., pp. 75, 83.

193. Ibid., pp. 87, 90.

194. Ibid., p. 91.

195. RIE, Minutes, 9 Apr. 1877.

196. Mathewson, "Sketch," pp. 95, 106.

197. The letter to her brother Arthur was dated July 19, 1877. See Goldman, *Lister Ward*, p. 102.

198. There were ladies which came regularly every Friday with baskets of flowers tied into bouquets and a precious text as well under the thread, and gave each patient a bouquet then went through all the Infirmary." Mathewson, "Sketch," pp. 34–36.

199. Mathewson, "Sketch," p. 116.

200. RIE, Minutes, 30 July 1877. An official letter of resignation dated August 1 was considered at the next weekly meeting. For Lister's departure, see Cheyne, *Lister*, p. 32.

201. "Hospital accommodation for infectious diseases in London," *Br Med J* 1 (1877): 311–12.

202. Turner, *Story of a Great Hospital*, p. 175.

203. Margaret remarked that "I felt it to be a special privilege given me to acquire useful knowledge which it seldom fails to one in my station of life to acquire." Mathewson, "Sketch," p. 172.

204. Mathewson, "Sketch," p. 168. Following his arrival at King's College Hospital, Lister collided with the institution's Anglican sisterhood because he personally insisted on dressing his patients' wounds, a chore previously carried out by the nurses. In retaliation, the St. John's House sisters imposed a series of rules on the movement of the surgical personnel. Cheyne, *Lister*, pp. 34–35.

205. Mathewson, "Sketch," pp. 166–67.

206. Ibid., p. 2. Goldman characterized it as an "evangelical tract meant to convert people to hospitals and her brand of Methodism" in *Lister Ward*, p. 147. Indeed, as described in her sketch, Margaret on several occasions brought the comforts of Christian religion to her Infirmary roommates.

207. Anon., "What is the use of a hospital?," *Edinb Med J* 23 (1877):181–83, based on article in the London *Times* of June 28, 1877. See also Henry C. Burdett, *Pay Hospitals and Paying Wards Throughout the World*, 1st American ed., Philadelphia, Blakiston, 1880. For funding issues see S. Cherry, "Accountability, entitlement, and control issues and voluntary hospital funding, c. 1860–1939," *Soc Hist Med* 9 (1996): 215–33.

208. See L. Granshaw, " 'Upon this principle I have based a practice': The development and reception of antisepsis in Britain, 1867–90," in *Medical Innovations in Historical Perspective*, ed. J. V. Pickstone, New York, St. Martin's Press, 1992, pp. 17–46. See also T. H. Pennington, "Listerism, its decline and its persistence: The introduction of aseptic surgical techniques in three British teaching hospitals, 1890–99," *Med Hist* 39 (1995): 35–60.

209. Editorial, *Lancet* 1 (Apr. 28, 1877): 614.

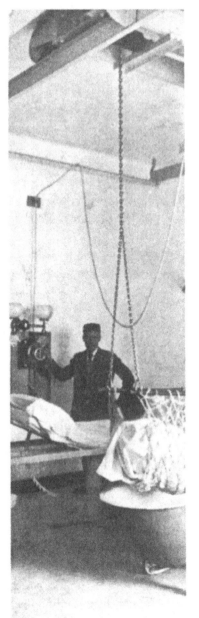

8

THE LIMITS OF
MEDICAL SCIENCE

Hospitals in Fin-de-Siècle
Europe and America

*TYPHOID FEVER AND
JOHNS HOPKINS
HOSPITAL, BALTIMORE,
1891*

The indigent sick of this city and environs without
regard to sex, age, or color who may require surgical or medical treatment . . . and the poor who
are stricken down by any casualty, shall be received
into this hospital without charge . . . you will also
provide for the reception of a limited number of
patients who are able to make compensation for
the room and attention they may require.

Johns Hopkins, 1873[1]

A bartender with fever

In the middle of February 1891, John S., a
bartender, suddenly fell ill at work. Originally
from New Jersey, John, who was 34 years old and single, lived in Baltimore at Patterson Avenue and Monroe St., in Ward 19. This small, mostly white neighborhood at the western fringes of town had sprung up recently between the Fulton
Station of the Western Maryland Railway, the Baltimore-Potomac tracks, and St.
Peter's cemetery. Surrounded by warehouses and tire and scrap metal companies,
this industrial area lacked the usual stores and markets, forcing its few dwellers
to seek their supplies as well as employment farther east.[2] Instead of the red brick
townhouses with white steps characteristic of other Baltimore neighborhoods, this

cul-de-sac featured low-rent, ramshackle dwellings placed between depots and factories. Open sewers flowed along the sides of most unpaved streets.

Little else is known about John S. He was one of countless young Americans who sought their fortunes in the expanding cities of the Eastern seaboard. We do not even know how long he had been living in Baltimore, a midway station between North and South since the Civil War. We can presume, however, that he was part of the great influx of people—an average of nearly 8,000 per year—that by 1891 had pushed the city's population to a record level: 442,000. More than 50% of Baltimoreans were under age 30, members of a multiethnic, segregated urban center. At this time, the city was burdened by a large population of uneducated, even illiterate workers, and lacked much civic cohesion.[3]

As John later recalled, he had enjoyed good health since childhood. During the previous fall, a flu-like fever prevented him from working for about three weeks. He only remembered suffering from colicky pains in the right side of his abdomen and back and having lengthy coughing spells, not surprising for someone who enjoyed drinking and smoking. He eventually recovered, but became sick again in February 1891, experiencing chills and fever, a bad cough, and pains on the right side of the abdomen as well as in his back. Feeling hot and dizzy, he was forced to leave his job and return to his quarters, where he remained bedridden for six and a half weeks. Although constipated, John later denied experiencing headaches or nosebleeds, but under the circumstances, this information could not be confirmed. Whether John was aware of the seriousness and nature of his acute illness remains unknown.[4]

Typhoid fever was then very prevalent in Baltimore, especially in the city's outlying areas. Drinking water was obtained from public pumps connected to shallow wells, now mostly contaminated by the myriad privies and cesspools located in backyards. Based on information from the city's annual *Health Reports*, mortality from typhoid fever in the city during the years 1888–1892 averaged around 229 cases per year, disproportionately affecting poor blacks and those of German and Irish extraction. This figure could be translated—given the disease's mortality of 12%—into a total of around 2,750 cases each year for its population of around 450,000. Throughout the 1880s, Ward 19 reported a significant number of typhoid fever cases and had the highest mortality rate in the city. However, except for a few articles in popular science journals, this febrile disease was mentioned only during sporadic epidemic outbreaks.[5]

Typhoid usually had an insidious onset, with headaches and progressive fever. John's respiratory symptoms might well have suggested a severe spring flu or bronchitis, particularly because of his heavy smoking. Most uneducated lay persons remained ignorant of the germ theory of disease, and particularly the nature of this fever.[6] Typhoid lacked dramatic symptoms, and with a spontaneous recovery rate of nearly 85%, there seemed little to worry about. After a steadily rising temperature during the first week, John should have noticed the typical but transient rose-colored spots on his abdomen, but perhaps he paid little attention or mistook them for a trivial rash. Even clinicians occasionally missed the spots.[7]

Events during the ensuing weeks went unrecorded. How sick was John? How did he react to his illness? Was he worried, being alone and bound to his bed at the very edge of town? Or, being in the prime of life and previously quite healthy, did he remain optimistic, trusting that his body would shake off whatever was causing the trouble? Moreover, who, if anybody, took care of this bachelor while he lay in his bed, probably confused and delirious, shivering under the blankets, thirsty, hungry, uncomfortable with his abdominal pains? Did some of John's friends take the trouble to visit him after work? Was he able to summon a neighbor or hire a nurse to take care of him? According to later statistics, a majority of Americans preferred to be treated at home for such fevers, even in protracted cases, possibly because many benefited from adequate family care networks, which were unavailable to single, newly arrived, and foreign-born immigrants.[8] In spite of such a preference, physicians argued that home care in typhoid fever was inadequate, since the desired physical and mental rest was difficult to achieve in such a setting. Moreover, strict cleanliness of the body and frequent changes of contaminated clothing could not be ensured, leading to one of the most common hazards of the disease: the development of bed sores. By the end of March, John was finally up, and within a week he supposedly returned to work. Was he really on the mend or just low on money after six weeks of serious sickness and unemployment?

On April 24, John began suffering from a relapse, with lack of appetite, vomiting, constipation, some coughing, renewed bouts of chills and fever, and slight nosebleeds. This time, the situation appeared to be more dangerous; after two days of escalating symptoms, either John or his friends finally decided to get him to a hospital. They chose the new Johns Hopkins Hospital located on a hill two miles east of the city, already said to be one of the best facilities in the country. Despite this reputation, many Baltimoreans remained unimpressed, and as the chief medical resident later recalled, there was no immediate bond between the institutional staff and the public.[9] Part of the tension was ascribed to the southern and somewhat clannish nature of the city's inhabitants, and to the fact that all department heads at Hopkins had received their medical training at northern universities. Moreover, rumors circulated among the local black population that physicians were "cutting up niggers" due to the pathological work conducted there even before the institution officially opened in 1889. In addition, since the hospital lacked segregated facilities, few black patients were initially allowed to enter unless separate rooms were available.[10]

Since Johns Hopkins had no ambulance service, John had to endure a four-mile ordeal in a horse-drawn carriage or railway car across the few cobbled city streets and the foul-smelling stream called Jones' Falls that carried garbage from nearby factories and slaughterhouses.[11] Following his arrival, the admitting clerks classified John as a paying patient—the stipulated fee was $ 5 per week—and had him transported by stretcher up the stairs to Ward A, which contained 13 beds.[12] The presumptive diagnosis was typhoid fever. The widely accepted cause of this fever was a bacillus discovered in 1880 by the German Carl J. Eberth, a finding later confirmed by bacteriologists Robert Koch and Georg Gaffky.[13]

Among those being admitted at Hopkins, John S. was a typical typhoid case. Nearly half of the patients were in their third decade of life; 90% were white and 81% were male, although only 37% were native-born Americans. The rest were foreigners, particularly Germans living near the hospital and said to be "without regular homes."[14] At certain times of the year, half of the medical service was occupied with victims of this disease.[15] Between 1888 and 1892, fully 75% of the typhoid patients came from the city of Baltimore.

Hopkins and Billings: Genesis and gestation of a new hospital

Johns Hopkins (1795–1873), founder of the hospital that bore his name, was a prominent new entrepreneur in mid-Victorian Baltimore. A native of Maryland and a Quaker, Hopkins was president of the Merchants Bank and one of the directors of the Baltimore & Ohio Railroad, another important economic player in the city.[16] Single and thrifty, Hopkins had amassed a fortune based on real estate holdings and shares of the railroad, but in the twilight years of his rags-to-riches career, he decided in 1867 to divide his impressive $7 million estate into two portions for the founding of a local university and a hospital linked to a medical school. Two separate corporations with overlapping membership, also composed of strict Quakers, were to implement Hopkins' wishes. A friend and adviser, Francis T. King, was selected as the president of the future hospital board of trustees.[17] In 1872, Hopkins purchased the site of the old Maryland Hospital for the Insane, where yellow fever cases and Civil War casualties had been treated. The site at Loudenschlager's Hill east of Baltimore's center had excellent drainage and its own springs. Because of its elevation, fresh breezes provided the ventilation still believed to be critical for sanitation.

In March 1873, Johns Hopkins articulated his vision of the new hospital.[18] First and foremost, the new institution was to be erected according to traditional charitable goals for "the indigent sick of this city and its environs, without regard to sex, age or color who may require surgical or medical treatment," a population group then being swelled by successive waves of immigrants. Like the Massachusetts General Hospital in Boston, the facilities would house "a limited number of patients who are able to make compensation for the room and attention they may require, "an obvious reference to the growing number of individuals now living in lodging houses and apartments, where the lack of caregiving family networks and space hindered home care.[19] Perhaps impressed by recent experiences in England with the Nightingale school and his own exposure as a cholera victim to the Sisters of Charity during the 1832 epidemic in Baltimore, Hopkins also demanded the creation of a training school for female nurses to provide the care.

The donor was quite aware that the "usefulness of this charity" would depend upon the building plan to be adopted by the trustees. Hospital construction and organization needed to compare favorably with arrangements at similar institutions in Europe and America. In Hopkins' view, the most desirable system would allow "symmetrical additions to the buildings" for housing up to 400 patients. Additional facilities were to be reserved "for the reception of convalescents" and surrounding hospital grounds "planted with trees and flowers to afford solace to the sick." Finally, Hopkins insisted that "the administration of the charity shall be undisturbed by sectarian influence, discipline or control," but he quickly added that "it is my special request that the influence of religion should be felt in and impressed upon the whole management of the hospital."[20]

Implementation of Hopkins' wishes began even before his death on December 24, 1873. Later, additional land purchases and the appointment of an architect, John R. Niernsee, led to discussions about the usefulness of pavilion versus temporary barracks hospitals, and further expertise was sought.[21] Five prominent medical experts were requested to present plans for the new hospital. Among them was John S. Billings (1838–1913), a medical officer familiar with the barracks system of military hospitals, whose experience battling hospitalism had recently drawn the attention of the British surgeon John E. Erichsen. As noted before, for more than a century, hospital architects and medical experts like Frank in Vienna and Tenon in Paris, had suggested breaking down the block-type hospital into separate smaller buildings.[22] Now these authorities debated the merits of building permanent pavilions or erecting temporary barracks to prevent institutional hospitalism. In the end, Billings' plan presented in November 1875, proved the most ambitious, although the trustees published all five invited essays to stimulate further discussion. A variation on the notion of small and separate building units, Billings' plan relied on a carefully designed ventilation system to combat contagion.[23]

Almost a year later, Billings was officially hired to supervise construction of the new hospital. His ideas about medical education and research in hospitals were also deemed by the trustees congruent with modern views on the subject in Europe, as well as with the aims of the new Hopkins University. Billings was asked to redraft his original proposal, and new but very expensive plans were approved. In fact, an estimate for the entire complex was $1.2 million, and if nothing but Hopkins' endowment income was to be available, completion would take several years. Aware of the danger that his plan could be drastically downsized, Billings pleaded with the trustees for full implementation of the original project. In his view, any reductions would compromise "the benefits of this charity" and hamper the planned scientific research with the help of adequate laboratory space.

The trustees agreed that grading at the site could be postponed until the spring of 1877 so that Billings would have an opportunity to obtain further information during a visit to Europe, as well as conclude ventilation experiments at the Barnes Hospital for soldiers in Washington, D.C.[24]

Billings now traveled to Europe to study ventilation and heating at prominent hospitals in London, Leipzig, Berlin, Vienna, and Paris. Not surprisingly, he failed to find a consensus regarding optimal construction and ventilation schemes, although experts agreed that institutional infections had to be reduced, in part through the employment of antiseptics. After his visits, Billings reported once more to the trustees in January 1877, stressing that the "prime importance in a hospital is minute care of and cleanliness in every part and person about it."[25] The experience of the new Nightingales in British hospitals had demonstrated that effective nursing personnel trained in principles of personal and institutional hygiene was also critical. Improved patient management and supervision were to be additional weapons against hospitalism.

For Billings, the new hospital was also to be a site for medical education, considered a boon to patients.[26] Clinical teachers would work in a fishbowl atmosphere where every diagnostic error and treatment failure would be immediately exposed and corrected. Teaching, however, was not enough. Billings believed that the new hospital also had a responsibility to foster medical research, to provide institutional support for such studies, and thus to create a community of investigators: "the hospital should not only teach the best methods of caring for the sick now known, but aim to increase knowledge and thus benefit the whole world by its diffusion."[27] Final plans were submitted to the trustees and approved in April 1877.

In June 1877, construction crews began excavating the foundations; hospital completion was tentatively scheduled for 1882. Yet as the separate buildings took shape a year later, their elaborate ventilation systems produced significant cost overruns and work slowed because of a lack of funds.[28] Should the building committee consider some shortcuts? Everyone agreed that no viable alternative existed. The hospital's future reputation depended upon a physical plant designed to ensure maximum fresh air and cleanliness. This was crucial to future patients, especially those who would occupy the paying wards and private rooms.[29]

The construction of the Johns Hopkins Hospital complex—eventually comprising 17 buildings and 600 yards of connecting corridors—thus proceeded at a slow pace over the next 12 years. The tempo was dictated by the cautious board of trustees and the limited income available each year. Billings insisted that only the best materials be employed, boasting that "I do not hesitate to affirm that these are the best built buildings of their kind in the world." The showcase of the complex was the central administration building facing west on Broadway Street. In fact, one-quarter of the total budget had been devoted to its construction and that of the two adjacent ornate structures flanking it. These Queen Anne-style buildings were built of pressed brick trimmed with stone. Their pitched roofs were covered with slate and some portions with copper. Flanked by two pavilions for paying patients, the administration building had three floors and was linked by a north-south corridor to a separate nurses' residence to the south and the kitchen facilities to the north. Furnished with all the comforts of home, the house for the nurses resembled a small hotel, away from the wards and ideal for rest and recreation.

Five separate pavilions, linked by a west-east corridor, rose in succession on the northern side of the complex. The octagonal surgical ward, a two-story building, held a general ward and two special wards, a central hall, lavatory, and closets, with a sun room at the south end. In each building, patients had to be carried on stretchers up the stairs to reach the connecting passage, especially if they were brought to the bathhouse located at the junction of the north-south and east-west corridors. All walls were curved at the ceiling and floor for easier cleaning.[30]

The various wards were rectangular, with all service rooms collected at the north end of the building and linked with an octagonal lobby at the entrance. Each general ward accommodated 24 beds, with provisions for two smaller rooms for special cases and greater privacy. The southern end remained fully exposed to the sun. A large bay window allowed ambulatory patients to look out to a central garden. Gas fixtures provided lighting. Since there was no running water, the wards were provided with wooden, movable wash stands, equipped with pitchers of hot and cold water for the use of all caregivers. All waste water was collected in slop jars and disposed of by the male attendants. Artificial ventilation was provided through individually adjustable ventilators located on the floor under the beds. Each building also had its own ventilation system, preventing foul air from spreading between buildings. These units were connected by corridors and underground tunnels to prevent staff and patient exposure to cold air, rain, and snow. Corridors ended at the basement level of each unit, from which the actual ward and roof were reached by an open stairway. This ingenious layout was designed to prevent any possible disease transmission through contaminated air. Unfortunately, it created considerable obstacles to the distribution of supplies, food, and medicines and hampered patient circulation.[31]

Finally, the hospital had a separate isolation ward. More than any other structure, this building's location and design were based on prebacteriological notions of contagion. It was situated at the eastern end of the complex to ensure that the wind would blow any disease-producing miasma in an easterly direction, away from all other structures. Like the other wards, it had a north-south orientation, but it also had double-thick walls and a capacity for 20 private rooms, each outfitted with its own chimney to assist in removing any possibly corrupted air produced by the patient's bodily vapors. Another constant current of air flowed from the basement through separate grates. In turn, all the individual rooms had access to a central corridor wide open on both ends to allow the passage of wind through the building. Billings continued to stress that heating was closely linked to proper ventilation and air supply. For him Baltimore was a special case. Its temperatures varied from a tropical 103°F during some summer days to −17°F during harsh winters. All buildings needed double walls with air spaces between them for insulation. The actual heating was to be accomplished by circulating nearly 80,000 gallons of hot water from central boilers through pipes placed beneath every building and connected to coils located under every other bed.

By 1883, the hospital's slow gestation was generating pressure on the hospital board to begin providing service. A proposal by trustees Garrett and Smith was to open the 56-bed octagonal ward, a dispensary, and a surgical amphitheater by the fall, but further construction delays seemed to frustrate such plans. With costs escalating and annual endowment income stationary, completion seemed uncertain. If Billings had to decide between early service and completion of the original master plan, he clearly preferred the latter. Indeed, he contended that the sick poor of Baltimore could afford to wait until what he believed to be the best hospital in the world was finished.[32] A new opening date was set: October 1, 1885. By that time, all ward buildings on the north side would be completed together with the necessary service facilities. Buildings planned for the south side were temporarily placed on hold and, in the end, never built.

In anticipation of the 1885 opening, planning for the medical school continued. In 1883 three faculty members—Henry N. Martin (physiology), Ira Remsen (chemistry), and John S. Billings (hygiene)—had already been appointed. During the following year, William H. Welch (pathology) was selected, although he assumed his post only in October 1885 after a tour of German laboratories and universities. Unfortunately, the scheduled hospital opening had to be delayed again, leading to new pressures on King and the trustees to open the institution before completion. Even the mayor of Baltimore made an appeal before the board of trustees, but to no avail. By January 1886, the upper story of a separate laboratory of pathology was ready for occupancy by Welch. These facilities were in a square, free-standing building located at the northeast end of the sprawling complex but still close to the future wards. Separate areas were planned for pathological and bacteriological investigation, pathological histology, and experimental pathology. An autopsy room, amphitheater, photo laboratory, and museum completed the installation. The complex was comparable to that of the Hygienic Institute in Berlin. With permission from the trustees, Welch gave his first course of lectures in microbiology in February–March 1886; in the fall, he taught two courses in pathological histology using cadaveric material from the City Hospital. Those enrolling were young Baltimore physicians eager to improve their meager knowledge of the subject.

Buildings and machinery were only the means to an end, tools to achieve the desired goal of a well-ventilated hospital. Equally important for Billings were organization and personnel. "A hospital is a living organism made up of many different parts, having different functions, but all these must be in due proportion and relation to each other and to the environment to produce the desired results," he argued.[33] Selection of the administrative and professional staff of the hospital had already started in 1885, carried out by a joint committee of university and hospital trustees. The buildings were practically finished, and everything pointed to an imminent opening. In 1887, however, Johns Hopkins University experienced a severe financial crisis after the collapse of the Baltimore & Ohio Railroad, on whose shares the endowment was almost exclusively based. When the company stopped paying dividends after May 1887, its stock plunged, shrinking the university's endowments by 75% and forcing the trustees to suspend their plans for the medical school indefinitely.[34] By contrast, hospital income remained unaffected, since it was almost entirely derived from real estate, and its trustees thus made new plans to open the institution by October 1888.

In the meantime, Billings, busy organizing the future hospital, declined an invitation to assume its directorship because of his obligations in Washington. The immediate task was to find and appoint chiefs of the hospital clinics and offer them professorships of medicine and surgery. But who would want to come to Baltimore now that the medical school was in limbo? This turned out not to be a problem. In October 1888, William Osler (1849–1919), then at the University of Pennsylvania, promptly accepted an offer from Billings to assume leadership of the medical service, and William S. Halsted agreed to take the surgical post in 1889. Both men represented selections made from a national pool of younger candidates, based on their qualifications as clinicians and investigators. As full-time chiefs, they were allowed to see only a few private patients. No Baltimore practitioners received staff privileges and hospital beds, as was usually the rule at other institutions, because of their inferior credentials and education.

For Billings, life at the Johns Hopkins Hospital was to be structured so that the institution "shall do as little harm as possible" in an attempt to overcome the centuries-old stigma of hospitals as gateways to death. The usual culprits of foul air and contagion would be avoided by the novel and ample ventilation system. Another old hazard, the "neglect or carelessness of its nurses or attendants," would be prevented by hiring a competent nursing staff.[35] While the goal to link the hospital to the university remained elusive—the medical school was on hold—hospital appointees who were to be also faculty members, were relieved by the repeated construction delays. The postponement provided Osler and others with an opportunity to get at least the hospital's own educational program off the ground before the inevitable burden of patient care became a reality.[36]

As completion of the entire hospital complex became imminent in early 1889, the president of the university, Daniel C. Gilman (1831–1908), was drafted by King to become interim director and complete the organization and staffing.[37] Gilman was quite interested in medical education. As president of the University of California before he came to Baltimore, he had already successfully incorporated a proprietary medical college in San Francisco and converted it into an important academic institution. Gilman now also made an extensive study of hospital organization and management by visiting a number of larger institutions. If Billings' primary concern had been the creation of an appropriate physical plant capable of facilitating hygienic care, clinical teaching, and scientific research, Gilman envisioned a management plan that would make the patients as comfortable as hotel guests. "Between an hotel and an hospital there is no difference," was Gilman's maxim.[38] Indeed, looking at department stores and hotels for institutional models, Gilman devised an administrative structure dividing the hospital into separate services with their own heads reporting to an overall director. A medical board was to be composed of all chiefs of services, including medicine, surgery, and pathology, together with hospital and university trustees. This board would make all personnel appointments based on nominations submitted by the individual departments. Unlike those in other American hospitals, Johns Hopkins' service chiefs were free to select their own patients and share power with the lay trustees, thus creating a setting favorable to the desired clinical research and teaching.

On May 7, 1889, the Johns Hopkins Hospital was formally launched with a number of speeches and functions. The first chief resident recalled that there was a "feeling of elation—one might even say of exaltation—that the structure which had taken twenty years to evolve, absorbing the energies and thought of so many able minds, had at last become a fait accompli."[39] First to open was the dispensary, where Osler spent most of his time until the hospital wards were full. Frantic efforts were made to purchase needed equipment, compose dietary lists, and create admission forms and other documentation for medical record keeping. By June, 50 patients had been hospitalized. The large wards were praised as luxurious and fresh, although the ventilation system was rarely employed correctly. The windows were too wide, and it was beyond the physical power of the nurses to open or close them or to operate the heavy blinds.[40] In the meantime, a new hospital superintendent, Henry M. Hurd, a medical graduate from the University of Michigan, had taken over the administrative duties. Formerly at the Eastern Michigan Asylum at Pontiac, Hurd possessed excellent administrative skills and medical training, and he fully supported the research and educational agendas espoused by Billings, Welch, and Osler.[41]

Osler, physicians, and nurses

From a distinguished Canadian family, William Osler had trained at Toronto and McGill universities before visiting clinics and laboratories in England, France, and Germany. Now in his early forties, Osler was a well-trained pathologist and anatomist with a strong interest in public health.[42] He followed the tradition of French medicine by studying the correlations between clinical observations and pathological anatomy, but he also strongly supported the new linkages between the basic medical sciences—physiology, biochemistry, and bacteriology among them—that now informed clinical events.[43]

When he arrived, the hospital complex had finally been completed, and its administrative structure was in place. Relieved of many administrative chores by the hospital's superintendent, Osler gladly concentrated on the activities of his medical department, especially the care of patients—their welfare seemed always his highest priority—together with the selection of his staff. At first, he lived on the second floor of the administration building, occupying comfortable quarters that overlooked the city and its harbor.[44] His hospital routine was said to be so predictable that other residents "set their watches at 10 PM by the sound of his boots as they dropped on the floor outside his door."[45] Unmarried, Osler briefly rented a house on West Monument Street, where he may have seen some private patients, but most of his income came from his salaried position. Although quite busy, Osler went abroad between April and September 1890, and upon his return began work on his textbook. At the time of John S.'s admission, Osler continued to live and see private patients in his house. Contemporaries described him as an attractive individual with a charming personality capable of bringing people together, a quality essential to starting a new hospital.

One of Osler's most salient innovations was to hire a staff of experienced resident physicians, their tenure to be indefinite. This appointment fulfilled the need to have young but experienced physicians in attendance who wished to spend a number of years studying and teaching, and thus acquire professional reputations in preparation for an academic career. As conceived by Osler, the position followed the German model of a first assistant, to be complemented by two or three assistant residents and several interns, an arrangement that differed from Gilman's more traditional plans. The first chief resident physician was Henry A. Lafleur, a French Canadian, who stayed for two years, from 1889 until 1891. After graduating in 1886 from McGill University, Lafleur had served for 18 months as house physician at the Montreal General Hospital and, like Osler, had training in pathology. He stayed at Hopkins until September 1891 before returning to his alma mater as a faculty member. Harry A. Toulmin, and later Charles E. Simon and D. Meredith Reese, were Osler's first assistant residents.[46]

During the academic year 1890–1891, a limited number of medical graduates—mostly from Baltimore—were permitted to accompany Osler and his assistants during their daily ward visits. Enough funds to open the planned medical school were still lacking. Characterized by Lafleur as a "motley group," the visitors received instruction in the methods of history taking, physical diagnosis, and the study of therapeutic actions, subjects completely neglected at the local two-year medical schools many of them had attended before receiving their MD degrees.[47] These doctors also went to the dispensary, where important cases were selected for study and demonstration—"caviar" for mental nourishment, according to Lafleur.[48] Moreover, Osler organized weekly clinics in the amphitheater featuring particular cases, or groups of cases, that illustrated points in diagnosis or treatment. Students were forced to follow up on such focused subjects while developing their own independent learning habits. Since it was impossible to convey the entire spectrum of medicine, common diseases such as tuberculosis, typhoid fever, and pneumonia were selected for in-depth study and analysis.

Osler and others were confident that, despite decades of medical controversy, typhoid fever could now be separated from a peculiarly American disease entity: typho-malarial fever. During the Civil War, the manifestations of malaria and typhoid fever remained merged into a single disease. A resolution of this problem began after the discovery of separate causal microorganisms—Laveran's parasite and Eberth's bacillus—in 1880. In fact, Osler and the Johns Hopkins Hospital became an ideal site for the bacteriological research necessary to make the differential diagnoses; both malaria and typhoid fever were still quite prevalent in Baltimore.[49]

Osler's conception of the medical clinic was described by one of his first residents as a synthesis of various European models, including the British ritual of "walking the wards," the French internat, and the German-Austrian method that combined the clinic with the laboratory.[50] Rather than employing a "military type" of organization, Osler created a team in which a group of physicians, led by the professor-in-chief and his associate professors, "visited" the wards, which were under the constant supervision of a resident staff headed by a chief physician, assistant physicians, and interns.[51] A second characteristic of Osler's approach was systematic instruction at the bedside, focused on obtaining information about the structural and functional disturbances afflicting individual patients. History taking, physical examination, and the laboratory examination of blood, urine, and other bodily fluids were the tripod on which these fact-gathering efforts rested. For laboratory tests, the house staff of all services utilized a small room, hastily outfitted on Osler's orders under Ward G.[52]

Medical school graduates residing in Baltimore were admitted free of charge to the lectures and clinics in the amphitheater simply by registering at the hospital's office, where they obtained a ticket of admission. To take a special course or make rounds, they had to pay a $50 fee and "give satisfactory evidence to the officers of the hospital that they are fitted to profit by the courses."[53] During these lectures, Osler's background as a pathologist readily emerged as he attempted to reconstruct clinical events from the pathological specimens. Here Osler revealed himself as a true disciple of the earlier Paris Medical School and its notable advocates Pinel, Bichat, and Laennec.[54] However, he was also a student of the new German scientific medicine, based on findings and understandings derived from research laboratories that were devoted to the study of human physiology and pathology at the cellular level.[55] At the hospital, courses in clinical microscopy and the examination of blood and urine were given by Dr. Lafleur at Welch's clinical laboratory, adjacent to the wards, consisting of four rooms provided with chemical, microscopic, and clinical apparatus.

In 1890, hospital board trustees tried to devise a plan for lectures without official approval from the university, following the example of certain London hospitals that had become de facto medical schools, but the plan was immediately rejected by Gilman. He insisted that all medical instruction needed to be under the control of the university.[56] Among the courses given during 1890–1891 were one in pathology by William H. Welch and his assistant, William T. Councilman; in bacteriology by Welch and Alexander C. Abbott; and in medicine by William Osler. Under Welch, an in-house medical society and a journal club held bimonthly meetings attended by members of the hospital and dispensary staffs.

After September 1890, Osler, for his part, became involved in a number of writing projects after attending the Tenth International Congress of Medicine in Berlin.[57] Perhaps this was a good time to write a textbook for the kinds of medical students Osler expected to instruct in the future. When an agent from the New York publisher D. Appleton and Company came calling and made an attractive offer, Osler signed a contract "selling my brains to the devil."[58] Little progress was made during the final months of the year, but after January 1891, just as John S. became ill, Osler began working in earnest on his book.

A training school for nurses had been part of Hopkins' original plans, based in part on Quaker traditions of humanitarianism and the equality of the sexes.[59] During a stop in London during the 1880s, King, president of the hospital's board of trustees, consulted Florence Nightingale on nursing education and obtained information about her renowned training school.[60] By this time, the success of Nightingale's elite nurses left no doubt about the importance of training young women as skillful caregivers. This fact did not escape the attention even of Billings, who originally was partial to male attendants. The plan to establish a school independent of the hospital, however, was unacceptable to him.[61]

By 1890, American nursing boasted 35 independent training schools but had fewer than 500 graduate nurses practicing their profession. During the final decade of the century, however, an extraordinary expansion took place: by 1900 there were 432 schools.[62] The principal justification for a training school was that it provided hospitals with competent caregivers, although it also trained others who worked in private homes or, as visitors, carried out preventive work. A consensus had emerged that this work could best be carried out by women of "superior attainments" on the basis on their physical fitness, moral strength, and social skills, including "sound sense, loving kindness, patience and tact."[63]

In April 1889, Isabel A. Hampton was appointed superintendent of nurses and head of the Hopkins Training School, considered by Gilman a subdivision of the hospital with equal standing to other departments. Canadian by birth like Osler, Hampton had graduated from Bellevue Hospital's Training School in New York before going to Chicago's Cook County Hospital. Tall, dignified, charming, and maternal, she was described as having a strong physique and "caryatid-like figure."[64] After her experience at Bellevue, where nursing students were exploited and received fewer educational opportunities than medical students, Hampton was determined to raise educational standards and thus eradicate the stereotype of nurses as untrained domestics.[65]

Since Hampton planned to assume her post in early October, an English nurse, Louisa Parsons, trained in Nightingale's school in London, was temporarily put in charge. To ensure proper care, a number of trained nurses known to Osler from the Philadelphia General Hospital were hired during the summer. Each ward had one trained nurse on duty from 7.30 AM to 7.30 PM, replaced by another who worked the night shift. Male patient wards, such as Ward A, where John S. was hospitalized, had an additional male orderly to assist with routine chores. Hurd, the hospital's superintendent, supported the notion that the new nurses needed to be better educated and trained, but he viewed their primary role more in traditional terms as a nurturing one, stressing the qualities of sympathy, feeling, enthusiasm, and personal interest. Osler was similarly inclined but had an additional educational mission. He seemed to recognize that, together with physicians, nurses could be partners in lessening human suffering while disseminating knowledge about health and disease. However, he condemned the nurses' penchant for getting married and quitting nursing—"bartering away [their] heritage for a hoop of gold"—and often expressed concerns about the nurses' "thin veneer of knowledge."[66]

Both the training school and the nurses' residence were officially opened on October 9, 1889.[67] Selected from a large pool of eager applicants, 19 students initially entered the school. The candidates were 23–25 years old and had to have at least completed their elementary education. Hampton's own vision of nursing also encompassed the traditional notion of woman's work, together with its nurturing function. Domesticity was institutionalized as student nurses were drawn into cooking classes linked to new dietary insights. At the same time, Hampton and others sought to stress the idea that nursing, far from being socially demeaning or emotionally hardening, created a new and exciting arena for the personal development of middle-class women. Opportunities to gain knowledge of modern medicine, hygiene, and dietetics were liberating, allowing young women to leave their homes and domestic tasks behind. As in Victorian Edinburgh, nursing was to be no longer just hard physical labor, largely devoted to housekeeping chores. For Hampton and other nursing leaders, like Lavinia Dock, who became assistant superintendent in November 1890, the new caregiving functions required "headwork," additional knowledge, and judgment.[68]

At the Hopkins school, student nurses learned the necessary skills—subject to a probationary period—within a strict hierarchical system that employed military metaphors to explain its goals. The new educational standards established by Hampton prescribed a two-year program of training that included laboratory courses, as well as special programs for dietetics and psychiatry. Two classes per week during the first year and one in the second year were mandatory. Hampton and members of the medical staff were the instructors. In 1891, the superintendent established a journal club to discuss contemporary issues, present new publications, and "promote a feeling of esprit de corps."[69] Yet, in spite of such efforts, the bulk of the students' time was spent rotating through the wards. Wearing pale blue uniforms with white aprons and caps, they were expected to work 12 hours daily from 7 AM to 7 PM, including Sundays. Half a day, usually one afternoon per week, the students were off duty and could relax in the adjacent attractive nurses' home, equipped with its own library.[70]

The early years of the Hopkins hospital experience were unique. Members of the medical and nursing staffs were drawn into an intimate, stimulating atmosphere created by significant bonding between idealistic, ambitious young middle-class professionals, many of whom lived on the premises. The dining room quickly became the meeting point as well as the informal launching pad for new ideas, initiatives, and personal friendships. During those close encounters, a camaraderie flourished that would henceforth transcend institutional confines. The atmosphere was relaxed and often festive, with the hierarchical distinctions temporarily suspended, as chiefs of service such as Osler mingled freely with the house staff and played pranks on unsuspecting victims. His boyish, fun-loving nature must have contributed to the atmosphere.[71] Student nurses received special attention. In the eyes of their male house staff members, their thinly veiled eroticism apparently was a frequent topic of conversation. Osler spoke of "the many love affairs of the early years."[72] He also told Gilman that Hampton selected probationers for their good looks, and therefore "the house staff is in a sad state."[73] Addressing the nursing class of 1897, Osler openly suggested that they "abstain from philandering during [their] period of training."[74]

Life in the hospital: The healing power of water

Described as stout and plethoric by the admitting house officer—probably Dr. Henry A. Lafleur—John indeed looked quite sick following his admission to the upper floor of Ward A on April 26, 1891. An initial physical examination disclosed a low-tension, dicrotic pulse of 120, respiration of 30–40 beats per minute, and a temperature of 103.2°F. The patient's tongue appeared slightly furred and his throat and tonsils congested, without an exudate, but his lungs were clear. There was no resonance over the sternum. John was initially rational, but toward evening he became delirious. His rectal temperature rose to 104.5°F, and the skin of his swollen abdomen was covered with the copious rose-red rash typical of typhoid fever. In spite of a thick panniculus, Lafleur distinctly felt the edge of John's spleen, but there was no tenderness. On percussion the liver was normal, and on auscultation the heart sounds were clear. Laboratory tests of blood and urine were quickly performed. An initial urinalysis revealed a specific gravity of 1026, and the sediment contained traces of albumin but no casts.[75] The Ehrlich's reaction was not present, and there was no record of a positive bacteriological culture.[76] A sputum sample disclosed some blood-stained mucus. The patient was probably placed on a liquid milk diet—up to three or four pints daily—or clear chicken or beef broth, even vegetable juices. The idea was promptly to provide proper, easily digestible foodstuffs with minimum residue.[77] Water or barley gruel were given freely on demand.

John was undoubtedly visited within the next few days by William Osler. After returning from his "quinquenial brain dusting"[78] in Europe, the physician-in-chief had now reduced his hospital visits to two days a week, preoccupied as he was with the writing of his textbook. However, Osler kept a very active daily schedule that included teaching rounds at 8 AM. Punctual and methodical, he would appear in the passage outside the ward, often humming a tune, to be formally welcomed by the nursing staff. "Spare in flesh, with a dark olive complexion and a slender figure,"[79] the chief was known as a "lark"—an early riser—and, with what was described as "a blend of easy informality, native poise and dignity," he strutted into the ward.[80] With the resident staff and visitors gathered around him, Osler made rounds by going from bed to bed. His routine was to position himself at the head of each bed, with the stethoscope hooked in the armhole of his vest, head cocked somewhat to one side, glancing down and attempting to ease the tension with a friendly word or joke.[81] Perhaps he also sniffed for the peculiar musty smell, characteristic of a freshly killed mouse, by which typhoid fever patients could be identified.[82] Through his blurry eyes, John may have vaguely distinguished the chief's "broad forehead, sallow complexion, good eyes and lively expression," together with a "rather long mustache, the position of the ends of which seemed to vary with his mood." "His clothes," a young pathologist remembered, "were always simple and worn well, and he fancied cravats of rather striking color."[83]

Osler was well known for what his first chief resident characterized as courtesy and the ability to mediate between apprehensive new arrivals and the caregiving staff.[84] His successor spoke of Osler's extraordinary "capacity of making you feel that he was interested in you and your personal welfare"[85] while at the same time priding himself on being detached and placing his emotions "on ice."[86] Osler was said to have possessed a fabulous memory, and he apparently retained even the smallest clinical details about those under his care.[87] When he later reported John's illness, Osler hinted at some discrepancies in the patient's story, but he eventually came to accept the fact that this was an unusually severe relapse of typhoid fever, interesting enough to be reported and published.[88] Perhaps John had gotten up too soon. Illnesses were considered relapses only if the patient had completely recovered from all previous symptoms and had been well for at least five days before the return of fever, an enlarged spleen, and eventually a new abdominal rash. Otherwise, practitioners considered the return of fever a very transitory phenomenon common during convalescence. To some extent, the differential diagnosis was not critical since most relapses were shorter, less severe, and less deadly than the original disease. With luck, the bartender's second illness would be brief and relatively uneventful, although Osler was to warn readers of his forthcoming textbook that "fat subjects stand typhoid fever badly."[89]

According to Osler, mortality in typhoid fever was often determined by the time the patient came to the attention of physicians. As he observed later, general hospitals became repositories of the more severe and complicated cases, contributing to a higher institutional mortality rate.[90] Osler's therapeutic strategy can be summarized by his statement that "the earlier he [the patient] takes to bed and is surrounded by all those accessories of nursing which have come to mean so much in fever cases, the better the chance in the prolonged fight of the *vis medicatrix naturae* against progressive toxemia."[91] Patients such as John were to remain in a recumbent position and avoid all physical or emotional exertion. After admission, John S. spent his first two days with continuous fever, fluctuating between 103° and 105°F. Readings were obtained every two hours and were carefully charted on a graph.[92]

To manage such typhoid fever patients, Osler insisted that "an intelligent nurse should be in charge."[93] Patients had to be kept clean to avoid the danger of bed sores and transmission of disease to auxiliary personnel. Rigid methods of disinfection were absolutely essential. Mattresses and pillows were protected through the use of rubber sheets and covers, and were changed daily together with bed clothing and blankets. These articles, including towels, were wrapped in carbolic acid-soaked sheets. Placed in containers, the sheets were shipped each day to the laundry for further soaking and rinsing in cold water. Linens, in turn, were boiled and washed with soap. Moreover, nurses collected and removed all feeding utensils and cups for cleaning in boiling water. Stools were collected in bedpans already filled with half a pint of carbolic acid, to be thoroughly rinsed and wiped dry before further use to avoid nasty chemical burns on the patients' buttocks.[94]

Osler's approach to therapeutics was that of a skeptic, although some of his opponents periodically tried to tarnish his reputation with the pejorative label of "therapeutic nihilist."[95] Caution at the bedside was imperative at a time when the pharmacological properties of most drugs had not yet been experimentally ascertained.[96] Variations in symptoms were still considered, in part, expressions of individual constitutions—according to Osler, the "personal equation."[97] Unfortunately, the amount of a typhoid poison already in the body could not be estimated, and its actions depended entirely on the virulence of the causative agent. Fortunately, most typhoid fever patients experienced spontaneous recovery, and the duration of the disease was believed to depend on the gradual production of substances that inhibited bacterial growth. The key was to intervene early and support the patient's natural healing forces, hoping that the individual constitution and immunological reaction would overcome the problem.

Contemporary practitioners seemed divided about whether there was a particular treatment for typhoid fever, and thus Osler's purported "armed expectancy" appeared justified.[98] Despite efforts to institute a specific therapy aimed at destroying the typhoid bacilli in the intestine through the administration of antiseptics, this approach remained controversial. In addition to the traditional measures used to support and strengthen the patient, prominent academicians such as I. Burney Yeo in England argued for an antiseptic treatment of typhoid fever. The gravity of the disease could be reduced through measures designed to neutralize and destroy the responsible microbe—"a living, propagating poison"—with the aid of local antiseptics ranging from chlorine water, eucalyptus and turpentine oil, calomel, carbolic acid, and iodoform to the newer remedy: naphtol mixed with bismuth salicylate. In the spirit of the classical poison model, these products were called specific "antidotes."[99]

Osler's statement that "with the diminished reliance upon drugs, there has been a return with profit to the older measures of diet, exercise, baths, and frictions, the remedies with which the Bithynian Asclepiades doctored the Romans so successfully in the first century"[100] was in harmony with contemporary views of typhoid fever management. Instead of intestinal antisepsis, this physician-in-chief had been impressed by the systematic method of cold baths developed by the German physician Ernst Brand in Stettin almost 30 years earlier. Cold water in the treatment of fevers had classical roots and was still in use in the 19th century. Brand's 1887 statistics, obtained from treating military personnel, persuaded Osler to adopt this treatment.[101] However, when the Johns Hopkins Hospital opened in 1889, organizational difficulties and a shortage of nurses forced him to follow a purely expectant plan of treatment. Finally, during Osler's visit to Europe, his assistant, Lafleur, started the cold-water treatment in mid-1890 after visiting the wards of Dr. J. C. Wilson at the German Hospital in Philadelphia.

Lafleur initiated the bathing routine with John S. on April 28. Cold baths were to be administered to typhoid fever patients each time their rectal temperature went above 102.5°F. The procedure consisted of wheeling a light tub made of thick papier-mâché material and filled with water at a temperature of 68°–70°F to the bedside, although others suggested a somewhat lower temperature of 65°F. Shielded by a screen for privacy, John was stripped of his heavier bedclothes and nightshirt, with a light sheet thrown over his body. Then he was given a small drink of whiskey before two orderlies lifted him into the bath, still covered with the sheet. In most cases, the tub was deep enough to cover the patient's entire body up to the neck. An icy cloth was placed on his head, or the attendants used a small sponge to moisten both the face and head. While in the tub for 20 minutes, John was subjected to systematic friction over his entire body, except for the abdomen, with a cloth or rubber massager. At the end, he was lifted out of the tub and placed on his bed, previously prepared for his reception with a rubber sheet and blanket. If his fever was still very high, the attendants delayed drying the patient and simply covered him with another sheet for five minutes. At the end of this ordeal, another temperature measurement was taken, with the patient receiving two ounces of milk with another shot of whiskey. In most instances, typhoid patients experienced a temporary drop in body temperature below prebath measurements. If at the end of three hours it rose again over 102.5°F, another bath was indicated.[102]

Osler's cold baths were expensive and labor-intensive. They required abundant fresh water, some ice, and considerable auxiliary personnel, although the water was renewed only every 24 hours.[103] Most men's wards at the Johns Hopkins Hospital had an average staff of seven nurses and assistants and two male orderlies. Working in shifts, they carried out bathing around the clock. Under supervision of the ward nurses, male attendants often struggled to lift tall, heavy patients such as John into and out of the tubs, the procedure marred by occasional accidents in which the patients' arms were scratched on the sides of the tub. More important, delirious patients were not always docile and cooperative when they were summarily plunged into what they perceived to be very cold water. Moreover, intense shivering was frequent when patients were placed in and taken out of the tub, and the attendants found that they had to quickly place hot water bottles near the feet and sides of the body as the patient was wrapped again in a blanket. Often, blue-faced patients loudly cursed their caregivers. Even Osler admitted that this shivering was "one of the most unpleasant features of the system," with nearly all patients complaining bitterly about the treatment.[104] Some patients also objected to the forceful friction administered while their bodies were submerged in the bath, fearing to catch a cold. As one editorial in a medical journal suggested hopefully, "American ingenuity may devise some less disturbing, cumbrous and barbarous mode of application than frequent 'tubbing'."[105]

The therapeutic rationale for these baths was, in part, to reduce the patient's fever, especially through heat dissipation by the cold water. Occasionally, patients were even sponged with ice water. However, proponents claimed that its primary aim, enhanced by bodily rubbings, was to act as a tonic to stimulate the circulatory and nervous systems. In that sense, the tonic effects of a cold bath were much more important than any modest decreases in bodily temperature. In fact, practitioners such as Osler and Lafleur believed that, if applied early in the course of the illness, these baths, by rallying the body's healing forces, would have a beneficial effect on the nervous system, diminishing delirium, favoring sleep, and promoting mental clarity. This method was also supposed to stimulate appetite, digestion, and general well-being. The primary contraindication to the baths mentioned by Osler was intestinal hemorrhage, for which absolute rest was deemed essential. In protracted cases, if the patient was too debilitated, these baths were omitted.[106]

By contrast, other physicians preferred to employ antipyretic drugs, eventually those of the coal-tar variety.[107] With the advent of systematic thermometry at the bedside, a link had been forged between high fever and mortality.[108] Higher temperatures seemed to exhaust and waste the patient's already flagging strength and energy. Initially very popular because of their thermic effects, antipyretics were soon noted to have a variety of serious side effects, including decreased urinary output, depressed breathing, cardiac irregularities, and the all too visible blue staining of the skin with aniline. Suppressing fever, whether with cold-water baths or antipyretic drugs, remained a priority of the therapeutic regimen, although some authors like Welch speculated that fever was nature's attempt to destroy disease-carrying substances and organisms.[109]

In spite of frequent baths over the next four days, John's temperature remained very high and his delirium persisted. In the meantime, new crops of abdominal spots erupted everywhere. Lafleur was very disappointed with his early results, stating that this was the first real failure he had experienced with the cold-water treatment. Like other patients, John was to receive a plethora of drinks like lemonade or orange juice. Although the progress notes remain silent on this issue, Osler's occasional rounds and his "remarkable gift of empathy," as well as personal visits by a clergyman, may have helped to lift John's spirits as he shivered and was bathed around the clock.[110] Visiting hours remained limited.[111] Like another contemporary patient, John perhaps took an interest in the zigzags of his temperature chart, which "looks like a coast-survey and was just mysterious enough to be amusing."[112]

Patients did not routinely receive medication except alcohol before and after the baths. But by May 3, the attending physicians noted that John had developed a fast, irregular pulse, 120–140 beats per minute. In this situation Osler was fond of giving strychnine or ether, but we have no record of such prescriptions. The next day, however, John was reported to be conscious, with good facial color but a slight tremor in his hands. His tongue was dry and respirations were more frequent—48 beats per minute—and labored. The abdominal rash persisted and the patient now also experienced diarrhea. Perhaps he was subjected to a course of bismuth salicylate powder or simply given an opium enema "to splint the bowel." On examination, John had wheezing sounds over the lungs in front and slight dullness at both bases, with feeble breathing and numerous fine rales. A blood analysis, however, revealed no leucocytosis; the white blood cell count was around 5,000 to 6,000, with slight anemia and lowered hemoglobin. At this point, Osler and Lafleur decided to continue the systematic bathing and sponging. It seemed especially important to rouse patients from their stupor. This system of stimulation and bathing, Osler maintained, was an intelligent approach toward ameliorating some of the cardinal symptoms of typhoid fever and thus decrease its mortality.

Three days later, overt clinical symptoms of pneumonia appeared, and another examination on May 7 disclosed dullness at the bases of John's lungs together with numerous fine rales. These new manifestations of disease, however, failed to derail the cold-water bathing. Osler insisted that "neither pneumonia nor bronchitis is regarded as a special contraindication, and pleurisy only if the pain is severe."[113] Then, a day later, the attendants detected blood in John's stool, presumably from hemorrhages in the small bowel. The abdominal rash was still plentiful. Moreover, nurses charting John's high temperature failed to detect any decrease, and his breathing remained labored. John had clearly taken a turn for the worse. His heart sounds were feeble and displayed a fetal rhythm. He was now also incontinent.

How much Osler remained involved with the case is unknown. He had just moved back into the hospital to concentrate on his writing project. On rounds, Osler rarely displayed his emotions about a clinical outcome, his face a mask concealing all anxieties and doubts.[114] In spite of unfavorable clinical developments, he always tried to be reassuring and cheerful, moving rapidly from one patient to another. Although not explicitly noted in the clinical chart, it is probable that Osler and Lafleur decided on May 8 to suspend the cold-water baths because of the patient's progressive weakness. Whether John was aware of his deteriorating condition remains unclear. We have no observations about his mental state or behavior. Like all patients, he must have hoped for a cure and thus went along with the treatments. The record shows that John S. received 67 cold-water baths in the course of 10 days of hospitalization, suggesting that the bartender had been bathed about every three hours around the clock, as originally prescribed.[115]

The next few days of John's hospitalization became critical. Did Osler remain optimistic in spite of the apparent failure of the baths? Perhaps intensive nursing, not medical interventions, could still turn the tide. Osler believed that good nursing saved lives and that the mortality from this disease in general hospitals was dependent on the number of persons attending the sick. John's slight intestinal hemorrhaging continued, but everybody watched for signs of massive bleeding and possible bowel perforation. The patient's pulse, meanwhile, remained extremely feeble and rapid, around 140–160 beats per minute. Did he receive hypodermic injections of ether or strychnine?[116] In spite of the cold sponging, his temperature at one point reached 107°F.

By May 14, John's rash was fading but the abdomen appeared considerably distended, with bowel tympany extending about 2 cm above the costal margin. Here some practitioners suggested the traditional employment of turpentine oil in an effort to heal the intestinal ulcers, but Osler was adamantly opposed to what he considered a dangerous empirical practice.[117] The patient's pulse was 144 and his respiration 44, with a temperature above 104°F in the majority of readings. No blood pressure readings were recorded, but the coldness of his hands and feet suggested progressive circulatory failure. We should also assume that John remained fairly quiet, since no notes were written about violent behavior or attempts to get out of bed.

Even to the most optimistic practitioner, the patient appeared to be gradually sinking. John had already been hospitalized for 18 days. His strong body appeared exhausted, its strength sapped by a slowly progressive toxemia. His heart sounds were weaker. Delirious, at times comatose, experiencing generalized tremors, John entered his "coma vigil," characterized by moving his head from side to side, with open eyes, twitching fingers, and attempts to pick at his bedclothes. These manifestations resembled an alcoholic's typical delirium tremens.

The next day, May 15, John S. died of progressive asthenia[118] after a 20-day stay, somewhat shorter than the four-week average for typhoid sufferers. His nearest of kin was notified. As Osler later remarked elsewhere, year by year, physicians seemed to be the "unwilling witnesses of an appalling sacrifice," sitting helplessly at the bedsides of thousands of chiefly young people "whose lives are offered up on the altars of Ignorance and Neglect."[119] According to Osler's favorite metaphor, John S. was another human sacrifice—in the "early years of vigor"—devoured by the Minotaur of infectious diseases, the dreaded typhoid fever.

Science and religion: Partners in healing

An autopsy was performed the next day by Welch's assistant, Councilman, probably with Osler and physicians enrolled in his course in attendance. John's body was described as large, strongly built, and well nourished, with numerous bluish marks possibly caused by hypodermic injections, either ether or morphine. Alternatively, they could have been injuries suffered during the frequent lifting required for the cold baths. The abdomen was tympanitic. Following an incision, the peritoneum was discovered to be smooth, with no signs of inflammation. The small intestine presented many points of extreme congestion, with the characteristic lesions—inflamed, swollen Peyer's patches—located in the jejunum, but no bowel perforation was found. The spleen adhered to the diaphragm and appeared much enlarged and semifluid, with all the mesenteric glands and the liver soft and swollen. Scattered areas of bronchopneumonia and a few old caseous and tuberculous nodules were found in the lungs. Finally, the heart muscle was pale, soft, and flabby, with extensive fatty degeneration. Councilman's anatomical diagnosis was typhoid fever with its characteristic ulcers, some of them older and thus suggestive of a relapse. In addition, John had suffered from catarrhal pneumonia and old tuberculosis of the lungs.[120] At a clinical lecture delivered on November 9, 1892, Osler praised his traditional cold-water baths as a treatment for typhoid fever, indicating that most hospital statistics revealed a significant decrease in mortality with this method, from 15–25% to 6–7%, adding that "our own more limited experience is also strikingly in favor of the method."[121] Indeed, those patients not treated with cold water before Lafleur's introduction of the baths had experienced a 25% mortality. Lafleur and Osler's first 100 patients receiving cold-water treatments had only a 7% death rate, an impressive statistic perhaps more reflective of Hopkins' empathetic nursing than of its medical care.

Osler, for his part, considered the Johns Hopkins Hospital a traditional shelter, or "place of refuge for the sick poor of the city," where caregivers dispensed hospitality without making moral judgments. He professed to be aware of the "positive assurance" patients could obtain in the hospital and its powerful contribution to recovery. Osler recalled that "without any special skill in these cases, or special methods, our results at the Johns Hopkins Hospital were most gratifying. Faith in 'St. Johns Hopkins', as we used to call him, an atmosphere of optimism, and cheerful nurses, worked just the same sort of cures as did Aesculapius at Epidaurus; and I really believe that had we had in hand that arch-neurasthenic of ancient history, Aelius Aristides, we could have made a more rapid cure than did Apollo and his son, who took seventeen years on the job."[122] Yet the "ceaseless panorama of suffering tends to dull the fine edge of sympathy with which we started," a fact of life limiting the usefulness of the caregivers and making the hospital less than a "fervent charity."[123]

But if Osler had reached back to pre-Christian and Christian models to characterize his hospital, he also shared the Enlightenment ideals of creating a medicalized facility that could foster clinical teaching and research.[124] The goal was to make the hospital "a place where new thought is materialized in research, a school where men are encouraged to base the art upon the science of medicine."[125] The Oslerian concept of the hospital as a clinical laboratory for the systematic observation and understanding of disease went back to late eighteenth-century European models in Edinburgh and Vienna. It further embraced the pathological documentation carried out at Parisian institutions, sites for establishing clinicopathological correlations. Moreover, Osler's notion of the hospital as an experimental therapeutic place highlighted a trend already quite visible in the development of modern surgery, as witnessed at the Massachusetts General Hospital and the Edinburgh Infirmary decades earlier. Now, however, the role of the hospital in testing the new tenets of human physiology and pathology, as well as the emergence of modern bacteriology, had expanded further.[126] Inevitably, Osler expected new tensions between the hospital's assistential and scientific roles, but he believed that hospitals such as Johns Hopkins could function as a modern Cos. If Hippocrates returned and met a class of modern students, Osler thought, he "would dwell upon this latter development of the science and of the art [of medicine] as the crowning benefit which the profession has bestowed upon the race, and he would repeat again those noble words which have found in this triumph their practical realization: to serve the art of medicine as it should be served, one must love his fellow man."[127]

Gilman, with his keen sense of public relations, was eager to enhance the institution's local and national reputation based on the excellence of its clinical teaching and research. However, Gilman also still respected the hospital's traditional role as a house of mercy for the feeble, the sick, the injured, and the dying. In October 1896, he officiated at the unveiling of a majestic statue of Christ the Consolator in the rotunda of the hospital's administration building. With His extended arms, the Divine Healer would henceforth comfort and inspire those being admitted to the institution.[128] In Gilman's view, Johns Hopkins Hospital was a modern Hôtel Dieu or House of God. For him, "the rule of sympathy for the suffering must govern everybody with a strictness of discipline as rigid as the rule of the Benedictines or the Carthusians. Those who walk these cloisters will be the wardens of life and health."[129] In fact, he reached back further in history, explaining that "there is an altar in one of the churches of Messina which bears an inscription to Aesculapius and Hygeia, the god of medicine and the goddess of health, and their statues are found together on the facade of Guy's Hospital. May they always be associated in Baltimore."[130] Science and religion remained partners in healing.

CHOLERA AND EPPENDORF GENERAL HOSPITAL, HAMBURG, 1892

I thought yesterday my time had come. I had a headache, nausea and feverishness. I was reeking of cholera. . . . Herr Doctor Herald is the name by which I have become known here. The place is quite a little world. Probably two thousand persons are in it but everybody knows everybody else. In the face of danger all are equal.[131]

Aubrey Stanhope (1892)

A frightful collapse

Stanhope's dispatch of September 25, 1892—he was the Paris correspondent for the *New York Herald*, who had deliberately exposed himself to cholera at the Eppendorf General Hospital in Hamburg—followed a 15–hour stay at the institution. Assigned to one of the makeshift wards, the reporter worked as an orderly, taking temperature readings, transporting the sick and dead, and resting on a cot recently vacated by another victim of the epidemic. The stunt, arranged with the approval of the famous French scientist Louis Pasteur (1822–1895), followed Stanhope's inoculation with a cholera preservative developed by the Russian bacteriologist Waldemar Haffkine (1860–1930) at the Pasteur Institute in Paris. An announcement in the newspaper was greeted by an avalanche of congratulatory cards and telegrams, and New Yorkers anxiously awaited the fate of its eager human guinea pig.

About three weeks earlier, Erika W.,[132] a resident of Hamburg, suddenly fell ill early on the morning of September 4, 1892, suffering from severe diarrhea. Although her exact address was not recorded, the 31-year-old woman could have come from the squalid tenements near the Steinstrasse, "gloomy haunts of disease," with decrepit houses lining narrow streets.[133] Here cholera had found some of its first victims in mid-August, especially among middle-aged and older adults weakened by malnutrition and disease. Later, when questioned by hospital physicians, Erika assured them that she had only consumed boiled water, since there had already been deaths from cholera in her house. Before the evening was over, she vomited twice and experienced muscle cramps. Her stomach and back were also hurting. Nothing else is known about Erika except that she brought along a child, about whom she inquired while hospitalized.[134]

Erika's case was typical. Most cholera victims had an explosive onset of symptoms, perhaps due to the virulence of the disease combined with preexisting debility, fatigue, and possibly poor nutrition. As the number of cases soared in Hamburg, popular fears about contagion became widespread, fueled in part by sensational press reports. Many upper- and middle-class citizens left town with their domestic retinues. Everywhere, vegetables and fruits were suspected of harboring germs, cheese and butter were prohibited, and fish was simply not served. In a replay of medieval responses, charity and altruism crumbled, replaced by denunciations and forceful removal of perceived victims of disease. Wrote a domestic servant, Doris Viersbeck: "The fear that a loved one could be affected by this terrible plague and also the worry that one might oneself fall ill and then be pitilessly carried off under suspicion of having cholera to lie in bed among the victims put one into a feverish state of anxiety."[135] Opponents of bacteriology suggested that such fears, fueled by the exaggerated role attributed to germs, were powerful contributors to the infection.[136]

Hamburg physicians extolled the virtues of immediate medical attention, even if the symptoms turned out not to be true cholera. Visits to the homes of suspected cholera patients and efforts to diagnose the disease were critical. In line with the new bacteriological tenets, it was imperative that those suffering from cholera be separated from the healthy and isolated in an institution, because they carried the responsible germs and were thus capable of contaminating water and food supplies with their stools and vomit. Early intervention provided some hope of success. Many of the first ambulatory patients had been seen by physicians of the *Krankenkassen* or sick funds established in 1883.[137] More important were the *Stadtphysici* (municipal physicians), responsible for the health of the population, who reported the presence of infectious disease in their districts and arranged transportation of the sick to hospitals. Prospective patients viewed these events with anxiety, even terror, fearing hospitals as death traps and vigorously resisting removal from their houses.[138]

At the Eppendorf General Hospital, Theodor M. Rumpf (1851–1934), formerly director of the polyclinic at the University of Marburg, had been in charge since April. Rumpf was aware of these popular feelings concerning hospitals, admitting that "there exists in Hamburg a certain antipathy towards the hospital because the doctors there are suspected of performing too many experiments on the patients."[139] Exchanging the small-town tempo of Marburg for metropolitan Hamburg's frenetic commercial activity seemed to overwhelm Rumpf. Lacking interpersonal and administrative skills, the new director soon realized that the supervision of three dissimilar and geographically separate institutions—the St. Georg and Eppendorf Hospitals and the Marine Hospital for seamen—was a *Gewaltleistung*, a veritable tour de force. A neurologist by training, Rumpf supported the tenets of the new bacteriology pioneered by Robert Koch in a city populated by medical men who opposed or were skeptical of the theory. After his arrival, Rumpf had been warned by the head of the Medical Board, the anticontagionist Casper T. Kraus (1826–1892), not to confuse Asiatic cholera with less significant diarrheal diseases and to avoid proclaiming an epidemic because of a few isolated cases.[140] Similar advice had been given to the municipal physicians.

A newcomer to Hamburg, Rumpf clearly lacked the professional authority and rapport with the city's health authorities enjoyed by Heinrich Curschmann (1846–1910), an internist from Berlin, who had planned and built the Eppendorf a decade earlier. To make matters worse, complaints about the excessive operating costs of the newer Eppendorf institution had already forced Rumpf to institute cost-cutting measures, although the establishment was rapidly becoming the home for individuals suffering from infectious disease such as smallpox, leprosy, and typhoid fever. In addition to his extensive administrative duties, the director was expected to lead one of the hospital's medical divisions and attend its patients.[141]

Before Erika's sickness, the Eppendorf had already considered the possibility of an epidemic. During the late spring and early summer of 1892, the hospital had been placed on a state of alert because of cholera's presence in Russia. Rumpf's assistant, Theodor Rumpel (1862–1923), now systematically cultured the stools of all individuals admitted with symptoms suggestive of the disease. Also from Marburg, Rumpel was familiar with Koch's bacteriological techniques, and, according to Rumpf, all cultures so far had been negative for the Asiatic cholera vibrio.

· Then, during the night of August 16, a seriously ill young mason working in the port was brought to the Eppendorf with cholera-like symptoms, dying there about 24 hours later. His autopsy findings and cultures, however, were equivocal. At the same time, a *Stadtphysikus*, Friedrich B. Erman (1845–1917), pathologist at Hamburg's prison and almshouse and an opponent of Robert Koch's ideas, initially conducted autopsies on persons suspected of having cholera without subjecting their intestinal contents to microscopic analysis.[142] Such fateful delays were caused partly by the official policy that only pure vibrio cultures grown in gel qualified for an official diagnosis of cholera. Physicians, both at the almshouse and at the hospital, struggled to master the proper bacteriological techniques, unfamiliar with them because of their age and lack of training. To complicate matters, the gelatin, left in laboratory rooms, tended to liquefy because of the summer heat wave affecting Hamburg.

Rumpf and his assistants, conscious of earlier warnings not to rush the diagnosis, hesitated for the next two days about whether to officially pronounce their findings compatible with Asiatic cholera.[143] Five individuals admitted to the St. Georg Hospital in the center of Hamburg and 10 more the following day quickly became the focus of further bacteriological studies. Summoned back from a vacation, Eppendorf's own pathologist, Eugen Fraenkel, examined a second patient on August 22, confirming the presence of the almost pure cholera vibrio in the stool. This observation prompted an anxious Rumpf to muster enough courage and immediately send a telegram to the Medical Board and Kraus, informing them of these findings.[144] Kraus, however, insisted on a pure culture, and the announcement of a bacteriologically confirmed presence of Asiatic cholera in Hamburg was thus delayed for another day until Fraenkel finally provided the required proof.[145]

At this point, the epidemic was already in full swing, with 55 individuals living near the Elbe River arriving at the St. Georg and Eppendorf hospitals. The decision to send all prospective victims to hospitals for isolation and treatment required additional beds, and members of both the medical and hospital boards decided on August 23 to activate a plan to erect temporary barracks at both the St. Georg and Marine hospitals located near the center of the outbreak. The number of cholera patients brought to Eppendorf increased dramatically in the following days, from 265 on August 25 to 432 on August 30. To provide sufficient processing time for the new arrivals, Rumpf instituted a rotating system of admissions between St. Georg and Eppendorf, whereby the sick were directed to one or the other establishment during a 12-hour period by the police. This decision created further mayhem, especially among drivers who kept shuttling between the institutions with their morbid human cargo. Since schools were still in summer recess, several were now outfitted as emergency lazarettos. Other makeshift facilities were assembled at St. Georg's vegetable garden, while the army sent a complete 500-bed field hospital together with its medical and nursing personnel to the Eppendorf.[146]

As people collapsed in homes, workplaces, or on the streets, their removal to institutions became a source of great anxiety to relatives and friends. In the first days of the epidemic, some of the sick often had to lie for up to 15 hours in police stations on cold floors. In one particular instance, a woman traveling in a crowded tramcar, perhaps with the intention of getting to a hospital, fell from her seat to the floor, seized with terrible cramps. As one witness recalled, a veritable stampede ensued, with passengers scrambling to escape the vehicle, leaving behind their bags, parcels, and umbrellas.[147] At the outbreak of the epidemic, Hamburg possessed only four horse-drawn ambulances and six drivers. This potential problem had been discussed during the construction of the Eppendorf Hospital in 1888, but no action had been taken. Regulations issued by the Hamburg Senate in 1890 further hindered the transportation of cholera victims by insisting on the transport of infectious patients by special ambulance, proscribing any movement in horse-drawn cars belonging to the public transportation lines that served the hospital from the city's center.

This lack of conveyances fostered the use of many private carts and carriages. Their drivers, recruited from among the crippled and vagrants who were so poor that they leaped at the chance to earn some money, were said to be moving around in an alcohol-induced stupor, since strong drink was popularly believed to be the best defense against cholera. Wearing rubber coats, these men carried corpses to the hospital's morgue, where they caroused with similarly inebriated employees while cleaning their vehicles and attire with sprays of carbolic acid solution.[148] In the rush and confusion of this haphazard transportation system, family members became separated, and relatives had a hard time locating those who had been hospitalized. As Karl Wagner, a Viennese journalist and volunteer ambulance driver, described: "The vehicles which were to be used were horse-drawn coaches from which the upholstery had been removed so that patients, whom we had to wrap in blankets, were carried on the bare wooden seat frames. Almost inconceivably, 5–7 large holes had been cut in the floor of the coach through which the patients' excretions flowed onto the street! To begin with I fetched a 14-year-old girl, an old woman, and a boy; the woman died on the way. . . . During my service I transported 132 patients of whom almost half died on the way." Wagner also mentioned that individuals collapsing in the streets with other ailments, such as strokes or heart problems, were also brought to hospitals together with the cholera patients."[149]

Initially, most patients were taken to St. Georg because it was closer to the city center and the locus of the outbreak. Under the best of circumstances, the ride to Eppendorf over rough pavement could last for up to three hours. As one witness recalled, one carriage after another stopped in front of the main building, usually with two or three people inside, some already dead, others clearly moribund, and a few who seemed healthy but had been forced by the authorities to join the macabre journey. By the end of August, the Eppendorf had already been forced to admit 1,576 new patients in one week, a number that exceeded its entire capacity. As ambulances transporting individuals such as Erika made a beeline for the hospital, hearses and furniture vans rumbled through the streets of the city in the opposite direction to the city cemetery located at Ohlsdorf. Working in shifts around the clock, hundreds of gravediggers buried the victims in mass graves.

Given the circumstances, an appeal was made for volunteer caregivers. In addition, the hospital administration gratefully accepted offers from 300 nurses, including a few Catholic Sisters of Charity and local (Protestant) Deaconess Sisters, as well as others from Bielefeld, Kaiserswerth, and Duisburg. Their welcome arrival quelled some of the panic and restored a semblance of order to hospital routines. An urgent appeal from the Hamburg Senate also brought a number of volunteer physicians and especially adventurous medical students to the Eppendorf—primarily from Berlin and Halle, since the hospital was not affiliated with a medical school.[150] They soon began working side by side with the official hospital staff. Prominent academics such as Ferdinand Hueppe (1852–1932) of Prague and Edwin K. Klebs (1834–1913) of Karlsruhe offered their services, with the intention of subjecting hospital patients to experimental methods of treatment. At first, Rumpf gratefully accepted these offers, but soon the Eppendorf became an arena for clashes between competing personalities and therapies.[151]

Eppendorf General Hospital: Model for the world?

The planning and construction of the Eppendorf had taken place under the threat of the 1883–1884 cholera epidemics affecting the Mediterranean region. Hamburg already possessed a large general hospital, the St. Georg, built in 1820 for about 1,300 patients, later expanded to nearly 1,600. Since Hamburg's urban growth had accelerated after its incorporation into the German Reich in 1871, more beds were needed. In the late 1870s, patients admitted to the austere St. Georg barracks were housed in cellars. Matters became more urgent following the passage of the German sickness insurance law in 1884, which expanded the population eligible for hospital treatment. By 1890, the *Krankenkassen* in Hamburg had already enrolled 282,775 members and began paying half of their hospitalization costs, thus becoming a major player in Germany's medical marketplace. In fact, after November 1, 1890, Hamburg's 27,000 servants, 98% female, were enrolled in this plan.

The idea of building a new general hospital represented an important shift in Hamburg's health care delivery system. The planned facility was definitely not to be a traditional *Pflegeinstitution* or shelter primarily for the care of paupers, but a medical institution devoted exclusively to the isolation and treatment of acute and seriously ill individuals of all social classes. For the first time, medical and sanitary agendas gained the upper hand in shaping hospital management. This was already the case at St. Georg, where a new position of medical director responsible for such issues had been proposed in 1877. Two years later, Curschmann, formerly in charge of the new Moabit Hospital in Berlin, assumed this post. Curschmann made clear distinctions between *Behandlungskranken*—sick persons in need of medical treatment—and *Verpflegungskranken*—those simply in need of care.[152] Spurred by insurance schemes and the promise of new modes of treatment, especially aseptic surgery, hospital care was increasingly envisioned as a medicalized activity reserved for acute and severe cases. An important secondary goal—operative since the time of the Renaissance lazarettos—was for hospitals to become the isolation facilities for individuals suffering from contagious diseases, thus preventing the dissemination of their ailments.

Curschmann's proposal for such a medicalized institution was presented in 1882 and found favor with Hamburg's Mayor Carl F. Petersen, but the timing was poor. Hamburg was building its free port facilities, and the city was short of funds to engage in another major project. Unlike British voluntary institutions, German hospitals were strictly a municipal responsibility, thus shielding the authorities from the vagaries of private financing.[153] Moreover, the city's welfare bureaucracy opposed the idea that the St. Georg Hospital was to be demoted to a *Verpflegungs* facility for patients with chronic and venereal diseases. For Curschmann, however, the deliberate separation between these two institutions was necessary to transcend the stigma attached to the older, fever-producing hospitals, shunned even by paupers.

In sharp contrast, an establishment capable of attracting individuals from all social classes had to be conceived as a *Heilstätte*—a place of healing—in every sense. The hospital complex was to consist of separate pavilions surrounded by gardens instead of the massive, forbidding buildings of yesteryear. The new design was intended to minimize the chances for institutional contagion and create a restful environment where patients could temporarily escape their social predicaments, including the miserable living conditions in Hamburg's notorious damp cellars. In an effort at social engineering rooted in Enlightenment values, Curschmann wanted patients to have the healing experience of a "garden house," strongly believing that pure air, light, and pleasant surroundings would have a favorable influence on mind and body. This was to be just as important as antisepsis and medical therapies. The emphasis on *Versorgung*—provision of care—involved plenty of rest, good food, and nursing. To this end, Curschmann strongly advocated the concept of a full-time medical director with enough power to make all necessary administrative decisions concerning the appointment of caregivers, as well as the admission and discharge of patients. Inmates were to be segregated according to their diseases. In large institutions, the medical directorship needed to be a full-time post without additional clinical responsibilities.[154] With regard to finances and supplies, a team comprising a general administrator, economist, accountant, medical writer, and an overseer of supply depots was to play an auxiliary role. According to Curschmann, such broad decision making was absolutely essential to ensure implementation of the new hygienic and medical goals. Without such leadership, he insisted, the institution would fail to attract patients from all social classes and to serve as an effective isolation facility in the event of an epidemic.

Planning of the new hospital occurred at the dawn of bacteriology and was therefore based on the miasmatic premises still quite popular among Hamburg's physicians, sanitary leaders, and even Curschmann himself. Great care was exercised in the selection of a suitable site with sandy, porous soil, ample space, pure

air, abundant light, freedom from noise and pollution, and opportunities for natural ventilation. Curschmann argued for a location inside city limits since hospitals traditionally belonged near their potential patient populations. However, land
prices in Hamburg were too high. In February 1883, the municipal senate decided
to buy land at a truly bargain price near the town of Eppendorf, a northern suburb almost three miles from the Rathaus at the city center. The high, slightly un-
dulating plot contained 136 acres, with 45 chosen for the building complex. Aptly
for Hamburg, the site resembled a ship, its prow proudly facing the prevailing
northwest wind. This site precluded the organization of outpatient facilities—the
ubiquitous German polyclinics—which were forced to remain at the St. Georg.
Overruled about the location, Curschmann pleaded for the early development of
an adequate system of transportation to the new facilities. He characterized as
naive the official view that prospective patients—especially those suffering from
contagious diseases—would avail themselves of existing modes of public transportation to reach the institution.

The authorities gave Curschmann a free hand in shaping the physical plant
and organization of the new institution according to prevailing architectural, sanitary, and managerial principles. At the 1888 annual meeting of the German Public Health Association in Frankfurt, the future director was emphatic in his preference for the pavilion system. Hospitalism could be avoided through optimal
ventilation, a guiding principle in the creation of Britain's eighteenth-century infirmaries and Billings' new hospital in Baltimore. Listerism, asepsis, and bacteriology, however, remained outside the basic planning and execution. In fac ,
Curschmann rejected the notion of some early Listerian enthusiasts that space and
general hygiene were no longer critical. Nevertheless, he was widely praised for
masterfully combining some of the prevailing environmental notions with practical considerations of economy and efficiency.[155] Experts insisted that one-floor
pavilions were hygienic and cost effective because of their simple construction,
avoiding expensive cellars and ceilings between floors, which demanded a more
complex arrangement of pipes and electric wires.[156]

In the end, Curschmann's monumental plan for Hamburg encompassed 83
separate blocks or buildings. As models for Eppendorf, Curschmann looked at a
number of modern German hospitals but especially Berlin's Moabit, whose plan
had been based on the experiences of the American Civil War and the Franco-
Prussian conflict. The construction of the Eppendorf took place during Germany's
late-nineteenth-century hospital-building boom that culminated in the erection of
the colossal Robert Virchow Hospital in Berlin. Following the selection of an architect, Carl J. C. Zimmermann, the final planning for a new 1,300-bed facility
proceeded quickly. Instead of the traditional west-east orientation of European
hospital pavilions, the director advocated a north-south axis that better distributed light and sunshine. Each 30-bed ward was to be surrounded at both ends by
a small number of bathrooms, toilets, and private rooms.[157] The hospital project

started in December 1884 with construction of a ward for infectious disease victims. A kitchen, laundry, and power plant were to be located on the west side of the complex instead of the traditional placement at the center. The arrangement would prevent kitchen smoke and odors from seeping into the wards. The first completed building was occupied by sick children and tuberculosis patients from St. Georg the following April.[158]

Between 1885 and 1888, Curschmann regularly traveled to Eppendorf twice a week and attended to every minute construction detail, including the shape of door handles. Following his suggestions, the wards were to be roomier than those in average pavilions, allowing more space around each bed, and thus better opportunities for nurses to check patients and collect specimens. Private rooms located in each unit were to be reserved for the nurses on duty, who were no longer required to sleep in patients' beds.

Eppendorf's large hospital complex could only be reached through the principal entrance to the administration building located at the southern end. A large carriage hall allowed the entry of ambulance wagons. Next to the main entrance were the receiving and admissions departments, where all prospective patients were subjected to a careful triage. Inside the compound, a paved northwest-southeast road intersected with six parallel streets. The premises were equally divided into an eastern sector for males and a western sector for females and children. The individual pavilions were arranged in rows along the streets, with the first two assigned to surgical patients, the next two for medical cases, and the remainder devoted to contagious diseases. All arriving patients suspected of carrying infection were isolated for 24 hours in four small pavilions. Four two-story buildings near the main street were reserved for paying patients.

At the highest point in the southwest corner stood the service buildings, including offices, kitchen, ice house, power plant, laundry facilities, and disinfecting house with a steam sterilizer, a typical German creation.[159] Nurses lived in the northwest sector. A morgue, chapel, pathology department with dissection rooms, laboratories, and museum occupied the northeast corner. In the back was a special building for the detention of patients suffering from delirium tremens and mental disorders. Located along the main axis were operating rooms and bathing facilities. The operating pavilion had both septic and aseptic operating theaters, the latter naturally lighted by an octagonal bow window. Gas illuminated the entire complex, but individual wards and other patient facilities possessed electricity. All buildings were in telephone communication with the administration.

Lawns and flower beds covered the 20-foot spaces created between pavilions to allow the flow of air and direct sun exposure. Indeed no trees, only lower shrubs, were planted initially because it was felt that trees could obstruct the wind currents. During good weather, the lawns held folding chairs and tents for convalescents. All rectangular one-story pavilions were built of brick, glazed tiles, and stone dressings. Each had wood-supported concrete roofs, an innovation recently adopted by the architect Walter Gropius in Berlin. The interior arrangement featured four small rooms at the northwest entrance reserved for nurses and the temporary isolation of difficult patients. Then followed the 30-bed main ward, which opened onto a glass-enclosed day room or verandah. Terrazzo or mosaic floors received steam heat through a system of tubing. To prevent the dreaded hospitalism, furnishings and equipment, including the bedsteads, were made of iron, glass, and porcelain for easy cleaning. Walls were covered with ordinary lime plaster, and all rough and absorbent surfaces were avoided, including pictures and ornaments.[160]

The most obvious disadvantage of this new hospital plant was the difficulty of transporting patients between pavilions during rain, storms, and snow. This included patients requiring surgery in the operating building. At times, the now much-maligned corridors that had traditionally protected patients from the elements were sorely missed. Further inconveniences were encountered in conveying food and other supplies to each pavilion, especially coal shipments needed during winter to fuel the individual heating plants, whose chimneys kept spewing out large amounts of polluting smoke.[161]

Max Schede (1844–1902), already appointed in 1880 on Curschmann's recommendation, was to head the new division of surgery. A student of Richard von Volkmann at Halle, Schede was an early supporter of Listerian antisepsis who in 1872 had visited the Royal Infirmary in Edinburgh. His early selection reflected the growing importance of surgery in modern hospitals, in part linked to the higher occurrence of trauma in urbanized and industrialized areas of Europe. Given the realities of better anesthesia, greater technical proficiency, and asepsis, indications for elective surgery were rapidly expanding. Finally, Curschmann also recognized the importance of pathology at Eppendorf. He created a separate section, including a new bacteriology laboratory, placing it under the direction of Eugen Fraenkel, who had demonstrated the pathogenic properties of typhoid fever bacilli in experimental animals.[162]

Some of Eppendorf's medical pavilions opened in 1887 under the direction of Carl Eisenlohr, an internist and neurologist. Curschmann's assistant, Theodor Deneke (1860–1954), was put in charge of the children's ward. Both men continued to argue for a separate water filtration plant. Curschmann himself had been less than pleased with the hospital's water supply, directly linked to the Elbe and thus lacking filtration, especially since he had demonstrated years earlier that Hamburg's typhoid fever could be traced to this polluted source. However, after initial approval of the plan by the Citizens' Assembly in June 1888, a sand filtration scheme was ultimately rejected by Hamburg's senate because higher water tariffs and taxes unpalatable to property owners became attached to the legislation.

Just as the project neared completion, Curschmann—perhaps soured by city politics—accepted an academic offer from the University of Leipzig and left Hamburg in September 1888. Since the vacated post required considerable administrative skills, the search for a successor involved most of the Eppendorf physicians. The final selection was Alfred Kast (1856–1903), a pharmacologically trained internist, who stayed on until April 1892. Kast's administration became a critical time for Eppendorf. In 1888, 500 patients were being cared for at the new premises, but most facilities were far from completion. Kast's management style differed radically from Curschmann's. Instead of functioning as an authoritarian leader, the new director advocated cooperation and cultivated personal contacts, an attitude perceived as weakness by the powerful chiefs.

The Eppendorf facility officially opened on March 1, 1889, two months before the inauguration of Baltimore's Johns Hopkins Hospital. By this time, 1,100 of the planned 1,340 beds were already occupied, and activities were in full swing. During an open house for foreign dignitaries and leading physicians including Rudolf Virchow and Ernst von Bergmann later in the year, Curschmann returned to proudly assess his creation. In an article published in the British journal *The Hospital*, the secretary of the Royal Free Hospital, Conrad W. Thies, characterized the Eppendorf institution as "a model hospital" and described it as "the best example of elaborate arrangements for the restoration of health which yet exists."[163] The medical division alone comprised 127 wards with 791 beds—394 for males, 325 for females, and 72 for children. An independent cholera station— Erika's future destination—had been readied in six wooden barracks divided into 10 wards with a capacity for 126 beds. This station had its own administrative facilities, pharmacy, kitchen, and autopsy room located at the northwest corner of the complex. It was designed to function independently in the event of an epidemic. In turn, the surgical division had 81 wards and 441 beds, with 251 reserved for males, 154 for females, and 36 for children.

At Eppendorf, another inaugural ceremony was held on May 19, 1889, this one attended by city officials, including the mayor of Hamburg, Carl F. Petersen. In his speech Petersen remarked that "Hamburg is not a city of palaces, it does not have many proud monumental buildings, but the old Reichsstadt is pervaded by a spirit of simplicity and solidity which looks less on the exterior than on those things which promote the welfare of the state. Among those traits is the one about never being frugal concerning matters of public welfare. This principle is confirmed by the furnishing of this house. We hope that such a spirit of responsibility, duty, simplicity, and love of mankind will remain in our beloved city."[164]

Cholera and hospital caregivers

Erika W. was one of more than 100 individuals brought to the Eppendorf on September 4. On admission, the overworked physicians practiced a quick triage system, classifying arriving patients as having mild, moderate, or severe cases. Since the hospital had opened in 1889, the average length of stay had been 30–45 days or even longer, but a majority of newcomers during this epidemic survived for only a few days.[165] A particularly lethal variety—cholera sicca—led to death well before the appearance of gastrointestinal symptoms. Clinicians distinguished four different stages in the evolution of cholera. The first displayed the well-known symptoms of vomiting and diarrhea, with its typical rice-water stools. The next stage was one of vascular collapse with hypothermia—*stadium algidum*—characterized by a barely perceptible pulse, cyanosis, and lack of urinary output. If death did not occur, a third phase of gradual recovery followed. Less fortunate patients entered a terminal period of progressive typhoid-like symptoms that included fever, delirium, and coma.[166] Erika's initial diagnosis was *cholera gravis* or severe cholera, probably near the *stadium algidum*, with total cardiovascular collapse. Her condition was critical, the prognosis poor.

Based on animal experiments, the prominent bacteriologist Robert Koch (1843–1910) explained that this clinical picture was due not only to fluid loss but also to a release of toxins produced by the causal agent of cholera that especially affected the heart and brain. Koch insisted in 1883 that he had identified the responsible agent in the diarrheal discharges of victims of the disease while working in Cairo and later in Calcutta.[167] In a report dated February 2, 1884—more than six months before the Hamburg outbreak—Koch officially announced that the cholera vibrio was the true cause of this disease, a discovery pivotal for establishing the germ theory of disease.[168] Although the vibrio failed to fulfill one of his own criteria—it could not be transmitted to animals—Koch presented compelling epidemiological evidence of an association between the cholera microorganism and urban water supplies. Following his return to Europe, he presided over two cholera conferences in 1884 and 1885 designed to discuss his findings and deal with its key implications: individuals were contagious only if they harbored the vibrio in their stools.[169] In the event of a cholera outbreak, Koch's findings now suggested avoidance of contaminated water supplies, detention and quarantine of travelers from infected regions, prompt isolation of all persons showing signs of the disease, and heat disinfection of their contaminated clothing. Such measures and the research findings supporting them seemed consonant with the aims of Germany's central government.[170]

During the last quarter of the nineteenth century, Germany was universally acknowledged as the cradle of modern scientific medicine. Students throughout the world, but particularly from America, flocked to famous German universities and their laboratories, clinics, and hospitals to learn about the basic disciplines underlying medicine, the exacting methods of laboratory science, and their possible applications at the bedside. Lavish government expenditures supported costly research and care facilities that were the envy of the world. As William Osler had observed in 1884, "there may be disadvantages in the paternal form of government under which our German colleagues live, but these are not evident in a survey of their university and hospital arrangements."[171] Osler's remarks hinted at the distinctive character of German medicine, its academic elitism, and its special relationship with the state. In Wilhelmine Germany, this ideology of medical science increasingly underpinned status and professional authority. Scientific medicine assisted Germany's goals of political unification, economic development, and cultural superiority. A stream of fundamental discoveries in biochemistry, experimental physiology, and, more recently, bacteriology had placed Germany at the forefront of a new understanding of the human organism in health and disease. Strongly supported by state authorities, universities became engines of scientific progress. Research flourished with the infusion of vast sums of tax money to build institutes and laboratories. Growing numbers of medical graduates opted for academic pursuits in a rapidly expanding academic market.[172]

Koch's ideas concerning the epidemiology of cholera, based on bacteriological research, were vigorously opposed by Max von Pettenkoffer (1818–1901), a prominent chemist and hygienist at the University of Munich,[173] because they were contrary to his popular environmentalist *Bodentheorie* developed decades earlier after a cholera epidemic in Bavaria. Pettenkofer insisted that unique local environmental conditions—especially contaminated soil—played a central role in generating the specific miasma responsible for cholera. This motion buttressed the cause of anticontagionism shared by many Hamburg politicians. Those who adhered to Pettenkofer's views—such as Hamburg's chief sanitary officer, Kraus—believed that the preventive measures advocated by Koch—filtering the drinking water to eliminate cholera vibrios—would be useless in stopping an outbreak of the disease, because they failed to address local soil conditions and poison transmission through the air. For Hamburg's liberal, laissez-faire governing elite, Pettenkofer's theories also meant savings in basic sanitary infrastructure and avoidance of harmful trade embargoes.[174] Weather and the state of the groundwater were, in their minds, the only important environmental variables, and thus, general cleanup campaigns would be sufficient to stem further outbreaks of cholera.[175]

Tensions also persisted between the views of the pathologist Robert Virchow (1821–1902), doyen of German medicine, and Koch. Virchow's emphasis remained on the sociopolitical explanation of epidemics, including nutrition, income, and housing, and German physicians had adhered largely to this approach since the 1860s. Although he gradually came to accept the tenets of bacteriology in the genesis of infectious diseases, Virchow, like Pettenkofer, felt that emphasizing the causative role assigned in the 1880s to germs detracted from other important etiologic factors such as human predisposition, immunity, environment, and social conditions.[176] Koch, who was not particularly interested in the pathology of cholera, insisted that although the disease began with the local infection in the small intestine, the critical event was the production of a toxin that quickly spread through the bloodstream. This poison affected all vital organs, including the heart, lungs, kidneys, and brain. Such a proposed pathogenesis, buttressed by

Koch's scientific reputation, eventually came to dominate all subsequent preventive and therapeutic efforts by the end of the century.[177]

In late summer of 1892, Hamburg had an estimated population of 600,000. The epidemic's most striking feature was its sudden, almost explosive beginning, with a large number of cases appearing almost simultaneously in many widely scattered areas of the city. Just as important was the sharp limitation of the epidemic to Hamburg, sparing neighboring cities such as Altona and Waldek that filtered their water supplies. Moreover, a pattern of cases widely distributed throughout the city had exempted Wandsbeck and the military barracks at Gündel, which derived their water from independent wells.[178] The facts suggested contamination of the city's water supply directly from the Elbe River, also the destination point of the main sewer. In fact, the cholera developments were a replay of frequent typhoid fever outbreaks in the city during the 1880s.

Now, Hamburg's entire sanitary setup, together with the nature and location of the new cholera outbreak, drew the attention of the *Reichsgesundheitsamt* (Imperial Health Ministry) in Berlin which had jurisdiction over the planned public health measures. This provided Koch and his cadre of bacteriologists working for the agency with an excellent opportunity to confirm their etiological and epidemiological views and press for reforms based on the newest scientific knowledge regarding cholera.[179]

As the Reich's official representative, Koch wasted no time traveling to Hamburg with a number of assistants after being notified of the outbreak. Arriving on August 24, he first conferred with Chief Medical Officer Kraus and then went on to visit the city's hospitals. Here, at the St. Georg, he had started his medical career in 1866 and become interested in cholera. At the Eppendorf, Koch met the director, Rumpf, who provided a census of cholera patients, as well as bacteriological and clinical proofs of the disease's presence. This prompted Koch to remark to one of his assistants that Rumpf was "the first man in Hamburg who is telling the truth."[180] Subsequent discussions with Kraus and the president of the medical board, Senator Gerhard Hachmann, led to further differences of opinion about the presence of cholera in the city. Hamburg's authorities were only slowly emerging from denial and had not made any contingency plans for an epidemic.

After a tour of the affected unsanitary areas in the city, a shocked Koch delivered a stinging indictment of Hamburg's political leadership with his sarcastic comment, quoted in the newspapers, "Gentlemen, I forget that I am in Europe."[181] The next day, Koch held a formal conference, lecturing municipal officials about the necessary steps to halt the epidemic. With his own scientific reputation somewhat tarnished by the recent failure to offer an effective remedy for the treatment of tuberculosis, Koch used the Hamburg epidemic as a golden opportunity to restore his image as the undisputed German authority in bacteriology and an expert in the design of rational methods of diagnosis and prophylaxis for infectious diseases.

While Koch unfurled the flag of laboratory science to claim victory over the hapless medical leaders of Hamburg, German medicine stood at the crossroads of conflicting ideologies of health and professional agendas. The new bacteriology enhanced the prestige of the academic medical profession, while ordinary practitioners continued to compete and struggle in an unregulated market where their authority was contested by lay groups, sectarians, and quacks. Threats to their economic and professional standing continued in spite of the creation of a national organization, the *Deutsche Aerztevereinsbund* (Union of German Medical Associations) in 1873. Unprotected by state regulations, the new scientific physicians were viewed with suspicion, especially since their therapeutic armamentarium was still largely based on traditional measures. The dramatically expanded knowledge of physiology and pathology obtained from laboratory research enhanced diagnostic precision and prognostic accuracy, but so far it had failed to produce the expected cures.[182] Moreover, scientific medicine, with its emphasis on the objective biological underpinnings of disease, neglected the individuality of the patients. These problems similarly affected hospital physicians, often accused of performing clinical experiments on their charges in blatant disregard for patient welfare.[183]

In early September 1892 the Eppendorf wards were still overcrowded, but a semblance of order was beginning to prevail. Nearly 60 patients were housed in several makeshift units, their cots crowded together, making it difficult for caregivers to circulate among them. Erika's institutional destination was most likely one of the cholera barracks under the direction of the aptly named Dr. Sick, one of the seven chiefs of service. The hospital's rather skimpy medical staff was composed of 25 full-time physicians expected to care for all 1,300 patients, but how many of them treated cholera patients is unknown. Based on the St. Georg model, there were four medical divisions, one supervised by the director, the other three by part-time chiefs as well as two assistant physicians. Another 17 assistant physicians worked in the wards, usually supplemented by 10–15 visiting volunteers. Rumor had it that, in general, German practitioners had less clinical experience than their British and American counterparts.[184] Since the hospital lacked an academic affiliation, no medical students roamed the wards.

Kast, Eppendorf's previous director, had stressed the importance of clinical research and instruction. Staff physicians were urged to publish papers based on studies done at the hospital in a series of *Jahrbücher*, as well as organize regular meetings to discuss scientific matters of mutual interest. Unfortunately, time for clinical research and writing was scarce. Each assistant or resident physician worked 12-hour shifts and monitored about 70 patients, a heavy load considering the fact that the needs of laboratory medicine were beginning to expand and complicate the clinical work. In larger 30-bed pavilions, rounds took place only every other day as harried staff physicians alternated between the male and female wards. Despite the volunteers, physicians and nurses were in very short supply during

the 1892 epidemic, and compliance with many of the carefully crafted ward regulations was nearly impossible.[185] Patients at the Eppendorf were subjected to a
strict, almost military discipline traditional in Germany since medieval times. Visiting hours were brief: Wednesdays and Sundays from 2 to 4 PM. Women were
often placed together with their children. According to the hospital's paternalistic rules, patients were not supposed to receive much information about their management and condition.[186]

At the Eppendorf, nurses were recruited from among the city's low-status servant population, with no prior qualifications or skills. In the beginning, this practice had been justified by the assertion that proletarian "attendants" would be
more effective because they came from the same social class as most patients.[187]
Pay was low, working hours long, and turnover extremely high. Predictably,
women were paid even less than men.[188] Attempts to attract young middle-class
women and widows were stymied by the miserable working conditions and stingy
salaries. Daily schedules included 18 hours of constant service plus night shifts
several times a month. Thirty to 40 hours of continuous caregiving were not unusual, leading to sleep deprivation and exhaustion. Doctors distinguished between
nurses displaying an idealistic "higher call" vocation and those categorized as cold,
calculating "wild nurses" bent on tricking a physician or grateful patient into mar-
rying them. Many nurses viewed the hospital as a marriage market, an opportunity to escape from an unattractive job and perhaps achieve upward social mobility.[189]

Out of *konfessionelle Bedenken*—denominational scruples—the Hamburg authorities continued to reject the hiring of more highly trained and skillful caregivers, including members of Protestant nursing organizations. Such decisions
were ostensibly based on city regulations supporting the strict separation of church
and state. These qualms about hiring religiously trained caregivers prevented the
Eppendorf from enjoying the highly skilled services of the Deaconess Sisters, the
Protestant nursing order that had profoundly influenced caregiving in 19th century Germany. Many nursing experts believed that the work performed by these
women was "bound up heart and soul with the Protestant Church in Germany
and deeply rooted in the life of our people."[190] In fact, the Deaconess Training
Institute, founded in Kaiserswerth in 1836, was considered the fountainhead of
modern nursing and the model for Florence Nightingale's famous London
school.[191] By the 1840s its leaders, Theodor and Friedericke Fliedner, had managed to systematize caregiving, linking it to the growing needs of contemporary
medicine. Since the Deaconess rank implied a role in church affairs, the Kaiserswerth pupils brought to their work a strong religious and moral character, and
they defined "true nursing" as a Christian "labor of love."

The asceticism and spirit of sacrifice displayed by Deaconess nurses were legendary. Their dark blue uniforms and snug-fitting caps gave them a dignified appearance, signaling occupational respectability and moral character.[192] As part of

their Christian ethos, many of these nurses quietly endured the many hardships of their vocation. Like traditional Catholic nuns, they showed little concern for personal health and forfeited all claims to a personal life; critics portrayed them as birds trapped in cages. Lack of rest often caused illness and depression.[193] While the reason for not hiring Deaconess nurses was supposedly financial in some institutions—they were paid more than their untrained sisters—there was also a question of control. In most German hospitals, nursing groups composed of Catholic nuns, Protestant Deaconesses, or Red Cross nurses were directly governed by their respective mother houses. Individual assignments to particular institutions were subject to immediate recall irrespective of a hospital's needs. Facing powerful and authoritarian organizations, hospital administrators and physicians frequently felt threatened. Sisters often criticized medical interventions. Conflicts with expert head nurses intensified as part of complex power struggles played out to the detriment of institutional harmony.

With its stress on institutional order and social control, Eppendorf's nursing staff still resembled a traditional hierarchical organization better suited for an almshouse environment than a modern hospital. There were 15 supervising male attendants (*Oberwärter*) together with 8 supervising female ones (*Oberwärterinnen*) working as station inspectors. The core caregiving staff consisted of 88 regular male attendants (*Krankenwärter*) and 99 female ones (*Krankenwärterinnen*). Only station inspectors were given higher salaries and lodging on the premises; they were even allowed to marry. Most male nurses continued to be recruited primarily from among army orderlies, and together with their female counterparts, they were selected mainly for their physical strength and endurance, their frugality, and their obedience. Dress identified caregiving status. The male attendants wore long brown robes, while the women were dressed in their street clothes—no caps—and merely donned small white aprons. Among their basic tasks were cleaning, scouring, and making beds. The daily routine began at 6 AM when the patients were awakened by a bell, and it ended 15 hours later at 9 PM, except for those who had night duties. This exhausting regimen took place seven days a week, with the nurses getting only half a day off during the week. Although by 1892 the number of patients per caregiver had been reduced to about five or six, the intensity of the work with cholera victims, the danger of contracting the disease, and the widespread exposure to strong disinfectants took their toll on those who ministered to the sick.

In 1892, the regular nursing staff had no specific training for managing contagious patients during an epidemic. To his credit, in 1889 Director Kast had organized a series of special classes attended by about half of the personnel as part of a four-month course in the theory and practice of nursing. Routines like making beds, tucking bed sheets, and fluffing pillows were deemphasized in favor of isolation techniques. During the cholera epidemic, many nurses came to resent the temporary presence of educated volunteers, especially a few sisters from various religious groups, who were allowed to take charge in some wards during the emergency and impose much stricter discipline.

Back to water: Managing cholera at the Eppendorf Hospital

Following the appearance of cholera, conditions in Hamburg's hospitals were characterized as chaotic. In most instances, there was not even enough time to obtain specimens and perform the bacteriological investigations required to confirm the diagnosis.[194] Patients admitted during the first two weeks of the epidemic endured terrifying experiences. The barracks housing cholera patients were crowded and impregnated with a chloroform-like stench emanating from the dying patients laying side by side on cots. In addition to the nauseating smell, the ward was filled with the screams of delirious patients, their shriveled hands flailing in soiled sheets and blankets. Many, like Erika, had dark faces with sunken eyes staring up. Others thrashed around, their husky voices constantly begging for ice water, complaining of terrible cramps and demanding painkillers.

Because of the virtually constant diarrhea and frequent vomiting of the patients, cholera was particularly hard on the nursing personnel, who desperately tried to keep their charges as clean as possible and attempted to neutralize all potentially contagious bodily fluids.[195] Only periodically could patients' bodies be with rags dipped in carbolic acid. As a result of this neglect, many patients soon displayed severe burns and ulcers around their buttocks caused by prolonged sitting on bedpans soaked in carbolic acid. Caregivers were overworked, exhausted, and depressed by events in their units. Many were terrified about the risk of infection associated with their chores, although only 12 nurses and 7 laundry workers officially contracted the disease, and only 4 died.[196]

Patients complained that the primary concern of the nurses was to ensure institutional disinfection, not to promote the comfort of the sick.[197] The patients' soiled clothing was disposed of in barrels containing disinfectant located at the entrance to each pavilion. Before being taken to a rather small, central steam-cleaning facility, these items lingered in and around their overfilled containers, risking contamination of caregivers. More exposed were the laundry workers, many of whom contracted mild cases of cholera in the early stages of the epidemic. Collected on wire shelves and placed in an oven, most clothing and bedding, contaminated or not, was literally baked at temperatures exceeding 600°F, which often destroyed the fabric.[198]

Among the most gruesome sights was the massive pileup of bodies awaiting disposal in the corridors. Those presumed dead were collected, their faces covered by a sheet. Some hands and legs could still be observed twitching periodically in the dim light.[199] Some were to be brought to the morgue for autopsies and studies. Others still lay in their excrement-covered beds, their skin "tinged

with blue," eyes wide open and faces distorted by pain. Busy porters, their fortitude periodically enhanced by gulps of brandy, splashed carbolic acid solution
over the dead and unceremoniously tossed them onto canvas-covered stretchers.
This routine was almost surreal, as the light, desiccated bodies, like gruesome toys
made of dry bark instead of flesh and blood, were stacked like lumber. Because
of the high mortality, removal took up to 10 hours. Corpses were placed outside
on the grass, where specially hired cabinet makers carried out the dreadful task
of nailing down the ready-made coffins or wooden crates stacked up by the hundreds in the adjacent gardens. Built of soft plywood and made in only one size,
they were popularly known as "nose-squashers" in a display of typical black humor.[200] By early September, however, the worst was over at the Eppendorf. Porters
had caught up with the demand for their services and were very prompt in removing the dead.[201]

On admission, Erika's examination revealed that she was nearing a complete
circulatory collapse. Apathy and insensibility were prominent features. Pale and
cold, with sunken eyes and a hoarse voice, she had a faint, irregular pulse, fast
breathing, and minimal urinary output. At about 8 PM her face turned gray and
cyanotic, and she began complaining of pressure in her chest, all typical manifestations of what medical experts characterized as *cholera asphictica*. The initial therapeutic approach was purely symptomatic and palliative, focused on providing
some circulatory stimulation in the form of hot beverages. German physicians
showed a predilection for warm blankets, hot water bottles, and *Glühwein*, red
wine heated with sugar, cinnamon, and other spices. At Eppendorf, however, a
strong, copper-tasting tea became the staple stimulant, often increasing the patient's nausea. For extreme thirst, ice chips were given, although nurses took pains
to limit their ingestion for fear of disturbing the stomach further and causing additional vomiting. If abdominal cramping was present, patients received hypodermic injections of morphine and small enemas with chamomile tea and opium
tincture.

At Eppendorf, physicians were aware of the great opportunities awaiting them
to test the efficacy of several therapeutic approaches. Powerless and often desperately ill, patients were seldom consulted about treatments. Gliding through the
wards in their flowing white linen coats, hospital physicians were notorious for
their autocratic behavior and indifference to the sick. Such research designs were
usually rationalized because of the extremely critical status of the patients involved—most were going to die anyway—and the lack of contemporary professional qualms regarding medical experimentation.[202] As a foreign observer from
the Edinburgh Infirmary pointed out, systematic postmortem examinations were
even carried out during the cholera epidemic in spite of the large number of admissions and the shortage of attending physicians.[203]

After the initial chaos, Eppendorf's medical staff developed a somewhat standardized approach in response to the aforementioned stages of cholera, eventu-

ally discarding a number of treatments that proved useless. In 1892, one strategy, based on the newest bacteriological knowledge, attempted to destroy the cholera germ selectively by intestinal irrigation with the help of acids or disinfectants. This approach contrasted sharply with the older "heroic" and depleting treatments attempted during the 1820s and 1840s, especially bloodletting—considered useful during the early stages of the disease but difficult to perform later because of circulatory collapse. The earlier rationale had been to reestablish circulatory balance, a goal also sought through the application of leeches, scarification, or dry cupping. Purgatives were administered to help nature clean the intestinal tract, while emetics—especially antimony salts—cleaned out the stomach. Subsequent cholera outbreaks from the 1850s to the 1870s witnessed a partial retreat from depleting therapies, especially bloodletting. They were replaced by the ingestion or injection of neutral salt solutions, designed to convert black into red blood again, and the administration of tonic remedies such as quinine, tinctures of iron, ether, and ammonia.[204]

The new, scientifically informed strategies employed agents that could specifically neutralize or destroy causal agents of disease.[205] Lister's example, eventually based on bacteriological theories, suggested that germs could be selectively poisoned. Unlike therapies in earlier historical periods, the late-nineteenth-century therapeutic rationale aimed at destroying the microscopic causes of a given disease became even more dependent on diagnostic precision. This approach, pioneered by Pasteur, pointed toward the use of sera as specific treatments. The concept of serotherapy promised the employment of substances designed to neutralize particular germs. Could scientists therefore achieve cures with specifically prepared blood sera or even chemical compounds capable of achieving similar results? Events surrounding the failure of Koch's tuberculin to cure tuberculosis in 1890 had led to a certain skepticism about the fruitful transfer of laboratory findings to the bedside.

Still, some of the physicians at Eppendorf were willing to attempt a causal therapeutic approach based on Koch's pathogenic notions, suggesting that cholera bacilli with their toxins could perhaps be removed from the body or rendered harmless through some sort of neutralizing compound or serum.[206] In one of the temporary barracks, Edwin K. Klebs, followed the same approach that Koch had employed with tuberculin by subcutaneously inoculating some patients with a product termed *anticholerin*, obtained from pure cultures of cholera bacilli.[207] Unlike tuberculin, however, anticholerin was believed to possess a specific toxic action that would affect only the cholera vibrio, a fact seemingly confirmed by earlier animal experiments. The thick, brownish material was periodically injected intramuscularly, later subcutaneously, using selected gravely ill patients, who were also receiving intravenous saline infusions, together with a control group. To Klebs' dismay, the results were unfavorable, with the small number of patients suffering a 67% mortality rate.[208]

While serotherapy failed, another etiologically based strategy was tried. Based on Listerism, this approach suggested the employment of diluted acids or newly developed disinfectants to kill the cholera vibrio outright and neutralize poisons in the gut. To achieve antisepsis, part of the intestine needed to be washed out by *enteroclysis*, a procedure pioneered by the Italian bacteriologist Arnaldo Cantani (1837–1893) during the 1884 epidemic in Naples. Cantani gave repeated enemas consisting of one to two liters of a hot, sterile 1% solution of astringent tannic acid supplemented with drops of laudanum and gum arabicum. Although partial absorption of the solution occasionally prevented circulatory problems and anuria, this method proved ineffective in the Eppendorf patients, perhaps because of the advanced stage of their disease, but more likely due to the drastic and destructive nature of the procedure.[209]

Meanwhile, Ferdinand Hueppe, a former army surgeon, also proposed intestinal washings with another disinfectant, tribromphenol (Bromol), combined with bismuth. This compound was also expected to kill the cholera vibrio specifically and neutralize the poison while protecting the intestinal lining, but once again the results were equivocal. For three weeks, the case-specific mortality rate in Hueppe's pavilions was 54%, somewhat higher than that of other cholera wards at Eppendorf. Faced with hospital physicians trying a plethora of compounds, including salol, a phenylsalicylate, Director Rumpf issued a warning against the indiscriminate use of newfangled pharmaceutical preparations—many developed from coal-tar or petroleum products such as benzene and cresol—that could prove harmful.[210] Hueppe, however, defended his results by suggesting that Rumpf had referred only very sick patients to his pavilion, also arguing that some of his patients were dying from other diseases.[211] Quite damaging to Rumpf's authority were Hueppe's public pronouncements that chaotic conditions at Eppendorf were detrimental to the proper conduct of scientific experiments.[212] Painting himself as a man of science, Hueppe questioned Rumpf's expertise in the cholera-induced emergency at Eppendorf and belittled him as merely a specialist in nervous disorders.[213]

Since the causal therapy—to kill the cholera vibrio—practiced by experimenting physicians like Klebs and Hueppe seemed dubious and ineffective, other Eppendorf physicians concentrated on making patients comfortable, with the expectation that close to half of them would recover naturally. Most important were attempts to rehydrate patients who had lost copious amounts of fluid. Such symptomatic treatments addressed a number of important problems, including the persistent thirst, vomiting, and diarrhea. The approach was not new—it had been employed since the 1830s—but nausea and frequent vomiting always limited the amount of fluid that could be ingested, and German practitioners did not link vascular collapse to excessive bodily fluid loss. *Gerolsteiner Sprüdel*—a mineral water—became the staple beverage, uncontaminated and carbonated to neutralize the nausea. Thirsty cholera patients consumed thousands of bottles. Ice chips cooled parched lips and ulcerated mouths, while the old standby, calomel, administered in low dosages to prevent mercurial poisoning, controlled diarrhea during the early stages. Pain, whether in the form of abdominal or leg cramps, prompted the use of morphine injections. Dietary indications were frequently ignored by the overworked physicians, and patients who tolerated food were treated to a fatty, almost indigestible bouillon lacking vegetables, omitted for fear of contamination with polluted water. White wine or claret—even the ubiquitous *Glüwein*—were recommended in the popular belief that they could kill the cholera vibrio nestling in the bowels.

Supplementing the drinks was a parenteral method of supplying fluid. Subcutaneous infusions of a 4% salt solution seemed beneficial, especially if they were warm. Employing a cannula and rubber tubing, the fluid was placed under the skin of both thighs and the abdominal wall, employing aseptic techniques to prevent secondary infection.[214] Another, faster method used to counteract severe dehydration was an intravenous infusion of saline solution, recommended since 1830, although published results found little support among the medical profession. Not surprisingly, air embolisms had caused strokes, while the thick needles employed at the time damaged veins and produced local infections. Better surgical techniques and equipment in the 1880s caused fewer complications.[215]

In 1892, repeated observations at Eppendorf made by attending physicians such as Chief Surgeon Max Schede and Director Rumpf suggested that on many occasions saline infusions seemed to save lives. By early September, hospital practitioners were told to employ the *Salzlösung* as soon as the patient's pulse and temperature began to fall, encouraging its subsequent use as long as there was still a chance for clinical recovery. Shortly after admission, this was done in Erika's case. Doctors ordered the subcutaneous infusion of two liters of a warm (40°C) saline solution, distributed with little discomfort under the right abdominal skin and other parts of her body. The favorable action of such infusions was attributed in part to their temperature and their stimulating effect on the heart. Moreover, based on bacteriological theory, the saline diluted the poisons introduced by the cholera bacillus into the blood, thus contributing to their elimination.

Used on some 1,659 hospital patients in Hamburg that year (average dose, 1,500–2,000 cc), the *Salzlösung* achieved limited success. It was agreed that saline solutions were not a cure for the disease but simply an aid to help the patient through its stages.[216] The quantities of fluids infused or provided orally could never compensate for the massive dehydration.[217] As observers noted, some patients periodically stumbled out of bed, desperately searching for something to drink. In spite of the infusion, Erika's condition failed to improve, and she remained very thirsty. Her pulse was no longer detectable, her respiratory rate was unchanged, and her hands were ice cold, all signs that she was slipping again into *stadium algidum*. Since Erika's condition remained critical, the attending physicians injected another 2,000 cc of warm saline solution during the following night—this time, however, intravenously. The sterile solutions were administered via a graduated one-liter glass irrigator with an attached rubber tube connected to a small, blunt metallic cannula. "What impressed me most," wrote one observer, "was the reliance the staff had in saline injections and the confidence with which they spoke of it."[218]

Because of the generalized vascular collapse, attending physicians usually encountered difficulties in finding a vein in the elbow to open and start an infusion. As in other situations, therapeutic decisions were made even at the risk of creating a subsequent infection—perhaps an abscess—at the point of needle insertion. Under current institutional conditions, nobody could guarantee aseptic techniques. In Erika's case, the saline fluid had an excellent effect, restoring her faint pulse and bringing her back to consciousness. She opened her eyes spontaneously and even made inquiries about her child. Throughout the next day, her condition remained somewhat improved, with a good pulse and less vomiting, but persistent diarrhea.

Trials of rehydration such as Erika's prolonged the lives of patients already in the *stadium algidum*. They reversed some of the symptoms associated with vascular collapse and decreased thirst and muscular cramps. Most individuals admitted to Eppendorf, however, were already in an advanced stage of the disease and thus too sick to obtain lasting benefits. Moreover, the amounts infused were clearly insufficient; even so, ignorance about true blood volume and failure to measure blood pressure[219] contributed to circulatory problems, collapse, and even death as infusions rushed into the bloodstream—one quart in 10 minutes. Lack of special needles caused injuries as the delirious patients thrashed around during the procedures.[220]

On September 6, two days after admission, observers recorded that Erika's face began to acquire the reddish hue typical of those patients whose condition was stabilizing. She was much quieter, but her pulse remained weak. Most patients in this condition were fed oatmeal gruel. However, diarrhea continued, and muscle cramps in Erika's legs required a shot of morphine. A decision was made to employ an antiseptic remedy—in this case, 40 drops of creosol—presumably mixed in a beverage in spite of the reservations expressed about this approach by Director Rumpf. Her condition remained fair.

By September 8, Erika still vomited and complained of stomach pains, prompting doctors to prescribe bismuth powders. Since most patients retained a weak pulse and felt extremely cold to the touch, another strategy was to warm the body by improving the blood circulation through massage, steam, or hot baths. These procedures provided relief from painful cramps and were popular with patients. Although not recorded, Erika may have been subjected to such baths, repeated about every six hours if enough nursing personnel were available. Attempts were also made to stimulate her heart through subcutaneous infusions of camphor oil and ether. Other stimulants included hot tea, coffee, and wine. In the wards, large bottles labeled *"potus hydrochloricus"*—a weak hydrochloric acid solution—were available together with mineral water for those who needed to quench their thirst.[221] When Erika seemed to rally the next day, the attending physicians ordered another intravenous saline infusion of 2,000 cc to promote further diuresis.

Erika reached a critical point in her clinical course on September 10. She definitely looked better and told the nurses that she felt improved—with no further vomiting and only minor diarrhea. However, Erika's pulse remained high and full, and her urine contained considerable albumin. More ominously, she now began to complain of pain on her left side. By evening her condition had deteriorated; fever (101°F) was present, and her breathing became more difficult and frequent, with rales detected over the right upper chest. She also complained of stabbing pains in her right lower abdomen. Physicians attending Erika interpreted her symptoms as representing the "typhoid" stage of the cholera and hesitated to continue the infusions. In truth, they gave up.

Erika was occasionally delirious during the next day, and her breathing became very frequent, although no cyanosis could be detected. Her facial expression remained calm. When physicians made their rounds and listened to her chest, her breathing was reported as bronchial and the sounds were muffled in both lungs. No doubt she was developing pneumonia, a common complication resulting from the aspiration of vomit in earlier stages of the disease.[222] Not surprisingly, Erika's case was now characterized by the attending physicians as *gravissimus*. A urine specimen contained more albumin, suggesting progressive kidney failure. On September 12, her condition continued its downhill course. She was now delirious; when measured, her temperature was 103°F and her breathing quite frequent. Attending physicians feared that the cholera poison was paralyzing her circulatory system and only prescribed another injection of morphine. The next morning, Erika W. quietly slipped into a coma and was pronounced dead at nine o'clock. No autopsy findings were recorded. As with John S. in Baltimore a year earlier, a fateful complication—pneumonia—was ultimately responsible for this outcome.

Later consensus among European medical experts was that none of the therapeutic approaches employed in Hamburg had any lasting value, except perhaps the subcutaneous and intravenous salt water infusions, considered purely symptomatic therapy.[223] In all, a total of 8,292 cholera patients were officially admitted to the various city hospitals, of whom 3,994—including Erika—died, a rate of 48.16%. The overall mortality at Eppendorf was somewhat higher—56.2%—perhaps reflecting a more compromised patient population debilitated by long waits, hazardous transportation, experimentation, and indifferent caregiving.[224] Officials, however, conceded that this was just an average and that the institutional mortality had fluctuated significantly during the first month, falling from nearly 80% during the first days in August to 25% later in September when Stanhope, the American reporter, tried to get infected.

Aftermath

"How is the Herr Dr. Herald getting along?," asked the medical attendants making their rounds in Eppendorf's notorious Pavilion F, the "ward of the hopeless," under the direction of Dr. Manchot, one of the full-time assistants. Following an examination in late September, Stanhope was pronounced in good health and sent to a private room in Pavilion 23. To further prove his acquired immunity, however, Stanhope insisted on drinking potentially polluted Elbe River water in the presence of witnesses while rubbing his contaminated hands over his mouth and pressing his lips on the edges of a mug previously used by a very sick cholera patient. He also repeatedly violated hospital rules by eating in the ward or with other caregivers without following proper disinfection procedures. Fortunately for Stanhope, the influx of new patients had slowed to a trickle, and many new arrivals had only mild cases of cholera. The epidemic was ebbing. After about 10 days in the institution, the reporter left Eppendorf with disinfected clothes and clutching a health certificate issued to him by Director Rumpf. Some medical students gave him a rousing farewell party. Stanhope's caper had achieved its original objectives: to advertise the postulated efficacy of Haffkine's cholera preservative and to make him an instant celebrity in Hamburg, where he granted interviews and was photographed by other reporters.[225]

As events in Hamburg reached their expected denouement, Koch presided in Berlin over six days of meetings. From September 26 to October 1, a commission of experts discussed the draft of a *Reichsseuchengesetz*—imperial legislation—to deal with future outbreaks of epidemic disease. Among the commission's members was none other than the old, stubborn hygienist Pettenkofer, who still vehemently opposed Koch's proposals for mandatory quarantine measures and isolation of cholera victims in hospitals. Pettenkofer's counterproposals suggested that such measures be applied only in towns and cities already known for their poor sanitary conditions, where the soil factor could also be operative. In a victory for Koch, the commission approved the proposed disinfection and isolation procedures, and a dejected Pettenkofer returned to Munich. Clean water, and especially the use of sand filtration for removal of bacteria, became the centerpiece of urban public health well into the next century.[226]

However, the controversy had not ended. In one last, desperate move that guaranteed his immortality, Pettenkofer requested a culture sample of cholera vibrios from Koch's associate, Georg Gaffky (1850–1918), who had stayed behind in Hamburg to complete the bacteriological studies. After its arrival on October 7, Pettenkofer gulped down a teaspoonful of the broth, teeming with organisms, together with a sip of sodium bicarbonate to neutralize the stomach's acidity, considered a possible barrier for the vibrio's spread. Within 48 hours he experienced cramps and diarrhea, and cholera microorganisms were cultured from his stools. These manifestations gradually abated by October 15, and Pettenkofer declared his theories vindicated: the cholera vibrio was not the sole agent of the disease! To further prove his point, the professor suggested a similar experiment to his assistant, Rudolf Emmerich, who experienced much more severe symptoms but also survived the ordeal. With much fanfare, both cases were presented at a meeting of the Munich Medical Society, triggering further debates with Koch and Gaffky and stimulating further opposition to portions of the *Reichsseuchengesetz.*[227] Far from becoming a decisive triumph for bacteriology, the events surrounding the cholera epidemic in Hamburg continued to justify the importance of environmental and individual constitutional factors in the genesis of this disease.[228]

Cholera exposed a number of weaknesses inherent in the "world's best hospital." Conceived on miasmatic premises, the Eppendorf needed to enter the bacteriological age with new and larger sterilization facilities for personal and bed clothing and to create separate facilities for the disinfection of human wastes following their removal from contagious disease pavilions. As Hueppe had suggested, the Eppendorf's administrative structures were also in need of reform, with reduced duties assigned to its overworked medical director, who needed to be above all an expert in hygiene, epidemiology, and management.[229] One central problem was the institution's water supply, provided by the city from unfiltered Elbe River water. In spite of recommendations from Curschmann and others, the construction of a sand filtration plant had been repeatedly postponed. During its construction, the hospital had already cared for typhoid fever cases from among the construction workers. Only after 1892 could the Eppendorf rely, at least in part, on its own well water.[230]

Another critical deficiency was proper nursing care. The use of qualified and disciplined Deaconess and Red Cross nurses during the epidemic persuaded Hamburg's health authorities to establish their own training facility. With partial funding from the private Schmilinsky Foundation, an independent teaching institute was set up with links to the Eppendorf Hospital in April 1895. Admission was restricted to local Protestant women between the ages of 20 and 35. The one-year course featured a three-month probationary period devoted largely to cleaning and bed-making chores, followed by a similar period of theoretical studies before a series of rotations through the various hospital departments. Higher salaries and a pension system that ensured lifelong care to invalids attracted a number of middle-class women.[231] The new graduates managed not only to improve significantly the social status of hospital nurses but also to introduce a measure of professionalism and clinical experience to their caregiving. As elsewhere, the status of the new nurses was nonetheless kept in check by medical professionalization and contemporary ideology concerning women's work.[232]

The cholera epidemic of 1892 was not hospital medicine's finest hour. The impressive physical plant at Eppendorf could not obscure its staff deficiencies or the organizational disarray caused by the sudden influx of thousands of cholera patients. The temporary institutional chaos renewed the distrust of institutional care

that Curschmann had worked so hard to erase with the construction of his monumental new hospital. Resistance to forcible isolation, as demanded by Koch and
the bacteriologists, persisted. Unfortunately, hospital care was no substitute for
prophylaxis and a comprehensive approach to public health, which was seriously
lacking in Hamburg. Although supported by the city, the hospital remained woe-
fully inadequate as a barrier against contagious disease. Medicalization meant more
accurate, scientifically grounded diagnoses—in this instance bacteriological confirmation of the presence of the cholera vibrio[233]—but, as at the Johns Hopkins
Hospital in Baltimore, therapeutics still lagged far behind.[234] Scientific medicine
could offer only limited remedies. Instead of treatments aimed at the eradication
of causal agents, both Osler and Rumpf had returned to traditional measures. As
one editorial commented, "the therapeutic lessons of the recent epidemic of
cholera that has played such havoc in the city of Hamburg are not very assuring.
In spite of modern methods of treatment and in the face of an enlightened hygiene, the mortality of the disease . . . does not reflect much credit upon our therapeutic resources and is not likely to inspire much confidence in them."[235] Could
hospitals become houses of cure?

NOTES

1. Quote from the letter of instructions given by Johns Hopkins to the trustees of the
Johns Hopkins Hospital, March 10, 1873. Reprinted in "A brief account of the Johns Hop-
kins Hospital," *Johns Hopkins Hosp Bull* 1 (Dec 1889): 4, and in Helen Hopkins Thom,
Johns Hopkins, A Silhouette, Baltimore, Johns Hopkins Univ. Press, 1929, pp. 87–90.

2. This section of Baltimore is now called Rosemont, and the patient's address placed
him across from the Fulton Station of the Western Maryland Railway. R. Ryon, *West Baltimore Neighborhoods: Sketches of their History, 1840–1960*, Baltimore, Institute for Public Design, Univ. of Baltimore, 1993.

3. Sherry H. Olson, *Baltimore, The Building of an American City*, Baltimore, Johns Hopkins Univ. Press, 1980, pp. 198–241.

4. W. Osler, "Treatment of typhoid fever," *Johns Hopkins Hosp Rep* IV (1895): 3. The
case of John S. was included by Osler among his fatal typhoid fever cases: W. Osler, "A
study of the fatal cases," in *Johns Hopkins Hosp Rep* IV (1895): 18–20. The original clinical chart could not be found in the Medical Records. Additional information was obtained
through the efforts of the Alan Chesney Archives personnel, including the Johns Hopkins
Hospital Admission Log and the original autopsy results. I am grateful to Nancy McCall
and her archival staff for their efforts and for those of a graduate student, Cynthia Ronzio,
who assisted with this research.

5. Terra Ziporyn, *Disease in the Popular American Press*, Westport, CT, Greenwood
Press, 1988, especially pp. 71–111.

6. For an overview see N. Tomes, "The private side of public health: Sanitary science,
domestic hygiene, and the germ theory, 1870–1900," *Bull Hist Med* 64 (1990): 509–39. Her
new book on the subject is *The Gospel of Germs: Men, Women, and the Microbe in American Life*, Cambridge, Mass, Harvard Univ. Press, 1998.

7. William B. Bean, ed., *Sir William Osler: Aphorisms from his Bedside Teachings and Writings*, New York, H. Schuman, 1950, p. 144.

8. W. Osler, "General analysis and summary of the cases," *Johns Hopkins Hosp Rep* IV (1895): 1–2.

9. H. A. Lafleur, "Early days at the Johns Hopkins Hospital with Dr. Osler," *Can Med Assoc J* X Sir William Osler Memorial Number (July 1920): 43.

10. M. J. Vogel, "Patrons, practitioners, and patients: The voluntary hospital in mid-Victorian Boston," in *Victorian America*, ed. D. W. Howe, Philadelphia, Univ. of Pennsylvania Press, 1976, pp. 121–38, and C. E. Rosenberg, "From almshouse to hospital: The shaping of Philadelphia General Hospital," *Milbank Mem Q* 60 (1982): 108–54.

11. Harvey Cushing, *The Life of Sir William Osler*, London, Oxford Univ. Press, 1940, p. 380.

12. No information is available about John S.'s financial status. Employed patients were usually considered capable of paying for their care. See H. M. Hurd, "Superintendent's report of the Johns Hopkins Hospital for the year ending January 31, 1891," *Johns Hopkins Hosp Bull* 2 (September 1891): 128.

13. For a discussion at the 40th annual meeting of the American Medical Association in June 1889, see *Boston Med Surg J* 121 (July 18, 1889): 63–64.

14. Osler, "General analysis of cases," 1–2.

15. W. S. Thayer, "The Osler clinic," *Bull Johns Hopkins Hosp* 52 (1933): 103–04.

16. See Hamilton Owens, *Baltimore on the Chesapeake*, Garden City, NY, Doubleday, Doran & Co., 1941, especially pp. 288–303.

17. For a brief summary, see "The opening of the hospital and medical school," in *A Model of Its Kind: A Centennial History of Medicine at Johns Hopkins*, ed. A. M. Harvey et al., Baltimore, Johns Hopkins Univ. Press, 1989, vol. 1, pp. 7–32, and also by Harvey et al., "A model of its kind: A century of medicine at Johns Hopkins," *JAMA* 261 (June 2, 1989): 3136–42.

18. John Shaw Billings, who would be largely responsible for designing the new hospital, later termed Hopkins' vision a "an ideal which was no doubt somewhat misty, but which did not correspond to any existing hospital." See J. S. Billings, "The plans and purposes of the Johns Hopkins Hospital," *Boston Med Surg J* 120 (May 9, 1889): 449.

19. Morris J. Vogel, "The transformation of the American hospital, 1850–1920," in *Health Care in America*, ed. S. Reverby and D. Rosner, Philadelphia, Temple Univ. Press, 1979, pp. 105–16, and his book *The Invention of the Modern Hospital, Boston 1870–1930*, Chicago, Univ. of Chicago Press, 1980.

20. "A brief account," 4

21. K. D. Young, "On recent progress in hospital planning and arrangements," *Am J Med Sci* 91 (1886): 441–49.

22. The first institution built according to this plan was the Royal Naval Hospital near Plymouth, completed around 1764.

23. J. S. Billings, "Hospital construction and organization," in *Hospital Plans*, pp. 11–25. See also G. H. Brieger, "The original plans for the Johns Hopkins Hospital and their historic significance," *Bull Hist Med* 39 (1965): 518–28. For a biography of Billings see Carleton B. Chapman, *Order Out of Chaos: John Shaw Billings and America's Coming of Age*, Boston, Boston Med Library, 1994. For the other proposals, see *Hospital Plans: Five Essays relating to the Construction, Organization, and Management of Hospitals, contributed by their Authors for the Use of the Johns Hopkins Hospital of Baltimore*, New York, W. Wood, 1875. For a review by Isaac Hays, its editor, see *Am J Med Sci* 71 (1876): 485–96.

24. Alan M. Chesney, *The Johns Hopkins Hospital and the Johns Hopkins University School of Medicine: A Chronicle*, Baltimore, Johns Hopkins Univ. Press, 1943, vol. 1, p. 30.

25. Billings, as quoted in Chesney, *Chronicle*, vol. 1, p. 56.

26. "The hospital should provide the means of giving medical instruction for the sake of the sick in the institution as well as those out of it." See Billings, "Plans and purposes," 450.

27. Ibid. See also Charles F. Withington, *The Relation of Hospitals to Medical Education*, Boston, Cupples, Upham, 1886.

28. The cost estimate was $1,028,500 for a separate pavilion system. Quoted in Jon M. Kingsdale, *The Growth of Hospitals, 1850–1939: An Economic History of Baltimore*, New York, Garland, 1989, pp. 101–18.

29. Details in Hugh Hawkins, *Pioneer: A History of the Johns Hopkins University, 1874–1889*, Ithaca, Cornell Univ. Press, 1960.

30. Thayer described them as "beautiful, large, fresh, a luxury with their famous ventilation system rarely put into correct practice but so good." "The Osler clinic," 103–04.

31. "The Johns Hopkins Hospital at Baltimore," *Lancet* I (Feb. 10, 1877): 216.

32. Kingsdale, *Growth of Hospitals*, p. 105.

33. See Billings, "Plans and purposes," 454.

34. For a brief history of the university see John C. Schmidt, *Portrait of a University*, Baltimore, Johns Hopkins Univ. Press, 1986.

35. Billings, "Plans and purposes," 450.

36. "The primary distinctive feature of the hospital which placed it at the foundation in a different class from all other hospitals in the country . . . is the close union with the university." W. T. Councilman, "Osler in the early days at the Johns Hopkins Hospital," *Boston Med Surg J* 182 (1920): 341–45.

37. For a brief biography see Abraham Flexner, *Daniel Coit Gilman*, New York, Harcourt, Brace, 1946.

38. Gilman's words were recorded by Osler after he was summoned by Gilman to New York City at the end of January 1889 to have breakfast at the Fifth Avenue Hotel and experience its excellent service. See Osler's manuscript "Johns Hopkins Hospital—Inner History of an Early Organization," ed. D. G. Bates and E. H. Bensley, *Johns Hopkins Med J* 125 (October 1969): 184–94. See also Cushing, *Life of Osler*, p. 303.

39. Lafleur, "Early days," 42.

40. Thayer, "The Osler clinic," 102.

41. Hurd also became editor of the *John Hopkins Hospital Bulletin*, first published in December 1889, and *John Hopkins Hospital Reports*, begun in 1890. For a biography of Hurd see Thomas Cullen, *Henry Mills Hurd: The First Superintendent of the Johns Hopkins Hospital*, Baltimore, Johns Hopkins Univ. Press, 1920.

42. Cushing, *Life of Osler*, pp. 183–84.

43. Ibid., pp. 3–310.

44. Cushing, *Life of Osler*, vol. 1, p. 317.

45. L. F. Barker, "Osler as chief of a medical clinic," *Bull Johns Hopkins Hosp* 30 (July 1919): 193.

46. H. M. Hurd, "Report of the Johns Hopkins Hospital, May 15, 1889–Jan. 31, 1890," *Johns Hopkins Hosp Bull* 1 (September 1890): 78. For details consult T. S. Huddle and J. Ende, "Osler's clinical clerkship: Origins and interpretations," *J Hist Med* 49 (1994): 483–503.

47. H. M. Thomas, "Some memories of the development of the medical school and of Osler's advent," *Bull Johns Hopkins Hosp* 30 (July 1919): 187.

48. Lafleur, "Early days," 44.

49. D. C. Smith, "The rise and fall of typhomalarial fever II: Decline and fall," *J Hist Med* 37(1982): 287–321.

50. Barker, "Osler as chief," 190. See Chesney, *Chronicle*, vol. 1, pp. 149–79, for information about the first years of hospital operation. Concerning the tensions between bedside and laboratory see R. C. Maulitz, " 'Physician versus bacteriologist': The ideology of science in clinical medicine," in *The Therapeutic Revolution*, ed. M. J. Vogel and C. Rosenberg, Philadelphia, Univ. of Pennsylvania Press, 1979, pp. 91–107.

51. Barker, "Osler as chief," 191. See also T. N. Bonner, "The German model of training physicians in the United States, 1870–1914: How closely was it followed?," *Bull Hist Med* 64 (1990): 18–34.

52. Thayer, "The Osler clinic," 102.

53. "Courses of instruction for graduates in medicine, 1890–91," *Bull Johns Hopkins Hosp* 1 (July 1890): 65–67.

54. T. McCrae, "The influence of pathology upon the clinical medicine of William Osler," in *Appreciations and Reminiscences of Sir William Osler*, ed. M. E. Abbott, Montreal, private issue, 1926, pp. 37–41.

55. For a useful synthesis see William F. Bynum, *Science and the Practice of Medicine in the Nineteenth Century*, Cambridge, Cambridge Univ. Press, 1994, pp. 92–117.

56. John C. French, *A History of the University Founded by Johns Hopkins*, Baltimore, Johns Hopkins Univ. Press, 1946, p. 106.

57. In September 1890, Osler set out to write about clinical aspects of typhoid fever for a projected two-volume text edited by William Pepper. Later, Osler translated into English a German text on the subject written by Heinrich Curschmann: *Typhoid Fever and Typhus Fever*, Philadelphia, W. B. Saunders, c. 1901.

58. Cushing, *Life of Osler*, p. 341.

59. Johns Hopkins: "I desire you to establish in connection with the hospital, a training school for female nurses. The provision will secure the services of women competent to care for the sick in the hospital wards, and will enable you to benefit the whole community by supplying it with a class of trained and experienced nurses." See "A brief account," 4.

60. The literature on Florence Nightingale is voluminous. Quite useful are her own *Notes on Nursing: What it is, and What it is not*, New York, D. Appleton & Co., 1860, especially pp. 7–12 and 105–36. See also Monica E. Baly, *Florence Nightingale and the Nursing Legacy*, London, Croom Helm, 1986, pp. 171–86, and also by Baly, "The Nightingale nurses: The myth and the reality," in *Nursing History: The State of the Art*, ed. C. Maggs, London, Croom Helm, 1987, pp. 33–46.

61. According to Billings: "of the difference between an educated, properly trained female nurse, and one of the old-fashioned sort, I can only say that in many cases a competent trained nurse is as important to the success of treatment as a competent doctor and that one of the greatest difficulties in treating well-to-do patients in their own homes in this city is the want of proper nurses. Affection and zeal may do much but they cannot take the place of knowledge." Billings, "Plans and purposes," 452.

62. May Ayres Burgess, *Nurses, Patients, and Pocketbooks*, New York, 1928, p. 35. For an overview see C. Davies, "Professionalizing strategies as time- and culture-bound: American and British nursing circa 1893," in *Nursing History*, ed. E. C. Lagemann, New York, Teachers' College Press, 1983, pp. 47–63.

63. An interesting contemporary sketch of nursing in New York can be obtained from M. Cadwalader Jones, "The training of a nurse," *Scribner's Magazine* 8 (November 1890): 613–24. For more details see Susan Reverby, *Ordered to Care: The Dilemma of American Nursing, 1850–1945*, Cambridge, Cambridge Univ. Press, 1987, pp. 39–59.

64. L. Dock, "Recollections of Miss Hampton at the Johns Hopkins," *Amer J Nursing* 11 (October 1910): 16–17.

65. For an important analysis of Hampton's place in American nursing see J. W. James, "Isabel Hampton and the professionalization of nursing in the 1890s," in *The Therapeutic Revolution*, pp. 201–44.

66. William Osler, "Nurse and patient," in *Aequanimitas*, 3rd ed., Philadelphia, Blakiston, 1932, p. 155. See T. Ingles, "The physician's view of the evolving nursing profession, 1873–1913," *Nurs Forum* 15 (1976): 123–64.

67. Isabel Hampton's opening remarks were reprinted in "Opening of the Nurses' Home and inauguration of the Training School for Nurses," *Johns Hopkins Hosp Bull* 1 (December 1889): 6–7.

68. See A. M. Carr, "The early history of the hospital and training school," *Johns Hopkins Alumni Mag* 8 (June 1909): 54–75.

69. "Nurses' Journal Club," *Johns Hopkins Hosp Bull* 2 (April 1891): 65.

70. "Training School for Nurses in the Johns Hopkins Hospital," *Johns Hopkins Hosp Bull* 1 (December 1889): 15.

71. Osler, who was still single, was remembered as a "buoyant factor in the development of student life." H. M. Hurd, "The personality of William Osler in Baltimore," in *Bull Int Assoc Med Museums* 9, Sir William Osler Memorial Number (Montreal, 1926): 263–65.

72. This included the romance between Isabel Hampton and Dr. Hunter Robb, Howard Kelly's first assistant in the Gynecology and Obstetrics Department. They were married in 1894. Another head nurse, Caroline Hampton, from the New York Hospital, married Dr. Halsted in 1890. Osler commented that "considering the fact that Miss Hampton was very strict in nipping early signs of flirtation in the nurses, her own conduct for a long period illustrated the axiom, Love is blind." See Osler, "Inner History," 187–88.

73. Osler to Gilman, March 6, 1890. See Cushing, *Life of Osler*, p. 325.

74. Osler, *Aequanimitas*, p. 156. For useful discussion of nurses' sexuality before and after Nightingale see Catherine A. Judd, "Hygienic Aesthetics: Sick Nursing and Social Reform in the Victorian Novel, 1845–1880," Ph.D. diss., Univ. of California, Berkeley, 1992.

75. Typhoid fever patients were subjected to periodic urine examinations. In most cases, their urine had higher than normal specific gravity. J. Hewetson, "The urine and the occurrence of renal complications in typhoid fever," *Johns Hopkins Hosp Rep* IV (1895): 113–55.

76. As a diagnostic test, Ehrlich's diazo reaction had received mixed reviews. C. E. Simon, "Ehrlich's test in typhoid fever," *Johns Hopkins Hosp Bull* 1 (November 1890): 93–95, and J. Hewetson, "The diagnostic value of Ehrlich's diazo reaction," *Johns Hopkins Hosp Rep* IV (1895): 5–8. At the hospital, the test had been positive in 22 of 26 patients initially treated. Since the patients arriving at hospitals had already been ill for several days, their blood cultures were usually negative, and the confirmatory bacteriological diagnosis was made from stool cultures.

77. "On the treatment of typhoid fever," *Am J Med Sci* 96 (1888): 178–79.

78. Cushing, *Life of Osler*, p. 328.

79. Hurd, "Personality of William Osler," 262.

80. C. B. Farrar, "Osler at Johns Hopkins," *Univ West Ontario Med J* 20 (1950): 130.

81. "Hilarity and good humor . . . help enormously both in the study and in the practice of medicine." Bean, *Osler: Aphorisms*, p. 81.

82. Ibid., p. 144.

83. Councilman, "Osler in the early days," 343.

84. Lafleur, "Early days," 44.

85. Barker, "Osler as chief," 193. Another witness recalled Osler's "unusual facility to make all patients feel that he was interested in them as persons." See G. T. Harrell, "Osler's practice," *Bull Hist Med* 47 (1973): 553.

86. Bean, *Osler: Aphorisms*, pp. 66, 68.

87. T. McCrae, "Osler and patient," *Bull Johns Hopkins Hosp* 30 (1919): 201.

88. Osler, "Study of fatal cases," 18–20.

89. William Osler, *The Principles and Practice of Medicine*, New York, D. Appleton & Co., 1892, p. 32.

90. W. Osler, "Five years' experience with the cold-bath treatment of typhoid fever," *Johns Hopkins Hosp Rep* V (1895): 321. At this point, the mortality rates from typhoid fever in patients treated with the baths averaged 7.3%.

91. Osler, "Study of fatal cases," 13. He expressed similar sentiments in his textbook when he declared that "the profession was long in learning that typhoid fever is not a disease to be treated by medicines. Careful nursing and a regulated diet are the essentials in a majority of the cases." Osler, *Principles and Practice of Medicine*, p. 33. For a contemporary overview of typhoid fever and its treatment see Karl Liebermeister, "Typhoid fever," in *Cyclopedia of the Practice of Medicine*, ed. H. von Ziemssen, trans. into English, New York, W. Wood & Co., 1874–1879, vol. 1, pp. 194–233.

92. Wrote Osler: "Typhoid fever has a Pennsylvania Railway-like directness, in distinction to the zigzag Baltimore-and-Ohio chart of aestivo-autumnal fever." Bean, *Osler: Aphorisms*, p. 129.

93. Osler, *Principles and Practice of Medicine*, p. 33. Osler linked nursing by trained personnel to lower mortality rates in hospitals. See Osler, "Treatment of typhoid fever," *Johns Hopkins Hosp Rep* IV (1895): 3. For Osler's approach to the treatment of typhoid fever see L. G. Stevenson, "Exemplary disease: The typhoid pattern," *J Hist Med* 37 (1982): 159–81.

94. Osler, *Principles and Practice of Medicine*, p. 32–33.

95. Osler wrote that "as an enemy to indiscriminate drugging, I have often been branded as a therapeutic nihilist. . . . I bore this reproach cheerfully, coming, as I knew it, from men who did not appreciate the difference between the giving of medicine and the treatment of disease." See Cushing, *Life of Osler*, p. 866. For a brief discussion of this issue see L. G. Stevenson, "Joseph Dietl, William Osler, and the definition of therapeutic nihilism," in *Festschrift für Erna Lesky zum 70. Geburtstag*, ed. K. Ganziger, M. Scopec, and H. Wyklicky, Vienna, Verlag B. Hollinek, 1981, pp. 149–52. The charge of nihilism proved to be groundless since Osler used a number of single and widely known drugs in his practice. See D. I. Macht, "Osler's prescriptions and materia medica," *Trans Am Ther Soc* 35 (1936): 69–85. This important study of Osler's prescriptions filled at a nearby pharmacy in Baltimore has been recently reprinted in the *Osler Library Newsletter* 76 (June 1994): 1–5.

96. "In the employment of such simple measures of treatment as were proven to be of value, in the intelligent use of rest and massage and other physical methods, especially in the all important treatment of the patient from the mental and human standpoint, Osler was an admirable therapeutist." See Thayer, "The Osler clinic," 103.

97. Osler, "Study of fatal cases," 12. According to Osler, each person had a different constitution and thus reacted differently to all stimuli, including those of disease, making it impossible to place therapeutics on "settled" scientific principles. See William Osler, *Teacher and Student*, Baltimore, J. Murphy & Co., 1892, p. 17.

98. "Imperative drugging is no longer regarded as the chief function of the doctor," Bean, *Osler: Aphorisms*, p. 102. For greater therapeutic activism see A. L. Mason, "Notes on typhoid from 6766 cases admitted to the Boston City Hospital in 1890 and 1891," *Boston Med Surg J* 126 (Apr. 7, 1892): 329–31, 340–42, and 357–59. See also "The treatment of typhoid fever," *Medical News* (Phila.) 61 (Sept. 10, 1892): 302–04.

99. I. B. Yeo, "The antiseptic treatment of typhoid fever," *Lancet* I (Apr. 11, 1891): 811–13 and 865–67, especially p. 866, for the specific poison-antidote reference. For a sum-

mary see *Am J Med Sci* 102 (1891): 77–78. An American view is presented in J. H. Musser, "The occasional danger of antipyretics in typhoid fever," *Am J Med Sci* 104 (1892): 586. For the German experiences with antiseptic agents see also "Naphtalin and typhoid fever," *Am J Med Sci* 98 (1889): 513–14.

100. William Osler, *Counsels and Ideals*, Boston, Houghton, Mifflin & Co., 1908, p. 88. This excerpt is from an address, "Teaching and thinking," that originally appeared in the *Montreal Medical Journal* in 1895.

101. E. Brand, "Ueber den heutigen Stand der Wasserbehandlung des Typhus," *Deutsch Med Wochenschr* 13 (1887): 4–7, 28–31, 45–47, 68–70, 89–90, 128–29, 149–51, 178–80, 217–20. A favorable 1889 report of 36 patients treated with cold baths was reported from France, and the results were reprinted in the section of medicine under the direction of Osler: "The treatment of typhoid fever with cold baths," *Am J Med Sci* 99 (1890): 73. In the United States, Frederick C. Shattuck at the Massachusetts General Hospital also abandoned antiseptics and relied on the cold baths: *Boston Med Surg J* 121 (Sept. 5, 1889): 221–24.

102. The procedure is best described in W. Osler, "The cold-bath treatment of typhoid fever," *Med News* (Phila) 61 (Dec. 3, 1892): 628–31.

103. There was a widespread belief that water had to be renewed, lest it turn infective and become a danger to the attendants. The question of cost was raised in Boston. The decision was that if cold baths did not substantially lower mortality from the disease, their expense could not be justified. See *Boston Med Surg J* 126 (Apr. 7, 1892): 341.

104. Osler, "Cold-bath treatment," 629. "To transfer a patient from a warm bed to a tub at 70°F and to keep him there twenty minutes or longer in spite of his piteous entreaties does seem harsh treatment and the subsequent shivering and blueness look distressing." Osler, *Principles and Practice of Medicine*, p. 35. For background see M. R. Currie, "The rise and demise of fever nursing," *Int Hist Nurs J* 3 (1997): 5–19.

105. "The treatment of typhoid fever," *Boston Med Surg J* 131 (Apr. 14, 1892): 374–75.

106. Hewetson, "Urine and the occurrence of renal complications," 120.

107. J. R. McTavish, "Antipyretic treatment and typhoid fever: 1860–1900," *J Hist Med* 42 (1987): 486–506. Beginning with salicylic acid, discovered in 1874, a veritable flood of new antipyretics descended on hapless practitioners, especially during the early 1880s.

108. Carl A. Wunderlich, *On the Temperature in Diseases, a Manual of Medical Thermometry*, trans. W. B. Woodman, London, New Sydenham Society, 1887, especially p. 433.

109. A. Vogl, "Zur Typhus-Therapie," *Deutsch Med Wochenschr* 14 (Nov. 29, 1888): 983–85 and (Dec. 6, 1888): 1008–11.

110. As one observer recalled, "there was healing in [Osler's] voice. The vocal tone, the facial expression, the chosen word all united to enhance the effect of treatment measures." Farrar, "Osler at Johns Hopkins," 131.

111. According to the hospital's by-laws, adopted in November 1889, visitors were allowed only for one hour, from 4:00 to 5:00 PM, on Tuesdays, Thursdays, Saturdays, and Sundays. See Chesney, *Chronicle*, vol. 1, p. 289.

112. A. B. Ward, "Hospital life," *Scribners' Magazine* 3 (June 1888): 700.

113. Osler, "Cold-bath treatment," 629.

114. McCrae, "Osler and patient," 202. The suggestion "Osler, drop your mask, let us know what you actually think of the situation," is quoted by the hospital's superintendent, Henry Hurd, in describing an emergency. See Hurd, "Some early reminiscences," 214. Osler himself spoke frequently about the virtues of taciturnity and silence.

115. Osler's reports indicate that some patients received between 75 and 120 baths during more extended hospitalizations. See Osler's "Five years' experience," 325.

116. Such multiple injections could be iatrogenic and cause local abscesses or pulmonary

emboli. See "The treatment of typhoid fever by cold baths," *Boston Med Surg J* 106 (June 9, 1892): 583.

117. The original article by H. C. Wood of Philadelphia had appeared in the *Therapeutic Gazette* and was summarized as "Turpentine in typhoid fever," *Am J Med Sci* 104 (1892): 459–60.

118. Osler quoted the description of an eighteenth-century physician, Thomas Huxham: "Now nature sinks apace, the extremities grow cold, . . . the sick become quite insensible and stupid . . . the delirium now ends in a profound coma and that soon in eternal sleep." See Osler, "Study of fatal cases," 14–15.

119. W. Osler, "The problem of typhoid fever in the United States," originally published as a pamphlet in Baltimore, J. Murphy Co., 1899, and reprinted in *Medical News* (NY) 74 (Feb. 25, 1899): 229.

120. The first distinct ulcer was discovered 20 cm from the ileocecal valve, with clean edges with a base on the muscular coat, with another series of such ulcers nearby. Following the autopsy, Councilman showed the specimens at a meeting of the hospital's medical society. Typhoid bacilli had been detected in the spleen, liver, and mesenteric glands, and samples of spleen tissue produced a pure culture. Osler, who was present at the discussion, took the view that the lesions might have been produced during the new attack, which had lasted for exactly three weeks and killed John S. A summary of the findings is also contained in Osler's "Study of fatal cases," 20

121. Osler, "Cold-water baths," 630.

122. Cushing, *Life of Osler*, p. 909.

123. Osler, *Aequanimitas*, p. 159.

124. Ibid., pp. 313–25.

125. Bean, *Osler: Aphorisms*, p. 47.

126. "To do justice to patients, to carry out modern lines of treatment, indeed, to diagnosticate skilfully, require now the assistance of trained laboratory workers who should form part of the staff." See William Osler, *Modern Medicine and Its Theory and Practice*, Philadelphia, Lea Bratner & Co., 1907, p. xxxii. For a recent analysis see J. H. Warner, "The fall and rise of professional mystery: Epistemology, authority and the emergence of laboratory medicine in nineteenth-century America," in *The Laboratory Revolution in Medicine*, ed. A. Cunningham and P. Williams, Cambridge, Cambridge Univ. Press, 1992, pp. 110–41.

127. Osler, *Modern Medicine*, p. xxxiv.

128. N. McCall, "The statue of the Christus Consolator at the Johns Hopkins Hospital: Its acquisition and historic origins," *Johns Hopkins Med J* 151 (1982): 11–19.

129. D. C. Gilman, "Charity and knowledge," in Chesney, *Chronicle*, vol. 1, p. 259.

130. Ibid., p. 263. Before taking a vacation in the summer of 1889, Osler reported on his "stewardship" to Gilman. "The machine works smoothly thanks to your manipulation," he wrote on July 19, 1889. See Cushing, *Life of Osler*, p. 319. For a brief but glowing report see "The most interesting hospital in the world," *The Hospital* 11 (Nov. 28, 1891): 100–01 and (Dec. 5, 1891): 111–12.

131. Aubrey Stanhope was a correspondent for the *New York Herald* who stayed at the Eppendorf Hospital in September 1892. See his dispatch of September 25, 1892, p. 17. I am indebted to Dr. Howard Markel for providing me with these newspaper reports.

132. This patient was simply identified as W. Her clinical history is summarized in C. Sick, "Die Behandlung der Cholera mit intravenöser Kochsalzinfusion," *Jahrb Hamburg Staatskrankenanst* III (1891–92): 107–08. See also Richard J. Evans, *Death in Hamburg, Society and Politics in the Cholera Years 1830–1910*, Oxford, Oxford Univ. Press, 1987, pp. 342–43.

133. A. Kennealy, "Some of the 'cholera streets' in Hamburg," *Scientif Am* 67 (December 1892): 387–88.

134. For basic information about cholera see R. H. Speck, "Cholera," in *The Cambridge World History of Human Disease*, ed. K. F. Kiple, Cambridge, Cambridge Univ. Press, 1993, pp. 642–49. Concerning the origins of this disease, see L. A. McNichol and R. N. Doetsch, "A hypothesis accounting for the origin of pandemic cholera: A retrograde analysis," *Perspect Biol Med* 26 (1983): 547–52.

135. Doris Viersbeck, *Erlebnisse eines Hamburger Dienstmädchens*, Munich, 1907, in Evans, *Death in Hamburg*, p. 346. For further information see Gunnar Stollberg, "Health and illness in German workers' autobiographies for the 19th and early 20th centuries," *Soc Hist Med* 6 (1993): 261–76.

136. E. Hueppe, "Zum persönlichen Gesundheitsschutze und zur Krankenpflege," in Ferdinand Hueppe, *Die Cholera Epidemie in Hamburg 1892*, Berlin, A. Hirschwald, 1893, p. 98.

137. For details see Alfred Grotjahn and Franz Goldmann, *Benefits of the German Sickness Insurance System from the Point of View of Social Hygiene*, Geneva, International Labour Office, 1928.

138. Medical care became a way to alleviate the physical consequences of low wages, unhealthy work, and poor food. For an overview regarding the financing of nineteenth-century German hospitals see R. Spree, "Krankenhausentwicklung und Sozialpolitik in Deutschland während des 19. Jahrhunderts," *Hist Zeitschr* 260 (1995): 75–105. Both Spree and A. Labisch also argue that the main roots of German hospital development and patronage during that century were local welfare schemes: A. Labisch and R. Spree, "Die Kommunalisierung des Krankenwesens in Deutschland während des 19. und 20. Jahrhunderts," *Münch Wissenscht Beiträge* 95 (February 1995): 1–37.

139. Evans, *Death in Hamburg*, 333.

140. Theodor Rumpf, *Lebenserinnerungen*, Bonn, Marens & Webers Verlag, 1925, p. 41.

141. Rumpf was ridiculed because he rode through Hamburg's streets in a small, open hunting carriage pulled by a heavy brown horse and guided by a formally attired livery man. See Max Nonne, *Anfang und Ziel meines Lebens: Erinnerungen*, Hamburg, Hans Christian Verlag, 1972, pp. 264–65.

142. This sequence of events was presented at a meeting of Hamburg's Medical Society on August 30, 1892. See *Deutsch Med Wochenschr* 18 (Sept. 15, 1892): 837–39. It differs in part from the events presented by Evans. See U. Weisser, "Die Cholera in Hamburg 1892: Nachbetrachtungen zur Diagnose der ersten Erkrankungen und zu den Therapieansätzen in den Krankenhäusern," in *Universität Hamburg*, ed. R. Ansorge, Berlin, D. Reimer Verlag, 1994, pp. 85–96.

143. For a description of the bacteriological studies at the Eppendorf, T. Rumpel, "Die bakteriologischen Befunde der Cholera im Jahre 1892," *Jahrb Hamburg Staatskrankenanst* III (1891–92): 49–64.

144. The diagnostic efforts at the Eppendorf have been described by T. M. Rumpf, "Die Diagnose der ersten Cholerafälle in den Staatskrankenanstalten zu Hamburg," *Deutsch Med Wochenschr* 18 (Sept. 22, 1892): 858. See also his report "Die Cholera in den Hamburgischen Krankenanstalten," *Jahrb Hamburg Staatskrankenanst* III (1891–92): 35–49.

145. E. Fraenkel, "Die Cholera in Hamburg," *Deutsch Med Wochenschr* 18 (Sept. 8, 1892): 818–19.

146. Hamburg at this time had a capacity for 3,820 hospital beds. Unfortunately, it took more than a week to assemble this portable lazaretto near the Eppendorf Hospital. Ironically, some hospital physicians believed that these tents, with their expanded sanitary fa-

cilities, proved superior to the much-touted Eppendorf Hospital pavilions with their scarce toilets. F. Hueppe, *Cholera Epidemie*, pp. 55–57.

147. D. R. O'Sullivan, "The Hamburg cholera epidemic, a retrospect of personal observation," *Med Press* (Dec. 14, 1892): 606.

148. Nonne, *Erinnerungen*, p. 96

149. Evans, *Death in Hamburg*, p. 329.

150. A British visitor noted that "the exceptional advantages afforded by this hospital for teaching purposes are entirely wasted, there being no medical school in Hamburg and therefore no students to avail themselves of this wealth of clinical material." See C. W. Thies, "A model hospital," *The Hospital* 11 (Nov. 28, 1891): 106.

151. "The Cholera," *Br Med J* II (Oct. 1, 1892): 759.

152. For a general overview of hospital developments in Germany see A. H. Murken, "Grundzüge des deutschen Krankenhauswesens von 1790 bis 1930 unter Berücksichtigung von Schweizer Vorbildern," *Gesnerus* 39 (1982): 7–45. For an examination of the political and economical issues see A. Labisch, "The role of the hospital in the health policy of the German Social Democratic movement before World War I," *Int J Health Serv* 17 (1987): 279–94.

153. For more details see A. Labisch, "Stadt und Krankenhaus: Das Allgemeine Krankenhaus in der kommunalen Sozial-und Gesundheitspolitik des 19. Jahrhunderts," in *Einem jeden Kranken in einem Hospitale sein eigenes Bett*, ed. A. Labisch and R. Spree, Frankfurt, Campus Verlag, 1996, pp. 253–96.

154. Such a proposal reflects the growing professional authority of physicians such as Curschmann who possessed special expertise in hygiene. See O. Schwartz, "Die hygienischen Aufgaben des Krankenhausarztes," *Deutsch Vierteljahrschr f. öffent Gesundheitspflege* 19 (1887): 147–53.

155. H. Curschmann, "Welchen Einfluss hat die heutige Gesundheitslehre, besonders die neuere Auffassung des Wesens und der Verbreitung der Infectionskrankheiten auf Bau, Einrichtung und Lage der Krankenhäuser?" *Deutsch Vierteljahrschr f. öffent Gesundheitspflege* 21 (1889): 181–203.

156. See the discussion of construction models in *Deutsch Med Wochenschr* 16 (13 Mar. 1890): 225.

157. For a brief historical sketch see G. Uhlmann and U. Weisser, "Grundzüge einer Geschichte des Eppendorfer Krankenhauses," in *100 Jahre Universitäts-Krankenhaus Eppendorf, 1889–1989*, ed. U. Weisser, Tübingen, Attempto Verlag, 1989, pp. 13–62. Additional information and iconography by the same authors is available in *Krankenhausalltag seit der Zeit der Cholera*, Hamburg, Kabel Verlag, 1992.

158. For details and copper engravings see C. J. C. Zimmermann and F. Ruppel, *Das Neue Allgemeine Krankenhaus in Hamburg-Eppendorf*, Berlin, 1892, W. Ernst & Sohn, 1892.

159. J. N. E. Brown, "A comparison between German and American hospital construction," *The Brickbuilder* 22 (April 1913): 73–77. A complete description of the facility can be found in T. Deneke, "Mittheilungen über das Neue Allgemeine Krankenhaus zu Hamburg-Eppendorf," *Deutsch Vierteljahrschrift f. Oeffent. Gesundheitspflege* 20 (1888): 549–88, and 21 (1889): 273–309.

160. W. Milburn, "Modern German hospital construction—II," *J R Inst Br Architects* 19 (Dec. 9, 1911): 97–102.

161. W. Milburn, "Modern German hospital construction-I," *J R Inst Br Architects* 19 (Nov. 25, 1911): 38–39.

162. E. Fraenkel, "Ueber Typhus abdominalis," *Deutsch Med Wochenschr* 12 (7 Jan. 1886): 13–14.

163. Thies, "A model hospital," 106.

164. *Jahrb Hamburg Staatskrankenanst* III (1891–92): VIII; see also Carl Eisenlohr, *Festschrift zur Eröffnung des Neuen Allgemeinen Krankenhauses zu Hamburg-Eppendorf*, Hamburg, Mauke, 1889. Another celebration took place a month later, attended by Curschmann, Virchow, and other prominent leaders of German medicine: *Deutsch Med Wochenschr* 15 (18 July 1889): 600.

165. Such scenes were repeated in hospital wards at the St. Georg and were widely reported. One volunteer nurse recalled that "in the large, airy rooms, there lay, in bed after bed in a row the poor patients, here contorted in powerful muscular convulsions, there begging the nurse for a bedpan or a drink; some had violent attacks of vomiting and befouled the bed and the floor in a nauseating manner; others lay in their last moments, a loud death-rattle in their throats, and many passed on in my very presence." Evans, *Death in Hamburg*, p. 332.

166. T. M. Rumpf, "Die sekundären Krankheitsprocesse der Cholera," *Jahrb Hamburg Staatskrankenanst* III (1891–92): 65–82.

167. For a brief biographical sketch see C. E. Dolman, "Koch, Robert," *Dict Scientif Biogr* VII (1973): 420–35. A recent biography is Thomas D. Brock, *Robert Koch, a Life in Medicine and Bacteriology*, Madison, WI, Science Tech. Pub., 1988, especially pp. 140–68.

168. H. Mochmann and W. Kohler, "The clarification of the etiology of Asiatic cholera by the German Cholera Commission under the direction of Robert Koch in the year 1883," *Indian J Publ Health* 27 (January–March 1893): 6–20.

169. R. Koch, "First conference for discussion of the cholera question," [1884], in *Essays of Robert Koch*, trans. K. C. Carter, Westport, CT, Greenwood Press, 1987, p. 155. See also W. Coleman, "Koch's comma bacillus: The first year," *Bull Hist Med* 61 (1987): 315–42.

170. The political and economic context of German bacteriology is succinctly described in Evans, *Death in Hamburg*, pp. 256–84.

171. W. Osler, "Notes of a visit to European medical centers," *Arch Med* 12 (1884): 170. See J. Harwood, "Institutional innovation in fin de siècle Germany," *Br J Hist Sci* 27 (1994): 197–211.

172. E. Shils, "The power of the state and the dignity of academic calling in Imperial Germany," *Minerva* 9 (1973): 571–632, and R. Paul, "German academic science and the mandarin ethos, 1850–1880," *Br J Hist Sci*, 17 (1984): 1–29.

173. For a useful biographical sketch see C. E. Dolman, "Pettenkofer, Max Josef von," *Dict Scientif Biogr* X (1974): 556–63. More information can be found in H. Breyer, *Max von Pettenkofer: Arzt im Vorfeld der Krankheit*, Leipzig, Hirzel, 1980.

174. The topic is treated in great detail in Evans, *Death in Hamburg*, especially pp. 1–179.

175. A. S. Evans, "Pettenkofer revisited," *Yale J Biol Med* 46 (1973): 161–76. The classic biography of Virchow is Erwin H. Ackerknecht, *Rudolf Virchow: Doctor, Statesman, Anthropologist*, Madison, Wis., Univ. of Wisconsin Press, 1953.

176. Ferdinand Hueppe, who attended patients at the Eppendorf Hospital during the epidemic, was also a supporter of Pettenkoffer's ideas. Ironically, he had been an early assistant of Koch's at the Imperial Health Department in Berlin during the early 1880s. See "Professor Hueppe on cholera," *Br Med J* I (Mar. 11, 1893): 540.

177. For a view of the relationship between Virchow and Koch see H. U. Lammel, "Virchow contra Koch? Neue Untersuchungen zu einer alten Streitfrage," *Charité Ann* 2 (1982): 112–20. For more details, see Byron A. Boyd, *Rudolf Virchow: The Scientist as Citizen*, New York, Garland, 1991.

178. A report about the suspected pollution of Hamburg's water supplies with the

Eberth's bacillus was presented by Curschmann on December 6, 1887, at a session of the local medical society. *Deutsch Med Wochenschr* 14 (3 May 1888): 361–62.

179. For a comparative overview of the political and social consequences of cholera see R. J. Evans, "Epidemics and revolutions: Cholera in nineteenth-century Europe," in *Epidemics and Ideas*, ed. T. Ranger and P. Slack, Cambridge, Cambridge Univ. Press, 1992, pp. 149–73.

180. Rumpf, *Lebenserinnerungen*, p. 43. The story and the details of Koch's visit to Hamburg are described in Evans, *Death in Hamburg*, pp. 311–14.

181. Quoted in Evans, *Death in Hamburg*, p. 313.

182. "The condition of the profession in Germany," *Lancet* I (May 25, 1889): 1049–50. For details, see C. Huerkamp, "The making of the modern medical profession, 1800–1914: Prussian doctors in the 19th century," in *German Professions, 1800–1950*, ed. G. Cocks and K. H. Jarausch, New York, Oxford Univ. Press, 1990, pp. 66–84, and G. B. Risse, "Patients and their healers: Historical studies in health care," in *Who Decides? Conflicts and Rights in Health Care*, ed. N. K. Bell, Clifton, NJ, Humana Press, 1982, pp. 27–45, and U. Frevert, "Professional medicine and the working classes in Imperial Germany," *J Contemp Hist* 20 (1985): 637–58.

183. P. Weindling, "Bourgeois values, doctors, and the state: The professionalization of medicine in Germany 1848–1933," in *The German Bourgeoisie*, ed. D. Blackbourn and R. J. Evans, London, Routledge, 1991, pp. 198–223, and M. H. Kater, "Professionalization and socialization of physicians in Wilhelmine and Weimar Germany," *J Contemp Hist* 20 (1985): 677–701.

184. See "Defective practical teaching in Germany," *Lancet* II (Nov. 2, 1889): 920, and Paul Güterbock, *Die englischen Krankenhäuser im Vergleich mit den deutschen Hospitälern*, Berlin, A. Hirschwald, 1883. A review of this book can be found in *Berliner Klin Wochenschr* 20 (July 9, 1883): 431.

185. One example were the Kenealy sisters, Henrietta and Annesley, who had offered their services to Rumpf by telegram. The director promptly replied that if they could speak some German they were quite welcome. Both wrote for the *British Medical Journal*: "In the cholera wards at Hamburg," *Br Med J* II (Sept. 17, 1892): 654.

186. For a copy of the rules approved by Hamburg's senate in January 1888 see "Aerztliche Hausordnung für das Neue Allgemeine Krankenhaus," *Jahrb Hamburg Staatskrankenanst* I (1889): xi–xxxi.

187. For a historical perspective on German nursing see Anna Sticker, *Die Entstehung der neuzeitlichen Krankenpflege*, Stuttgart, Kohlhammer, 1960, that covers the period from the early 1800s to 1850, and Claudia Bischoff, *Frauen in der Krankenpflege. Zur Entwicklung von Frauenrolle und Frauenberufstätigkeit im 19. und 20. Jahrhundert*, Frankfurt, Campus Verlag, 1984.

188. As reported in *Deutsch Med Wochenschr* 14 (Mar. 29, 1888): 257–58, there were officially only 8,271 nurses in Germany, with 4,305 identified as brothers and sisters belonging to Catholic orders or congregations, another 2,429 Protestant Deaconess sisters and brothers, and 805 lay male and female nurses.

189. For details see Eva-Cornelia Hummel, *Krankenpflege im Umbruch (1876–1914)*, Freiburg, Schulz Verlag, 1986, especially pp. 57–65. The author reveals that the number of German nurses nearly doubled between 1887 and 1898, largely among the nondenominational lay groups.

190. At the time, the order had 60 establishments with a total of 6,000 members throughout the world. For a summary see "The work of the Deaconesses in Germany" in *Hospitals, Dispensaries and Nursing*, ed. J. S. Billings and H. M. Hurd, Baltimore, Johns Hopkins Univ. Press, 1894, pp. 477–80.

191. For details see Irene Schuessler Poplin, "A Study of the Kaiserswerth Deaconess Institute's Nurse Training School in 1850–1851: Purposes and Curriculum," Ph.D. diss., Univ. of Texas, 1988.

192. I. S. Poplin, "Nursing uniforms: Romantic idea, functional attire, or instrument of social change?" *Nurs Hist Rev* 2 (1994): 153–67.

193. See Anna Sticker, *Agnes Krell*, Wuppertal, Aussaat, 1977, especially pp. 10–13.

194. W. Russell, "Some practical results of the investigation of cholera in Germany," *Edinb Med J* 82 (1892–93): 521–25.

195. Most of these observations were made by E. Hueppe, "Krankenpflege," pp. 104–07.

196. E. Ratjen, "Bericht über die Choleraerkrankungen im Marienkrankenhause in Hamburg," *Deutsch Med Wochenschr* 19 (1893): 12.

197. E. Hueppe, "Krankenpflege," p. 117. Although the patient's voice was seldom recorded in this period, a number of autobiographies from workers provide useful glimpses of German hospital life at the turn of the century: B. Elkeles, "Das Krankenhaus um die Wende vom 19. zum 20, Jahrhundert aus der Sicht seiner Patienten," *Hist Hospitalium* 17 (1986–87): 89–105.

198. E. Hueppe, "Krankenpflege," pp. 57–58.

199. Such dramatic descriptions are taken from the accounts of Stanhope in the *New York Herald* in September 1892. Stanhope was in the Eppendorf for about 10 days following Erika's hospitalization. See especially "Night of horror in the death ward," Sept. 23, 1892, p. 7.

200. Evans, *Death in Hamburg*, p. 332.

201. Kenealy, "In the cholera wards," 654.

202. B. Elkeles, "Die schweigsame Welt von Arzt und Patient. Einwilligung und Aufklärung in der Arzt-Patienten-Beziehung des 19. und frühen 20. Jahrhunderts," *Med Gesell Geschichte* 8 (1989): 63–91, and Risse, "Patients and their healers," pp. 38–41.

203. W. Russell, "Cholera in Germany," *Edinb Med J* 82 (1892–93): 525.

204. For a review see N. Howard-Jones, "Cholera therapy in the nineteenth century," *J Hist Med* 27 (1972): 373–95, and C. C. J. Carpenter, "Treatment of cholera—tradition and authority versus science, reason, and humanity," *Johns Hopkins Med J* 139 (1976): 153–62.

205. W. F. Bynum, "Chemical structure and pharmacological action: A chapter in the history of 19th-century molecular pharmacology," *Bull Hist Med* 44 (1970): 518–38.

206. F. Reiche and M. Wilckens, "Die therapeutischen Bestrebungen während der Choleraepidemie 1892," *Jahrb Hamburg Staatskrankenanst* III (1891–92): 140–52. See also Weisser, "Die Cholera in 1892," 96–109. The enterotoxin was isolated only in the twentieth century: R. A. Finkelstein, "Cholera enterotoxin (choleragen): A historical perspective," in *Cholera*, ed. D. Barua and W. B. Greenough, New York, Plenum Med. Book Co., 1992, pp. 155–87.

207. E. Klebs, "Zur Pathologie und Therapie der Cholera Asiatica," *Deutsch Med Wochenschr* 18 (Oct. 27, 1892): 975–78 and (Nov. 3, 1892): 999–1003.

208. C. Manchot, "Ueber die Behandlung der Cholera mit dem Klebs'schen Anticholerin," *Deutsch Med Wochenschr* 18 (Nov. 11, 1892): 1050–52 and F. Reiche, "The cholera in Hamburg in 1892," *Am J Med Sci* 105 (February 1893): 118. See also the editorial "The limitations of bacteriological therapeutics," *Ther Gazette* 15 (June 1891): 397.

209. A. von Genersich, "The complete washing-out of the intestinal tract as a treatment for cholera and allied conditions," *Lancet* 2 (Oct. 14, 1893): 926–27. William Osler also referred to Cantani's approach. See "Notes on the diagnosis and treatment of cholera," *Med News* (Phila) 61 (Sept. 10, 1892): 290–91.

210. T. M. Rumpf, "Die Behandlung der Cholera im Neuen Allgemeinen Krankenhause zu Hamburg," *Deutsch Med Wochenschr* 18 (1892): 877–79. See also D. D. Stewart, "The prevention and treatment of cholera by naphthols," *Am J Med Sci* 105 (1893): 388–93. For an overview see E. Hickel, "Das Kaiserliche Gesundheitsamt (Imperial Health Office) and the chemical industry in Germany during the Second Empire: Partners or adversaries?" in *Drugs and Narcotics in History*, ed. R. Porter and M. Teich, Cambridge, Cambridge Univ. Press, 1995, pp. 97–113.

211. F. Hueppe, *Cholera Epidemie*, pp. 95–96. See also "Professor Hueppe on cholera," *Br Med J* 1 (Mar 11, 1893): 540–41.

212. Nonne, *Erinnerungen*, p. 97

213. Evans, *Death in Hamburg*, p. 336.

214. R. Kutner, "Die subcutane und intravenöse Infusion bei der Cholerabehandlung," *Deutsch Med Wochenschr* 18 (Sept. 1, 1892): 794–95. See also Osler, *Principles and Practice of Medicine*, p. 124.

215. See J. E. Cosnett, "The origins of intravenous fluid therapy," *Lancet* 1 (April 1989): 768–71.

216. As one British observer, T. W. Hime of Bradford, wrote: "undoubtedly the transfusion is like the rope thrown to the drowning man: it enables him to be saved from his immediate peril." "The cholera in Hamburg," *Br Med J* II (Oct. 15, 1892): 865.

217. Kutner, "Cholerabehandlung," *Deutsch Med Wochenschr* 18 (Sept. 1, 1892): 795.

218. Russell, "Cholera in Germany."

219. Scipione Riva-Rocci's sphygmomanometer became available only in the late 1890s.

220. For a summary see D. Heyse, "Mitteilungen zur Choleratherapie," *Deutsch Med Wochenschr* 18 (Nov. 24, 1892): 1074–77. See also Weisser, "Die Cholera in 1892," 96–109.

221. As described by the Kenealy sisters in "In the cholera wards," 710.

222. See T. Rumpf, "Die sekundären Krankheitsprocesse der Cholera," *Jahrb Hamburg Staatskrankenanst* III (1891–92): 65–82.

223. Discussions were held among the leading Hamburg hospital physicians at a meeting of the Hamburg Medical Club on September 30, 1892, *Deutsch Med Wochenschr* 18 (Oct. 6, 1892): 906–08.

224. Based in part on the Eppendorf experience, British experts recommended the use of makeshift facilities—so-called cholera camps—in parks and other suitable open spaces if an epidemic were to break out. G. A. Heron, "Cholera from an urban point of view," *Lancet* I (May 27, 1893): 1246–48.

225. *New York Herald*, Sept. 24, 1892, p. 7; Sept. 25, p. 17; Sept. 28, p. 9; and Sept. 29, p. 9. Stanhope's dare was severely criticized in several German newspapers.

226. Evans, *Death in Hamburg*, pp. 494–96.

227. For a report of the Munich meeting see Max von Pettenkofer, "On cholera, with reference to the recent epidemic in Hamburg," *Lancet* II (1892): 1182–85, and R. H. Firth, "Some reflections upon the more recently expressed views of von Pettenkofer concerning the causation of cholera," *Practitioner* 50 (1893): 221–27. See also Emmerich's comments in *Deutsch Med Wochenschr* 18 (Dec. 15, 1892): 1153–55. For an excellent summary see Evans, "Pettenkofer's last stand," *Death in Hamburg*, pp. 490–507. Sources for Pettenkofer are presented in Ellen Jahn, *Die Cholera in Medizin und Pharmazie im Zeitalter des Hygienikers Max von Pettenkofer*, Stuttgart, Steiner, 1994.

228. A letter to the editor of the *Lancet* a year later sought to clarify the role of Koch's comma bacillus in the genesis of cholera, questioning the (as he put it) fin de siècle finality of the bacteriological findings as opposed to the more contextual and environmental considerations so dear to Virchow and other social reformers. "Means directed against bacilli—quarantine, notification, and protective inoculations—may be good, but sanitary

reforms which shall make the soil safe against invasion by raising the standard of comfort and health are better." W. J. Collins, "What is the criterion of cholera?" *Lancet* II (Sept. 30, 1893): 837–38.

229. F. Hueppe, *Cholera epidemie*, p. 53.

230. Regarding the linkage between drinking water and cholera see Koch's conclusions, dated May 26, 1893: R. Koch, "Wasserfiltration und Cholera," *Zeitschr f. Hygiene u. Infektionskrankheiten* 14 (1893): 393–426.

231. T. Rumpf, "Die Gründung eines Schwestern-Vereins für die Hamburgischen Staatskrankenanstalten," *Jahrb Hamb Staatskrankenanstalten* 4, pt. 2 (1893–94): 3–6.

232. As one author declared, "it would be impossible to efficiently cope with cholera emergencies without properly trained nurses in sufficient numbers." Heron, "Cholera," p. 1247.

233. R. Koch, "Ueber den augenblicklichen Stand der bakteriologischen Choleradiagnose," *Zeitschr Hyg Infektionskrankheiten* 14 (1893): 319–38, and T. Rumpel, "Die bakteriologischen Befunde der Cholera im Jahre 1892."

234. "Although we know that cholera is caused by bacilli, we are no more able to cure it than we were before. . . . If one looks at these discoveries only from the perspective of the practicing physician, as yet there are no visible uses," R. Koch, "The cholera question," p. 169.

235. "The cholera in Hamburg," *Medical News* (Phila) 61 (Nov. 5, 1892): 524.

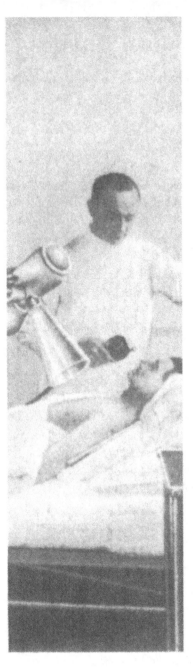

9

MAIN STREET'S CIVIC PRIDE

The American General Hospital as Professional Workshop

The last thirty years have witnessed the most spectacular building of hospitals by a hopeful people that has ever taken place in the world's history. Instead of being dreaded, hospitals are now looked at with confidence and even affection as places wherein most can be done to cure disease and alleviate suffering.

Nathaniel W. Faxon, 1930[1]

An automobile accident in 1930

On June 14, 1930, at exactly 4:15 PM, Paula S. of Madison, Wisconsin, was brought into the Emergency Room of Madison General Hospital (MGH) by Carl L., a resident in the nearby town of De Forest. This young man was later identified as the driver of a brand-new Ford sedan that had struck the middle-aged woman sideways on Roth Street. The accident had occurred near the Oscar Mayer meatpacking plant in the northeastern part of the city earlier that Saturday afternoon as she was walking along the road returning to her home. According to the police report, Carl had two passengers, Mr. and Mrs. Clarence N. of Waunakee. When she was hit, Paula was returning from the Pierre Lorillard Company's tobacco warehouse that had employed her sporadically for the past 16 years. Newspapers reported that Saturday had been a warm day, with temperatures in the high 70s and thundershowers. Winter had suddenly turned into summer without much of a transition, and 10,000 people took advantage of the summery weather to attend the First Wisconsin Air Show at the Royal Airport, making city traffic worse than usual.[2]

In Madison at this time, all injured patients were being admitted to MGH because the University of Wisconsin Hospital did not take emergency cases. Accidents comprised nearly 10% of all hospital admissions in the city, placing MGH—an independent (nonsectarian) private institution—in a financially advantageous position, with a busy emergency room. Its nearest competitors in the city were St. Mary's Hospital, a Catholic institution, with 125 beds and a 96% occupancy rate, followed by Methodist Hospital, with 110 beds and a 71% occupancy rate. With 154 beds distributed among 66 private rooms and 6 solarium wards, MGH, however, reported only a 59% occupancy rate in 1930.[3] The city's directory boasted that, with a total of 1,013 hospital beds, Madison's medical facilities were among the best in the country, serving not only the metropolis but all of south central Wisconsin.[4]

Clutching her bloodstained head cap, "Pauline," the petite patient of Austrian nationality—she was only about five feet tall—appeared somewhat confused and dizzy as she was carried into the Emergency Room on a cart. Mixing English and German words, she complained of tenderness over her right hip extending to the right side of the abdomen. She also had multiple bruises and pain over the right side of the chest. A laceration at the right side of her head and forehead was causing a bad headache. More severe were her lumbar stiffness and back pain. At MGH, newcomers such as Paula encountered well-lit rooms fully equipped with diagnostic instruments, drugs, and supplies in nearby cabinets. The carefully planned facilities were close to the X-ray department and operating rooms. Blood transfusion equipment was on hand, conveniently located near the ambulance entrance, together with a list of universal donors from among members of the hospital staff. Admitting clerks, physicians, interns, and orderlies on call were urged to follow institutional checklists designed to obtain all pertinent information relative to injured persons, including the names and addresses of relatives. Those admitted also had to be checked for excessive alcohol consumption and mental status. To assist the police, witnesses, the time, place, and nature of accidents, and details about the persons involved needed to be ascertained. In 1930, statistics indicated that accident cases constituted nearly 23% of all hospital deaths.

On admission, Paula claimed to be 44 years of age; she was actually 48 but no longer celebrated her birthdays. Originally from the town of Vojnik near Zagreb in Croatia, she had emigrated as a young woman with her family to Milwaukee. Following her marriage to Victor S., another immigrant from Prague, Paula and her husband went to live in Minnesota before coming to Madison after 1914. At the time of the accident, she had recently obtained a divorce and was living alone with her 12-year-old son, Peter.[5] Her current job was probably menial, sorting and grading tobacco leaves delivered by local farmers.[6]

Routinely, the first person to deal with patients admitted to the Emergency Room was an intern on call. In Paula's case, Dr. Michael P. Ohlsen from Chicago, who was two weeks away from completing his internship, was assigned to the case. Indeed, MGH had a full complement of four interns, all completing one year of hospital duty. Seeking guidance from their mentors, the interns were said to be well trained in the medical sciences but lacking in the "art" of medicine.[7] They received a meager salary of $50 per month and were widely considered a cheap and thus welcome source of labor.

Paula, who spoke English with a noticeable German accent, was next seen by the staff physician "on service." Dr. Thomas W. Tormey was a surgeon and one of the hospital's attending physicians. Ten years earlier, he had been the institution's first chief of the medical staff. He and his brother, Albert, were considered the hospital's leading surgeons. As in organizational and financial matters, medical practitioners at this time easily controlled their relationship with patients, a relationship built upon trust and accountability. Physicians considered patients to be child-like, dependent, and ignorant of science, and expected them to be respectful and deferential and to comply with physicians' orders without question. Practitioners earned the confidence of the sick through a display of scientific know-how and dazzling technology instead of quaint exchanges of "pleasantries" and what they called the "human touch."[8] Surgeons such as Tormey were willing to assume the sympathetic, paternalistic role of "father knows best" while displaying the necessary "affective neutrality" consonant with scientific objectivity, thus sharply distancing themselves from the more emotional approach they thought characteristic of quacks and fringe healers.

Shaping this new relationship were the settings in which the encounters between patients and physicians took place. Medical care had shifted since the early 1900s to offices and hospitals, and neither party shared previous cultural meanings and spaces for the development of personal bonds. "You are given but little occasion to feel that you are in any other respect regarded as a human entity," complained one contemporary hospital patient, adding that "you are merely a patient, known in hospital parlance by the number on the door of your room."[9] Such personal estrangement had already led to more impersonal bureaucratic relationships in which the outcome and the financial bottom line played an increasingly great role. The famous and rarely followed dictum "The secret of the care of the patient is in caring for the patient" was coined at the time precisely in response to the depersonalizing aspects of American hospital practice.[10]

Ohlsen, supervised by Tormey, took a brief history and performed a physical examination of the patient. Paula seemed lucid but complained of pain. Her pulse was rather weak, her blood pressure 120/72. A scalp wound was located over the right side of her forehead, and she also had a bruised cheek. The neck was normal, including the thyroid gland, but the chest showed multiple bruises and probable fractures from the sixth rib down. The lungs were normal, and there were no rales. The heart tones disclosed no murmurs. Paula's abdomen displayed no scars, and on palpation, Ohlsen detected no masses. There was, however, significant tenderness over the right hip extending to the right side of the abdomen, with discoloration but no rigidity. A neurological exam was normal. A large bruise discolored the right thigh, but Paula was able to move her legs. A urine specimen contained no blood. Given her complaints, the initial treatment consisted of administering one-quarter of a grain of morphine subcutaneously. Ohlsen debrided, cleaned, and sutured the scalp wound and placed a rubber brace on it. Paula also received 500 cc of normal saline intravenously and a shot of tetanus antitoxin. Her injured cheek was cleansed with the application of a solution of 5% mercurochrome. Then Ohlsen and Frank A. Gruesen, another intern, ordered X-rays of the skull, chest, and pelvis.

Paula was therefore taken to MGH's new diagnostic department, where X-ray and laboratory work could easily be performed. In 1930, a total of 169 patients had already been cared for there.[11] Radiologists now played a prominent role in hospital care. Although older practitioners continued to be skeptical about the value of X-rays in the diagnosis and treatment of disease, the American Medical Association (AMA) had recently launched efforts to standardize radiology departments. This work could not be left to mere technicians. The AMA stated that, even for routine examinations, the radiologist needed to interact personally with the patient. The new model envisioned that radiologists would be specialists and consultants, recruited from a pool of versatile general practitioners. However, this newly sanctioned image and status created tensions as hospital boards sought to enhance the profits from their X-ray services by hiring young, inexperienced individuals at low salaries.[12] In Madison, the costs of MGH's new laboratory addition and equipment forced the hospital administration to raise the rates for rooms and operating services.

Somewhat later, the radiological reports concerning Paula, signed by the hospital's radiologist, Dr. Lawrence Littig, confirmed some of the clinical impressions. The skull films showed a small linear fracture, two inches long, in the midregion of the right parietal bone, but fortunately, no depression was noted. The chest X-ray disclosed fractures, extending on the right side from the 4th to the 12th rib, with some pleural damage and the production of a small amount of subcutaneous emphysema in the right axillary region. Paula's pelvis also showed a chipped fracture of the right iliac crest.[13] The most serious lesion was observed in the spine: a compressed fracture of the first lumbar vertebral body. This was the most common lower spine injury, an increasingly frequent consequence of industrial and automobile accidents.[14] In Paula's case, only the vertebral body was involved. As Paula returned to the Emergency Room for further disposition, her blood pressure had fallen dangerously to 70/48. She immediately received half an ampule of coramine and was kept under close observation. Fear of accident complications such as traumatic shock or loss of consciousness often delayed or canceled radiological examinations.

In injury cases, nurses routinely gave antitetanus injections as part of a detailed protocol. The issue of standardized management or *treadmill medical practice*, especially involving the use of drugs, was still vigorously debated at this time. Doctors feared that any regimen would hamper their freedom to individualize treatments based on professional assessments involving special knowledge of the particular patient. Mental factors were believed to foil all standardization efforts. On the other side of this discussion were accusations of abuse, polypharmacy, and the continued employment of useless remedies still stocked in hospital pharmacies. Institutional formularies generated similar discussions about individualizing versus standardizing therapies.

In emergency care, however, certain precautionary treatments were essential, and they needed to be instituted well before a final diagnosis became available.[15] For the first 24 hours, head injuries demanded periodic measurements—every two hours—of blood pressure, pulse, respiration and pupil size. In addition, an ice cap was placed on Paula's head that was immobilized between two sandbags. For the rib fractures, expected to heal spontaneously in about five weeks, the intern applied adhesive plaster straps around the whole chest to minimize the pain due to pleural and muscular involvement. As she lay on a gurney waiting for transfer to a room, Paula must have wondered about her future. Was full recovery possible? How would she pay for all her care?

"A public undertaking": American hospitals after 1900[16]

At the time Paula was being attended to in MGH's Emergency Room, private voluntary hospitals had become firmly entrenched in American communities. Indeed, nearly 65% of all births and half of all deaths occurred within their walls. According to U.S. Census Bureau estimates, Wisconsin had the best ratio of population to hospital beds in America—154—with the national average being around 270.[17] The American hospital, so recently a partially medicalized, mostly charitable shelter, had been rapidly transformed into an institution organized on scientific and business principles. This transformation had markedly accelerated after 1900, only to be temporarily halted in the late 1910s as the United States entered World War I. Dramatic changes in mission, patronage, staff, patients, and treatments could be seen as efforts to cope with shifting health conditions and profound social and economic changes. Recovery and cure were the goals, to be achieved on the basis of scientific principles by a cadre of professional nurses and physicians with the assistance of increasing medical technology. In the process, American hospitals became institutions of first resort, not only for the poor, but also for members of the rapidly expanding middle and upper classes of society who became ill and were willing to pay for their care. Endowed with a favorable new image, hospitals were henceforth praised as monuments to humanity and science.[18]

Since the 1870s, America's industrializing cities had fostered an ecology of disease influenced by social factors such as rapid growth and overcrowding. New opportunities in the industrializing centers of the country contributed to the shift from farm to city and the arrival of successive waves of immigrants. Recurrent epidemics of infectious diseases and trauma associated with manufacturing, transportation, and crime afflicted vast sectors of the public. In fact, by 1900, trauma accounted for 75% of the most common surgical diagnoses. At that time, nearly 40% of the population was already urban, composed of a large number of single individuals such as our previously discussed patient, John S. of Baltimore. Many were travelers and immigrants. This transient, uprooted population needed attention and care for illness. Without family, community, or financial means for home care, they turned to institutional care. For this process to include middle-class individuals who could pay for their care and thus financially support hospitals, institutions needed to be transformed into appealing home substitutes where routine medical and surgical care could be delivered with efficiency and success. As the medicalization of society progressed, hospitals were selected as the primary locus for fighting acute and potentially curable conditions. This status contrasted sharply with the previous emphasis on the chronic and incurable conditions linked to charity and dependency, not rehabilitation. Moreover, human experiences such as birth, childhood, old age, and death also became hospital-bound, leading to the development of separate facilities in obstetrics, pediatrics, surgery, and medicine.[19]

America's cultural diversity was critical in constructing the voluntary hospital's new mission. Religious rivalries and charitable goals remained but were deemphasized in favor of medical ones. To be sure, private religious institutions retained the notion that the hospital symbolized hope and pious benevolence based on the Scriptures. However, the welfare role narrowed at the expense of physical rehabilitation in a cultural atmosphere that sought to foster personal responsibility and economic self-reliance. Most new voluntary hospital foundations in America came to be components of local networks of prominent and influential citizens. Faced with waves of new and recently arrived immigrants, many religious, ethnic, and national communities sought to provide welcome settings to protect the newcomers' cultural identity. Among these facilities were churches, schools, service clubs, mutual aid societies, and hospitals. Much more than temporary shelters, American voluntary hospitals became sources of civic pride, embodiments of local philanthropy, and displays of economic power. Sponsors were determined to assist members in need and then encourage them to realize their individual potential.

A hospital's social space contributed to a community's identity, unity, stability, and security. Framed narrowly for a given constituency, volunteer service in such establishments came to be seen as both a charitable and a civil duty. As a result of such community linkages, hospitals acquired a strong sense of institutional personality and autonomy. Their "inward vision" was trained solely on their own administrative and financial needs, priorities of the medical and nursing staffs, and expectations of patients. "Outward glances" addressing broader community issues of public health and education remained sporadic in spite of periodic efforts that turned out to be mostly public relations ploys. Indeed, given their private character, there was little or no incentive for individual hospitals to cooperate with other local or regional institutions. A hospital ethic of self-sufficiency and competition usually energized its corporate life and shaped its business practices.[20]

Another powerful component of the hospital's new mission was the ideology of science. America's growing belief in the power and progressivism of science aided the hospital's goal of aggressive physical intervention and the expectation of total recovery. Public expectations about the hospital's healing capacities had already been changing, especially the promise of surgical success based on antiseptic and aseptic methods. New skills and abilities to penetrate bodily cavities such as the chest and abdomen vastly increased the scope of surgical interventions. Appendectomies, removal of tonsils and adenoids, and, later, caesarean sections constituted a sizable percentage of admissions. The promise of bacteriology in diagnosis and treatment suggested changing criteria for admission. Hospitalization at earlier stages of illness now made sense instead of waiting until the bitter end when death was near.

The new health challenges and caring needs were thus eagerly met in America by a vast decentralized system of private, voluntary hospitals, all competing for resources within their own constituencies and communities. This panorama reflected the nation's laissez-faire capitalist economy and a culture focused on local initiatives to solve problems. Indeed, local political and corporate leaders such as municipal officials and businessmen became the main sources of hospital patronage and sponsorship, followed by religious orders, ethnic groups, and women's groups, along with the assistance of a growing and increasingly powerful medical profession. Hospital building and provision conferred prestige on the sponsors.[21]

The American quest for paying patients brought significant changes to the hospital's physical plant. Following acceptance of the germ theory of disease, there was no further need for pavilion-type hospitals. Fresh air and constant ventilation were now seen as less critical than the use of chemical disinfectants and the isolation of contagious patients. Given the competition for urban space, new and remodeled buildings were compact and multistoried. In the name of institutional efficiency and decreased maintenance costs, architects went back to design vertically expanded monoblocks, even high-rise buildings, taking advantage of developments in steel construction. A basic pattern was a six- or seven-story structure with a basement containing X-ray and storage facilities, a laundry, and a kitchen. The first floor was reserved for administration and laboratories, even outpatient clinics, and the second and third floors featured the medical wards. The fourth and fifth floors were reserved for surgical wards and operating rooms, and the sixth floor contained obstetric and pediatric units. The top level usually had quarters for house staff and nurses on call. By the 1920s, the era of the big high-rise hospital was at hand, pioneered in the United States, the land of skyscrapers. The designs of the period sought to reproduce the eighteenth-century block hospital, often stacking a series of Nightingale pavilions on top of each other.[22] They were arranged like medieval cross-shaped buildings: four separate arms connected to a central core or tower containing stairs and elevators. The importance of efficiency seemed to transform the hospital into a recovery factory.[23]

Like modern homes, hospitals took advantage of new standards of construction and the desire for more privacy. Most wards were converted into single and double rooms.[24] Kitchens were enlarged, and parlors and solariums were lavishly outfitted for socializing convalescents. To ensure rest and comfort, the interiors were equipped with central heating, ventilation, and cooling. Emphasis on hygiene created good housekeeping and laundry services, with floor and wall materials designed to facilitate cleanliness. Glistening operating and delivery rooms and a gigantic steam sterilizer signaled progressiveness and a determination to guarantee aseptic surgery. Prodded by the demands of medical staffs and patients, hospitals also followed the technological imperative of providing state-of-the-art laboratory facilities for the examination of bodily fluids and tissues, as well as purchasing new diagnostic devices and machines such as X-ray and electrocardiography machines.[25] Indeed, technology was instrumental in providing the broad range of services envisioned by an institution caring for all sectors of the population while also widening the distance between patients and their caregivers.[26]

A troika composed of a board of trustees or directors, a professional medical staff, and an administration governed private voluntary institutions such as MGH. Volunteer trustees represented the sponsoring community and handled development, fiscal matters, and community relations. Generally leaders in banking and manufacturing, the trustees considered institutional growth as its own reward. Such activities conferred an aura of charity, prestige, and social status on all involved in this work. The medical staff was responsible for all professional affairs and issues related to the delivery of medical care, including the quality of their services. Members were autonomous and usually enjoyed working in hospitals. This setting allowed physicians to employ new technology and satisfy the demands of their patients while acquiring greater clinical experience and specialization. Trustees and doctors were separated by what was dubbed the "gauze curtain," a barrier between the worlds of politics and healing that prevented linkages between the costs and quality of care but led to constant budget overruns and demands for new capital.[27]

Finally, the third leg, which increasingly bridged the gap between the trustees and physicians, were the administrative officers emerging from America's managerial revolution. Competition for patients and the need for larger capital expenditures, especially in the 1920s, demanded professional business skills. Charged with management issues, including finance, maintenance, and auxiliary personnel, a new position of superintendent or administrator became necessary as hospitals became complex and bureaucratized. In time, this third locus of power grew at the expense of both trustees and medical staffs, replacing the traditional gauze curtain with an expanding layer of financial accountability and planning. Administrators took control of key hospital functions dealing with purchasing, supplies, and the hiring of nonmedical personnel. This development was aided by organized efforts to standardize numerous hospital functions and improve efficiency.[28]

Voluntary American hospitals were indeed economic hybrids, proclaiming a charitable mission while operating like a business. They generated income from patients and made capital investments based on donations, endowments, and private gifts. Given their perceived need to attract more paying patients, hospitals' appetite for capital was voracious and constant, fueled by the development, maintenance, remodeling, or expansion of existing physical plants and the updating of medical technology. In spite of higher construction costs, voluntary hospitals tended to overbuild in anticipation of expected demands and lucrative admissions. New space and equipment, in turn, required additional staff. If the anticipated demand failed to materialize, the administrators struggled with chronic low occupancy rates. Room charges had to be increased, while hospital workers received lower wages. Since traditional sources of funding—endowments and donations—became insufficient, the push was on for even more revenue from paying patients. Like other corporate structures, voluntary hospitals experienced classic boom-and-bust cycles. During the latter, they frequently requested government aid—subsidies or land leases—to fulfill their charitable obligations. In 1930, hospitals represented a $3 billion investment and constituted the largest American industry after iron and steel. While the U.S. population had nearly doubled since 1880, the number of hospitals had increased by 2,500%.[29]

In the competitive economic climate of the 1910s and 1920s, American hospitals realized that they needed to change their patient mix by reducing the number of charity patients and attracting more paying ones. As early as 1904 in Wisconsin, 77.6% of hospital expenditures were covered by funds obtained from paying patients, the highest percentage in the Midwest. Scientific medicine concentrated on acute care and the consequences of shorter hospital stays, and rapid turnover demanded an even higher patient volume. In 1904, the average length of stay in nonsectarian institutions was already down to 19 days. Financially profitable services such as maternity, pediatrics, surgery, and emergency medicine were to be expanded together with the newest diagnostic facilities offered by the X-ray department and the clinical laboratory. Moreover, it was time to create effective "pull factors" to lure patients into particular institutions. There was no longer any pretense: health had simply become another commodity to be purchased. Marketing strategies suggested that hospitals improve their appeal by offering all the amenities of a home or hotel.

As already envisioned by the founders of the Johns Hopkins Hospital in Baltimore, American hospitals became the primary workshops for the professionalization of medicine.[30] Indeed, scientific medicine became a basis for claims of professional authority, and access to modern hospitals was crucial to physicians in private practice.[31] Optimism about controlling disease remained high; many surgical procedures such as the removal of infected tonsils and adenoids, inflamed appendices, and uterine tumors were believed to be highly effective, even lifesaving. Relieved of fund-raising, which was conducted by trustees, and free of administrative chores now handled by superintendents, physicians exercised complete control over clinical work in hospitals, now their professional workshops. They improved their skills while fostering training, research, and ultimately specialization, activities central to educational and licensing requirements. At the same time, the scientific and often specialized physicians could charge additional professional fees, while most of the care was dispensed by their surrogates, nurses and house officers. Hospital access also bestowed on members of the medical staff a reputation for charity since they still provided free care to low-income patients, a practice increasingly neglected after 1910. With physicians joining hospital staffs, local medical staff organizations remained flexible, awarding admission privileges to both general practitioners and specialists who could attract paying patients. "Open staff" policies were designed to increase the number of referring private physicians, and community hospitals competed fiercely for their patronage.[32]

During the 1920s, American voluntary hospitals became indispensable instruments in the modern practice of medicine.[33] Fueled by generous investments of private capital, a second wave of foundations and expansions occurred to accommodate new technical facilities such as operating rooms, X-ray facilities, clinical laboratories, and physical therapy departments. As a result, workloads increased, particularly in obstetric and pediatric care, emergency treatment, and elective surgery. Because of improving living standards, an ever-larger number of individuals took advantage of the available institutional facilities and paid for services they received as a measure of self-respect. By 1930, fully 23% of all American hospital beds were semiprivate. To cover at least half of the escalating costs, competition for paying patients ensued; the supply gradually outpaced the demand for beds. More endowments or other types of subsidies were urgently needed.[34]

In June 1929, America hosted the first International Hospital Congress in Atlantic City, New Jersey. Participants from 43 nations exchanged experiences and engaged in a series of comparisons. Their comments—while general and sometimes tinged with envy—provide a useful gauge to assess the status of American—

mostly voluntary—hospitals in relation to their European counterparts on the eve of the Depression.[35] Not surprisingly, foreign observers concluded that a much broader spectrum and number of American citizens sought hospital care than in Europe and that the facilities were more extensively used for clinical education.[36] Seventy percent of American hospitals were private institutions, as opposed to only 12% of those in Europe. Most were nonprofit organizations, obtaining nearly 70% of their expenses from patient fees and collecting the rest in the form of bequests and donations through an independent board of trustees. In spite of competition, both administrative and care costs were much higher in America, where hospitals were said to spend about $13 per person per year, but no figures were given for European institutions.[37]

American hospital buildings were judged impressively spacious by European standards. Most consisted of several buildings, each of them multistoried, together with supporting structures such as power plants, laundry facilities, storage houses, and nurses' residences. To ensure better supervision, all services seemed to be in close physical proximity. Since many American hospitals were several stories high, vertical transportation by elevators—involving long waits and mechanical failures—became necessary. For their part, Europeans criticized American hospitals because they lacked separate isolation facilities for patients suffering from contagious diseases[38] and consistently segregated their facilities based on race.[39] Large wards with 24–30 beds, still typical in Europe, were being abandoned in favor of smaller rooms containing 1–4 beds and separated by long, low corridors. In the minds of European visitors, the pressure to create private or semiprivate rooms reflected the higher living standards of the American people, as well as their exaggerated individualism.[40] Also noteworthy in American institutions were the greater number of operating rooms, medical records departments, larger kitchens, and expanded laboratory facilities.

American hospital staffs were also found to be, on average, 10 times larger than those serving comparable European establishments. A 10- to 20-fold increase in the space devoted to administrative and social services compared to their European counterparts raised eyebrows. In the eyes of European administrators, the amount of paperwork generated in American hospitals was truly staggering. On the other hand, Europeans approved of the number of social workers present in many U.S. establishments, since their contacts with patients could expose links between disease and the domestic environment.[41] Instead of the sharply divided spheres of external and in-house medical practice common in European countries, most medical care in American hospitals was rendered by private practitioners who had secured admission for their patients. To exert some institutional control, medical staffs created committees to deal with issues of credentials, admissions, quality control, and education. The resulting administrative complexity and instability required frequent staff meetings to negotiate and achieve consensus. While European hospitals were usually staffed by full-time practitioners, their American counterparts made only brief visits to their patients. Considerable responsibility for patient care was delegated to nurses and house staff, requiring extensive written progress notes and telephone communications between them. The American patient charts recorded confidential impressions of caregivers and were thus zealously kept from patients. Their growing size demanded the creation of separate departments with clerical personnel trained to transcribe, file, and retrieve this information.[42]

In America, food, furnishings, and service resembled those of first-class hotels, a fact the foreign observers considered psychologically harmful. Europeans felt that hospitals should not become convenient places for the care of trivial conditions where patients could be pampered with the help of every possible technical convenience. Establishments needed to remain functional enough to provide only the simple routines necessary for recovery, a view shared by American surgeons trained in earlier, more spartan times.[43] People needed to care for their health but not blindly worship it. Americans—in European eyes—apparently believed that health was "divine," and they constantly fretted about losing any of it, whereas in other parts of the world, people simply viewed health as a means for achieving life's various goals. Thinking thus, the European visitors felt that medical criteria should have greater weight than patients' comfort. The conclusion was that more institutional discipline was needed in America, with less catering to patients' whims. After all, hospitals needed to be distinct from a patient's home or a hotel.[44]

Despite the relative luxury of their accommodations, American hospitals were accused of neglecting the emotional needs of their inmates. Because of their disease orientation and increasing laboratory work and paperwork, physicians had less personal contact with their patients. Modern hospitals on both sides of the Atlantic had the duty not only to provide essential physical caring and sheltering services, but also to restore mental balance to those admitted in a state of fear, anxiety, and worry. A sympathetic approach, felt the visitors, could support the healing process. In accordance with American cultural values, the planning and organization of nursing services emphasized the patient's individual responses and wants. However, in the opinion of European observers, American nursing was routine and "mechanical," not taking into account the patients' emotional needs. By contrast, they argued, personal care remained at the center of all hospital routines across the Atlantic, an idealized generalization. American critics admitted that pre–World War I nursing had been more patient friendly in the United States. Nurses' hours in those days had been long, extracurricular time was brief, and caregivers were less optimistic about their patients' recovery, thus showered them with tender, loving care. Nurses trained during the war had improved their education and technical abilities but were apparently less intimate with their charges. Finally, those trained after the war were even more educated and procedure oriented, and their professionalism created a distancing effect from their patients similar to that observed among physicians. For the American nurse subjected to a system of written medical orders and progress notes, case presentations, and daily conferences, professional tasks remained fragmented.[45]

To be sure, American nurses received a substantial theoretical education and enjoyed better hospital training facilities than their European counterparts, but their exposure to scientific knowledge was believed to be shallow and unsuitable. In Europe, the focus was still on practical training, stressing the vocational aspects of the profession and instilling in students strong feelings of compassion and service. Foreign observers wondered whether American nurses were only interested in education or still cared for their patients as human beings. Could they at least learn to create the illusion of personal interest? The visitors were concerned that American nurses were spoiled, living in lavish homes, while at the same time lacking job security and a pension system. With their negotiated salaries, graduate nurses in the United States indeed had a greater range of knowledge and skills, but they could easily be laid off if the hospital census went down.[46]

At the 1930 American Hospital Association (AHA) convention, Julius Rosenwald, a prominent American businessman and philanthropist, observed that the country's voluntary hospitals were not repaying their huge investment in buildings and equipment. Current economic conditions, however, demanded restraint and greater accountability. Indeed, public duty required higher use of existing facilities before new expansions were to be planned. Rosenwald demanded that hospitals change their policies to meet the new economic order. Charity no longer represented the bulk of hospital service, and free care was to be curtailed further in favor of fee for service. The pay-as-you-go method of medical care was more in accord with current American ideals and would provide income no longer available from charitable gifts. For those who could not afford medical services, either the state would have to assume this responsibility or interested individuals and groups had to find other ways to provide good medical care at a fair price.[47]

Madison, Wisconsin, and its general hospital

Paula's destination already had a proud history, extending back to the first years of the twentieth century. An early president of the MGH Association, E. J. B. Schubring, explained in November 1919 that "Madison General Hospital is not a 'city hospital.' This hospital is owned and controlled by the people of this community. It belongs to them and is merely held in trust for them by the board of directors. Its expenses are paid by its earnings and contributions from philanthropic persons."[48] More than two decades earlier, Madison's most prominent citizens had come together for the purpose of establishing a general public hospital. The institution was to be free of religious influence, operated "according to the most approved principles of hygiene" and with the participation of physicians adhering to all current medical doctrines.[49] The city's only facilities at the time were a private 10-bed home, the state mental hospital at nearby Mendota, a small municipal isolation hospital, and the city jail. When the MGH Association was organized in 1900, its voluntary membership broadly represented Madison's religious, social, and business communities.[50] Members pledged to pay a yearly subscription that gave them the right to shape policy through attendance at annual meetings and the election of officers to the board of trustees. A year later, the group rented and remodeled a double house with accommodations for 16 patients. However, these quarters on the Mound Street Hill soon proved inadequate because of the growing local demands for medical care, particularly surgical and obstetric services. This prompted the Association in 1902 to purchase its own site between Mound and Chandler Streets on the main route leading to the downtown area.

Like similar institutions across America, MGH started as a nonsectarian, voluntary establishment. Since private efforts failed to provide sufficient funding, progressive community leaders argued that the city had a responsibility for the health of its citizens and should enter into partnership with the MGH Association. Health care was to be another municipal service provided to taxpayers, and the hospital was to be a source of civic pride. In fact, a well-equipped general hospital was viewed as a magnet attracting business and population. In reaching an agreement with the city, the hospital association pledged to give up its rights and privileges and run MGH as a quasi-public hospital. In return, Madison's municipal authorities pledged to contribute funds for the hospital's maintenance and repair, as well as to seek bond issues for future remodeling and expansion. To have a voice in decision making, two city council members joined the Association's board of directors.[51] A new 30-bed MGH opened in 1903, thanks to a $15,000 grant from the city, which kept title to the property, supplemented by public subscriptions and donations. The institution welcomed patients from all social classes to its nine private rooms and five four- to six-bed wards. Paying patients could choose between private rooms and ward beds, and received food, medical supplies, and nursing. Since MGH gave preferential admission to surgical cases, it also featured an operating and anesthetizing room and quarters for nurses on the third floor. Not surprisingly, the demand for private rooms quickly exceeded the supply, prompting calls for developing further facilities, especially for obstetric care.

These auspicious early developments occurred against the backdrop of a strong community effort to develop Madison into an important metropolitan center. Widely known in the nineteenth century for its university, and as the seat of state government, Madison had failed to industrialize. With fewer than 20,000 inhabitants at the turn of the century, the former village was rapidly falling behind other Wisconsin cities in population and economic growth. Located at the center of an agricultural region, the city was nevertheless an important railroad hub, with nine lines radiating in all directions. As the local chamber of commerce pressed for greater "advancement," efforts began in 1909 to turn over the control of the hospital to the city. Madison was viewed as a natural hospital center since there was scarcely another institution worthy of the name within a radius of 75 miles. "This large territory looks naturally to Madison for its hospital facilities and the city should be prepared to properly meet such requirements," declared a local medical leader.[52] Faced with opposition from the mayor, the proposal was rejected. City Hall was quite concerned about the dangers awaiting the municipality if hospital management became politicized. Shared responsibility between local government and the private sector seemed ideal.

In the meantime, overcrowding at MGH had forced authorities to double the number of beds in the available space and to have patients bedded in halls and corridors. The small hospital was in dire need of more medical, obstetric, and pediatric facilities. In 1910, the city council supported the needed expansion and provided additional land at the rear of the existing hospital. Granting temporary title to part of the land and an additional $33,000 for construction costs, the municipality set the stage for a new building, planned with the aid of an advisory medical board. In doing so, the city fathers subscribed to the notion, prevalent at the time, that communities should have excess hospital facilities in the event of disasters and emergencies. The move was part of a coordinated effort to create the necessary infrastructure for Madison's impending industrialization, concentrated in a new factory district on the east side of Capitol Hill. Connecting to the existing structure at the north end, a fireproof building (the east wing) with a capacity for 60–70 beds opened in January 1912. The facility also had a solarium, roof gardens, and a hydrotherapeutic department.

Financing for the new hospital also came partly from Dr. Reginald Jackson, a prominent local surgeon, who paid for the construction of a private operating room on the fourth floor, reserved for his exclusive use. The staff was reorganized into three divisions of medicine, surgery, and laboratory, headed by a chief physician, surgeon, and pathologist. As anticipated by the planners, MGH in 1913 already depended financially on fees from paying patients, who arrived from the city as well as from adjacent villages and farms. The growing demand for beds occurred primarily in surgery and obstetrics. Hospital births nearly doubled from 1915 to 1916, doubling again in 1918 as part of a wartime baby boom. When the flu epidemic hit the city in late 1918, 328 patients were hospitalized at MGH, with nearly a 50% mortality. However, few of the patients could afford the $3 per day hospitalization charge. A call for municipal subsidies went out, and Madison's city council authorized the necessary appropriations to cover expenses. Remission of street and water taxes was also approved. The hospital's growing expenses covered primarily personnel, food, laundry, and coal. To save money for food purchases during World War I, vacant lots across from the hospital were converted into vegetable gardens. By the end of the decade, the institution had acquired separate buildings for a laundry and a heating plant.[53]

Buoyed by the collection of fees from its paying patients, MGH, like other American community hospitals, turned rapidly into a business. However, this aspect was downplayed by the hospital's spokesmen, since it could hamper donations to the endowment fund. As the president of the Association declared in 1924, "the hospital must furnish a very large amount of free service and it has always been the motto of MGH that all who applied for admission, regardless of race or creed, would be given the best possible service."[54] To protect itself from losses incurred in treating charity cases, MGH had already made arrangements in 1922 with Madison's Community Union, a central clearance house for charitable giving and forerunner of the United Way. Henceforth, instead of conducting its own charity drives, MGH would receive periodic allocations from the Community Union to defray expenses incurred in caring for indigent patients. As before, private bequests and endowments supplemented these expenditures. To provide better accountability in this burgeoning bureaucracy, the board of directors created the post of hospital superintendent in 1924.

Chosen for the position was Grace T. Crafts, a rather quiet but well-respected member of the nursing staff. Crafts had a long association with the hospital dating back to 1911, when she came to the institution as a night nursing supervisor. Gradually rising through the ranks, Crafts became head of the nursing training program in 1918 before assuming the new post of superintendent. She was described as a very frugal individual who ran her institution as a tight ship. By the late 1920s, nearly 20% of the hospital superintendents in the United States were females with a nursing background, said to be "adapted by nature for household affairs."[55] Their homemaking instincts and sense of cleanliness were believed to ensure the salubrity and orderliness of their institutions, coupled with common sense, sympathy, and the tenacity of a bulldog. Craft micromanaged MGH to the point where even the surgeons had to see her if they wanted to obtain new rubber tubing for transfusions when the older ones became useless.[56] Her willingness to continue to provide personal services to patients—a reflection of her vocational nursing background—even extended to notifying the next of kin in the event of a death, sometimes by venturing into outlying areas on horseback.

Unlike other institutions, MGH's board of directors was always willing to play a central role in management. In 1920, an executive committee led by the Association's president was given general oversight and superintendence of all hospital matters, including rules for patient admission. Reporting to the board of directors, this committee featured the Association's secretary and treasurer, trustees, the mayor of Madison, and the medical chief of staff. During the 1920s, its president met weekly with Miss Crafts to discuss all matters, even to the extent of reviewing advertised sales of groceries in newspapers. As one former administrator recalled, if rutabagas were selling well that week in Madison, Grace Crafts would personally go downtown to the farmers' market and do the shopping, condemning both patients and caregivers to eat a lot of rutabagas.[57]

MGH was never governed by a single core group of practitioners. From its inception, the attending physicians had labored hard to attract a small professional staff of well-trained individuals, most of them surgical specialists, who could lure an expanding clientele of paying patients. Surgeons on the staff competed fiercely, bringing their own instruments to surgeries and adopting a proprietary attitude toward the hospital. In fact, the arrangement in place since 1912 reserved one of the two operating rooms for the exclusive use of Dr. Jackson, while the other one had to be shared by everyone else. The effect of such special privileges created constant tensions and scheduling battles, prompting Jackson to actually place a padlock on his operating room to keep everybody else out. Confronted by other medical staff members, Jackson relented but eventually left MGH to establish his own clinic and hospital nearby.[58]

With the cancellation of the private operating room agreement in 1920, MGH limited its formal medical staff to 26 members "in the interests of better service and increased efficiency."[59] The primary goal was to bring the hospital's physicians and surgeons into closer cooperation and allow them to speak with one voice when dealing with the board of directors and the executive committee. Two separate departments, medical and surgical, were created under the umbrella of an executive committee charged with formulating rules for medical and surgical practice. The committee banned fee splitting and surgery without patient consent, except in emergency cases. Rules required the staff to attend at least seven meetings a year and enjoined them to assist in the education of interns. This voluntary service elevated the status of medical and surgical professionals attending MGH. In the 1920s, the medical staff created standing committees, including committees on diet, laboratory and X-ray work, records, surgical procedures, and interns. Next came the appointment of a resident pathologist and a director of the X-ray department in the mid-1920s following recommendations made by the laboratory and X-ray committee. The former was to be responsible for examining all tissues removed by members of the surgical staff. In 1924, the medical staff got the board to restrict admission privileges to physicians who were members of the Dane County Medical Society. By 1930 the group was still limited to 30 individuals, but expansion efforts were underway.

Given Madison's population growth and demand for medical services, MGH's 110 beds became inadequate by 1920, and plans were drawn to build yet another addition. In 1922, the old hospital was converted into an administrative center with offices and classrooms for the nursing school. A new wing opened in May 1923. It consisted of four floors "with the most modern equipment and furnishings."[60] Initially, only 28 of the private rooms were to be used for paying patients; the other 25 were assigned to the nurses to live in until other facilities became available. Each fire- and soundproof room had a telephone, a night light, and fan service; 12 had private baths. The rooms, furnished with sofas, wooden dressers with large mirrors, rugs, and flowered drapes around the windows, projected a true home-like atmosphere. All walls were painted in light colors instead of the regulation white. Much of the $250,000 earmarked for this addition was used to equip the fourth floor under the guidance of Walter J. Meek, an assistant dean of the University of Wisconsin Medical School. Most of the space was devoted to X-ray and fluoroscopic facilities painted black and protected with lead. Every examination room had its own dressing room. There was also a separate fracture room, a viewing room for radiographs, and several treatment rooms. These facilities were connected with the operating rooms still located in the old building. Taking charge in 1925 was Lawrence V. Littig, appointed hospital radiologist.

Like similar institutions, MGH had organized a nursing training program as early as 1898, before the hospital even opened. Until 1909, the authorities offered only a two-year course, but the school expanded after the First World War. Since 1905, arrangements had been made with the University of Wisconsin to include one year of academic education in the prescribed training, including classes in chemistry, physiology, bacteriology, materia medica, and domestic science. Five years later, the program was lengthened to three years. After 1917, nursing students lived in a modern four-story residence at Rest Harrow, a former nursing home located nearby and deeded to the Association, with an annex for the faculty. Scene of "many a lively frolic," the house was alive with piano or phonograph music, and relaxing occupants danced the Charleston.[61] Eventually, further dormitory facilities were provided on the first floor of the new East Wing.[62] When Grace Crafts became superintendent of the school in 1922, the emphasis shifted from service to more education. After 1923, applicants needed to be graduates of an accredited high school. By 1930 the school had a total of 90 student nurses, and the hospital had hired more general duty nurses to relieve the students and thus provide them with more time for study and recreation.[63]

Under Superintendent of Nurses Ida A. Collins, MGH's Nursing School had consistently ranked among the nation's upper 25%, but the Depression now made it difficult to find money for further operation. Training schools in America were the handmaidens of hospitals that sponsored and financed them. By the late 1920s, however, growing economic difficulties had contributed to a paucity of applicants. In spite of reforms, the remaining nursing students at MGH still defined their training as a "voyage of service,"[64] continuing to live in cramped quarters and to enjoy limited recreation time. When not on call, the students tried to have a good time, gathering in their rooms to talk, play bridge, or listen to the radio. Instructors warned them not to fraternize with the interns and to avoid two seemingly disreputable entertainment venues: a dance hall at Lake Monona and the French Villa in Middleton.[65]

Because of their financial plight, many hospitals were increasingly unable to hire their own graduates and secure a competent caregiving staff. In spite of economic difficulties, demand grew for skilled nurses with broader educational backgrounds, a rationale for pursuing even higher standards and providing better education in nursing schools. Besides lack of instructional facilities, especially laboratories, there was a national perception—dubious at best—that nurses were being overproduced, and many new graduates were in danger of unemployment after graduation. However, there seemed to be no surplus of good nurses at the end of the decade; in fact, experts spoke of a real shortage during the previous five years. Many nurses continued to work hard in daily 10-hour shifts, which were considered inefficient. They also functioned as administrators and medical deputies, taking vital signs measurements, sterilizing instruments, and even dispensing anesthesia. Most caring, however, was entrusted to inexperienced probationers.[66]

In 1927, the board of directors proposed to the city administration another six-story addition to be funded by a municipal bond issue. The wing would hold 75 patients, and the first floor would be a dormitory for 25 nurses. The plan included extra space for the X-ray department, two new operating rooms, a fracture room, and a cystoscopic facility. Special quarters were to be erected for housing X-ray films outside the building (exposed film constituted a fire hazard). MGH's authorities argued that fire doors, automatic sprinklers, and extinguishers would reduce fire insurance. Also by this time, the clinical laboratory had experienced significant growth with 21,730 specimens examined in 1928 (an average of five tests per admitted patient).

MGH's central wing was completed in May 1929 at a cost of $225,000; the city of Madison provided $200,000 in bonds, and the balance came from private gifts. To upgrade its emergency services, the hospital greatly enlarged the radiology unit and added rooms for setting fractures.[67] Similar developments occurred elsewhere as the American hospital, already in full flight, sought to stretch its wings even further. In 1930 Wisconsin witnessed its most dramatic increase in hospitals: 65 more institutions. There were now 225 registered hospitals in the state with a capacity of for 24,393 beds, one for every 277 inhabitants, a figure close to the national average. Short-term needs dictated successive expansions, branching out in several directions and creating labyrinthine circulation patterns that after the Second World War prompted their characterization as "spaghetti hospitals."[68]

At the time of Paula S.'s arrival, MGH also had an "A" rating from the American College of Surgeons and was qualified by the Council on Medical Education and Hospitals to provide instruction to interns. It was also one of only 10% of U.S. hospitals accredited by the Council on Medical Education and Hospitals to give a course of instruction to their interns. Weekly clinicopathological conferences were held on Fridays under the direction of the chief of staff, Dr. Hugh P. Greeley, with the assistance of a full-time pathologist, Lester McGary, and the radiologist, Littig. These meetings were open to all attending physicians, as well as the house and nursing staffs.[69]

At MGH, the new facilities and services caused further rate increases for rooms and operating room use. However, as the superintendent reported for 1930, "an integral part of any hospital is a well-organized and efficient laboratory service and X-ray department."[70] The same year, the Association's elected officers proudly revealed in their reports the creation of a Social Services Department to assist patients. The number of individual subscribers had tripled to 309, an impressive development during a period of uncertainty and gradual economic decline. In their traditional fiduciary role, the officers explained that "this is an encouraging indication of the increased interest in the hospitalization of the community shown by the citizens of Madison."[71]

Who pays? "Hospital-hotels" face the Depression

Paula's automobile accident had occurred at a bad time for her and for MGH. Regardless of its ability to obtain reimbursement for services, providing first aid to the sick and injured was a duty of virtually every hospital. However, the sustained economic malaise that had been plaguing the country since October 1929 now threatened not only to halt decades of expansion, but also to force cutbacks, as the pool of patients able to pay for their care dwindled. Private hospitals such as MGH depended on patient income for more than half of their operating expenses. A sharp, sustained decrease in demand had already reduced occupancy rates from 64% (1929) to 59% (1930). As conditions deteriorated, some people postponed elective surgery and avoided hospital care altogether. Not surprisingly, lower occupancy rates created even higher per capita costs while curtailing services. Salaries for nurses and other auxiliary personnel were cut, and maintenance was deferred.

At the same time, the growing Depression forced some welcome adjustments. European critics had already pointed out the widespread practice of unnecessary hospitalizations. This custom was a product of the private patient revolution, prescribed for the convenience of practitioners and their well-to-do patients. Like physicians in other voluntary institutions, MGH's staff charged separate professional fees. Much of the diagnostic work and treatment monitoring that they performed in hospitals could be handled more economically in physicians' offices. Given the availability of the pertinent technology, X-rays, electrocardiograms, and laboratory tests were being used excessively as supplements and even substitutes for clinical examinations.[72] To control the deteriorating situation, hospitals in 1930 considered requesting more public subsidies, personnel layoffs, and greater support from subscribers and volunteers. At the same time, the trustees continued to invest in new medical equipment, hoping to bolster income from lucrative departments, including the Emergency Room.[73]

The voluntary hospital-hotel concept harked back to the late nineteenth century and was epitomized by the Johns Hopkins Hospital in Baltimore. Most institutions insisted that every effort be made to eliminate the traditional hospital atmosphere and surround paying patients with the comforts of a home. This was a ploy to attract middle-class individuals and provide them with some of the amenities they were accustomed to while they mended. These included private, well-appointed rooms, tasty meals, and private duty nurses. Plush lobbies greeted patients and visitors; the private rooms were spacious, painted in light colors, and furnished with tables, easy chairs, radios, and telephones. Some rooms had ice boxes and featured air conditioning. The steady supply of clean, snow-white laundry was also key.[74] Before Paula's arrival, MGH's superintendent had even ordered the installation of Simmons Beauty Rest spring mattresses for the comfort of the remaining paying patients. For convalescents, sun rooms with rocking chairs beckoned. Others could read or socialize by playing cards and games. Patients were no longer categorized as *inmates*—a term suggesting forced confinement and punishment. Once more, as in the Middle Ages, hospital patients were elevated to the rank of guests who could overcome their sickness in an environment far better designed and staffed than their own often cramped living quarters.[75]

The high-rise monoblock model served the interests of the medical profession and the paying public. Modern designs recognized the need for privacy and acute care tasks. The multiplication of single rooms signaled the influx of fee-paying patients who cared very much for their own privacy. Public spaces for social interaction dwindled. Not surprisingly, the kitchen became the center of the modern hospital-hotel geared for the middle class. It was generally under the direction of a competent dietitian with a degree in home economics. "Wooing the patient's appetite" with meals advertised as "delicious" gave institutions a competitive edge.[76] One of the cardinal rules of the dietary department was to avoid repeating any bill of fare for at least three weeks. Special menu cards were distributed for the holidays. Food trays had to look attractive, enhanced with distinctive china and colored glassware. When in season, fresh fruits and vegetables were important, and complimentary nuts or mints provided an extra touch. Above all, meals had to be served hot. Critics of this increasingly narcissistic trend—"physicians and nurses particularly should follow the hotel plan of serving,"[77]—joked about the creation of a hospital etiquette including new dress requirements, as well as the impulse to bring along one's own bedclothes, sheets, pillows, and knickknacks. Perhaps an interior decorator could appoint the room before the patient's arrival with lamps and flowers, drapes, and soft carpets to create a cozy atmosphere.[78]

But who could afford such luxury, particularly in bad financial times? At MGH, the daily hospital charge was not excessive; it fluctuated in 1930 between $4 and $6, including lodging, nursing, food, and ordinary drugs. However, special fees for laboratory and X-ray work, anesthesia and surgery, as well as orthopedic casts and oxygen supplies, could significantly increase the total charges.[79] Additional employment of special duty nurses at an extra $6 to $8 per day was possible, although most hospitals already had an adequate supply of staff working around the clock. Even before the Depression, patients resented large, itemized bills and often wondered, appropriately, whether they were subsidizing the hospital's charitable cases. Given the public perception that the cost of sickness was not equally distributed, hospitals tried to institute flat-rate services and offer packages that included drugs and dressings. Whenever possible, the cost of charity cases was passed on to the local authorities.

In spite of the growing costs, hospital rooms had been hard to get in the late 1920s, particularly for elective admissions. The wait for surgical beds often stretched to four to six weeks. By 1930, however, occupancy rates had plummeted. Patient revenue now became critical, with administrators fearful of being stuck with a large number of unpaid accounts. Bill collection was aggressively pursued in many hospitals. Before care was provided, the widely recommended procedure consisted of first demanding from accident victims or their relatives a detailed explanation of the financial arrangements they were capable of making to ensure full payment. In view of accusations that hospitals were "money grabbers," this first contact and interrogation was to be conducted by a "tactful, competent, and trained" person.[80] However, there is no evidence that by June 1930—the time of Paula's arrival—MGH had adopted what critics labeled a downright commercial attitude. In its 1930 report, the Social Services Department at MGH admitted that "during this past year of unemployment it has been exceedingly difficult to ascertain economic conditions in many homes because of the general hysteria as to what the future would bring. Families who have always been independent are now needing aid, and whether they can make reimbursement later depends on how long they are forced to live on inadequate incomes and what their income will be when it again becomes stabilized."[81]

To minimize friction, many hospitals provided "attractive little cards" on admission in lieu of a potentially embarrassing personal discussion. The cards listed the hospital's room rates and contained statements requesting one week's advance payment of the charges. Upon leaving the institution, moreover, full settlement of unpaid accounts was expected. Credit ratings were instituted, and some hospitals even teamed up with local banks to float loans. Impressions of patients at the time of admission and any remarks concerning financial matters were to be recorded by admitting clerks and transmitted to the business office after the patients had been escorted to the ward or private room. In accident cases, clerks were instructed to impress upon their arrivals the notion that the hospital would not "under any circumstances, look to any insurance company to pay the bill but to the patient only."[82]

Although the American middle class rejected the notion of free health care as undeserved charity, as the Depression deepened they became more conscious of their own financial vulnerability. In an era of solo medical practices entirely supported by out-of-pocket payments from patients, the escalating cost of medical care, a concern since the mid-1920s, quickly became the topic of the hour: "I do not think I exaggerate when I say that the high cost of sickness, at least among the middle classes, is as potent a cause for social unrest as poverty among the poor," wrote one observer.[83] Henceforth, Americans would worry about the affordability of health care and its perennially escalating costs. One serious illness in a family could threaten their financial solvency for years to come. "Many people are struggling under a mountain of debt and worry to pay slowly the mounting costs of private practice."[84] Hospital bills could be equally disastrous. An editorial in the *Journal of the American Medical Association* indicated that "the hospital takes the patient, like a bride, for better or worse, and from the hospital point of view it is usually for worse. The patient's delusions of grandeur on entrance are soon dissipated by rapidly mounting bills for a variety of necessary services, and he soon finds himself confronted with a situation demoralizing to both his pride and his pocketbook."[85]

Medical writers recognized that "tradition has taught the layman that he is not expected to question his physician as to the cost of his service."[86] Money talk was taboo in American medicine. Physicians attempted to build a fire wall between the caring and business aspects of their practices. Financial matters were believed to threaten the patient–physician relationship built on personal trust and the ideal of a selfless healer acting primarily as the patient's advocate. This standard harked back to earlier times when doctors were family friends, dispensing free advice or bartering for other goods or services. Fee-for-service care was America's practice of choice. However, the fee was seldom discussed in advance, and its collection was left to surrogates to avoid letting money interfere with what was believed to be a therapeutic relationship.[87]

To stem any criticism of earning excessive income, physicians argued that they deserved at least a decent living. An earlier attempt to solve this problem in America had been the establishment of fixed fees, prominently displayed in fee bills. However, given the rapidly changing nature of medical care in the 1900s, this approach was no longer feasible in an increasingly dynamic marketplace for medical care dispensed with the aid of various technologies. Moreover, while patients hesitated to place a dollar value on health, they also believed that payment of medical and hospital bills, mostly unexpected, was a low priority. Physicians, for their part, were no longer as informed as they had been about a patient's ability to pay and were reluctant to jeopardize the budding relationship with the patient by inquiring at the first visit about financial matters.[88]

If during the Depression the middle-class public was concerned about paying for medical care, the physicians delivering medical services were equally worried about income, together with a potential loss of prestige and confidence. The high cost of medical services had already been forcefully expressed before the financial downturn of 1929. " 'But, doctor, I simply can't afford it.' The tragic significance of these seven words to many an American family has bitten deeply into their hearts and minds," wrote one member of the Committee on the Cost of Medical Care. He added that "to middle class Americans—that large group too proud to accept medical care offered as charity, yet too poor to pay for the type of treatment now considered adequate—one need only to mention the cost of medical care to hear a great outpouring of the unfortunate experiences of themselves and their friends."[89]

While Paula remained hospitalized at MGH, writers dealing with medical care characterized the period as one of "financial astringency."[90] Doctors feared that "if the hospital is too expensive, somebody will have to wait for his money, and it requires no Ph.D. to guess who that somebody is going to be."[91] Moreover, practitioners also insisted that they were no more obligated to provide free care to the indigent sick than were their fellow citizens.[92] At MGH in 1930, the social worker expressed her concern that physicians seemed to have forgotten the original concept of charity care, whereby a needy person was afforded free or partially free care. The American medical profession seemed to be betraying their hard-earned public trust.

In an era of growing commercialization, the medical profession had to take control of developments and launch a public relations campaign lest the public react and demand some governmental regulations based on emotions and economic pressures.[93] Physicians defended their fees by stressing their expertise as the product of an expensive medical education, recast as "capital investment." Moreover, new technology and the bureaucratization of office practice—designed to achieve greater efficiency—created a significant overhead to be paid for by the treatment of more patients. At this time, the average net income of the American physician was estimated to be about $5,000 per year, a statistic that included a large number of rural practitioners still bartering their services. This sum represented well over twice the annual income of the average family in the United States at the time.[94] In the end, physicians argued that there was indeed a relationship between the cost and value of medical service and hospital care: "The rise in the cost of medical care is a reflection of the increased knowledge that has come to the practice of medicine."[95]

Confronted with cold-hearted financial considerations, physicians vigorously defended their traditional philanthropic image. In Wisconsin, for example, in the fall of 1930, the Medical Economics Committee of the Medical Society of Milwaukee County issued a report documenting the scope of charitable work performed by its members. On the basis of a questionnaire sent to all practitioners, the Society proudly concluded that in 1929, 57,000 patients had received free treatments, valued at $680,000, by private practitioners in their offices. Additional work performed in free dispensaries, clinics, and hospitals amounted to another $620,000, for a grand total of $1,300,000.[96] Since a larger number of individuals were unemployed or underemployed, attempting to pay their bills by borrowing money at high interest rates, practitioners were told not always to expect full payment. In response, the doctors contended that their fees were only a small portion of the hospitalization costs compared with the cost of nursing services, specialized laboratory tests, and X-ray films.

As the Depression deepened, the charitable veneer of many voluntary American hospitals splintered, exposing a less attractive business side. Stories appeared about patients being turned away from hospitals simply because they had too little money. Although some found this practice outrageous, others defended it as realistic. After all, were not homeless people turned away from hotels and hungry people refused food at restaurants? This was not a medical but a social and economic problem, and the solution was in the hands of local and state governments.[97]

Faced with the worsening Depression, some voluntary hospitals sought to run their establishments more efficiently through better purchasing practices and cuts in personnel. "We are living in a commercial age. Standardization, efficiency, solvency, are words to conjure with, to strain to compass, to mourn in absence," wrote one nurse, pleading, however, that such "efficient administration and joy-giving solvency" still needed to take into account the real purpose of a hospital: taking care of patients.[98] To preserve their own charitable image and activities, hospitals also attempted to improve the status of their endowments with the help of more aggressive trustees. In 1924, MGH's board of directors had already declared that the chief need of the hospital was the establishment of an endowment fund, "the income of which is sufficient to cover the cost of hospital service furnished to those unable to bear the burden of hospital charges."[99] Trustees were to establish more contacts with their local business community and secure the loyalty of the medical staff. The appeals often fell on deaf ears: "They want you to contribute all the time but when you have to go to them they want you to pay full price for everything" was a popular complaint.[100] The truth, however, was that public contributions were leveling off, and private philanthropy could no longer bear the burden of caring for indigent patients. One solution was to demand additional supplements from local governments.

But how could private hospitals convince the public that their services were still essential? To counteract any unfavorable views, hospitals launched their own public relations campaign. Testimonials from grateful former patients were publicized, together with charitable and educational deeds involving the community and a frank exposé concerning the reasons for their rising expenses. Inside the institutions, improvements in staff behavior were sought. Nurses were told to be friendly and tactful, make frequent visits or rounds, and respond promptly to emergency calls. Discretion and respect were to be maintained at all times. Unnecessary staff discussions within earshot of patients needed to be avoided and their charts kept confidential. Dying and very sick patients were to be removed to separate rooms. [101]

Another tool created before the Depression to neutralize the growing criticism of American hospitals was the plan to celebrate an annual National Hospital Day. The proposal, formally adopted by the AHA in 1925, involved several thousand institutions, and the observance was held each year on May 12, the anniversary of Florence Nightingale's birthday. Although no active fund-raising was attached to the celebration, Hospital Day provided an opportunity to foster public under-standing by showcasing hospital facilities. Each participating institution developed a full program of activities with the help of staff members and volunteers. An open house of high-tech facilities such as operating rooms, X-ray and laboratory facil-ities, and the kitchen was combined with pageants and fairs. Radio programs, sem-inars, and displays provided health-related information and educated the com-munity about the hospital's needs. A yearly reunion of babies born in the hospital and their mothers served as a visible reminder of the hospital's success in pro-viding excellent obstetric care and launching the lives of the community's newest members.

As a needed public relations tactic, National Hospital Day in 1930 assumed greater importance and was endorsed by President Herbert Hoover and former President Calvin Coolidge. In their messages, these men conveyed the notion that the hospital enriched the life of the community. As a house of health, the hospi-tal sought to make the community healthier, safer, and more productive. In the contemporary consumer-oriented society of America, hospitals were extolled as "a vibrant, pulsing factor in the standards of better living."[102]

A new national epidemic: Automobile accidents

Even before Paula's dreadful injury, an article in the *Chicago Evening Post* stated that "the most appalling problem confronting the American people today and which so far has baffled solution is the automobile accident situation."[103] The predicament was characterized as a slaughter, a devastation, or a "war of attri-tion" in which 33,000 persons, or 4 persons every hour, had been killed by auto-mobiles in 1929. Another million suffered either minor or serious injuries.[104] Fig-ures released by the American Motorists Association disclosed that about 218,000 persons had been killed in automobile accidents during the past 13 years, in-creasing from 9,000 in 1917 to over 30,000 in 1929.[105]

At the time of Paula's accident, traffic in Madison was indeed thought to be out of control, with people recklessly driving down Main Street at 40 miles per hour and endangering pedestrians. On the day of her misfortune, the Madison newspapers disclosed that four additional people had been injured in the city dur-ing the same afternoon in three unrelated automobile accidents.[106] A contempo-rary newspaper editorial complained about the lack of road signs in Madison and the "speed mania" of its drivers. The city—population 50,000 in 1930—was said to be orderly and friendly[107] but ignorant of its traffic dangers and flow of auto-mobiles.[108] Apparently neither arrests nor warnings were given to violators.[109] To compound the problem, many of Madison's thoroughfares were in a sorry state, since the local gas and electric company was tearing up the streets to lay under-ground wires.[110]

No longer promoted as machines providing needed exercise and pure air,[111] automobiles had become agents of injury and death in the 1920s. Estimates disclosed that serious auto accidents in the United States happened at the rate of 2,000 a day, the highest in the world. By 1911, 1 out of every 40 accidental deaths had been caused by automobiles, but in statistics supplied by the National Safety Council, the ratio in 1927 was 1 out of 4. Mortality statistics based on information routinely supplied by 78 large American cities to the U.S. Department of Commerce listed automobile accidents as 26.4 per 100,000 population in 1930. This figure represented a 13% increase over the previous year.[112] However, available statistics remained unreliable, and the escalating "war" on automobile accidents was more of a media event than a reality. Accident rates were actually declining in proportion to the total number of cars on the road, and the National Safety Council's annual tabulations were presented within the context of significant decreases in mortality from infectious diseases. As auto wrecks became a fact of American life, information about casualties was widely circulated.[113]

Not surprisingly, this new "epidemic" attracted the attention of insurance companies, safety experts, traffic and transportation agencies, and local and state governments. Fully 60% of the accidents involved automobiles striking pedestrians—almost a third of the victims were under the age of 15—while less than 20% of the fatalities were due to cars colliding with each other. The most common accidents happened when distracted pedestrians crossed streets between intersections or at intersections lacking signals. Other frequent victims were children playing on the streets. In Wisconsin, 2,441 automobile crashes (1,038 involving intoxicated drivers) killed 721 people during 1929 and 790 in 1930, which was equivalent to half of the deaths reported by the state for tuberculosis.[114] "Speed mania appears to be as much of a disease as any recognized ailment, but its cure must come from the public itself," commented one Madison newspaper.[115]

Most of this pestilence was caused by the growing number of cars in operation. At this time, Americans owned about 80% of all the automobiles in the world. According to the 1930 federal census, there were now more than 23 million cars on America's roads. In a nation with a population of 122.7 million, this represented about one passenger car for every 5.5 persons. The proliferation of automobiles had begun after 1907, with the introduction of the inexpensive Model T Ford runabout. Following a national trend, by 1916 cars had come to outnumber horses on Madison's streets. In 1930, on the eve of Paula's accident, Wisconsin had 734,700 automobiles registered, more than double the number 10 years earlier.[116] Before the stock market crash of October 1929, cars had been selling in record numbers. Because of their low price and the practice of installment purchasing, automobiles had become an integral part of American life. Closed-bodied models were no longer used strictly for transportation but became all-weather vehicles for pleasure drives.

Given the growing number of vehicles and roads, the mid 1910s signaled the beginning of a new era of mobility and freedom in America, creating opportunities for suburban residential expansion and direct competition with urban streetcars and railway systems. Just as important, the new conditions allowed unfettered leisure travel from coast to coast. In 1919, thousands of visitors touring in their automobiles poured into Madison. During the following summer there were nearly 40,000 guests, attracted by the city's lakes and recreation facilities, the foundation for a prosperous tourist industry. By 1929, Madison's city directory boasted that "miles of concrete pavement are being added each year to the county highways, and soon a network of concrete will cover the county of Dane."[117] Newspaper editorials continued to discuss the need for paving additional roads, especially concrete trunk lines into northern Wisconsin to stimulate tourism further. At this point it was estimated that about 1,500 "foreign" automobiles went through the county each day. Madison found itself at the crossroads of eight separate highways, three of them national thoroughfares. No wonder its busy streets had become veritable death traps for its pedestrian population, especially during summer weekends, as residents from Chicago and other Illinois towns funneled through the city in search of the cool lakes and woods to the north.

The growing presence of the automobile in Wisconsin made the issue of control and education of drivers urgent. A law had been in effect since January 1927 requiring all individuals who operated an automobile, not just owners, to obtain a driver's license.[118] By 1930, about half of the 1,037,145 licensed drivers in Wisconsin were indeed nonowners, but there were still no rigid requirements for obtaining a license in the state. Enforcement of rules governing the operation of automobiles also expanded. In 1929, 1,950 people had been convicted in court for traffic violations and had had their licenses revoked.[119] Excessive speed and traffic density were blamed for most accidents. However, driver education and posted speed limits failed. There was need for more "motor-cop brigades," but hiring them was very expensive.[120]

By the late 1920s, the legal and financial implications of automobile accidents were being increasingly discussed. Did the injured parties or their families have a right to compensation? Should funeral bills, medical expenses, loss of wages during recovery, and so-called pain and suffering be reimbursed? The law prescribed that persons injured through the agency of another had the right to hold the offending person liable for damages if negligence could be proven in a court of law. However, proof of negligence was not enough, particularly if defendants were incapable of paying. Most motorists, like Carl L., who had purchased their vehicles on the installment plan, had nothing of value except their automobiles. Their financial status made it almost impossible to pay liability insurance premiums. "She could be lame for the rest of her life but receive no compensation because the owner of the car which struck her was uninsured," declared one critic in reference to a case similar to Paula's.[121]

In 1929, only 27% of all American motor vehicles were covered by public liability insurance. Should the wages of the guilty drivers be garnished until they had made proper restitution? Another basic injustice prevailed. If a motorist was insured, victims with temporary disabilities would usually receive enough money from the insurance company to settle their immediate medical bills. For persons such as Paula, however, who had sustained serious, long-term injuries, the final settlements often failed to cover both medical expenses and loss of income. Thus, whether the driver carried car insurance or not, seriously injured individuals and their dependents became the real victims of the system.

As a result of highway accidents, an estimated 250,000 patients were cared for annually in American hospitals. Although accident patients provided a welcome boost to occupancy rates, their complicated injuries and long-term institutional stay hindered patient turnover while leaving behind large, often unpaid bills. In fact, hospitals increasingly approached such cases with great caution, since many of the victims became entangled in legal suits and thus deferred payment. Until arrangements had been completed with a relative or the insurance company, administrators assigned these patients to their least expensive wards. It was also important to keep adequate medical records for future insurance claims and lawsuits for the protection of both the hospital and the patient: "records are necessary to the real function of a hospital, serving humanity by alleviating not only the pain but the anxiety of the sick and injured."[122]

Faced with their own financial woes, hospital administrators became increasingly concerned about the impact of automobile accidents on their institutions. The number of unpaid hospital bills stemming from such accidents was growing, especially the reimbursement for emergency services. Failure to place the responsibility for the accident or the insolvency of the responsible parties was often to blame. Moreover, many accidents involved nonresidents who became injured near the institution. Thanks to the presence of ambulance-chasing lawyers, these cases could be exploited for their profit. But, what could be done? Suggestions included passing state laws diverting a portion of automobile licensing fees to pay for hospital care. States such as Massachusetts had required motorists since 1927 to take out liability insurance, but the rates were too low and not lucrative enough for insurance companies underwriting the policies. Hospitals, meanwhile, urged the passage of legislation giving them the same legal protection against fraud or nonpayment of bills already accorded to hotels.[123]

The cost of hospital care for highway accidents in the United States amounted to over $15 million in 1929, with hospitals forced to absorb nearly half of this amount as a loss because of nonreimbursement. Since insurance companies paid compensation to the injured person, not the hospital, accident victims delayed or even withheld their payments, especially if they lived outside the county or the state. Local communities like Madison supporting their hospitals found themselves bearing the brunt of this financial burden, which compounded the increased cost of charity cases. Could hospitals force the person responsible for an accident to assume the hospital bills of those they had injured? Again, the approach was problematic since it was not always clear who was at fault. Unfortunately, existing laws contained no mandatory features. The best solution was to demand that, under state control, all auto licensees should automatically carry compulsory liability insurance. With a structure similar to that of the existing Workmen's Compensation Bureau, the adjudication of claims and a division of the funds among accident victims, hospitals, and physicians could thus be made.[124] Some contemporary hospitals took a more aggressive stance and placed the entire responsibility for payment of services on the patients receiving treatment. To protect themselves fully from losses incurred in accident cases, hospitals required incoming patients to sign an agreement in the event that they could not pay their bills. This document gave the hospital the right of lien and assigned any proceeds obtained from a legal judgment or insurance payment to the hospital covering the amount previously billed for services rendered.[125] No wonder Paula was worried.

Efficiency versus humanity: Hospital life at MGH

After the initial diagnostic workup and first aid were completed, Paula S. was wheeled by an orderly to the elevator that would take her to the third floor and a private room located near the maternity ward. A sheet with Ohlsen's written orders accompanied them, alerting the night nurse about Paula's condition and the need for close monitoring. This private unit was one of a handful of rooms set aside by the board of directors for patients returning from surgery or other seriously injured patients who, by the nature of their condition, would be disturbing other patients on the wards. In spite of reassurances from her caregivers, Paula had not yet been told that her back was broken, a diagnosis that would only have increased her fears by conjuring up notions of permanent disability and possibly a painful, bedridden existence. Surgeons expressed great concern about the mental condition of patients with spinal injuries, "perhaps the most important single factor in treatment."[126] Moreover, the patient needed rest. At this point, reassurances about a gradual recovery may have rung hollow to Paula. Although a devout Catholic, she distrusted priests—she had cooked for some as a child—physicians, and strangers in general.[127] To her great relief, Tormey had decided against surgery to reduce the fractures or fix the deformed spine. In spite of vast improvements in operating techniques and aseptic methods, surgeons at MGH still employed ether as their anesthetic of choice. Paula, like many patients, seemed to fear ether and its complications more than surgery, especially the choking and prolonged postoperative nausea and vomiting.

Thanks to the newly available diagnostic employment of X-rays, Paula's compression fracture was not only detected early but could be subjected to more aggressive management. Experts acknowledged that the treatment of such lesions by simple bed rest on fracture boards was most unsatisfactory, leading to permanent deformity and pain. Failure to reduce the fractures by forcible hyperextension doomed those so afflicted to a future as helpless, often bedridden cripples. For Paula, a permanent spine deformation with its accompanying postural problems would have meant chronic back complaints, muscular weakness, nasty bed sores, and neurological symptoms. She therefore required hyperextension of the lumbar spine to correct the deformity produced by the wedge-shaped bone. Contemporary statistics suggested that surgically and medically treated patients had about the same degree of disability.[128] By contrast, Paula's pelvic lesion required a conservative approach, since the very common fracture at the right ilium—the thinnest portion of the bone—did not affect the continuity of the pelvic ring and would heal quickly in six to eight weeks.[129] In any event, doctors knew best.

Although it was not mentioned in the clinical notes, the patient was probably placed on a Bradford frame or its equivalent, attached to the bed and provided with spring steel bands and canvas stretched tightly across. With Paula placed in the dorsal position, the frame could be initially left in a concave position, but in the following days, the ends had to be lowered across a fixed crossbar, gradually stretching the body and spine. This system of traction and countertraction could be assisted by the use of weights until complete reduction of the fracture had been achieved.[130] To monitor the patient for possible concussion and circulatory shock, all vital signs were to be checked every three hours and the room kept dimly lighted. Paula also received eight grains of aspirin for her headaches, and 1,000 cc of a normal saline solution was administered intravenously. She was allowed to drink water and to be catheterized every eight hours if necessary. An ice bag was placed on the sore groin. Whether a private duty nurse was hired to monitor the patient is unknown.

Why the Madison surgeons failed to apply a body cast immediately remains unclear. Certainly, some of their colleagues in Milwaukee treated crushed vertebrae by manipulation and the application of a posterior and anterior plaster shell to maintain the hyperextended position.[131] The traction system, on the other hand, allowed for gradual multiple spinal displacements that could be monitored by X-rays. Moreover, the body cast—to be worn for six to eight weeks—was not only heavy and restrictive of arm movements, but also caused some patients to have difficulty sitting up. Perhaps Paula refused, afraid of the inconvenience and concerned about the costs involved. In any event, the patient's personal hygiene would remain significantly compromised, with a high risk of bed sores and ulcers. These complications could be avoided only by frequent changes in position and scrupulous hygiene provided by a cadre of dedicated and knowledgeable nurses.[132]

After a number of contacts with nurses and students who checked her vital signs, Paula may also have been visited by hospital superintendent Grace Crafts, who tried to see all in-patients daily. Crafts was a kind, low-key, "positive" person who apparently could establish good rapport with virtually anyone. Perhaps somewhat reassured, Paula must have looked forward to rest and quiet. The light-colored room was nicely furnished with easy chairs and a dresser, although it conveyed a certain sanitized impersonality. Its ample window provided a view of Monona Bay, separated from the rest of the lake by a railroad trestle. Although it was still light outside, the last visitors took their leave at 8 PM. Once more, blankets were smoothed, patients turned, and backs rubbed before the lights went out a half hour later.

Sleep for Paula may have been problematic, with her aching body grotesquely extended and firmly strapped to the bed frame. This may have been very difficult for a person who prided herself on being independent and resourceful. Before the accident, Paula had supplemented her income as a tobacco worker by taking in roomers, preferably Croats or Serbs, with whom she could speak in her native language. Unfortunately, one of them had been recently taken to a sanitarium after being diagnosed with tuberculosis.[133] After single-handedly running her own household and boarding house, Paula suddenly found herself totally dependent on strangers.

Although Paula spent her first night in a single room meant to offer privacy and rest, her sleep had to be regularly interrupted by the night nurse checking her vital signs. Notes indicate that by 2 AM she felt panicky enough to ring for the nurse and request another sleeping pill. Perhaps her neighbor, Lillian Rafferty, had been allowed to stay with her in an attempt to quell some of her initial anxiety and loneliness. Unfortunately, the vigil was short-lived. As one observer commented, "every department of the hospital is set to the tune of early rising."[134] Although perhaps annoying to some inmates, hospital routines at this time in many hospitals consisted of waking patients by 6 AM. This allowed for morning care chores, including washing and grooming, and a final personal inspection before nurses ended their shift at 7 AM. Breakfast trays followed. Most administrators felt that later rising would involve more personnel and increase the cost of care. For Paula, this early grooming routine may have been similar to the one she followed in her own home, but she found herself immobilized on a bed frame and the recipient of some light sponging by the student nurses on call. The early meal—just sips of juice for her—was immediately followed by visits from often still sleepy house staff members, who checked surgical dressings before the attending surgeon made official rounds at 9 AM. The only patients exempted from this early house routine were private patients who hired their own nurses.

In contrast to similar institutions relying solely on student service, MGH in 1930 had a small contingent of 12 staff nurses, all dressed in crisp white uniforms with perky caps. There were also three head nurses, two extra night nurses, an assistant to the night supervisors, two extra relief nurses, and four extra floor nurses. Since the attending physicians and surgeons visited daily for only a few hours before returning to their offices, the nurses virtually controlled the hospital. At the time of Paula's hospital stay, MGH was reputed to have the best nurses in Madison. Each floor had its own nurses' station with a repository for medications, including narcotic "hypo" trays. Ward chores were divided among various caregivers, preventing any continuity, either personal or professional. Some nurses made the beds, others took patients' temperatures, and still others gave baths and administered medications. Given such expanding responsibilities, service was frequently delayed, and the overworked nurses spent most of their time implementing the physicians' written orders.[135] While nurses paid a great deal of lip service to personal relationships with patients, these contacts were no longer emphasized as before. The sheer amount of work made some nurses appear harried and indifferent, although those paying for a private room received treatment commensurate with their social status. The old familiarity was vanishing, and patients were often formally addressed. "In a hospital one soon learns to obey everyone," observed one contemporary patient, "for every attendant, even down to the meanest orderly, is clothed with an authority not to be questioned by any invalid intruder."[136]

Patient passivity—being a "humble milk-fed subject"—was expected, especially during the daily ceremonial of physicians' rounds.[137] The sick remained children cared for by their surrogate parents, the nurse-mother and the physician-father. Moreover, the code of deferential behavior exhibited by nurses in Osler's time still prevailed. In a reenactment of the familiar ritual, the head nurse solicitously accompanied the doctors from bed to bed, carrying the clinical charts. Socialized into subservience since their training days, certain nurses never dared to question the physician's superiority. However, as a measure of their increased professionalism, some staff nurses were occasionally praised by practitioners for their thorough reports and intelligent comments, in sharp contrast with the condemnation heaped by physicians on so-called paper nurses, bureaucrats who had less patient contact because of their administrative work.

Nursing continued to be an art, combining feminine domestic services such as feeding, massaging, bathing, and cleaning with a basic understanding of the principles of health and disease. The latter knowledge allowed nurses to claim a marginal, junior partnership with physicians and to become their extended hand, a strategy that demanded greater education but also promised more respectability and status—although always within the context of subservience to the physician. One female observer, writing in the July 1930 issue of *Harper's*, observed: "The days when women gave up their lives to nursing as they would to a sisterhood have passed. The best of the nurses today are animated by the same high ideals, but they see very clearly that the profession must be reorganized on a sound educational and economic basis."[138] In contrast, the public still expected caregiving to be a calling, not simply a career.[139]

Paula interacted mostly with student nurses from the hospital's training school who worked eight-hour shifts. The new "probies," with their blue dresses, graduated to striped uniforms with white aprons, bibs, cuffs, and collars one month after their admission in September.[140] For 15 minutes each morning, they were required to sing Christian religious songs before going to work. Since the nursing personnel were still organized in a hierarchical, almost paramilitary fashion, the students did all the menial bedside work. This included cleaning bedpans and rectal tubes, administering enemas before and after surgery, and dragging bags of soiled linen to the laundry. They also fluffed pillows, swept floors, watered plants, and made cotton balls and swabs. Some of the student nurses were so afraid of hospital physicians that they often hid in bathrooms during daily rounds.[141]

On Wednesday, June 18, Paula's condition had sufficiently stabilized to allow her transfer from the third-floor private room to a first-floor ward. Her destination was a surgical unit with four beds recently enlarged to allow more light and air. The reasons for Paula's transfer were unclear. Perhaps the private room was needed for another very ill patient, but given the hospital's low occupancy rate, this was unlikely. A more plausible reason may have been a request from Paula or her friends to have her placed in "steerage," the least expensive facility. Perhaps the move represented an administrative decision based on reports from the hospital's social service worker, Mary L. Taylor, who took care of all dubious payment cases and may have alerted the business office that the patient complained of having limited funds.[142] At this stage, institutions such as MGH tried to determine the financial status of their emergency admissions. Relatives were usually summoned to the hospital's business office to provide details to the person in charge of collections. Unlike a private room, costing $4.00 per day, a ward bed went for $3.50. In addition to daily room rates, the hospital charged a $3.00 laboratory fee on admission, followed by $3.00 per week for drugs and dressings during the first week and $2.00 thereafter. There were separate charges for the X-rays. Paula herself may have already been classified as a part-pay patient, meaning that she did not have enough money to pay her bill in full at the time of her discharge.

Transferred to the ward, Paula must have been somewhat reassured as she was greeted with good or clean aromas. Such odors came from the use of chlorine compounds, iodoform, phenol, and creosote preparations, a tribute to MGH's good nursing and housekeeping, in sharp contrast to the usual fetid ward smells in larger institutions.[143] Paula was reported to be alert, with no signs of serious concussion, although her severe headaches persisted. Stretched out on her bed, the diminutive patient may have reflected on the value of money and what it bought in a hospital. Her new surroundings were much more spartan: gone were the easy chairs and dresser, as well as the lake view, and the nurses were less friendly. The ward displayed a haphazard mix of patients and diseases, from a teenager who had just had her appendix removed, to an older widow suffering from incurable cancer, to a middle-aged housewife with a hematoma on her forehead. To ensure some privacy, ward beds could be surrounded by curtains, but modesty inevitably suffered. Paula's constant recumbency must have been quite stressful, although new balloon pillows were in use, advertised as being just as cozy as down. Given her enforced immobility, Paula depended totally on the nurses to turn, wash, and feed her.

On June 23, the intern removed all adhesive bandages covering Paula's ribs, taking out the scalp sutures two days later. As a patient, it was difficult for Paula to obtain information from tightlipped caregivers. On principle, practitioners rarely volunteered information that had the potential to impede their patients' progress. Tormey seemed pleased with Paula's progress and ordered her to exercise her legs gently to avoid unnecessary stiffness. This was probably not the time to reveal the long months of immobility and physical rehabilitation Paula still faced. Student nurses were instructed to turn Paula sideways, thus preventing adhesions in her chest from the rib injuries. The customary bland diet may have been supplemented by brand new entries into America's food pantheon: sliced Wonder Bread, Hostess Twinkies, and perhaps even a Snickers candy bar. According to the nurses, Paula continued to complain of headaches, and her spirits began to sink. Docility and passivity were not her traits. She worried about the effects of the accident on her ability to resume normal activities and return to work. A Catholic priest may have visited Paula in the hospital—despite her aversion to men of the cloth—heard her confession, and administered the Eucharist.

According to the physicians' progress reports, Paula's general condition seemed much improved by July 8, although it was still difficult to bathe and feed her. The wounds appeared well healed, but Paula was still marooned on the hyperextended canvas. Such passivity must have been very stressful. Who was willing to communicate with Paula and pay attention to her comfort while she was restrained and stretched out on the small ward? Ohlsen, the intern, was too busy to pay social calls and mostly relied on the nurses' reports. Tormey spent most of his time in the operating room. The few nurses were occupied with administrative routines and following doctors' orders. Paula's predicament—common to many hospital patients—was eloquently expressed by another sufferer, who suggested that "since modern science has seemed to reach the zenith of its efficiency, let common sense take a hand in lessening the weariness, the aches, and the sharp suffering of patients in our hospitals."[144] Perhaps one of the student nurses wheeled her bed to the solarium for a few hours so that she could see the garden and feel the warmth of the sun. Moreover, social workers were encouraged to make frequent visits and run errands for their patients. They also acted as interpreters and educators, explaining the institutional rules to their clients and communicating the patient's wishes to the caregivers.[145] Maybe the visiting librarian provided her with some magazines and books.[146] Perhaps Paula's son and some of her neighbors had a chance to be with her, although visiting hours were strictly enforced so as not to interfere with hospital routines.

Paula's abdominal muscles were still tense, so she tried to perform the prescribed leg exercises with help from a student nurse. This was quite difficult and stressful since her head was still kept somewhat lower than her body, but the nurses insisted. As another contemporary patient recalled, "the harassment of my body and mind was such that I sometimes wondered if I had become an inmate instead of a patient."[147] The four-bed ward arrangement, of course, allowed for companionship. Perhaps one of her roommates even had a radio, thus somewhat relieving the monotony and loneliness of her situation. According to the chart, Paula's doctors had left standing orders to give her Luminal tablets for pain and sleeplessness. On July 9, Ohlsen ordered further laboratory work. There was now a presumption that the patient suffered from a bladder infection caused by previous catheterizations, a common occurrence but possibly also a reflection of deficient hygiene and poor nursing care. Paula's white blood cell count was reported to be elevated, but her clinical symptoms of urinary frequency and pain fortunately subsided.

Paula, however, must have gradually come to suspect that the spinal damage, with its long-term disability, could handicap her for the rest of her life. Fear of the unknown gripped this otherwise energetic, hardworking, and intelligent woman, who used to get up every morning at dawn to brew her strong coffee, using eggshells to settle the grounds. An excellent cook, she occasionally treated her family and boarders to a thin pancake or *polacsinta*. She also raised chickens, vegetables, and grapes, and even canned her own produce and made wine. Perhaps in moments of privacy and reflection, Paula may have worried about accumulating a mountain of unpaid hospital bills. She was known to be honest and was always eager to pay her own way. As a recently divorced, single parent with meager monetary reserves—the hospital reported that she only had $200 in savings and drew a small salary—she was financially vulnerable. Moreover, would she ever hold a job again?[148] Characterized by the hospital's social worker as "extremely frugal," she was making payments on her small house on Hoard Street.

Paula was discharged on July 14, exactly two days after a body cast in the form of a plaster jacket from her neck to her pelvis had been applied by Tormey, presumably to preserve the hyperextension and ensure further healing of the crushed vertebra. She went home with strict instructions to remain confined to bed for at least three months. Experts predicted that total recovery would take six to eight months, with the last three spent in an ambulatory state wearing a spine brace, corset, or removable jacket. Moreover, physicians stressed the need for physical therapy to achieve total rehabilitation. Paula was told to carry out a number of directed exercises to prevent joint stiffness and muscular weakness. However, the key to a patient's recovery was mental status. Surgeons worried about depression and inactivity.[149]

How Paula left MGH went unrecorded. What must have gone through her mind as she departed? Was she relieved or frightened about her future prospects? The hospital stay had not been particularly happy, partly because of her immobility, dependence, lack of privacy, and financial worries. Perhaps she also had a nagging feeling that some of her care had been influenced by her financial status, such as the early transfer from the private room to a ward. Did she know that earlier placement in a plaster jacket would have allowed ambulation? Since she remained prone in traction, why was her spine alignment not periodically checked with the aid of X-rays? Even if she knew the questions, Paula would not have dared to ask them of her surgeons. Did the financial aspects of these procedures shape the surgeon's decision-making or did she refuse them herself, in part because they would add to her growing debt? In a replay of the money taboo, her hospital physicians deliberately left all money matters in the hands of administrators and social workers who, in their periodic visits, inquired about the precise details of her life circumstances, bank account, and future prospects.

The road to financial health

Once home, Paula must have faced new problems. Who would take care of her? Both Paula's son and her remaining roomer and close friend, a Croatian named Mike B., apparently played important roles in her recovery. Perhaps her neighbor, Lillian, from across the street, looked in on her as well. One can only speculate about the subsequent involvement of the visiting nurse. Her condition certainly justified the need for home visits, but lack of money may have been an obstacle.[150] Already saddled with her unpaid bill, would the hospital have provided further services? The social worker was supposed to follow up on particular patients and function as their advocate, easing Paula's adjustment after discharge. The paradox of her situation could not have escaped Paula's mind. Modern science had provided her with a chance to heal her back and possibly resume a nearly normal life, but lack of funds threatened her full recovery.[151]

Regarding the legal issues of Paula's accident case, a claim was filed against both the driver and the owner of the automobile, but neither was insured, and it was highly questionable whether they would meet her hospitalization costs voluntarily or compensate her in any other way. The driver of the car, Carl L., was the son of a De Forest bank cashier of modest means. Shaken, Carl had been taken to nearby Mendota Hospital, a psychiatric institution, for observation the day after the accident because he complained of "extreme nervousness." The physicians who examined him detected the presence of a small goiter—very common at the time in Wisconsin—that was promptly blamed for his symptoms. Observed the hospital's social worker: "It is cases of this kind that clearly illustrates the need for compulsory automobile insurance which all hospitals are beginning to feel is necessary to finance hospital care which they are now having to give free."[152]

Paula's case provides a context for the strong contemporary criticisms of mismanagement, unfairness, and general heartlessness hurled by the public at the American voluntary hospital. On the other hand, MGH followed a successful strategy to consolidate its position in the local market and portray itself as a genuine public utility and community institution. At first glance, it would seem difficult to understand why, in the early throes of the Depression, MGH would add another six-story wing to its building, mostly with taxpayers' money raised through a municipal bond issue. This project was completed precisely at a time when institutional expenses were escalating and occupancy rates declining. The evidence, however, shows that the diagnostic center was not just a new boon for physicians, surgeons, and radiologists, but was undertaken as an important hospital marketing tool for outpatient and emergency medical care that attracted more patients. In fact, the new wing, with its modern equipment, made it possible for the hospital to raise its income in 1930 as well as change its patient mix. The percentage of those preferring private accommodations—usually well-heeled patients who could pay their bills—increased from 47% in 1929 to 52% in 1930, a significant shift that allowed a reduction in the admission of those who could become potential credit risks. Based on this success, in December 1931 Littig requested the purchase of additional radiographic equipment, including a 200,000-volt X-ray therapy machine. Another money maker under Littig's jurisdiction was MGH's physical therapy department, a facility that not only treated inpatients but also attracted many paying outpatients, perhaps even Paula, who may have returned for recommended massage and ultraviolet treatments.

But could the hospital collect the increased fees for all these new services and equipment? In 1930, well over half of MGH's income was derived from room and board fees, supplemented by X-ray charges, city appropriations, and interest on the endowment. The answer, therefore, was simple: the hospital could afford the capital investments and obtain reimbursement, but only from those who could afford to pay the charges. Complaints of unfairness and inhumanity had indeed a basis in fact, with critics claiming that the hospital sought to increase its income at the expense of the suffering working class. Even in the eyes of Superintendent Crafts, hospital care was a product, a commodity for sale, with patients envisioned as willing consumers of services. In spite of her frugal instincts, Crafts was persuaded to provide the growing number of paying customers with all sorts of amenities, including comfortable mattresses, new rubber-tile flooring, an electric toaster, and electrically heated food carts.[153]

During 1930, MGH treated 4,608 patients, with a daily average of 102 patients (slightly higher than in 1929), a 53% occupancy rate. The average stay was 8.24 days. However, operating expenses began to move beyond the costs of food, heat, light, and nurses' wages, threatening the financial status of the institution. Rigid economy in hospital purchases and control of other expenses made it possible to continue to pay the fixed interest and principal on the bond issue that had financed the new wing. In her own quiet way, Crafts rationed the hospital's resources and kept the institution afloat in spite of its second annual loss. MGH's monopoly on emergency services gave it a decisive competitive edge with paying patients, although denominational Madison hospitals, both Catholic and Protestant, experienced higher occupancy rates because of their religious affiliation and charitable cases.

Fortunately, in contrast to other industrialized states, Wisconsin had been less severely affected by the Depression. Still, the tough times placed increased demands on the institution's benevolence. MGH was able to provide increasing care to charity patients: $37,780 in 1931. In an era devoid of social safety nets, recipients were not strangers or welfare cheaters, but average Madisonians with no work or savings. According to the statistics, 328 cases had been referred that year to the hospital's social services department, including 282 inpatients. The collection of accounts payable was getting ever more difficult due to growing unemployment, in spite of President Hoover's modest emergency job program instituted a year earlier. Nearly 1 in 10 former patients claimed to be unable to pay all or part of their hospital bills. At the same time, the Wisconsin legislature drafted a proposal for an automobile accident compensation law similar to its industrial legislation for injured workers. Failure to enforce liability and provide insurance had financially harmed people like Paula. With automobile accidents increasing three times faster than industrial mishaps, this law was designed to provide for people injured or killed in motor car accidents. They or their next of kin would get compensation regardless of the legal determination of negligence.[154]

On March 31, 1931, MGH's social worker acknowledged that it was often very difficult for unemployed and penniless patients to accept public assistance even though financial anxieties hindered their recovery. Others in dire straits had created their own difficulties through excessive reliance on credit, with their unexpected hospital bills remaining a lower priority as they tried to settle their debts. The tendency to pay hospitalization charges in small installments over an extended period of time—sometimes years—forced hospital authorities to carry many accounts receivable for the remainder of the decade.[155] There was no question that the deepening Depression was taking its toll at MGH. A large number of transients began arriving in Madison, many in acute need of medical care and with nowhere to go. Hoover blankets—newspapers used by the homeless to shield themselves against the cold on park benches—were no substitute, particularly during Wisconsin's winters. To complicate matters, relations between Madison's hospitals and the county welfare agencies were strained. Dane County could offer only $4.00 per day in hospital costs, but MGH reported a per capita expense of $7.18, a fact that contributed to the institution's growing deficit. If county welfare clients were in need of hospitalization, these governmental bodies could only send the sick poor to institutions that were willing to take them.[156] By 1932, the county was forced to lower the payment to a flat daily rate of $2.50. Worried MGH board members decided that it was "unwise to acquiesce to this request."[157]

Given this state of affairs, MGH adopted a new set of rules for admission of patients on October 2, 1931. The first rule stated that physicians who wanted to hospitalize certain patients first had to apply to the business office and select those accommodations "most suitable to the financial condition of the patient." Moreover, the doctors were to "accurately inform the patient concerning the hospital charges and terms of payment." Another regulation prohibited the admission of any charity patients except those who were Madison residents. Physicians whose patients needed free care were enjoined to notify the hospital superintendent or the social services department, if possible, before admitting the patient so that "some financial plan can be worked out to the best advantage of the patient, the doctor, and the hospital."[158] Moreover, nonresident patients were now expected to pay their hospital bills in advance. If they could not, physicians had to make arrangements with county officials and obtain an affidavit that they assumed responsibility for the anticipated costs. Madison physicians, however, were told to render medical services "without charge to patients admitted as Dane County, General Charity, or Madison Community Union patients and to any case when free hospital care is given." However, the latter would not be "allowed to remain in the hospital longer than six weeks except by permission of the Association's President or the Executive Committee."[159]

In spite of its difficulties, MGH weathered the year 1931 fairly well; its operating deficit was only $3,500, compared with $5,211 a year earlier. But a drop in the patient census of nearly 20% over the next three years and a 56% increase in charity expenses severely affected the hospital's finances. Comments were heard nationwide that some communities had permitted the building of too many hospitals and that public-spirited citizens should discourage the further construction of large, expensive facilities. Perhaps the critics were right: America was over-hospitalized. If typical Darwinian marketplace dynamics were indeed at play, one official remarked, "the time is fast approaching when poorly endowed and weakly staffed hospital parasites must close their doors or unite their resources with stronger and more deserving institutions."[160]

In 1932, MGH's superintendent once more complained to the board about the increasing difficulties of collecting bills and generating income. Additional charity aid from the county was requested because voluntary contributions were slow. The collection of accounts of patients injured in automobile accidents continued to be a serious problem and a financial burden throughout the decade. Perhaps Paula was among the patients still behind on their bills. Stooped over—probably the outcome of her spinal fracture—this hardy, energetic woman briefly returned to work at the Lorillard Tobacco Company in 1931, but later she supported herself mainly by taking in pensioners in her small house on Hoard Street. After the death of her former husband in 1935, she continued to live at that address with her son Peter and eventually his family, tight-lipped about her MGH experience. Paula came from a European milieu of almshouses in which social stigma was still attached to hospitalization.

Even before Paula's admission, the president of the AHA had characterized health insurance as the salvation of American hospitals, physicians, and patients provided that the latter retained their freedom of choice concerning institutions and practitioners.[161] By the mid-1930s, the Great Depression favored the creation of new funding schemes organized by prepayment insurance systems to keep hospitals solvent.[162] As early as 1932, MGH's board of directors examined the concept of health insurance. As the board of trustees observed, "the idea of developing some sort of insurance program whereby persons in good health might guarantee to themselves certain hospital attention upon payment of a small annual fee was already employed in a good many places."[163] When the Committee on the Costs of Medical Care issued its final report that same year, a key recommendation centered on the need for group health insurance, with the additional suggestion that voluntary hospitals such as MGH were to be reimbursed for care rendered to patients such as Paula who could not meet their own expenses and who were not included in insured groups. In such cases, local or state taxes were to be used for the payments.[164] Some of these insurance schemes, including Blue Cross, arrived in Wisconsin only in the second half of the decade. In time, the public became attracted to health insurance to avoid sudden, often major expenditures for which they were ill prepared. The additional bonus was their freedom to choose hospitals within their insurance plans.

Eventually, the burgeoning health insurance industry did rescue the American hospital system. Hospital administrators were delighted to support a scheme that guaranteed revenues in advance. Premiums could be set above per diem costs, and the nonpaying ward patients could generally be avoided or shunted to municipal institutions. Insurance income would also insulate the hospital from fickle philanthropists, local politicians, and the vagaries of America's medical marketplace, and it would finance the acquisition of new technology. Physicians, in turn, were quite pleased to discover that they no longer needed to worry about obtaining their fees. However, they pleaded for multihospital plans to preserve their patient–doctor relationship while also making sure that they could collect fees from patients distributed among various institutions where they had admission privileges. Given the desire for complete freedom of choice among physicians and hospitals, so-called closed-panel plans remained unpopular. This fact, of course, led some doctors to enter the insurance field themselves. However, the trade-off for physicians in the development of open-panel insurance plans was that attending physicians lost control over their patients as an economic asset with which to bargain with the hospital authorities, a scheme in place at least since the 1890s.

During the next decade, MGH admissions stabilized, slowly rising from about 4,500 to 5,352 by 1939. Total hospital income, in turn, grew from $262,000 in 1930 to $364,000 in 1939, the first year the hospital actually reported a gain. American hospitals like MGH remained autonomous local monopolies, resisting repeated calls to become community medical centers offering a broad range of services, including office, clinic, and home care. In spite of such policies, they continued to attract public support, community endorsements, insurance reimbursements, and eventually government subsidies, thus achieving financial security. Writing in 1935, the American surgeon Hugh Cabot (1872–1945) singled out the hospital as providing the "physical equipment which the modern physician must have at his disposal if he is to offer to his patients a really first-class article in diagnosis and treatment."[165] The role of hospitals as professional workshops had become firmly established. As for Paula S., she survived the Depression and the Second World War, dying on October 22, 1958, from a heart attack at St. Mary's Hospital in Madison.

NOTES

1. N. W. Faxon, "John Howard, J. R. Tenon and some eighteenth-century hospitals," *Bull Am Hosp Assoc* 4 (July 1930): 96.

2. *Wis State J*, June 14, 1930, p. 2, and *Capital Times*, June 15, 1930, p. 2.

3. This information is contained in "Hospitals registered by the American Medical Association," *JAMA* 94 (Mar 29, 1930): 931. At this time, average occupancy rates were around 70%, somewhat higher than a decade earlier (67%).

4. *Wright's Madison City Directory, 1929*, Madison, WI, 1929, pp. 9–12. For more information about the city see David V. Mollenhoff, *Madison: A History of the Formative Years*, Dubuque, IA, Kendall, Hunt, 1982. On health care in Madison, see especially pp. 384–407.

5. Information about Pauline S. was obtained from her hospital chart and through a series of interviews with living relatives. See also Henry A. Behrnd, "A Chronology of the Madison General Hospital," Historical Files, 1898–1987, MGH Archives, pp. 98–99.

6. Southern Wisconsin produced class five tobacco for cigar binding. See Joseph C. Robert, *The Story of Tobacco in America*, New York, A. A. Knopf, 1949, pp. 193–207.

7. H. L. Foss, "The hospital training of interns," *JAMA* 96 (Mar. 28, 1931): 1004–07, and N. P. Colwell, "The requirement of an intern hospital," *JAMA* 92 (Mar. 30, 1929): 1031–33. For more information see K. M. Ludmerer, "The rise of the teaching hospital in America," *J Hist Med* 38 (1983): 389–414.

8. For a summary see G. B. Risse, "Once on top, now on tap: American physicians view their relationships with patients, 1920–1970," in *Responsibility in Health Care*, ed. G. J. Agich, London, Reidel, 1981, pp. 23–49.

9. A firsthand account of hospitalization at the Mayo Clinic is Henry H. Harper, *Merely a Patient*, New York, Minton, Balch & Co., 1930, p. 73.

10. F. W. Peabody, "The care of the patient," *JAMA* 88 (March 19, 1927): 877.

11. The superintendent, Grace Crafts, stressed that "originally the hospital's mission was care of the sick but today it must be a laboratory for diagnosis and to give surgical, medical, and obstetrical service." See *The 1926 Litahni*, a booklet produced by the MGH School of Nursing, Madison, 1926, p. 30, MGH Archives.

12. F. M. Hodges, "The section on radiology," *JAMA* 95 (Sept. 20, 1930): 833–34. For the profound impact of Roentgen's rays, discovered in 1895, in shaping a new concept of health and disease see Joel D. Howell, *Technology in the Hospital*, Baltimore, Johns Hopkins Univ. Press, 1995.

13. Nearly 75% of all pelvic fractures in women were then caused by automobile ac-

cidents. See L. Noland and H. E. Conwell, "Acute fractures of the pelvis," *JAMA* 94 (Jan. 18, 1930): 174–79.

14. F. Christopher, "Compression fractures of the spine," *Am J Surg* 9 (July–Sept. 1930): 424.

15. W. C. Stoner, "The chaos of institutional drug therapy and management of patients," *JAMA* 93 (Nov. 23, 1929): 1630–32. See also George Rosen, *The Structure of American Medical Practice, 1875–1941*, Philadelphia, Univ. of Pennsylvania Press, 1983.

16. The characterization of American hospitals as a "public undertaking" appeared in the 1904 U.S. Census, and is cited by Rosemary Stevens in *In Sickness and in Wealth: American Hospitals in the Twentieth Century*, New York, Basic Books, 1989, p. 18.

17. For a summary see P. Shoemaker and M. V. Jones, "From infirmaries to intensive care: Hospitals in Wisconsin," in *Wisconsin Medicine*, ed. R. L. Numbers and J. W. Leavitt, Madison, Univ. of Wisconsin Press, 1981, pp. 105–31.

18. For a brief overview see G. B. Risse, "Hospital-modern history," in *Encyclopedia of Bioethics*, ed. W. T. Reich, rev. ed., New York, Simon & Schuster, 1995, vol. 2, pp. 1163–68. For essential details see C. E. Rosenberg, "The origins of the American hospital system," *Bull NY Acad Med* 55 (1979): 10–21, and Stevens, *In Sickness and in Wealth*, pp. 17–51.

19. S. Landefield, "The rise of the modern hospital idea, 1900–1913," *Synthesis* 1 (1973): 16–40. Although focused on Baltimore, another valuable source is Jon M. Kingsdale, *The Growth of Hospitals: An Economic History in Baltimore*, New York, Garland, 1988. For more details see Frances S. Hanckel, "American Hospitals in 1910," Sc.D. thesis, Johns Hopkins Univ., 1985.

20. The concept was expressed by Charles E. Rosenberg. See his "Inward vision and outward glance: The shaping of the American hospital," *Bull Hist Med* 53 (1979): 10–21. His book *The Care of Strangers: The Rise of America's Hospital System*, New York, Basic Books, 1987, is the best secondary source on this subject for the period 1800–1920.

21. See M. Vogel, "The transformation of the American hospital, 1850–1920," in *Health Care in America*, ed. S. Reverby and D. Rosner, Philadelphia, Temple Univ. Press, 1979, pp. 105–16.

22. Albert J. Ochsner, *Organization, Construction and Management of Hospitals*, Chicago, Cleveland Press, 1907, pp. 465–525.

23. Consult Edward F. Stevens, *The American Hospital in the Twentieth Century*, New York, Architect Record Pub. Co., 1918.

24. By the late 1920s, single-bed rooms made up 48% of hospital space, followed by semiprivate facilities (23%), small wards (21%), and large wards (7%). See also "The growth and development of the hospital field," *The Modern Hospital Year Book*, 9th ed., Chicago, Modern Hospital Pub. Co., 1929, pp. 77–86.

25. L. Barker, "The organization of the laboratories in the medical clinic of the Johns Hopkins Hospital," *Johns Hopkins Hosp Bull* 18 (1907): 193–98, and J. D. Howell, "Early use of X-ray machines and electrocardiographs at the Pennsylvania Hospital," *JAMA* 255 (May 2, 1986): 2320–23.

26. J. D. Howell, "Machines and medicine: Technology transforms the American hospital," in *The American General Hospital*, ed. D. E. Long and J. Golden, Ithaca, Cornell Univ. Press, 1989, pp. 109–34.

27. For details see Charlotte A. Aikens, *Hospital Management: A Handbook for Hospital Trustees, Superintendents*, Philadelphia, W. B. Saunders, 1911. See also D. Rosner, "Doing well or doing good: The ambivalent focus of hospital administration," in *American General Hospital*, pp. 157–69, and M. J. Vogel, "Managing medicine: Creating a profession of hospital administration in the United States, 1895–1915," in *The Hospital in History*, ed. L. Granshaw and R. Porter, London, Routledge, 1989, pp. 243–60.

28. F. D. Donoghue, "Medical competence and hospital efficiency," *Boston Med Surg J* 178 (1918): 594–98. One of the classical texts on this subject is Ernest A. Codman, *A Study in Hospital Efficiency*, Boston, n.p., 1915. For a useful analysis see G. Rosen, "The efficiency criterion in medical care, 1900–1920," *Bull Hist Med* 50 (1976): 28–44.

29. For more information see *American and Canadian Hospitals, A Reference Book of Historical, Statistical, and Other Information*, Chicago, Physician Record Co., 1937.

30. W. H. Welch, "The relation of the hospital to medical education and research," *JAMA* 49 (Aug. 17, 1907): 531–35.

31. Stevens, *In Sickness and in Wealth*, pp. 52–79.

32. S. S. Goldwater, "The medical staff and its functions: A study in hospital organization," *Am J Med Sci* 133 (1907): 501–21.

33. For Wisconsin see C. R. Bardeen, "Hospitals in Wisconsin: A historical survey, 1816–1925" *Wis Med J* 24 (1925): 235–67. For a background overview see G. B. Risse, "From horse and buggy to automobile and telephone: Medical practice in Wisconsin, 1848–1930," in *Wisconsin Medicine*, pp. 25–45.

34. For details and a sociological analysis of change since 1900 see Edith M. Lentz, "The American Voluntary Hospital as an Example of Institutional Change," Ph.D. diss., Cornell Univ., 1956.

35. W. H. Mansholt, "What can European and American hospitals learn from each other?," *Nosokomeion* 1 (1930): 185–232.

36. "Prof. Tandler's impressions of America—foreign letter Aug 8, 1929," *JAMA* 93 (Sept. 7, 1929): 784. For German conditions see E. Steinitz, "Ueber Entwicklung und Probleme des modernen Krankenhauswesens," *Klin Wochenschr* 9 (September 1930): 1685–89. For Britain consult Steven Cherry, "Accountability, entitlement, and control issues and voluntary hospital funding c. 1860–1939," *Soc Hist Med* 9 (1996): 215–33, and his book *Medical Services and the Hospital in Britain, 1860–1939*, Cambridge, Cambridge Univ. Press, 1996.

37. For other information see R. Lang, "Nordamerikanische Krankenhäuser," *Klin Wochenschr* 9 (1930): 312–19. Another detailed comparative analysis of Britain and the United States is Daniel M. Fox, *Health Policies, Health Politics: The British and American Experience, 1911–1965*, Princeton, Princeton Univ. Press, 1986, especially chaps. 1–3.

38. A. J. Ochsner, "Important practical points in hospital construction for American cities with special arguments favoring many storied buildings," *Clin Rev* 23 (1905–06): 389–412, and E. Stotz, "High hospital building proves a success," *Mod Hosp* 14 (1920): 1–9.

39. Julius Rosenwald Fund, *Negro Hospitals: A Compilation of Available Statistics*, Chicago, Rosenwald Fund, 1931. For details see Vanessa Northington Gamble, *Making a Place for Ourselves: The Black Hospital Movement, 1920–1945*, New York, Oxford Univ. Press, 1995. pp. 3–34.

40. G. Goldin, "A review of the hospital literature on the private room in England and the United States during the past century," *Episteme* 4 (1970): 37–76. See also John D. Thompson and Grace Goldin, *The Hospital: A Social and Architectural History*, New Haven, Yale Univ. Press, 1975.

41. R. C. Cabot, "Some functions of social work in hospitals," *Mod Hosp* 4 (1915): 188–91, and Ida M. Cannon, *Social Work in Hospitals: A Contribution to Progressive Medicine*, New York, Survey Association, 1913.

42. M. Roemer, "General hospitals in Europe," in *Modern Concepts of Hospital Administration*, ed. J. K. Owen, Philadelphia, W. B. Saunders, 1962, pp. 17–37.

43. J. E. Jennings, "The mental attitude of the patient," *Nosokomeion* 1 (1930): 56–59.

44. For more information see Stevens, *American Hospital in the Twentieth Century*. The

author was quite impressed with the facilities of the 2,000-bed Rudolf Virchow Hospital in Berlin and the European emphasis on outdoor convalescence in special arbors and gardens.

45. E. M. Jamieson, "An experiment in segregating nursing orders," *Am J Nurs* 30 (January 1930): 83–84. See S. Reverby, "A legitimate relationship: Nursing, hospitals and science in the twentieth century," in *American General Hospital*, pp. 135–56.

46. "Heartless nurses," *Am J Nurs* 29 (February 1929): 221–227, and "How do we look?" Ibid. 30 (May 1930): 647. See also Committee On the Grading of Nursing Schools, *Nurses, Patients, and Pocketbooks*, New York, COGNS, 1928, pp. 521–43.

47. "Do less free work and more for pay, Rosenwald tells hospitals," *Hosp Manag* 30 (November 1930): 27. See also C. Rufus Rorer, *The Public's Investment in Hospitals*, Chicago, Univ of Chicago Press, 1930. However, efforts to enact a compulsory health insurance program had failed in the 1920s. See Ronald L. Numbers, *Almost Persuaded: American Physicians and Compulsory Health Insurance, 1912–1920*, Baltimore, Johns Hopkins Univ. Press, 1978.

48. Fund-raising plea published in Madison's *Capital Times*, November 1919, and reproduced in MGH's newsletter *General Scope* VI (August–September 1980): 4.

49. C. A Harper, "Efforts by the citizens of Madison toward obtaining hospital facilities," Madison, WI, 1949 (Pamphlet 93–2336, State Historical Society of Wisconsin). The doctrinal eclecticism included so-called orthodox physicians, as well as homeopaths and eclectics. For a summary see Mollenhoff, *Madison*, pp. 400–06.

50. A brief overview of Wisconsin history can be found in J. D. Buenker, "Wisconsin as maverick, model, and microcosm," in *Comparative Histories of the Midwestern States*, ed. J. H. Madison, Bloomington, Indiana Univ. Press, 1988, pp. 59–85. More details can be found in Robert C. Nesbit, *Wisconsin, A History*, Madison, Univ. of Wisconsin Press, 1973.

51. Behrnd, "Chronology," p. 17. For the early developments, R. Kosmer, Jr., "The establishment of a hospital," MGH Archives.

52. Quotations from Dr. C. S. Sheldon, a local Madison physician in *Wisc State J*, Nov. 24, 1909.

53. For the influence of women in these developments see J. Kresge Secord, "The role of women's organizations in the development of health institutions and public health programs in Madison, Wisconsin, from 1890–1920," MGH Archives.

54. Behrnd, "Chronology," p. 79.

55. A. D. Rosenthal, "The success of the woman superintendent," *Trained Nurs Hosp Rev* 81 (July 1928): 58. For details concerning administration see Michael M. Davis, *Hospital Administration, a Career: The Need of Trained Executives for a Billion Dollar Business and How They May Be Trained*, New York, 1929.

56. Interview with Gordon Johnson, July 24, 1981, transcript, MGM Archives.

57. Ibid.

58. Ibid.

59. Constitution, by-laws, and rules and resolutions of purpose of the staff and diagnostic department of the Madison General Hospital, Madison, Wisconsin, adopted July 6, 1920, MGH Archives.

60. Excerpt from the *Wisconsin Democrat*, April 1923, in *General Scope* VI (August–September 1980): 9.

61. The well-known hospital expert Edward F. Stevens defended the provision of attractive living quarters for nurses: "The more alluring it can be made to the young woman who is taking up nursing, the better will be the class of women who will come to it," he wrote in *The American Hospital in the Twentieth Century*, p. 175.

62. "The Nursing School stages many parties and entertainments for the pleasure of the nurses, and the nurses themselves prove to be good boosters." *The 1926 Litahni*, p. 35, MGH Archives. See B. J. Kalish and P. A Kalish, "Slaves, servants or saints? An analysis of the system of nurse training in the United States, 1873–1948," *Nurs Forum* 14 (1975): 222–63.

63. See details in Marilyn E. Flood, "The Troubling Expedient: General Staff Nursing in the 1930s, A Means to Institutional, Educational, and Personal Ends" Ph.D. diss. Univ. of California, Berkeley, 1981, especially pp. 148–80.

64. "Senior story," in *The 1926 Litahni*, p. 17, MGH Archives. For subsequent developments see D. Wagner, "The proletarianization of nursing in the United States, 1932–1946," *Int J Health Serv* 10 (1980): 271–90.

65. Personal interview with former MGH student and nurse Mildred Green, October 1993.

66. For details see S. Reverby, "The search for the hospital yardstick: Nursing and the rationalization of hospital work," in *Health Care in America: Essays in Social History*, ed. S. Reverby and D. Rosner, Philadelphia, Temple Univ. Press, 1979, pp. 206–25.

67. E. J. B. Schubring, "Report of the President," in *Thirtieth Annual Report of the MGH and School of Nursing, for the Fiscal Year Ending December 31, 1929*, Madison, WI, 1930, pp. 24–25.

68. Isadore Rosenfield, *Hospital Architecture and Beyond*, New York, Van Nostrand Reinhold, 1969, p. 37.

69. Behrnd, "Chronology," pp. 100–01. See also "Hospitals approved for intern training by A.M.A.," *Hosp Manag* 29 (January 1930): 41, and J. A. Curran, "Internships and residencies: Historical backgrounds and current trends," *J Med Ed* 34 (1959): 873–84.

70. G. Crafts, "Report of the Superintendent," in *Thirty-First Annual Report of the MGH and School of Nursing, for the Fiscal Year Ending December 31, 1930*, Madison, WI, 1931, p. 27.

71. E. J. B. Schubring, "Report of the President," in ibid., p. 22.

72. E .E. Irons, "Telescopic vision and medical economics," *JAMA* 95 (July 26, 1930): 244. For an earlier view see W. H. Allen, "Hospital efficiency," *Am J Soc* 12 (1906): 298–318.

73. R. Stevens, "A poor sort of memory: Voluntary hospitals and government before the Depression," *Milbank Mem Fund Q* 60 (Fall 1982): 551–84.

74. "If the linens are grayish instead of snowy white, if a shower of lint comes from the shaking of a fresh laundered sheet or pillow case, if the linens have an odor, feel harsh or irritate the skin, patients are quick to perceive these imperfections and become discontented with the hospital generally." From an advertisement appearing in *Hosp Topics Buyer*, 8 (September 1930): n.p. For details, Frank E. Chapman, *The Care of the Patient of Moderate Means*, New York, Hospital Social Service, 1929, and Niles Carpenter, *Hospital Service for Patients of Moderate Means*, Washington, DC, Community Costs of Medical Care, 1930.

75. Editorial, "Inmate is no longer in the hospital lexicon," *Hosp Manag* 29 (April 1930): 49.

76. "The house diet, unalterable as the laws of Medes and Persians, and garnished with a prune, apparently is planned for its calories and vitamins but with little regard, if any, for individual taste, much less national appeal." W. S. Goodale, "The patient; some of his reactions to hospital administration," *JAMA* 94 (Mar. 29, 1930): 906. See also "Come into the kitchen," *Hosp Manag* 30 (September 1930): 67–70.

77. W. S. Goodale, "Is the patient usually right,?" *Hosp Topics Buyer* 8 (September 1930): 74. See also M. E. Stout, "Hospital versus hotel, as seen by the doctor," *Hosp Manag*

33 (January 1932): 38–39, and J. Collins, "The patient's dilemma," *Harper's Monthly* 159 (September 1929): 514.

78. "Funny business," *Hosp Topics Buyer* 8 (September 1930): 11–12, and E. H. Lewinski Corwin, "Hospital with a soul," *Nosokomeion* 1 (1930): 17–24.

79. A typical example was the Baker Memorial unit opened at the Massachusetts General Hospital in Boston with the support of the Rosenwald Fund Committee. See M. O. Foley, "A hospital for patients of moderate means," *Hosp Manag* 30 (August 1930): 42–46, and W. F. Wood, "Financing and administration of wards for persons of moderate means," *Bull Am Hosp Assoc* 4 (January 1930): 9–13.

80. "Careful routine needed for accident service," *Hosp Manag* 27 (February 1929): 67.

81. M. L. Taylor, "Social Service Department Report," in MGH's *Thirty-First Annual Report*, p. 29.

82. G. J. Sivers, "Definite routine is of great importance in the Admitting Department," *Hosp Manag* 30 (October 1930): 29–30.

83. E. A. Filene, "Autocare versus medical care," *JAMA* 93 (Oct. 19, 1929): 1247.

84. Anon., "A patient looks at doctors," *Harper's Monthly* 161 (November 1930): 718.

85. Editorial, "The cost of hospitalization," *JAMA* 94 (Jan. 18, 1930): 186.

86. A. T. Holbrook, "Hospitals and the cost of medical care," *JAMA* 94 (Mar. 29, 1930): 904. For details see George Rosen, *The Structure of American Medical Practice, 1875–1941*, ed. C. E. Rosenberg, Philadelphia, Univ. of Pennsylvania Press, 1983.

87. For a thoughtful study of this issue see H. F. Stein, "The money taboo in American medicine," *Med Anthrop* 7 (1983): 1–15.

88. For details about the development of the American profession see Paul Starr, *The Social Transformation of American Medicine*, New York, Basic Books, 1982, and Rosemary Stevens, *American Medicine and the Public Interest*, New Haven, Yale Univ. Press, 1971.

89. A. B. Mills, *Trained Nurs Hosp Rev* 81 (November 1928): 565.

90. Editorial, "Ebb and flow," *Hosp Topics Buyer* 8 (August 1930): 11.

91. Editorial, "The cost of medical care," *JAMA* 94 (Jan. 11, 1930): 106. For details see Maurice Leven, *The Incomes of Physicians: An Economic and Statistical Analysis*, Chicago, Univ. of Chicago Press, 1932.

92. This premise is contained in a report submitted to the AMA's board of trustees during their 81st annual meeting in Detroit, June 23–27, 1930.

93. C. A. Harper, "President's page," *Wis Med J* 30 (September 1932): 744.

94. *Historical Statistics of the United States, Colonial Times to 1970*, Washington, DC, U.S. Bureau of the Census, 1975, pp. 176 and 301.

95. Editorial, "Doctors of medical practice and the cost of medical care," *JAMA* 93 (Aug. 10, 1929): 459. Details are available in S. Kunitz, "Efficiency and reform in the financing and organization of American medicine in the Progressive era," *Bull Hist Med* 55 (1981): 497–515.

96. "Charity in private practice," *JAMA* 95 (Sept. 27, 1930): 943.

97. This was, of course, anathema to organized medicine. See "A doctor's advice to his critics," *The Forum* 87 (June 1932): 353–58. See also Howard R. Brill, "Producing Health: The Making of the Hospital as a Business, 1929–1946," Ph.D. diss., SUNY Binghamton, 1994.

98. I. C. Anderson, "The humanity of the nursing profession," *Trained Nurs Hosp Rev* 81 (October 1928): 463. For later developments see H. Frey, "How can the hospital increase its receipts and decrease expenses without impairing its efficiency?," *Nosokomeion* 8 (1937): 14–33.

99. Behrnd, "Chronology," p. 79.

100. This complaint is taken from an article written by John A. McNamara, editor of the journal *Modern Hospital*, titled "Mr. Brown pays his hospital bill," which appeared in *Scribners Magazine* in March 1930. For a commentary see *Am J Nurs* 30 (March 1930): 370.

101. S. S. Goldwater, "The correction by administrative methods of undesirable mental states in hospital patients," *Nosokomeion* 1 (1930): 70–7.

102. C. J. Garrison, "Getting it over to the public," *Trained Nurs Hosp Rev* 80 (March 1928): 309.

103. Quoted in "Widespread interest shown in problems arising from auto mishaps," *Hosp Manag* 27 (February 1929): 44.

104. D. D. Bromley, "After the automobile accident," *Harper's Monthly* 164 (March 1932): 477–87. See also Edgar Sydenstricker, *Health and Environment*, New York, Mc-Graw-Hill, 1933.

105. "Automobiles kill 218,000 in thirteen years," *JAMA* 95 (Sept. 6, 1930): 736.

106. *Wis State J*, June 15, 1930, p. 1.

107. For a comparison between Madison and New York see E. L. Meyer, "The lure of the provinces," *The Forum* 86 (July 1930): 40–44.

108. *Wis State J*, June 30, 1930, p. 3.

109. Ibid., June 16, 1930, p. 3

110. Ibid., June 20, 1930, p. 4.

111. "Automobile rides as a consumption cure," *Horseless Age* 13 (1904): 522.

112. Medical news: "General: mortality from automobile accidents," *JAMA* 94 (June 7, 1930): 1850.

113. See Anedith J. B. Nash, "Death on the Highway: The Automobile Wreck in American Culture, 1920–40," Ph.D. diss., Univ. of Minnesota, 1983, especially pp. 33–37.

114. *Wis State J*, July 14, 1930, p. 1.

115. *Wis State J*, July 10, 1930, p. 1., and *Wis Med J* 30 (April 1931): 301. For an overview of the influences of the automobile on rural areas of the United States, including Wisconsin, see Michael L. Berger, *The Devil Wagon in God's Country*, Hamden, CT, Archon Books, 1979.

116. *Wis State J*, June 27, 1930, p. 1.

117. *Wright's Madison City Directory, 1929*, pp. 9–12.

118. *JAMA* 89 (Nov. 5, 1927): 1616.

119. *Wis State J*, July 3, 1930, p. 1.

120. B. M. Parks, "Reducing automobile accidents by municipal control of operators," *Am City* 46 (April 1932): 92–94.

121. D. D. Bromley, "After the automobile accident," *Harper's Monthly* 164 (March 1932): 480.

122. V. R. Bosworth, "Providing for emergency cases," *Hosp Topics Buyer* 8 (July 1930): 24.

123. "Auto mishaps," *Hosp Manag* 27 (February 1929): 45.

124. "Who should pay hospital bills of traffic victims?" *Am City* 42 (January 1930): 153.

125. "Auto mishaps," 45.

126. F. Christopher, "Compression fractures," *Am J Surg* 9 (July–September 1930): 427.

127. Personal communication from Paula's relatives, 1996.

128. R. W. Harbaugh, "Fractures of the spine with or without operation, a statistical study," *Calif West Med* 32 (May 1930): 325–30, and A. G. Davis, "Fractures of the spine," *J Bone Joint Surg* 11 (January 1929): 133–56.

129. See Henry H. Kessler, *Accidental Injuries*, 2nd ed., Philadelphia, Lea & Febiger, 1940, pp. 231–33.

130. W. A. Rogers, "An extension frame for the reduction of fracture of the vertebral body," *Surg Gynecol Obstet* 50 (1930): 101–04. See also J. Dunlop and C. H. Parker, "Correction of compressed fractures of the vertebrae," *JAMA* 94 (Jan. 11, 1930): 89–93.

131. L. D. Smith, "Crush fracture of the spine; immediate treatment by manipulation with report of cases," *Wis Med J* 30 (August 1931): 639–42.

132. For an extensive discussion see Lorenz Böhler, *The Treatment of Fractures*, trans. E. W. Hey Groves, 4th ed., Baltimore, W. Wood & Co., 1935, pp. 117–32.

133. M. L. Taylor, "Social Service Department Report for June 1930," p. 2, MGH Archives.

134. See M. Constantine, "How early should we awaken our patients?" *Mod Hosp* 35 (July 1930): 97–99, and "What can be done about waking patients before the break of dawn?" *Hosp Manag* 29 (March 1930): 23.

135. Green interview, October 1993.

136. Harper, *Merely a Patient*, p. 53.

137. Ibid.

138. D. D. Dunbar, "The crisis in nursing," republished from *Harper's Magazine's* July 1930 issue in *Am J Nurs* 30 (1930): 913–14.

139. Details are presented in Marion L. Vannier and Barbara A. Thompson, *Nursing Procedures*, Minneapolis, Univ. of Minnesota Press, 1929. For a panel discussion of the historical importance of nursing see E. W. Hook, "Is there a feminist disdain for nursing?" *Pharos* 57 (Summer 1994): 36–40.

140. I. S. Poplin, "Nursing uniforms: Romantic idea, functional attire, or instrument of social change?," *Nurs Hist Rev* 2 (1994): 153–67.

141. Green interview, October 1993.

142. On the interplay between nurses and social workers see E. Slater, "Nurse and social worker," *Am J Nurs* 30 (May 1930): 598–600.

143. Green interview, October 1993.

144. C. R. Conover, "What's wrong with the hospitals?" *Hosp Topics Buyer* 8 (Apr. 1, 1930): 70.

145. B. C. Lovell, "The function of the hospital social worker," *Hosp Social Serv* 21 (1930): 104–14, and E. M. Baker, "Medical social worker as interpreter between patient and hospital," *Mod Hosp* 42 (1934): 65–68. For details see Elsie Wulkop, *The Social Worker in a Hospital Ward*, Boston, Houghton Mifflin, 1926.

146. N. M. Panella, "The patients' library movement: an overview of early efforts in the US to establish organized libraries for hospital patients," *Bull Med Libr Assoc* 84 (1996): 52–62.

147. Harper, *Merely the Patient*, p. 65.

148. Since 1929, tobacco prices had been dropping and the market remained quite unstable. About 135 Wisconsin tobacco dealers had just met in the town of Cambridge to oppose a bill banning imports from Sumatra. *Wis State J*, June 27, 1930, p. 2.

149. R. B. Osgood, "Compression fractures of the spine, diagnosis and treatment, *JAMA* 89 (Nov. 5, 1927): 1563–68.

150. MGH's social services department reported at the end of 1930 that "intelligent working out of plans for the post-hospital care are steps towards the physical and mental restoration of the sick person who is in the hospital, thereby making his illness as constructive a thing as possible," MGH's *Thirty-First Annual Report*, p. 28.

151. The Wisconsin state legislature passed the first state unemployment compensation act in 1932. See R. I. Vexler and W. F. Swindler, *Chronology and Documentary Handbook of the State of Wisconsin*, Dobbs Ferry, NY, Oceana Pub., 1978, p. 18.

152. Taylor, "Report for June 1930," p. 2.

153. G. Crafts, "Report of the Superintendent," in MGH's *Thirty-First Annual Report*, p. 26–27.

154. "Medical News: Wisconsin proposes compensation for automobile accidents," *JAMA* 95 (Nov. 22, 1930): 1434.

155. Behrnd, "Chronology," p. 102.

156. Personal interview with Earl Thayer, former secretary of the Wisconsin State Medical Society, October 1993. See also E. Wisner, "Can patient pay? And will he? Ask the social worker," *Mod Hosp* 37 (August 1931): 59–62.

157. Behrnd, "Chronology," p. 105.

158. "Rules for admission of patients," *Thirty-Second Annual Report of the Madison General Hospital Association for the Fiscal Year Ending December 31, 1931*, Madison, WI, 1932, p. 14a

159. Ibid.

160. R. F. Armstrong, "Effects of present economic conditions on hospital operations," *Trans Am Hosp Assoc* 33 (1931): 695–710, and M. T. MacEachern, "Some economic problems affecting hospitals today and suggestions for their solution," *Bull Am Hosp Assoc* 6 (July 1932): 58–67.

161. C. G. Parvall, "Let's give some thought to the question of the cost of illness," *Hosp Manag* 29 (May 1930): 58–60.

162. G. H. Agnew, "Possible effect of health insurance upon our hospitals," *Trans Am Hosp Assoc* 33 (1931): 586–92. See R. L. Numbers, "The third party: Health insurance in America," in *The Therapeutic Revolution*, ed. M. J. Vogel and C. Rosenberg, Philadelphia, Univ. of Pennsylvania Press, 1979, pp. 177–200.

163. Behrnd, "Chronology," p. 107. See also G. H. Agnew, "Possible effect of health insurance upon our hospitals," *Trans Am Hosp Assoc* 33 (1931): 586–92.

164. Committee on the Costs of Medical Care, *Medical Care for the American People*, Chicago, Univ. of Chicago Press, 1932, pp. 120–23. For an analysis see I. S. Falk, "Medical care in the USA 1932–1972: Problems, proposals and programs from the Committee on the Costs of Medical Care," *Milbank Mem Fund Q* 51 (Winter 1973): 2–13.

165. Hugh Cabot, *The Doctor's Bill*, New York, Columbia Univ. Press, 1935, pp. 19–20.

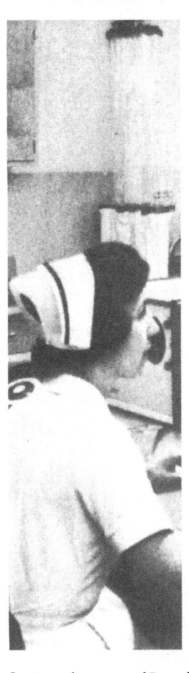

10

HOSPITALS
AT THE
CROSSROADS

Government, Society, and
Catholicism in America,
1950–1975

A hospital, particularly a Catholic hospital where
Christ dwells in the chapel tabernacle, is another
Holy Land where the workers from the Sister Administrator to the least of the maids are doing in
part and in a humbler way what our Savior did
long ago in Palestine. Its product is a happy death
for the few; for the many, health so necessary in
all walks of life.

Mercy Hospital, *Mercy's Fifty Years*, 1954[1]

A sudden heart attack

Periodically sounding its siren, a hospital ambulance made its way through a veil of snow
flurries on the evening of December 20, 1954, in South Buffalo. Inside the vehicle, lying on a stretcher, was Joseph O'H.,[2] a 67-year-old retired Irish engineer,
who had worked all his life for the Pennsylvania Railroad. His terror-stricken wife
sat at his side, clutching his hand. Outside it was cold and blustery, a typical early
winter night in a city getting ready for Christmas. After a short ride, the patient
arrived around 10 PM at the Emergency Room of Mercy Hospital, the nearest institution with such a facility.[3] The hospital was run by the Sisters of Mercy, an order of Irish American nuns with deep roots in the community.

The Sisters were a common sight, visiting families, asking for donations, and teaching in the schools. Joseph's first contact with these nuns had occurred long ago while he was a student in St. Brigit's parish school before going to South Park's high school. A native of South Buffalo and one of seven children of an immigrant Irish family, Joseph lived on Louisiana Street near the Buffalo River, a close-knit, predominantly Irish community and the city's first ward. Most inhabitants were devout Catholics and pro-labor Democrats. Catholicism and parish membership preserved their national identity. Indeed, the parish church constituted the social, religious, and political center for the community. To avoid discrimination in the predominantly Protestant public school system, most families in the neighborhood sent their children to the parish school, where the Sisters of Mercy taught.[4] Throughout his youth and adult life, Joseph's neighborhood had been "saturated" with Sisters of Mercy. He and his wife were quite comfortable with the Sisters, respecting them as both educators and health care providers. Their hospital had a good reputation in the neighborhood as a friendly, informal, and less bureaucratic institution. "Mercy Hospital has always been there for us if we needed it," insisted Joseph's wife.[5]

Located in the hospital's recently expanded wing, the Emergency Room was now staffed around the clock by interns and nurses. Advances in accreditation and standardization of health care facilities, especially after World War II, had been hailed as important factors in guaranteeing the physical recovery of patients. Indeed, the hospital construction boom triggered by the federal Hill-Burton Act had caused a dramatic surge in admissions. While a somewhat disoriented Joseph was being wheeled into a room, his wife anxiously provided most of the personal and financial information. Next door in the lobby, somebody at the reception desk, staffed by volunteers, quickly entered the data in a rotary Kardex file containing lists of current patients and clergymen who came to pay visits to their parishioners. Receptionists were familiar with many of the newly arriving patients, and Joseph was no exception. Joseph's chief complaint: chest pain suggestive of a heart attack.[6]

As Joseph was wheeled on a cart into Mercy's Emergency Room, his troubled mind fleetingly recalled earlier anxious moments linked to the birth of his last two children in this institution nearly four decades ago. Catholic hospitals prided themselves on being institutions where the patients' spiritual and social needs were recognized. In February 1954, a message from Pope Pius XII called the sick "precious jewels of the Church of Christ." Caring for them displayed a key quality: "Charity possesses a dignity, an inspiration and a strength that is lacking in mere philanthropy." Where nuns worked, a more solemn atmosphere prevailed: "virtue works wonders which technical aids and medical skills alone are powerless to accomplish."[7] Perhaps Mercy Hospital would be an ideal refuge, mused Joseph, who like other Irish males believed that sharing one's suffering meant weakness. Loss of physical strength threatened social status and even suggested punishment for some sinful behavior.[8] Here the hospital's "sweet influence of religion dispelling the nervous gloom of the patient, so dangerous to physical recovery," might be helpful.[9]

Catholic hospitals as well as nondenominational institutions were concerned about their public image.[10] The importance of patients' first contacts with hospitals—like those in emergency facilities—were deemed critical.[11] Joseph remembered Mercy Hospital's reputation as a good place to come for heart troubles. On the medical staff was a veteran internist with cardiology training: Dr. Robert E. DeCeu, an 1899 graduate of the University of Buffalo School of Medicine, who had practiced in South Buffalo for six decades. In the 1920s, DeCeu, who was also a member of the Western New York State Heart Association,[12] had studied with Dr. Paul D. White at Harvard and devoted himself to the practice of cardiology, an emerging subspecialty in both Europe and America.[13] To Joseph's surprise and peace of mind, a member of his parish working as a volunteer greeted him as he rested on a cart waiting for the physician on call to see him.

Buffalo's holiday mood, meanwhile, was marred by a fierce battle to scuttle the St. Lawrence Seaway legislation. Citizens feared that the new canal planned through Canada would be a disaster to the local waterfront economy. Already there had been cuts in the factory workforce, and unemployment was the highest in the state. In spite of gloomy statistics, however, Buffalo remained optimistic that the traditional nexus of steel and automobiles, together with the availability of inexpensive electric power from the Niagara Falls, would continue to preserve the local economy. Buffalo's chamber of commerce optimistically proclaimed in 1954 that "no area has a greater opportunity to grow than the Niagara Frontier."[14]

While economic problems preoccupied the citizens of western New York State, tensions between physicians in general practice and a growing number of specialists, especially in surgery, were mounting. At a time when medical education and practice were inclined "to concentrate upon disease rather than the understanding of the whole person,"[15] general practitioners were especially coveted by Catholic hospitals, but their numbers were dwindling. Erie County had 447 registered general practitioners in 1950 but only 371 in 1953, a drop of nearly 20%, despite efforts by the American Academy of General Practice—founded in 1947— to improve the standards of its more than 100,000 members nationwide.[16] For their part, general practitioners sought to protect their status by strictly following the policies and by-laws of the hospitals they were affiliated with.[17] Mercy's current chief of the medical staff was Dr. Matthew L. Carden. He, like many of the staff members, was a busy general practitioner of Irish descent, earning a modest living in the blue-collar neighborhoods surrounding the hospital. Mostly trained before World War II, only a few of the general practitioners at Mercy Hospital had completed an internship or taken further training other than wartime service. Pious Catholics, they strongly supported the Sisters of Mercy's philosophy of caring and were quite deferential to the nuns.

General practitioners were on the losing end of the struggle with the specialists. Since the American College of Surgeons had established hospital standards in 1917, admission privileges were extended only to competent and ethical practitioners. Although they still rendered more than 85% of medical care in their communities, many older general practitioners found their hospital privileges curtailed, even canceled. In response, the American Academy of General Practice sought to expand postgraduate training for younger general practitioners and thus allow them to compete successfully for hospital staff privileges and a portion of the medical marketplace. To ensure a better quality of medical care, even Mercy Hospital had just approved a three-year residency in general practice.

As at other institutions, the medical staff, together with the Sisters, tried to monitor the performance of all attending physicians to protect Mercy's accreditation. Concerns about the quality of surgical practice at the hospital were referred to the hospital's Tissue Committee. In 1954, this group found glaring examples of organ removals—tonsils, appendix, uterus—showing no pathological changes. Medical staff members needed to be monitored closely about correlations between their diagnoses, surgical interventions, and pathology of the removed tissues. Chief of Staff Carden and others also grappled with deficiencies detected in the hospital's medical records. Lack of progress notes, incomplete diagnoses, and omission of consultations were frequent. Narcotic orders were not being signed. Busy practitioners gave entirely too many verbal orders, either in person or via telephone, a practice forbidden by the staff's by-laws but frequently violated as the doctors hastily made their rounds before heading to their office appointments.[18] Another concern was the low autopsy rate—about 30%—allowed, remarkably enough, by attending physicians who tried to please their patient clientele by siding with relatives in opposing such examinations.[19]

In the company of Sister M. Victorine, the nun in charge of the Emergency Room, Joseph O'H. waited for the physician on call to arrive. He later admitted that a "whole atmosphere of caring permeated the institution."[20] The environment at Mercy Hospital was like an extension of Joseph's own neighborhood. A sense of solidarity and even familiarity began in the Emergency and Admission Rooms and spread to all wards. These facilities were populated by friendly and familiar faces, often relatives or friends who worked in the institution, and, of course, the nuns themselves, known from school functions and bazaars. The patients were mostly Catholics of Irish, Italian, and German descent. In carrying out their tasks, the Sisters of Mercy relied on a traditional Irish matriarchal model, widely represented in urban settings in both the old and new worlds. The authority of these Sisters was bolstered considerably by their religious status, which conferred additional respect and social prominence. Indeed, since their early days in Ireland, sisterhood had been a most successful strategy for women who desired respect, independence, and social mobility without losing their traditional identity and kinship.[21]

Summoned to check Joseph was Dr. John J. O'Brien, another internist with cardiology training, who was also in charge of house staff education.[22] Providing a history of the events preceding his acute attack, Joseph insisted that in recent years he had been active and in good health. During the past few months, however, he admitted having several similar transient episodes of "indigestion." He denied ever having had high blood pressure, but in recent months he had observed a slight swelling of his ankles and difficulty breathing on exertion, as well as some coughing. Joseph's account of the events immediately preceding his admission was not atypical for sufferers of heart disease. After shoveling some snow on his driveway, he had noted a dull, constricting substernal pain around 4 PM. This aching lasted for about half an hour, radiating into both shoulders and arms. When he finally sat down, the pain subsided. However, the symptoms returned around 9 PM after he had had his supper and was watching television with his wife. Slightly nauseated, he took some Bromo-Seltzer and then walked outside into the cold night, feeling somewhat relieved. After returning five minutes later, however, Joseph began to sweat profusely. He finally called his private physician, Dr. Louis F. Manze, a surgeon, who promptly arrived at the house, gave him a shot of morphine, and called the ambulance.

Physical examination disclosed an obese, pale, and apprehensive individual, now sweating profusely and breathing with some difficulty. His skin was wet and clammy. Despite his immobility, Joseph still complained of chest pain. The chest was resonant, but a number of fine rales could be heard in the posterior right base. His blood pressure was 180/110, with a heart rate of 92 beats per minute. His slight tachycardia also disclosed approximately 12–16 extra systoles per minute, but there were no pericardial rubs. Joseph's abdomen was soft; the liver, spleen, and kidneys were not palpable. He had slight but not pitting edema in both extremities, but the pulses were good and there was no tenderness or obvious varicosities. A heart attack and mild congestive heart failure were suspected. In 1954, Erie County was to report 3,675 cases of cardiovascular disease, the highest rate outside of New York City.[23] The first therapeutic objective was to prevent death, shock, or cardiac failure. At this point, Joseph's chances of dying from myocardial infarction were about one in three.[24] An oxygen mask was placed over his face, and he received an intravenous injection of morphine in the expectation that this would diminish the occasional extrasystoles. Close to midnight, Joseph O'H.—his face covered by an oxygen mask—left Mercy's Emergency Room on a stretcher for the third-floor medical ward.

Serving the community: Buffalo and Mercy Hospital

At Mercy Hospital, the authorities had been busy celebrating the institution's golden jubilee in September. Even before this event, plans had been filed for an

addition to the nurses' home at Choate Avenue, a three-floor structure now under construction that would include a 300-seat auditorium.[25] In 1954 alone, the
hospital cared for 12,300 inpatients and witnessed 200 births a month. With another 2,929 institutions in the United States and Canada, it was accredited by the
Joint Commission of Accreditation sponsored by the American Hospital Association and appeared on its first list, published in 1953. This listing was based on
a set of organizational and administrative criteria for efficient patient care.[26]

The early activities of the Sisters of Mercy in Buffalo went back to the year
1858, when the first bishop of the Buffalo diocese, John Timon, recruited three
members from a newly founded convent in Rochester to teach at St. Brigit's parish
school on the Irish south side of Buffalo.[27] The roots of this ministry went back
to Ireland and Catherine McAuley (1778–1841), daughter of a noted builder, who
in September 1828 had established a House of Mercy in Dublin to shelter the
poor, especially orphans and young women, as well as the sick.[28] Before her death,
McAuley managed to found 11 more convents in Ireland and 2 in England before members of her congregation crossed the Atlantic for America in 1845.[29] Because of conditions in Ireland during the 1830s, Mercy spirituality had an eminently activist bent; it was an apostolate of service toward the needy both in the
mother country and later in America. Indeed, Sisters of Mercy were "walking"
nuns, working outside their convents in the wretched tenements and alleys of metropolitan areas, bringing succor, hope, and education to the poor and sick. In
time, this congregation became the largest English-speaking religious order of
women in the world.[30]

After establishing their own convent in Buffalo in 1861, the Sisters of Mercy
began visiting the homes of parishioners, offering to assist with spiritual and physical care. Dressed in long black cloaks with a black bonnet covered by a gauze
veil, the Sisters moved about St. Brigit's carrying brown baskets filled with food
and clothing for the poor. A critical factor in their gradual success was their capacity to adapt to local conditions and make contact with lay members of the district. Following the Civil War, the Sisters of Mercy expanded their ministry in
Buffalo, creating a House of Mercy shelter and training school for young women
"of good character but out of situations" attached to their convent, the Academy
of the Immaculate Conception of Our Lady of Mercy. This community orientation and the desire to be educators set them apart from other Catholic orders seeking opportunities to carry out missionary work in America.[31]

The origin of the Sisters' hospital grew out of the same concerns. With typhoid fever reaching epidemic proportions in residential areas surrounding the
steel mills still under construction—especially among Italians—the need for a voluntary hospital in South Buffalo became acute in 1903. Mother Superior Mary
Dolores Clancy of the Sisters of Mercy thus commissioned another nun, Sister M.
Catherine Monahan, to procure a place for the establishment of such an institu-

tion. The result was the purchase of a large house on Tifft Street and South Park, strategically located south of the Buffalo River and near the edge of town, as well as in close proximity to Lackawanna and its expanding industrial facilities. The new 28-bed sectarian hospital opened its doors to the public on the day of the feast of Our Lady of Mercy, September 24, 1904, thanks to local fund-raising activities and a group of 100 women who formed the Mercy Hospital Aid Society. According to the hospital's by-laws, however, no specific ethnic group was to be favored or admission denied to non-Catholic patients. Legally, the institution belonged to the Sisters' mother house and, with Sister M. Camillus Stafford at the helm after 1905, it operated under the auspices of the Buffalo dioceses.

Soon thereafter, a training school for nurses opened its doors next to the hospital, an obvious outgrowth of the Mercy Sisters' traditional educational activities with young women. As in most other contemporary schools, the emphasis was on service following the Nightingale model, with an opportunity to learn basic skills and reside in a protected environment. Emphasis on Christian principles and obedience to the Sisters in charge made this training somewhat akin to a novitiate. Both hospital and training school were examples of a wave of similar sectarian foundations that occurred in America's large cities and small towns in the East and Midwest.[32]

Equipped with an X-ray machine and its own horse-drawn ambulance, Mercy Hospital combined caretaker and medical functions, quickly becoming the destination point of poor patients from the immediate area. Its very presence in South Buffalo became a symbol of Catholic identity, as well as a workshop for Catholic practitioners and nurses. Funds to sustain the institution came from the community and diocese, supplemented by donations given to the tireless roaming nuns who visited local steel plants, rail yards, and factories. As in most similar institutions throughout the land, it became obvious in the 1910s that the original facilities had become totally inadequate to cope with the local demands for care, prompting the purchase of a larger tract of land located a few blocks away on Abbott Road and Choate Avenue. Adjacent to the Mount Mercy convent and only a few blocks away from the Tifft Street facility, the future location ensured the continuous presence of the Sisters of Mercy in the neighborhood.[33]

When the well-known public health expert Haven Emerson reported on Buffalo's health care facilities for New York State's Department of Hospitals and Dispensaries in 1921, he stated that South Buffalo, with a population of 75,078, had the most industries and fewest hospital beds of any neighborhood in Buffalo. This revelation stimulated renewed efforts to build a new facility. In September 1923, a number of influential citizens met to discuss plans for a citywide fund-raising campaign in behalf of Mercy Hospital. The goal was to create a nonsectarian institution by raising an estimated $500,000, a decision endorsed by Buffalo's chamber of commerce, the mayor, Frank X. Schwab, New York State's Governor, Alfred E. Smith, and clergymen of all denominations.[34]

Although the general solicitation fell far short of its goal, further appeals were made by various citizens and church groups, including the Knights of Columbus, labor unions, and women's associations.[35] Brochures emphasized the increased automobile traffic, asking "Where would you go in case of accident?" An economic argument based on the active participation of many unsalaried Sisters of Mercy suggested that the new institution would be able to function at an average cost of $ 2.50 per day as opposed to the $ 4.60 per day typical at other hospitals.[36] Although ground was broken in 1924 for a new 165-bed hospital, and although a Men's Sustaining Society was created in 1926 to assist with a loan to proceed with the construction, the new cream-colored, six-story brick building trimmed with Indiana limestone did not open its doors until February 2, 1928. The monoblock hospital faced the vast, heavily forested Cazenovia Park with its creek. It was not quite the modern facility that had initially been envisioned. Because it lacked elevators, the sick had to be carried up the stairs on stretchers. Transferred to the third floor of the adjacent convent, the Nursing School was also reorganized and registered with the Board of Regents of the State of New York.[37]

As in other American cities, the Depression devastated Buffalo's economy, creating widespread unemployment and straining local welfare efforts, including Mercy Hospital's efforts to treat indigent patients. Before the advent of Social Security, the blue-collar population of South Buffalo, composed mainly of railroad employees, grain millers, and steel mill workers, found a welcome shelter for their sick, regardless of their religious affiliation, at the hospital. During its first decade of operations at the new location on Abbott Road, Mercy Hospital, under Sister M. Gerard Kennedy, served over 100,000 individuals, including 40,000 inpatients. When the industrial area in the Buffalo-Niagara Falls region became involved in the World War II effort, plans were made to expand the hospital's rectangular building by attaching wings to each side. The project, prompted by the presence of a larger workforce, did not get underway in earnest until 1947, when South Buffalo and its adjacent communities experienced a postwar boom. The goal was to build three new wings, increasing the hospital's total capacity to 325 beds and 75 bassinets.[38] Financing this expansion involved another grass-roots effort to attract a multitude of small donors like Joseph, who clearly had a stake in their neighborhood institutions.[39]

On February 2, 1949, the hospital's new "wings of mercy" were solemnly dedicated by the bishop of Buffalo. The western wing was dedicated to St. Joseph, the east wing to St. Camillus. The printed program for the ceremonies revealed that "more than 40 sisters work 14–16 hours in the hospital each day without worldly compensation."[40] In 1950, Mercy created a physical rehabilitation center with whirlpools, a gymnasium, and electrical machines, a veritable "muscle factory" certified by the state and designed to service a growing number of patients receiving workmen's compensation.[41] In October 1953, the hospital also opened a 28-bed geriatric facility to house the chronically ill, sometimes for years, since there were few nursing homes in the area and many of these patients were destitute. At the same time, the increasing role of Mercy's business functions required an expansion of the main office facilities, including separate sections on admissions, accounting, insurance, and bookkeeping, as well as credit and social services.

At the time of Joseph's admission, Mercy Hospital was still staffed primarily by busy general practitioners. To assist them in upgrading their medical knowledge and skills, the Sisters now looked for an academic affiliation to upgrade hospital practices and provide further educational opportunities to attending physicians and the house staff. Given the new advances in medicine, Mother General Sister M. Manuela investigated the possibility of establishing a link to the University of Buffalo, but her efforts failed. Mercy Hospital was a small community institution far away on the other side of the Buffalo River, and the local medical school already possessed a number of linkages with larger hospitals in the downtown area. Instead, the Sisters reached out to another private Catholic institution: Georgetown University School of Medicine, located in the nation's capital.

After several meetings and discussions with Dr. Harold Jeghers, a recently appointed professor of medicine at Georgetown, a formal contract was signed on March 20, 1951. Jeghers was particularly interested in providing continuous medical education to practitioners working in nonuniversity affiliated community hospitals, believing that such institutions could eventually become their own graduate and postgraduate teaching centers.[42] On July 23, Dr. Irving Brick, a gastroenterologist and professor at Georgetown University, inaugurated the newly organized affiliation, coming to Mercy Hospital to lecture and conduct rounds with house and attending staff physicians. The presence of famous physicians such as Proctor Harvey—a former president of the American Heart Association—and kidney specialist, George Schreiner lent prestige to Mercy's educational efforts to attract more competent physicians.[43] To coordinate this program and provide further guidance, John O'Brien—Joseph's physician—was appointed full-time director of medical education.[44] The program centered on the daily morning report about the condition of patients in various wards provided by house staff members under O'Brien's direction. Such day-to-day interactions were more important than the biweekly conferences with Georgetown professors. However, at Mercy, rounds, case presentations, and critiques of patient management created tensions and friction with the attending general practitioners, who had trouble accepting suggestions from interns and residents primarily headed for specialties. Here O'Brien's role as mediator was indispensable and frequently quite effective. In the early 1950s, improvements in medical care at Mercy were attributed to this formal affiliation. Celebrating its silver jubilee in February 1953, Mercy Hospital was characterized in the press as "an inspiring example of the teamwork of science, Christianity, and humanitarianism."[45]

Catholic hospitals and their nurses:
"The fairest flowers of missionary endeavor"

Pope Pius XII's characterization of Catholic hospitals in his 1951 encyclical "Heralds of the Gospel" implied that these institutions also had a role to play in drawing other Christians to the faith.[46] In consonance with the papal recommendation, the American Catholic Hospital Association (CHA) had dramatically expanded its headquarters in St. Louis and developed a complex bureaucratic structure. Special divisions were created for programs devoted to medical ethics, legislation, and education. Another area of professional services featured departments of nursing, hospital administration, public relations, and financial management. Moreover, Catholic hospitals were told to seek injunctions against fee splitting, create accurate and complete medical records, and establish tissue committees like those at Mercy. All patients were to receive a routine examination on admission and sign a consent form before surgery. Active consultation among medical staff members was to be required in all major cases, and all physicians' orders needed to be documented. At the same time, the CHA took the first steps toward reshaping the role and education of the religious women whose organizations sponsored a majority of Catholic hospitals. There was a growing feeling that these nuns needed to develop both their spiritual and professional lives. Decades of teaching and hands-on nursing had made these sisters more sophisticated and conscious of their limitations. Through the creation of the Sister Formation Conference, members were to meet regionally throughout the country and plan a more effective and organized system of postnovitiate education.[47]

The CHA traced its roots back to 1915, when the Rev. Charles B. Moulinier, a Jesuit and regent of Marquette University Medical School in Milwaukee, convened a meeting attended by 35 sisters from the upper Midwest committed to the hospital apostolate. The concern, articulated a year earlier, was that existing Catholic hospitals were not keeping pace with the rapid advances in medical science and technology required to maintain their accreditation and provide adequate services. During World War I and sponsored by the CHA, a summer school at Marquette had already sponsored courses in clinical pathology and radiology for nuns working in hospitals, although doubts were raised concerning the propriety of religious women attending them. At the CHA's 1918 convention in Milwaukee, Father Moulinier reminded his audience that previous assemblies had already repudiated the idea that Catholic hospitals were mere boardinghouses. In his opinion, these institutions were also places for surgeons to operate and internists to prescribe medicines. The danger was that recent advances in medicine threatened to separate caregivers from their patients. Administrators should never forget that, in Catholic hospitals, service to the patient remained the great fundamental, ethical principle. Patients had a right to the most enlightened and scientific care together with philanthropic, self-sacrificing, and conscientious religious services.

In Moulinier's view, the vitality of the Catholic hospital depended on its ability to set and maintain standards by submitting to the criteria of a secular agency, the American College of Surgery. But fears were expressed that such a commitment to standardization would erode Catholic morality. To counter criticism, Moulinier urged the adoption of a code of ethics, officially approved in 1921. This document dealt with a number of issues, including the protection of the fetus and the mother's life in surgical emergencies.[48]

By the end of the Second World War, there were approximately 700 Catholic hospitals in the United States, with a capacity of about 100,000 beds. Most institutions had become integral parts of their local communitys' health care systems and began to participate actively in community planning and service. The relationship between the Catholic hospital's religious and medical missions again demanded careful scrutiny. The CHA responded in 1949 with a revised code of ethics. The result was the publication of *Ethical and Religious Directives for Catholic Hospitals*, a summary of basic Catholic principles applied to medicine. Directed to hospital administrators and physicians, both Catholic and non-Catholic, the code, covering such practices as contraception and abortion, became an official document only after formal adoption by local bishops.[49]

At its 38th annual convention in Kansas City in 1953, the CHA addressed issues surrounding the rapid transformation of Catholic hospitals into businesses. Sound financial procedures were still lacking. Since these institutions now became increasingly involved with federal agencies and third-party insurers, their success depended upon adequate budgetary planning and the employment of uniform accounting principles in the areas of purchasing, personnel, and in-service training.

Another critical issue was the status of Catholic training programs for nurses, threatened by the new emphasis on university education for professional nurses. A proposal to reduce the work week of hospital sisters—who still kept a busy 70-hour schedule seven days a week—generated intense discussion. Since hospital work increasingly produced significant strains and tensions, CHA leaders insisted that the Sisters decrease their service to six days and a maximum of 60 hours in deference to their physical and emotional health. But, as one nun commented, what would the Sisters do with a whole day off if this activity was their vocation and entire life? This dedication now stood in sharp contrast to the 40-hour-per-week schedules of lay nurses, who opposed split shifts and resented weekend duty. While everyone agreed that the old-fashioned nurse had almost disappeared, expectations for personal service and the highest standards of medical and nursing care remained. But how, in the face of continuing shortages of nursing personnel in hospitals, could a more old-fashioned service attitude be returned to nursing? Unfortunately, the American hospital environment was rapidly changing. The hospital was no longer part of a monastery, but reflected the cultural and social practices of society. Modern nurses were no longer recluses or institutional captives, but active citizens, often wives and mothers, with lives outside the hospital.[50]

Following World War II, the growth in the number of professional nurses apparently had kept up with the increase in hospital beds across the nation, although shortages were periodically reported. In recent years, nursing personnel composed of nonprofessional workers such as licensed practical nurses, aides, orderlies, and ward maids had doubled to comprise nearly half of the caregiving staff. Hours were now shorter, with Mercy's eight-hour shifts—7.30 AM to 3.30 PM, 3.30 PM to 11.30 PM, and 11.30 PM to 7.30 AM—being typical. Nurses now also spent more time supervising all ancillary personnel. Moreover, with shorter patient stays and increasing illness of the patients admitted to the institution, these nurses found themselves spending more time with their patients.[51]

Mercy Hospital's Nursing School offered a three-year diploma program under the direction of Sister M. Ethel, and local affiliation with Canisius College provided a preclinical year of general studies. Several additional links to regional asylums and sanatoria allowed students to obtain specialized training in psychiatry and care for tuberculosis patients. Mercy strongly competed for the best and mostly Catholic high school students, providing financial aid. In the mid-1950s the school was located in Marian Hall, living quarters for 150 students. As elsewhere, the probationers—many of whom would join the nursing staff at Mercy— were primarily trained for hospital work, learning at the bedside and thus obtaining hands-on experience and training. The Sisters of Mercy also stressed philosophy and medical ethics. As one publication explained, "inspired with its cherished ancestry and guided by the spirit of Mercy, the school endeavors to combine the teaching, tradition and culture of Catholicism with the best in scientific developments."[52]

At the hospital, the commanding presence of the Sisters of Mercy, with over 45 members employed during the early 1950s, could hardly be ignored. If the building was the actual body of the hospital, the nuns were its soul, converting "the lifeless structure of brick and steel into a living, loving organism."[53] One witness recalled that the Sisters "automatically had a position of authority," extending from the superintendent, director of nurses, chief dietitian, librarian, and chief X-ray technician to the head of the surgical and laboratory technicians. At least one or two Sisters worked in each hospital department. Their high profile set the tone for all personal relationships in the hospital. Willingness to help others was deeply ingrained in the Sisters' family background and reinforced by living in a religious community. They greeted each other, the rest of the personnel, and patients with a friendly smile. Although they were protected from the burdens of ordinary life, their commitment and dedication were deemed absolute: "when they say mercy they mean mercy."[54]

Hospital life at Mercy Hospital, 1954

Joseph O'H. arrived on the ward accompanied by an orderly who carried his chart and medical orders. Confined to his oxygen tent, he tried to relax. The hospital overflowed with patients, often accommodated in extra beds placed in cubicles and hallways. Joseph was assigned to the "big" nine-bed male ward. Together with a similar unit for females, several semiprivate rooms, and the geriatric ward, these facilities completed Mercy's medical service, still the Cinderella of the house because it failed to produce as much income as other specialties such as surgery and obstetrics. Reflecting upon his recent lifestyle, Joseph tried to find reasons for his predicament. Since his retirement two years earlier, he had felt increasingly bored and useless. Tense, he relished his nips of brandy. Joseph admitted being homebound and inactive, smoking and eating too much, condemned to stare at a small television screen delivering slapstick comedy and canned laughter. He glanced at the crucifix on the wall, a lonely but somewhat inspirational figure, and vowed to change his ways if he survived this ordeal. At least, he thought, he was not alone in his suffering. He eventually settled down to sleep after receiving some Seconal or chloral hydrate capsules.[55]

The head of Joseph's bed had been elevated with blocks placed under the headposts to prevent pulmonary congestion and possibly edema, both common but potentially lethal complications. Additional pillows propped up his head and shoulders. The immediate objective was strict bed rest to avoid all physical and mental stress. With the help of a technician, the floor nurses took another 12-lead electrocardiogram (EKG) with a portable machine, and the new tracing—read by O'Brien—showed typical RS-T elevation and Q waves confirming the suspected myocardial damage. Joseph's initial, rigidly enforced confinement had the effect of converting him into a virtual prisoner in his own bed. He was ordered not even to lift a finger and, like a baby, he was spoon-fed a low-calorie, low-salt liquid diet together with subcutaneous injections of morphine for pain administered every six hours. The nurses began turning him routinely every hour to prevent bed sores. Joseph was eventually encouraged to turn by himself. He was also provided with elastic stockings and had his legs massaged to avoid the dreaded thrombophlebitis.

Early the next morning, Joseph was awakened by the night nurse making her final rounds, dressed in the uniform worn by all Mercy nurses: a white cap with black band, starched white uniform, and stockings and shoes of the same color. Catholic nursing remained strongly vocational, implying a calling, although physicians grumbled about a decline in dedication, excessive mistakes, and a less reverent attitude toward the medical profession. "From the physician's 'handmaiden' of bygone days, the graduate nurse of 1953 has blossomed into a much more respected member of the professional health team," wrote one author.[56] Despite their expansion in duties, nurses found it necessary to fight for a better social and economic position, complaining about the doctors' persistent "feudal" attitude that sought to condemn them to a subservient role.[57]

Most ward nurses were led by Mercy's Sisters, who believed that "God gives talents, and they should be used," and that a "Christlike devotion to the sick has contributed immeasurably to an enviable record of early and complete patient recovery."[58] The key purpose of its dedicated practitioners was "to identify with everyone you take care of as someone that could be you or a member of your family."[59] In the spirit of Mercy, the nurses' vision of patient care stressed the dignity of the human being. They acted as family surrogates, paying special attention to the very sick. Some nurses ended up staying beyond their shifts to complete workups and perhaps socialize with their charges. In a few instances, nurses even became conservators if the patients had no relatives or were disowned by their families. "Once you talked to them and they knew what you knew, you helped relieve the anxiety," one nurse recalled, adding that "the whole focus was patient-centered care, whether physical or spiritual; you were just engraved with the idea that the whole person was your responsibility."[60] Contributing to the team of caregivers were student nurses proudly wearing their blue and white uniforms. Most of them had already been "capped" after completing their college year.[61]

Cardiac patients were "treated like mummies,"[62] with placement of pillows between either arm, under the knees, and under the shoulders, as well as behind the back. Joseph's legs were kept straight by being supported against an adjustable foot board. To provide further back support, another board was placed between the spring and mattress. Rolls supported the hands and fingers in functional positions. Nurses even brushed the patients' teeth to avoid any exertion. Joseph was told never to raise his arms above the level of his shoulders: "Think about your bed as making your heart immobile just as a cast would do to your broken arm" was the nurse's recommendation. Conventional wisdom suggested that it took four to six weeks to convert an infarct into a scar. Like most patients, Joseph struggled with the bedpan and looked forward to using a bedside commode soon.

At the end of the first day, Joseph's condition remained unchanged. His blood pressure was still 185/90, pulse frequency 90, and respiration 20. He complained of minor chest and epigastric pain; the heart tones were normal, and no further extrasystoles could be detected. The electrocardiogram suggested myocardial damage in the heart's posterolateral area. The patient's legs were not tender, but he experienced some cramping in both feet. Laboratory data revealed a hematocrit of 37.5% and a white blood cell count of 6,200; the sedimentation rate was 50, and he had a prothrombin time of 56 seconds. Because of his symptoms, age, and lack of a history of peptic ulcer or bleeding, Joseph was considered a candidate for anticoagulants.[63] Thus, the patient received oral Dicumerol instead of intravenous heparin for the prevention of mural thrombi and systemic pulmonary emboli, a complication in almost 40% of all cases.[64] Everyone in the ward was aware that most fatalities from cardiac arrest—ranging in the 1950s from 20% to 60%—and other problems occurred during the first week of hospitalization.

Also checking Joseph's vital signs and supplementing O'Brien's management was a member of Mercy's current medical house staff, a Filipino intern selected by O'Brien and Assistant Director Dr. Carol Shaver. Mostly males, Catholics, and foreign graduates, these house officers were expected to be the eyes and ears of the attending physicians. A few were Americans who came from Georgetown University, but the majority hailed from predominantly Catholic areas of the world, including the Philippines, Puerto Rico, and Latin America. Some candidates for internship positions in Catholic establishments were pressed about their religiosity with requests for references from their parish priests. All were therefore presumed to possess a philosophy of care and a value system congenial with that promoted by the Sisters of Mercy. Because the American hospital system was currently undergoing a dramatic expansion, interns and residents were eagerly sought, and some hospitals even put out attractive recruitment brochures. To complete their prescribed year of medical services, interns rotated every three months through wards devoted to medicine, surgery, pediatrics, and obstetrics/gynecology. Lack of proper supervision during their so-called training was common.[65]

Working in 36-hour shifts and sometimes over 100 hours a week, these house officers merely fulfilled service roles while the attending physicians were busy seeing private patients in their offices. Stipends remained very low—$200 a month—but room and board were provided. On occasion, attending physicians emphasized the private status of their patients, requesting that house staff members maintain a hands-off attitude, especially concerning treatment orders. Occasionally patients refused to be examined by anyone except their own physicians. At Mercy and elsewhere, lack of dialogue and proper communications between patients, house staff, and attending staff—there were also occasional language barriers—hampered the educational role of the internship despite frantic efforts by O'Brien to bring all parties together. Interns were frequently bypassed by attending physicians, who simply phoned in their orders directly to the nurses and made unannounced rounds during late evening hours.[66]

At Mercy, interns and residents thus came to rely on the ward nurses for building relationships with private patients and their physicians. Some foreign house staff members even attempted to understand the prevailing Irish culture by attending community functions and religious services. Romances and marriages between doctors and local nurses and technicians were not unusual, although such liaisons were discouraged by the Sisters since they tended to distract the caregivers and could compromise service. After internship or residency, a handful of these men even settled in Buffalo. At a time when experienced nurses appeared to be in short supply, marriage became the "frustrating opponent of hospital administrators."[67] Marriage in 1954 was still viewed as a full-time occupation, and many of the nurses who married quickly had a number of children. Those who returned to work part-time were usually viewed as less dedicated and skillful.

In the presence of the Mercy Sisters, Joseph's fears seemed to ebb. These "girls" were sisters or daughters of his neighbors and work mates. Many had entered the novitiate after high school since their financially strapped families placed a lower priority on college education for their female offspring. Like family, the nuns had been strict disciplinarians in the parish schools and still acted now with the same firmness but kindness. Some of the matriarchal atmospherics were subtle, but Joseph and other devout Catholic patients found themselves immersed in a religious environment pregnant with symbols and rituals. Sister M. Bon Secour was the official visitor of patients admitted to the medical department, and she frequently made her rounds alone or in the company of the head nurse. In a display of humility, Sister M. Sacred Heart, the current superintendent of the hospital, personally visited each patient during evening hours, inquiring about their needs and often reaching for a bedpan or glass of water to assist individuals such as Joseph. The night visits were particularly important since this was a lonely and fearful time. It was good for Sisters and nurses to engage in small talk with their patients: "people's feelings are important," remembered one of the nuns, adding that "nurturing and fostering human dignity" was their ultimate goal.[68]

Shortly after admission, Joseph also received a visit from Mercy's chaplain, Rev. Francis A. Krupa. Although the priest's primary duty was to conduct religious services and administer the sacraments, Krupa was always on call and relished his role of spiritual counselor, providing hope and courage. His tenure at Mercy was no cushy sinecure. He prayed, heard bedside confessions, provided communion, and anointed the very sick. Krupa's frequent presence at hospital baptisms and funeral masses made him one of the most popular personalities in the hospital. For him, the problem of suffering remained a riddle and a concern, perhaps an evil in itself. Yet the time of sickness was also a time of grace. Suffering, dignified by Christ's own affliction, was honorable for Krupa, a device to remove shame: "Christ has made suffering fruitful, and helps sufferers return to God."[69] For many, Mercy's chaplain was also the consoling "sentinel at the death bed."[70]

This special home-like atmosphere at Mercy shaped the lives of nurses, house staff, attending physicians, and patients like Joseph. There was an implicit assumption that most were Roman Catholics or basically needy Christians whose spiritual well-being was a priority. Sisters used a religion rich in rituals and ceremonies to re-create in the hospital a daily and weekly rhythm of life that aimed to provide meaning to suffering and promote healing. The hospital had a beautiful chapel, walled in white marble, with an ample balcony and a capacity for 200 worshippers. This church was at the center of hospital life, a place for quiet meditation and prayer, where mass was celebrated daily and graduation ceremonies for the nurses took place. Early each morning, caregivers and ambulatory patients received the Eucharist, the traditional celebratory meal.[71] For those unable to attend, the day began at 7 AM with a three-minute morning prayer coming over the hospital's loudspeaker. The Angelus, a blessing before the meal, was also heard at noon and at 6 PM throughout the hospital. The day ended with another prayer at 9 PM. Sunday mass was also transmitted over a number of speakers. As one

CHA leader explained, "prayer is the Church's greatest accessory. The success in healing accomplished by it, as an adjunct to medicine proper, lends the art of medicine that prestige and dignity which have become allowed in the lapse of time."[72]

On December 23, Joseph lay still and somewhat confused in his oxygen tent. His vital signs had stabilized, and the laboratory results, especially the prothrombin time, urinalysis, sedimentation rate, and blood count, were within the expected ranges. By now Joseph was receiving daily visits from his wife and some friends. They all brought holy cards from other neighbors and a sacred heart badge that was pinned to his hospital gown. Everybody was praying for him. A number of nurses and students hovered over him, performing regular grooming, bathing, and bed-making routines. There was also an impressive parade of nurses' aides at mealtimes carrying trays. Hospital care in 1954 was labor intensive—Mercy had 700 lay employees, excluding the nurses and nuns—and given the length of stay of most patients, caregivers spent a lot of time with them. Employees were united by their vocational motivation to help the sick and sought satisfaction in their jobs through their loyalty to the Sisters of Mercy; salaries were usually quite low. However, there was already concern about the high operational costs following the reduction in working hours for the nurses from the traditional 48–44 to the contemporary 40-hour schedule.[73]

Three days after admission, Joseph was finally removed from the oxygen tent, although he still had a "light" feeling in the epigastrium. Perhaps God had answered his prayers. His heart tones sounded stronger, his pulse was 88 and regular, and his lungs appeared clear. A new EKG tracing was ordered and the patient brought to a special room on the fifth floor of the hospital. Located on the east wing, the Department of Electrocardiography was specially screened to eliminate the 60-cycle electrical interference. EKG tests were becoming more popular at Mercy, with over 2,000 recordings ordered in 1953, up from only 205 such tests 10 years earlier. Working in monthly rotations, physicians with cardiology training like DeCeu and O'Brien read the tracings.

With the EKG findings suggesting that his heart was on the mend, Joseph was now allowed to use the commode and comb his own hair, although he still received bed or sponge baths and could not shave himself. The risks were too great. Since he was on anticoagulants, any small cuts could trigger serious bleeding. Christmas was always festive at Mercy Hospital. Several choral groups, from college students to third graders, visited the hospital wards. They sang Christmas carols, chatted with and cheered up the patients, and fostered a special spirit for the holy season. A volunteer dressed as Santa Claus distributed small gifts to every patient. Then members of the Mount Mercy Academy ensemble sang at the annual Christmas Eve mass in the chapel, and their voices reverberated throughout the entire building.

Even before New Year's Day, Joseph began his gradual adjustment to "dormitory life." Like other ward patients, he frequently feigned sleep to preserve his privacy. His bed was surrounded by curtains, but they were frequently drawn back as the student nurses made their checks. Joseph remained on a bland diet and, because of his inactivity, required frequent enemas. Nitroglycerine was given as needed if he had any chest discomfort. He was also given a regular dose of digitalis and received a mercurial diuretic. His maintenance anticoagulant doses were carefully adjusted according to the rising or falling clotting times.[74] By January 6, Joseph managed to get transferred to a semiprivate room to counter his anxiety and lack of privacy. For the caregivers, it was always awkward to have a small number of acutely ill patients scattered about the ward. Like Joseph, many passed sleepless nights, still terrified of having their heart rupture like a worn tire. In Joseph's case, another EKG showed improvement. His heart seemed to be on the mend.

Along with commode privileges, Joseph was allowed to rest in an armchair instead of staying exclusively in bed.[75] Absolute bed rest was usually prescribed for a minimum of two or three weeks, but recent experience suggested the need for earlier ambulation. Many physicians were reluctant to give such orders since there was a widespread perception that doctors would receive greater blame if ambulatory patients died. However, the new approach had been gaining adherents since the early 1950s. Sitting up in a chair seemed to prevent dizziness and pulmonary edema, pneumonia, urinary retention, and infection, especially decubitus ulcers. A cardiac chair also neutralized depression and contributed to a better mental outlook in patients. On the first day, January 6, Joseph was allowed to sit up for only a few hours at mealtime and dangle his legs, thus preventing muscle and joint stiffness.

Over the next few weeks of forced inactivity, Joseph concentrated on a number of diversions to counter his boredom. Almost without fail, a friendly volunteer appeared each afternoon with stacks of books from the hospital library, and Joseph, in his boredom, devoured mystery novels, especially those of Agatha Christie. The daily panorama of sounds emanating from the frequently employed hospital paging system also held his attention. A nasal voice belonging to one of the switchboard operators tirelessly summoned attending physicians, house officers, Sisters, and nurses. Interestingly, one could hear more Italian names than Irish ones, while those of foreign interns were routinely mispronounced. An occasional frantic request to move vehicles blocking the emergency entrance revealed to the patients that there was still an outside world, populated by thoughtless or panicked drivers. The welcome call for visiting hours to commence and end was another routine distraction. Then there were the daily prayers, particularly meant "to soften the hearts of several black sheep,"[76] a category of Catholics who had wandered away from the sacraments.

By January 14, Joseph displayed signs of ascites—fluid in the abdomen—presumably a sign of congestive failure promising an extended hospital stay. His new roommate tried to break the monotony of hours in bed by reciting the rosary during the afternoons following a nap.[77] On weekends, the sounds of sacred music and an occasional choir at high mass radiated from the chapel, wafting through hospital corridors and lifting the spirits. On January 20, Joseph was wheeled in his chair to the chapel and allowed to attend mass in person. Longer hospital stays made the patients more conscious about the functioning of their bodies. Joseph kept listening to his heart, especially at night, checking every twinge and worrying about every pain. In spite of some movements from bed to chair to commode, his joints were stiff, his muscles weak. On the medical floor a whole patient subculture flourished, involving chronic and convalescent patients eager to exchange small talk and thus lessen the alienation of their hospital experience. With the participation of nurses, students, and aides, this socialization facilitated the establishment of deeper relationships between patients and their caregivers.

On January 28, 1955, O'Brien and Joseph's private physician decided to discharge the patient from the hospital and send him home by ambulance. Joseph had been hospitalized for 39 days, but he still complained of occasional chest pains, probably a reflection of coronary insufficiency, although the clinical signs of congestive heart failure were receding. Return to work was not an issue, but any resumption of physical activities had to be approached with great caution. How did Joseph feel about his future life? As both nurses and physicians explained, the prospects for a slow rehabilitation were good. He was alive, reborn, and eager to make amends for previous sins. He felt healed, thanks to God and the saintly Mercy Sisters.

Several months after Joseph's discharge, President Dwight D. Eisenhower suffered a similar episode of "indigestion" that turned out to be a myocardial infarction. This event triggered a flood of newspaper and magazine reports about the condition and its sequelae, with emphasis on the question of whether and when patients who had suffered heart attacks could return to fully active lives. The current view was that all individuals afflicted by heart disease were bad risks for any further employment.[78] Another effect of the president's malady was accelerated support from the National Institutes of Health for medical research in all aspects of arteriosclerotic heart disease. In spite of Joseph's wife's comfort and continued physician assistance—he repeatedly suffered bouts of congestive heart failure after his first visit to the hospital—he died suddenly three years later at home.

Another heart attack, 1974

At 7.45 PM on November 18, 1974, almost exactly 20 years after Joseph O'H.'s odyssey, another patient with a presumed heart attack arrived in an ambulance at Mercy Hospital's Emergency Room. Formerly from Lackawanna, the 55-year-old Albert F.,[79] a recent widower, was an accountant working in a downtown law firm. Albert's choice of Mercy Hospital was not based on any personal preference or religious affiliation; he was a Lutheran of German descent. With an influx of patients from the expanding southern suburbs, Mercy's inpatient population now included more people of different ethnic backgrounds and religious affiliations than it had in 1954. High state income taxes, high wages, a unionized workforce, bad weather, and a declining population had accelerated the industrial exodus from Buffalo, forcing Albert to resettle in the southeastern suburbs near East Aurora. Mercy was the logical destination point for him because of the availability of cardiologists on the medical staff, specialized nurses, and a coronary care unit said to have saved countless lives through its sophisticated monitoring systems and resuscitation procedures.[80] Like Joseph before him, Albert and his paramedic team viewed Mercy as the specialized site for cardiac care, but the religious dimension of the institution no longer consciously entered their minds as the ambulance sped to the hospital.

After his arrival, and after speaking to the Emergency Room resident on call, Albert insisted that he had been in good health until about two days prior to admission, when he developed chest pains while watching evening television. The next day, following a snowstorm, Albert had noticed some recurrence of these symptoms as he attended to his car, changing to snow tires—a yearly Buffalo ritual—before starting his daily commute. Although the pains were crushing and severe, they lasted for only a few minutes and gradually disappeared. On the day of admission, the mild pain returned while Albert was driving to work, and it recurred once more as he walked through the blustery weather near his office during his lunch break. Concerned, he decided to return home and rest, but he felt unusually tired after a brief nap. The symptoms persisted even after Albert walked around the house, making him sweat after he sat down to watch television. By now he was increasingly worried. Although he knew a private physician who for years had successfully managed his mild diabetes, Albert quickly summoned the Rescue Squad.

Albert had good reason to be concerned. It was not so much the degree of physical discomfort that made him decide to call for help. Because he lived alone within a loosely knit suburban community, the specter of a possible heart attack scared him. Both of his parents had died of heart attacks, his father in 1968 and his mother two years later. Even his younger brother had experienced a mild attack at age 45. According to national statistics, Buffalo still had a high incidence of fatal heart disease; Erie County had slipped only slightly behind Nassau County in reporting the highest number of cases after New York City.[81] In fact, in spite of $80 billion spent yearly on American's health care, fatal ischemic heart disease had declined only modestly in the United States between 1958 and 1969.[82] Moreover, widowers seemed to have higher death rates than married men. Medical experts, however, were dubbing the early 1970s the golden age of cardiology, now a rapidly evolving specialty with sophisticated diagnostic methods including cardiac catheterization and coronary angiography, as well as lifesaving procedures such as cardiac resuscitation and bypass surgery.[83] If the symptoms truly represented a heart attack, Albert was less likely to die—about one chance in five—than Joseph O'H. had been in 1954.[84]

By the early 1970s, Americans no longer went to community hospitals for just a rest or, at the convenience of their physicians, for diagnostic procedures and treatments available on an outpatient basis. A decade earlier, they had been forced to travel to distant academic medical centers, but now they sought sophisticated, technologically assisted specialty care near their own communities.[85] Mercy's Cardiac Care Unit (CCU) was a typical case in point. It had a reputation for space-age technology such as telemetry and special laboratory tests. Mercy's Men's Sustaining Society had presented a check for $10,000 to Sister M. Annunciata in October 1972, and she had unveiled plans for a new 17-bed coronary care unit designed to replace the existing 6-bed unit in the old hospital and attract more specialists to its staff. At an estimated cost of $500,000, this was to be Mercy's high-tech entry into the financially competitive arena of cardiac care in an era when expensive procedures were generously reimbursed by Medicare and private insurance plans. The center had already been approved by the Comprehensive Health Planning Council of Western New York. To avoid duplication of services and thus contain the ever-escalating costs of hospital care, however, a certificate of need was required on the basis of pioneering state legislation adopted in 1966.[86]

As an extension of the new CCU, the hospital also planned a new mobile life support unit to transport and treat the heart attack victims of South Buffalo and West Seneca. According to Dr. James E. Ehinger, an Emergency Room physician and long-time member of the Western New York State Heart Association, this was a typical coronary-prone community composed of middle-aged workers and the elderly. Ehinger hoped that this unit would put a local dent in national statistics that showed that half of all heart attack victims died before ever reaching a hospital. Available 24 hours a day, this life support vehicle was the only unit of its kind in the city of Buffalo. In Ehinger's view, patients could now be treated during those four or five critical minutes before arrival at the hospital. While transporting the patient to the Emergency Room, trained attendants monitored vital signs including EKG readings and, if necessary, performed cardiopulmonary resuscitation, external cardiac massage, and defibrillation while keeping in constant radio contact with the hospital.

On October 28, 1974, Mercy Hospital's new CCU was blessed by Buffalo's Bishop Edward D. Head and formally opened in a space previously slated for a laboratory on the second floor of the modern McAuley Building. As reported in the *Buffalo Evening News*, the spacious unit ended up costing more than $800,000 to build and equip. In addition to the patients' rooms and nurses' stations, the facility included a large waiting room, and separate rooms for pharmacy, dietary, and supply activities. The unit was placed under the supervision of Mary Ann

Gottstine, assistant director of nursing services for the hospital and head of the American Heart Association of Western New York. At the inauguration, Mercy's CCU boasted seven beds in private rooms categorized as "Phase 1" acute care, with seven additional beds in semiprivate rooms for "Phase 2" care involving individuals who had already passed through phase 1 and were now in need of "progressive care." A central nurses' station constantly monitored the heart rate of all patients in the unit and produced continuous EKG printouts. Ten beds had telemetry, and seven were hard-wired. While patients in phase 1 were directly monitored by bedside machines, those in phase 2 wore portable battery-operated units while they were ambulatory.

Following the development of such a facility in Kansas City during the early 1960s,[87] CCUs had rapidly proliferated throughout the country, stimulated in part by generous grants from the major manufacturers of monitoring equipment, including oscilloscopes, defibrillators, and alarm systems.[88] This development was part of nursing's progressive patient care begun in the late 1950s at selected larger hospitals and designed to achieve more efficient utilization of nurses' traditional observational skills.[89] Mercy Hospital had followed the suggestions of O'Brien and created its own CCU in 1965—the first in western New York State—under the direction of Sister M. Ethel, using the original nine-bed medical ward—Joseph O'H.'s original destination. Mercy's first CCU had six separate cubicles facing an enclosed, central monitoring station. Electrodes were fastened to individual patients and connected to an oscilloscope. Monitors at the nurses' desk checked the heart rhythm and sounded an alarm if arrhythmia appeared. Rather than a triumph of technology, this CCU was an organizational and economic innovation in the face of a shortage of well-trained nurses. In addition, its proponents believed that patients would be greatly impressed and reassured by the separate facilities and frequent monitoring. Relatives and friends were kept away by short visiting hours based on the belief that their presence would delay the patients' recovery.[90] However, the opposite occurred. For many patients sent to a CCU unit, the wiring caused considerable panic. Some individuals became quite upset, believing they were soon going to die, and brief visits by their families provided the only reassuring link to the outside world. Although some cardiologists had argued that special monitoring facilities could prevent heart rhythm disturbances, questions about the usefulness and cost effectiveness of CCU units lingered well into the early 1970s, with frequent calls for more randomized clinical trials to prove their efficacy.[91]

At Mercy Hospital's Emergency Room, meanwhile, Albert F. spent the next two hours under close observation. He was first seen by a female medical resident from India who rechecked his vital signs: heart rate 55, respiration 22, blood pressure 110/40. Hospitals like Mercy continued to expand their pool of residents and interns, in part to save labor costs. These physicians still worked about 100 hours per week, but their 36-hour shifts were much more demanding and stressful than in previous decades. Sleeplessness adversely affected the doctors' performance and their attitude toward patients. In contrast to previous decades, Mercy now had fewer Filipino interns and residents, replaced by arrivals from Pakistan, India, Turkey, and South Korea, a reflection of shifts in the origin of foreign medical graduates seeking training in the United States. Catholic identity was no longer a priority, although traditionalists believed that foreigners diluted the hospital's religious tone, "the Mercy spirit."[92]

Albert's history and physical examination were followed by a visit from Dr. Salvatore V. Cavaretta, then chief of Mercy's Emergency Room. Like his associates, Cavaretta was very busy practicing triage, focused on making tentative diagnoses and deciding paths of management. Albert's initial chest X-ray displayed no evidence of cardiopulmonary disease, but the EKG showed sinus rhythm with changes suggestive of an acute anterolateral infarct. Like Joseph before him, the patient was ordered not to move while a resident applied a nasal catheter for the delivery of oxygen and administered an intravenous shot of morphine. The events of the past hours had frightened Albert, who vividly remembered the death of his parents. Far from blaming his genetic background, he pinned the attack on his recent widowerhood. After a lifetime of companionship he felt rundown and lonely, missing his wife's cooking and caring. Albert suddenly felt tired and abandoned. Given the frantic pace and crisis atmosphere in the Emergency Room—every cubicle seemed to be filled with somebody in pain—nobody approached him to discuss his feelings.

Between Joseph O'H.'s arrival in 1954 and Albert's in 1974, conditions at Mercy Hospital had changed radically. While bed capacity had remained about the same, total admissions had increased to around 16,000 per year. This nearly 20% increase had been achieved through higher patient turnover because of shorter stays for acute cases and transfer of convalescents and chronic patients to other custodial care facilities. Now the average hospitalization lasted about a week instead of the two it had during the 1950s. By now, Mercy possessed a modern physical plant capable of housing the most up-to-date technology, operated by an expanded staff of caregivers and technicians with specialized skills and an extended cadre of bureaucrats to cope with the complexities of reports and audits required for federal and state reimbursements.

The impact of Medicare

Until the late 1960s, Mercy Hospital had experienced an unprecedented period of expansion. An inpatient survey of actual hospital usage for the years 1960 through May 1962 revealed that the principal users of the facility were wage laborers at the area's industrial plants and their dependents. Sixty-one major industries were represented among the 13,308 inpatients seen in 1961. Not surprisingly, overcrowding of diagnostic and rehabilitation facilities, as well as the maternity ward, prompted calls for another expansion of existing wings. However, it soon became apparent that the spatial needs and latest technological developments demanded construction of a brand new building. Another radical alternative, supported by many attending physicians, was to move Mercy Hospital to suburban Orchard Park. Movement of the city's Polish American communities to the southeastern suburbs of West Seneca and Orchard Park had already created additional health care needs in those areas. In the end, however, the institution's religious leadership decided to remain in South Buffalo but expand the hospital's service area to include residents of southern Erie County.

Meanwhile, implementation of Medicare in the late 1960s increased the number of older patients at the hospital. Mercy's administrators viewed the program as a godsend, allowing reimbursement for care provided to many elderly patients previously considered charity cases and carried at hospital expense. Assured that their costs were covered by Medicare, those who qualified now flocked to private voluntary hospitals instead of remaining in less attractive public institutions. At Mercy, the newcomers created further competition for beds. Since the most serious and complex cases usually won out, American hospitals gradually acquired a new patient population of sicker elderly patients with multiple and repeated breakdowns of their organ systems. These conditions demanded significant changes in patient management, including more intensive nursing care and the invention of technological devices to keep these patients alive.[93]

While the federal government, through Medicare and Medicaid, now provided significant resources to Catholic institutions, the downside of such provisions was a growing federal and state regulatory influence on the financial and operational aspects of American hospitals, including sectarian institutions such as Mercy. A growing forest of stringent federal, state, and local regulations—frequently contradictory—began to encroach on the hospital's planning, generating a number of internal "utilization" committees charged with determining current institutional needs and anticipating future ones. Bureaucratic snafus and utilization reviews sometimes denied expenditures, forcing institutions to return money already collected. Because of the large amount of paperwork required to process claims, the hospital's business bureaucracy expanded rapidly, and for the first time in Mercy Hospital's history, an assistant administrator had to be hired.[94] In 1967, the increased length of stay for complicated geriatric cases and the growing demand for broader, more comprehensive hospital care made expansion imperative because of an acute shortage of beds. In fact, the institution's own Utilization Committee became quite busy transferring convalescent patients from the hospital to their homes or to a number of extended care facilities. In Buffalo, however, the few qualified nursing homes were overcrowded, forcing Mercy to open its own Extended Care Unit.

By early 1967, Phase I of the planned addition to Mercy Hospital was ready for bids. The cost of this four-floor building with a nine-story central utility tower of fire-resistant concrete, steel, and masonry had risen from $4 million to $8 million and then to nearly $11 million. Most supplies were to be delivered by a monorail conveyor system housed in the service tower with its elevators, pneumatic tubes, dumbwaiters, and trash and laundry shafts. Mercy Hospital was the first institution in the country to employ this system.[95] The basement would be the operating core, consisting of a loading dock, receiving area, storage facilities, sterilization and processing areas, X-ray and medical records archives, a pharmacy, and a laundry. The main lobby and the admitting, administrative, and business offices were located on the ground floor. In addition, this floor provided special services such as dental care, eye, ear, nose, and throat care, the X-ray department, and eight surgical suites. Clustered nearby to complete a single functional unit were an orthopedic unit for setting fractures and recovery rooms with special ancillary services, including electroencephalography, EKG facilities, and cardiopulmonary and similar testing sites.

According to the plan, the first floor was to be shelled in for later conversion to a dietetic department with a kitchen, cooking and dishwashing areas, coolers, and freezers, together with a cafeteria, dining rooms, and a so-called cafetorium— a combined dining room and auditorium where physicians could simultaneously dine and participate in educational programs. Finally, the second floor was conceived as a complete obstetric department with 30 semiprivate rooms for 60 patients, together with 8 private labor rooms and 60 bassinets in 12 nurseries, including 2 for premature infants and 2 for isolation purposes. A recovery room, four delivery rooms, and lounges for physicians and nurses completed the arrangement.

In June 1967, ground was broken at Mercy for this addition, to be known as the McAuley Building in honor of the order's founder. At the same time, the hospital's School of Nursing finally closed its doors after 39 years, replaced by a 2-year nursing program and an associate degree at Trocair College, also under the sponsorship of the Sisters of Mercy. According to its director, Sister M. Ethel, "there is a trend that the teaching of nursing be taken out of the hospital, and, like other professions, be put into strictly education-oriented institutions."[96] Following national trends to beef up its ambulatory and emergency facilities, the hospital also established a new intensive care unit. Efforts to improve communications with the community, employees, and patients led to the creation of a public relations committee and the hiring of a local advertising agency. In 1968, Sister M. Sacred Heart Kreuzer's 20-year tenure as Mercy Hospital's chief administrator came to a close.[97] Her successor, Sister M. Annunciata Kelleher, looked forward to an ongoing process of institutional modernization that promised to create a new physical plant capable of housing the latest medical technology and delivering a wide array of high-quality medical services with greater efficiency.[98]

One feature of the new Mercy Hospital, recognized nationally, was the introduction of a jet-age food service system. With the employment of precooked convenience foods, together with sterile disposable dishes and eating utensils, conveyor belts scattered through the hospital delivered the food on trays to 16 microwave ovens. Meals were thus brought piping hot to patients throughout the institution. Another successful pilot project sought to decentralize the hospital's pharmacy, providing better and faster service. As in most institutions, drugs had previously been dispensed from a central pharmacy, always a time-consuming activity that often kept patients waiting. Relieved of some of their bureaucratic burdens by this decentralization, pharmacists could function better as members of the health care team, tracking possible drug incompatibilities and monitoring optimum dosages.

If Mercy's physical plant and patients such as Albert had changed dramatically since the 1950s, so had the nature of the caregivers. Rejecting their previous roles of domesticity and subordination to medicine, nurses had made great strides in their quest for a new professional identity, acquiring expanded individual and social responsibilities. They now demanded a voice in making the educational and managerial policies governing hospitals, lobbying for decentralization of authority and the creation of unit managers and team leaders. Indeed, since the mid-1960s, both Medicare and Medicaid regulations had placed more emphasis on nurses' educational credentials than on their clinical experience, a policy that altered dramatically the character of nursing personnel, especially for nurses who had only gone through a training program such as that provided by the now defunct school at Mercy Hospital.[99] Professional autonomy became very important; nurses now defined themselves as members of a caregiving team, demanded higher compensation, and threatened to unionize. Even their green scrub gowns worn in the Emergency Room made them less distinguishable from physicians and other caregivers.

The trend toward specialization among house staff members and attending physicians gained further momentum in the 1960s. Mercy Hospital's connection to the Georgetown University School of Medicine had finally ended in 1968, after years of threats by the academic institution to cancel the long-distance affiliation begun in 1951. Jeghers' original goals to upgrade the quality of medical care were obsolete. Nationally, the trend for academic medical centers was to associate with nearby community hospitals and create referral-producing networks. The Buffalo connection, created in an earlier era of hospital development and financing, had clearly become obsolete. Toward the end, Georgetown professors had to be cajoled to come to Buffalo, especially during the city's Siberian winters.[100] With further expansion of specialized services, Mercy hired a number of additional full-time, salaried medical staff members to supervise critical areas of care. Among them was Dr. Milford Maloney, full-time chief of a newly created Department of Medicine. Thanks to this nucleus of salaried individuals who were allowed only a small private practice within the institution, internship and residency programs in medicine, surgery, obstetrics, pediatrics, pathology, and plastic surgery received a boost. Moreover, Mercy's Department of Medical Education sponsored newly emerging fields such as nuclear medicine. O'Brien's earlier goal of educating generalists had been abandoned to promote specialization and even subspecialization.

Despite their dedication to their private practices, many of Mercy's attending physicians had traditionally volunteered to train house staff members, in part for the opportunity to keep professionally up to date and the added prestige that teaching offered. By the mid 1960s, this new generation of specialized attendings offered the hospital an even higher level of education and skills. Following the loss of the Georgetown connection, the hospital also negotiated a new affiliation with the State University of New York-Buffalo School of Medicine, a competent, somewhat blue-collar medical school, ranked 24th in the nation. Unfortunately, few of its 150 annual graduates wished to stay in the area for their postgraduate training.

Mercy and other community hospitals in western New York thus found themselves in an uphill battle to secure an adequate number of house staff members drawn from outside the area. Fortunately, shortly before Albert's admission in 1974, O'Brien reported that Mercy had had the best recruitment year for qualified house staff since the creation of the Department of Medical Education in 1951. Linkages with the local medical school had finally borne fruit, and plans were underway to stress issues of primary care during the training for internal medicine. In the end, O'Brien highlighted the importance of student participation in raising the level of medical care at the hospital. "If there is anything that tends to keep a staff man on his toes, it is the daily give and take with his house staff and more importantly with his assigned junior or senior medical students."[101] In the final analysis, the rotation of medical students, interns, and residents remained the link between Mercy Hospital and other health care institutions, private and public, within western New York State.

Mercy Hospital's new McAuley Building was dedicated in December 1969 during ceremonies attended by the bishop of Buffalo. Most diagnostic and therapeutic hospital facilities, including radiology and nuclear medicine, were relocated to the street level of the new facility to accommodate the steadily increasing number of outpatients and emergency patients such as Albert F. Soon, a Data Processing Department helped computerize inpatient billing, accounts receivable, and the institutional payroll.

According to local newspapers, the McAuley Building was designed to make Mercy the most completely automated hospital in the area. The *Buffalo Courier* characterized the structure as "the most modern in western New York," stressing its attractive design and kaleidoscope of room colors, "from soft mauves, pinks, and greens, to vibrant shades of hot pink, chartreuse, and orange." Patient rooms also displayed ultra-service features, with slivers of hand soap sliding from special dispensers, while electrically equipped bedside tables had a console with push buttons for signaling the nurse or tuning in radio and television programs. Shower rooms had heat lamps for quick drying. "It is more like deluxe hotel living than hospital confinement," declared the newspaper. Echoing traditional values, a small garden was planted in front of the new building to make Mercy beautiful.[102]

Catholic hospitals: Identity crisis and ethical guidelines

The two decades separating Joseph O'H.'s and Albert F.'s heart attacks witnessed Mercy Hospital's increasing struggle to preserve its traditional philosophy of care. On the religious front, momentous changes had occurred following the death of Pope Pius XII in 1958 and the election of his successor, Pope John XXIII. For the first time in almost a century, the new pontiff convened in 1962 an ecumenical Council of the Roman Catholic Church, known as the Second Vatican Council or Vatican II. Its stated goal was *aggiornamento* or renewal of the Church, a plan to make the institution less authoritarian and more responsive to contemporary needs and problems. This objective resonated with the American Catholic community, especially younger Catholics living in a more enlightened and technologically advanced modern society, who were already questioning the Church's authoritarian structure.[103] In anticipation of these proceedings, the executive board of the CHA sought to reemphasize in 1962 the main philosophical tenets guiding Catholic hospitals. These institutions were seen as an integral part of the work of the Church and extensions of Christ's mission of mercy. Total care was said to embrace the physical, emotional, and spiritual needs of each patient.

The primary objective of Catholic hospitals was to maintain and restore health, serving everybody, regardless of race, creed, or financial status. Addressing contemporary perceptions, the executive director of the CHA, Father John J. Flanagan, observed that selfless hospital service—identified with a religious vocation—was being portrayed as being at odds with the new professionalism in medicine and nursing, in fact, as "something demeaning."[104] Since the Catholic healing ministry had been traditionally based on such notions of service, the national leadership sought to emphasize the compatibility of dedication and mercy among Catholic physicians and nurses who would also be familiar with the latest developments in scientific medicine and medical technology. From a theological point of view, the healing apostolate was simply an expression of charity—love of God and God's love, to be practiced by both religious and lay staff members.

By the mid-1960s, other debates about the role of lay persons in hospital life were increasingly held against the background of deliberations and decrees emanating from the Second Vatican Council. The decree *On the Appropriate Renewal of Religious Life* asked religious institutions to review their by-laws and constitutions and to create more egalitarian relationships among their members. For women, there were calls to reevaluate the meaning of religious service, with emphasis shifting from cloistered, contemplative lives to more engaged, apostolic ones. In response, many Sisters, especially younger ones who had worked in hospitals, decided to leave these highly structured "corporate" ministries. To fill their place, a number of lay persons began moving into the system, performing roles traditionally reserved for priests and Sisters. In time, the departure of many religious women from Catholic hospitals would lead to a profound transformation of the traditional Catholic health ministry.[105] The Council significantly broadened the perspective of those engaged in such activities. At the 1966 CHA convention, priests, nuns, and lay persons carefully reevaluated their respective roles and officially began the process of rethinking their philosophy and goals. As the mother general of the Sisters of St. Francis in Maryville, Missouri, declared, "we are advocating a departure from the past not only in our thinking, but also in the actual workings of what we know as sisters and hospitals. I mean specifically the partnership of laymen and religious as opposed to a subservient role on the part of the layman."[106]

In sharp contrast to conditions prevailing in 1954, both the availability and visibility of the Sisters of Mercy had markedly diminished by the time Albert came to Mercy's Emergency Room. Many of the nuns had officially retired. Those continuing to work as volunteers viewed the profound changes in hospital care with resignation, meekly acknowledging that "the Lord is in charge."[107] Among those remaining and spending time with patients and their families was Sister Elizabeth Welch, patient relations coordinator at the hospital. All new arrivals—including Albert—received advice about the spiritual comfort and support available at the institution. Welch's creed that "caring is important; without it, the spirit sickens and the body refuses to heal" was directly in line with the traditional "Spirit of Mercy."[108]

There was no question that the Roman Catholic tone had been diluted since the time of Vatican II. Still, the grace of a vocation was an individual phenomenon, a tremendously uplifting and special experience for those who were thus blessed.[109] But even those who found that vocation expressed it differently than they had in the 1950s. Many of the younger Sisters did not wear habits, thus—in the eyes of their elders—failing to "give witness" to their faith and status. Although religious principles were still considered important, the spiritual environment at Mercy was much more ecumenical than before, with a proliferation of ministers, rabbis, and lay healers sometimes even holding joint services.[110]

At the same time, convents experienced a noticeable drop in novices following the Vatican II reforms. In the structured life of their cloister, the remaining Sisters of Mercy continued to live physically close together, but they were now quite independent people from many walks of life instead of the once close-knit Irish community. However, although outwardly more cosmopolitan, the religious Mercy leadership remained inherently conservative, reluctantly accepting change and thus perpetuating the perennial tensions between the hospital's charitable caring and its rapidly expanding specialization. The result was that Catholic hospitals such as Mercy were forced to hire more lay nurses based on educational credentials and technical expertise rather than character and a willingness to follow the hospital's religious philosophy.[111] In spite of such trends, Mercy sought to preserve its tradition of compassion and hospitality, as well as its commitment to medical excellence. In 1970 the hospital's administrator, Sister M. Annunciata, had insisted that the institution was still striving for "an atmosphere of dignity and compassion for the patient and family who are experiencing the joy of birth, the pain of sickness, the sorrow of death."[112]

With the passage of Medicare, new financial, legal, and social concerns complicated the reformulation of a clear mission for Catholic hospitals. A true Catholic identity in postconciliar American society needed to be established. In view of the proposed partnership between the government and private health care enterprises, how would a religious hospital fare in the legal world of Church-state relations? Catholic hospitals would be at odds with public policy regarding such issues as sterilization and euthanasia, not to mention birth control and, later, abortion. Their boards of directors still operated under the corporate structures established by their founding religious communities.[113] Clearly, a conflict between federal authorities and Catholic hospitals loomed, since the new relationship demanded a nonsectarian policy regarding patient admission and treatment. Perhaps even crucifixes would have to be removed from rooms housing non-Catholic patients, and religious ceremonies as well as visits from Sisters and chaplains discontinued, replaced by a multifaith Department of Religion. With regard to personnel, many of the Sisters, already provided with salaries and fringe benefits, now projected an image of employment rather than calling.[114]

In December 1966, Dr. Edmund D. Pellegrino, director of the Medical Center at the State University of New York at Stony Brook, spoke at a CHA conference on the topic "What makes a hospital Catholic?"[115] The crucial question was whether religious institutions could remain Catholic and continue to make unique spiritual contributions. Pellegrino readily admitted that American Catholic hospitals confronted "the most serious dilemma in their long and distinguished history," namely, the need to adapt to the profound changes occurring in America's scientific and social milieus. Catholic institutions had distinct sets of duties, encompassing a commitment to a specific philosophy that allowed the fullest expression of personhood, especially during an individual's loneliest moments when facing disease, disability, and death. Reflecting the new theological tone of the Vatican Council, Pellegrino pointed out that hospitals had far too long applied a rigid moral code instead of focusing on the experiential dimensions of human suffering.[116]

The CHA continued to debate the problems of religious hospital ownership, governance, and service within the new context created by the federal government's ever greater intrusion into the health care field.[117] These issues needed to be addressed within the framework of the traditional separation between public and private, state and religion, albeit in a more legalistic rather than simply a theological fashion. This change in emphasis was due in part to the leadership of CHA's new executive director, the Rev. Thomas J. Casey, a former practicing attorney. The issue of Church-state separation came to a head in a Maryland Court of Appeals case in 1966 in which the court refused the claim that loans to Church-related hospitals under Maryland's Hospital Construction Act of 1964 would be "in whole or in part an establishment of religion." The issue continued to be hotly contested in hospital circles.[118]

At the same time, a CHA commission studying revisions of the 1949 Code of Ethics tackled other legal questions by asking whether a Catholic hospital's board of trustees, as a corporate entity, could prohibit or restrict certain medical services and procedures otherwise legally and medically acceptable in society at large. This inquiry became even more pertinent after Pope Paul VI issued his encyclical *Humanae Vitae* in 1968, reaffirming the Church's prohibition of all artificial means of birth control, a prohibition that inspired many Sisters, Brothers, and priests to engage in various forms of social protest and ecclesiastical dissent. According to Casey, strict adherence to the existing guidelines caused serious moral dilemmas in contemporary Catholic hospital administration. In his report to the 1969 CHA convention, Casey pointed out the changing culture of the times and how it was prompting a "reexamination of the purposes and structures of institutions and organizations, especially those committed to public service."[119]

Renewal and reform were not confined to the Catholic Church but also affected the CHA. For nearly 20 years, this organization had devoted its resources primarily to educational and service issues, but with the passage of Medicare, its members now sensed that they needed to refocus their mission and turn to public policy matters within the framework of post–Vatican II reforms.[120] Perhaps a broader membership that would include administrators, physicians, nurses, planners, and others holding positions of leadership in the health field was essential to accomplish the new goals. Looking into the future, Catholic hospitals needed to address the growing health care burdens in American society, affected by the urban crisis, the specter of universal health insurance, a managerial revolution based on automation, and consumer activism. How could these institutions balance such multiple and often conflicting issues, including their traditional role of caring for the whole patient?[121]

Catholic health care facilities, while still private corporations, were increasingly being asked to recognize their public accountability. Broadened obligations necessarily involved changing relationships with the community, responsibilities for medical practice, and efficient management of the hospital's widening operations. Boards of trustees were asked to make decisions within the context of health care needs identified in the community at large, not for a particular parish or diocese. Many institutions, located within inner-city ghettos, were being subjected to the effects of a growing urban health crisis. Buffalo's urban population had steadily declined from 532,000 in 1960 to about 450,000 in 1970, with those remaining generally elderly or poor, and Mercy had to accept the challenge of meeting the needs of their declining communities. Indeed, at this critical juncture, Catholic hospitals were encouraged to step forward and respond to the Church's call for renewal by demonstrating their social conscience and speaking out on important contemporary issues such as civil rights and equal opportunity, universal health insurance, and environmental pollution.[122]

This key shift also called for a reassessment of the historical practice of excluding lay administrators and physicians from the governing boards of hospitals, particularly at a time when the leadership of the various religious orders sponsoring hospitals was dwindling rapidly. Absentee governing boards called into question the Sisters' grip on their institutions. A narrow interpretation of canon law, however, dictated that hospitals could only be Catholic if religious personnel were in charge. Moreover, in a technical sense, a Catholic hospital also needed to remain a property of the Church to retain its legitimacy as a moral space.

The contemporary goals of the American health care system, as defined by society, were now based on the premise that access to health care was a right, not a privilege based on ability to pay, and thus that every citizen should be assured of that access. Therefore, voluntary, nonprofit hospitals such as those with a religious affiliation and a right to determine their own admission policies were becoming increasingly unacceptable to the communities they were supposed to serve. Under such circumstances, fears were expressed that Catholic hospitals would lose their identification as charitable institutions. In the competitive climate of the late 1960s, institutional planning became mandatory, including mergers, satellite affiliations, and other cooperative arrangements designed to "enhance the apostolate."[123] From a peak of 850 institutions in 1968, Catholic hospitals began a gradual and steady decline, with nearly 200 abandoned by their congregations by the 1980s because of decreasing numbers of Sisters available to manage them.

Despite national developments, however, the Sisters of Mercy retained their firm control of the hospital at Cazenovia Park, creating in 1970 a new board of directors still largely composed of nuns but with the participation of a few selected lay persons. However, the regional mother house of the order remained the ultimate source of authority. At Mercy, a motion for greater medical representation on the board of directors had been tabled in May 1974, apparently because the Sisters perceived that physicians were reluctant to sacrifice their own professional interests for the sake of primary allegiance to the institution. As it turned out, the increasing technological and financial complexity of hospital operations was bound to shift power to the administrative sector—increasingly composed of qualified managers—at the expense of the trustees and medical staffs. In an age of renewal, what really was at stake was a new "apostolate of management"—a partnership between religious and lay persons committed to Christian values.[124]

The creation of a strong consumer movement in America's health care field also affected all hospital operations and increasingly brought patients into conflict with management as the gap between promise and reality widened. Cost assumed ever greater importance compared to the issues of quality and reputation. Like other voluntary institutions, Catholic hospitals such as Mercy were told to organize their resources, establish priorities, improve internal management, shift to automation and computers, engage in cooperative buying, and lease expensive equipment. This structural renewal of the Catholic hospital continued to be the central issue debated throughout the early 1970s.

Since the mission, resource allocation plans, and financial performance of voluntary Catholic hospitals were inextricably linked to local demographic, economic, and ethnic factors, Mercy Hospital in the late 1960s found itself in the enviable position of actually formulating expansion plans, in contrast to similar institutions located elsewhere, especially in some decaying inner cities. In conformity with national trends, Mercy and other voluntary hospitals now consolidated their position at the center of the American health care delivery system, with extension into ambulatory service, nursing homes, and convalescent care. Generously financed by the federal and state government and by private insurance companies, Mercy Hospital remained economically healthy. Drawing Medicare patients from its core constituency in South Buffalo and the growing "crabgrass frontier" of its suburbs, Mercy indeed followed the "graying" of America, caring more for the aged, with proportional decreases in obstetrics and pediatrics. Somewhat sheltered in a stable, still predominantly Catholic neighborhood, Sister M. Annunciata did not share the widely discussed angst about Mercy Hospital losing its religious identity.

A major event in 1971 was the publication of a revised edition of the *Ethical and Religious Directives for Catholic Hospitals*, finally approved by the National Conference of Catholic Bishops and distributed by the CHA. Unlike its 1949 predecessor, this document was to be subjected to further revisions when ongoing research concerning advancing medical and moral knowledge justified modifications. Bishops, in consultation with scientists, physicians, lawyers, economists, and political scientists, would set future policies. The twenty-two guidelines mostly echoed fundamental Christian values already articulated more than a millennium ago. Promotion of health and wholeness were central. The Church pledged to continue its prominent role in health care, extending "Christ's healing love to people whose lives have been disrupted by sickness, injury, or death." As before, the hospital was to remain an extension of the patient's religious and moral community, providing compassionate physical and spiritual support.[125]

The 1971 Directives were criticized for again placing undue emphasis on matters of human reproduction and reverence for life while ignoring the realities of the contemporary American health care system, especially the need for cooperative planning and the medical needs of the poor. Moreover, the ambiguities surrounding the impact of Vatican II on the Church were reflected in these Directives. Were Catholic hospital patients and staff bound collectively to follow the norms, or could they individually follow their consciences and simply be guided by such precepts? At Mercy, the Sisters had to insure that employees were aware of their responsibility to contribute to a Catholic environment with "loving care and respect for personal dignity." The patient was again characterized as "an integrated whole" with Catholic health care institutions once more affirming the centrality of patients in health care decision-making.[126]

Sensitivity toward patients required treating them with respect, dignity, and personal attention, particularly in an era of greater depersonalization created by technology and specialization. Regardless of status and condition, everybody was judged worthy. Given the inherent passivity and sense of helplessness of many patients, the provision of respect and decisin-making power were important items to bolster autonomy. Finally, one of the precepts stipulated that "health care personnel should be trained and available to help patients find meaning in their experirence of suffering and dying."[127] Readers were reminded that Catholic theology had always viewed suffering and dying within the larger context of a redemptive process. Hospitalization remained a period of grace and transformation aided by the sacraments, a time for sharing Christ's own sufferings and preparing for the resurrection and eternal life.[128]

Wired for survival: Life in Mercy's CCU

By 9.30 PM, Albert F. was finally placed on a narrow stretcher and wheeled from the Emergency Room down the corridor to a private, hard-wired "slot" in Mercy's new CCU for further observation and treatment.[129] Each room was equipped with a digital clock next to the doorway, prompting Albert to ponder whether his time was up: what were his chances of ever leaving this place? His room was relatively small and confining, full of strange equipment that only heightened his anxiety. Albert could see neither a toilet nor a television set. Thank God, he thought, that the room had a glass door facing the nurses' station. This configuration was specifically designed to prevent patients from feeling isolated; being able to observe the comings and goings of their caregivers might prove reassuring. As Mary Ann Gottstine, the head nurse of the CCU, observed, "coronary disease affects a person emotionally as well as physically. That is why every detail of the new unit is designed to create an atmosphere that's serene, yet alive."[130]

Conversely this arrangement allowed staff members to check on their patients instead of simply staring at the monitoring equipment and observing the tracings of their vital signs. But would it foster a personal relationship? Patients arriving at the CCU were initially placed in Phase 1 beds and told that their condition was to be routinely called "critical" for the first 24 hours.[131] Not surprisingly, this status only increased many patients' feelings of anxiety and doom. Because of his family experiences, Albert remained keenly aware of the potentially lethal outcome of a heart attack as he was carefully lifted onto the bed and told not to move. The patient felt locked in as nurses immediately raised the side rails of the bed for safety reasons. If he died in this position, he thought, the undertaker would have no trouble placing him in a coffin.

Soon Albert was virtually in terror as nurses began connecting the three light, disposable chest leads to a bedside cardioscope placed behind him. As in the Emergency Room, his chest was scrubbed for placement of the electrodes. He was repeatedly warned not to touch the wires because any movements would touch off an alarm system. "Hands were everywhere," Albert later recalled; they were touching, rubbing, and pricking his body without asking permission, including a frantic search for a good vein and placement of an intravenous line for the administration of morphine. To prevent arrhythmia, a bolus and a continuous infusion of lidocaine with atropine were started in a solution of dextrose. Albert continued to receive oxygen, and a Foley catheter was inserted into his bladder to monitor urinary output. Blood samples were drawn to measure electrolytes, enzymes, and blood gases.[132] Another EKG tracing confirmed the previous finding of a myocardial infarct. For Albert, all the hustle and bustle of the nursing staff working on him heightened his sense of crisis, and the wires and tubes further limited his mobility.[133] To facilitate relaxation, the patient was sedated with sodium amybarbital. Since it was near the end of the evening shift and Albert was getting sleepy, this was probably not a good time for him to ask questions. In fact, one of the nurses promised to give him a fuller explanation the next morning. Everything seemed to be happening in a fog, the eerie atmosphere in Mercy's CCU.[134]

CCU nurses were well aware of the emotional impact of myocardial infarction on patients.[135] In fact, one nurse wrote that "to me, nursing is giving complete care to the patient—physical, emotional, personal, whatever—to the best of one's ability. I felt I could do this best where the care required was most intense." However, she quickly admitted that "we nurses become so engrossed with machines that we neglect nursing."[136] Technical demands, like watching the oscilloscopes and EKG printouts, checking alarms, and concentrating on the patient's vital signs tended to displace attention from the actual person. As in other hospitals, there was at Mercy a constant struggle among the CCU nurses to retain their caring attitude in the face of a relentless technical emphasis. The unit predisposed caregivers to spend a disproportionate amount of time gathering data as opposed to providing information to patients and their relatives. The frequency of dangerous, even fatal arrhythmias and the opportunity to prevent death through prompt defibrillation procedures left the nurses with little choice. After a fitful night of sleep—further samples for enzymes were obtained every four hours together with blood pressure readings—Albert woke up, still anxious, disoriented, and exhausted. The frequent question "Where am I?" was answered by Nurse Gottstine, who was the first to visit him. At this point, Albert was also asked to sign a permission slip authorizing the nursing staff to perform a number of procedures, including resuscitation.

Work in a CCU represented a new nursing specialty.[137] It was in some ways a return to the late 1960's *primary nursing*, a one-to-one nurse–patient relationship, but arranged within a more complex context of care.[138] Here nurses, in fact, assumed major responsibilities ordinarily reserved for physicians: they gave intravenous medications, adjusted pacemaker rates, and used defibrillators in cases of cardiac arrest. Since the senior house staff members assigned to a CCU were usually unfamiliar with this equipment, they received training from the specialized nurses. Like other intensive care nursing, CCU work was challenging; it required more knowledge and skills, but the nurses in these units were also rewarded with more autonomy and responsibility for what often were lifesaving interventions.[139]

Nurses working in a CCU in the 1970s exemplified the changing pattern of care delivered since the days of Joseph O'H.'s hospitalization in the 1950s. Thanks to the women's liberation movement, nursing had shifted from a purely service function to one that included sophisticated caregiving and educational activities. Nurses were no longer "trained like seals" to smile, make beds, and fluff pillows; they had assumed administrative tasks, obtained advanced training and degrees, and even conducted clinical research. Among the prototypes revolutionizing patient care was the *clinical nurse specialist*, whose in-house training occurred in a particular specialty area, and who had more independence and less supervision. Another was the *primary care nurse*, writing her own care plans and directly responsible for a smaller, specific number of patients.[140]

At Mercy's CCU, in addition to the nursing staff, board-certified cardiologists like Anthony Bonner and William Breen were usually brought in for consultations. Mercy's earlier unit had already attracted nine cardiologists, and the unit also served as a recruitment tool for house staff members. This space was truly their special domain. Although many cardiologists were primarily oriented toward complex, technically assisted diagnostic procedures such as cardiac catheterization and coronary arteriography, the emphasis at Mercy was still more on providing high-quality cardiac care than on state-of-the-art diagnosis. Patients requiring these invasive tests needed to be transferred to Buffalo General, Meyer Memorial, or Millard Fillmore hospitals near the downtown area, a somewhat risky undertaking given the hazards of postinfarction.[141] For their part, cardiologists at Mercy Hospital employed echocardiography, an ultrasonic examination of the heart popularized in the 1960s to detect pericardial effusions and possible aneurysms.[142]

During his first morning in the CCU, Albert had a repeat chest X-ray showing a small left basilar, plate-like atelectasis in the lung. A portable echocardiogram suggested that a small aneurysm involving the left ventricular apex was already forming. In addition, the atrium was enlarged. A myocardial scan showed a gated blood pool image, with normal total circulation but a low ventricular ejection fracture of 23%. There was also global hypokinesis with apical aneurysm of the left ventricle. "When will all this testing end?" wondered Albert, and "Why are the nurses and doctors mostly talking this techno-gibberish among themselves?" In this confined environment, it seemed difficult to get a chance to rest.

But how could a CCU be quiet and relaxing? Its social system was made up of several groups, including cardiologists, nurse clinicians, senior residents, patients, and anxious family members interacting around the clock during shift changes, dramatic emergencies, and frequent deaths. Constant support from a skilled supervisor such as Gottstine was essential in dealing with scheduling issues, administrative snafus, equipment failures, anger between patients and caregivers, and problems with relatives. Given the numerous monitoring tasks, there was little time left for providing emotional comfort to the patient, and no one was specifically responsible for proper family communications. However, in spite of professional fragmentation and specialization, most nurses still attempted to focus on the patients' needs, not on the body systems they needed to monitor. Although often viewed as pampered prima donnas with an abundance of staff and equipment, the CCU nurses worked very hard in a pressurized atmosphere that frequently produced burnout.[143]

On his first full day in the unit, Albert F. also received a somewhat reassuring call from his minister, while the hospital's chaplain, Father Krupa, anointed another patient in the adjacent room.[144] Still upset about the extreme confinement, and wrestling with the bedpan, Albert was found to have low blood pressure. Sips of tea and a few mouthfuls of Jello were now allowed. The nurses also performed passive exercises to prevent excessive stiffness in his joints. By now some of his intravenous needles were hurting, and the noisy hiss from the oxygen flow became more than annoying. The buzzing sounds emanating from the monitor and Albert's entanglement with various wires created a surreal and oppressive climate. He felt trapped, scared to move, as if laid out alive in the viewing room of a funeral home. Ironically, anxiety among patients suffering from myocardial infarction increased the risk of developing more arrhythmias.[145] Indeed, Albert suffered a temporary episode of atrial fibrillation that was quickly detected. As the CCU supervisor explained to him, this was precisely the reason for placing him in such a unit: to detect and promptly treat all arrhythmias before they led to potentially lethal complications, especially the dreaded cardiac arrest. Fortunately, Albert's arrhythmia was promptly controlled by the administration of intravenous ouabain, designed to provide digitalis to the patient. The drug was to be administered around the clock for the next two days.

"Cardiac patients always have more fear. You can tell them that their heart is healing but they want to know if they will ever have that pain again," recalled Gottstine. She was fond of explaining to patients that the heart needed to mend slowly, just like a broken bone, but that it was much harder to heal the heart. To alleviate some of the anxiety, she also attempted to explain the spatial orientation of the unit and the purposes of its machines. This usually made patients feel a little better and more secure. Being told that their vital signs were being monitored constantly by diligent nurses available at the central station could be reassuring. At Mercy, morning and evening prayers were still heard through the paging system. A Brahms lullaby played each time a baby was born. Rather than religious ceremonies, however, technical procedures now structured most of Albert's hospital sojourn.

As hospitalization proceeded, turning and positioning cardiac patients was essential. Every nurse in the unit also performed her own bathing and caring routines. The importance of the daily nurse-assisted bath had not diminished since earlier times. It still provided cleanliness and increased circulation, but above all, it allowed for personal touching, feeling, and communication. Skin care remained a priority, with the generous employment of body lotion. Intubated patients initially receiving oxygen but nothing else by mouth frequently had dry mouths with sores. Here nurses could provide comfort by both wetting the mouth and removing debris. Moreover, to maintain each patient's comfort, soiled linen needed to be changed and secretions wiped away.

Albert continued to receive visits from the consulting cardiologists responsible for coordinating his care. Brief rounds with the medical residents and students conducted by Dr. Milford Maloney also provided a welcome human presence. Since canceling its affiliation with Georgetown, Mercy Hospital had been trying to break out of its traditional insularity, becoming part of a consortium of community hospitals in western New York. This new dialogue between institutions hitherto virtually isolated within Buffalo's metropolitan area allowed sophomore and junior medical students from the local university to rotate through the hospital in medicine, pediatrics, orthopedics, and physical and nuclear medicine. Both O'Brien and Maloney believed that Mercy Hospital was also a perfect setup for future family medicine practitioners, who could gain some understanding of and experience with sophisticated specialized technical procedures such as those performed in the CCU.

As in earlier times, the central mission to provide excellent medical care continued to depend on Mercy's educational resources. In July 1964, the hospital had appointed Dr. Joseph Prezio assistant director of medical education. A graduate of Georgetown University and former house staff member himself, Prezio rescued Mercy's internship and residency programs from their gradual demise. Both he and O'Brien had long given up on the dream that the Georgetown affiliation would attract more American graduates. In an increasingly competitive market, they were now forced to accept only foreigners, whose qualifications could not always be determined. However, the issue of house staff competence was now more important than ever. By 1974, interns and residents were no longer monitoring only private patients. Because of federal Medicare payments, there was now a widespread desire to educate and train house staff members properly as surrogate caregivers. In contrast to their predecessors, residents were given responsibility for complex medical decisions and even procedures. Instead of obtaining education in general

medicine, most foreign physicians now received specialty and subspecialty training, turning them into direct competitors in the American health care marketplace.
Because of their cultural backgrounds, many foreign house officers working at
Mercy were still considered exotic and alien. Some of them even displayed blatant chauvinism toward nurses and technicians, who were now full-fledged members of caregiving teams.

On the third day, Albert was finally placed on soft food and was given a silver
tray at breakfast with cereal and half a slice of bread. He was also encouraged to
perform some active exercises such as moving his feet, thighs, and arms under the
supervision of a physiotherapist. The patient now had commode privileges, and his
Foley catheter was removed. Although he was still on intermittent oxygen and intravenous therapy, Gottstine and the other nurses seemed pleased by his progress.
They had a great desire to see their patients get well and return home: "By everything we do, we insist that the patient display hope"[146] was a commonly expressed
sentiment in the CCU. Albert was still somewhat disoriented, although his room
had a view of the hospital's backyard. Visiting hours in Phase 1 were limited to periods of 15 minutes and only for close family members. Most CCU caregivers agreed
that at this stage family support was crucial. Albert's only son, living nearby, was
initially allowed to stay overnight in the room. At Mercy's CCU, visitors had a special waiting room provided with blankets and pillows. However, even as things
seemed to be looking up, Albert accidentally caused a dramatic and embarrassing
episode. While scratching his dry skin, he knocked loose one of his wires, and a
code 9 call brought the cardiac arrest team, composed of several nurses, a physician and a "crash cart," rushing into the room for a possible resuscitation attempt.

On November 25, Albert's condition was deemed stable and he was transferred to a Phase 2 semiprivate room in the CCU with a television set, where he
was provided with battery-operated telemetry instead of the confining wires. Daily
visits by his pastor provided companionship and reassurance. Having a roommate
was also a potentially positive development, somebody to talk to instead of the
loneliness of a private room.[147] Henceforth, Albert was not to be watched as closely
as before, and he was encouraged to walk around the room and the entire unit
two or three times a day. Soon, Albert came to know all the caregivers and ambulatory patients in this small 14-bed unit. This new familiarity and sense of intimacy helped to restore a feeling of dignity and personality to someone who until
a few days earlier had been a prone lump of flesh with a damaged ticker emitting
closely monitored electrical impulses. Finally, three days later, Albert was reclas-
sified to a Phase 3 facility outside the CCU and summarily transferred upstairs to
the hospital's medical floor without advance warning. This was quite a contrast.
He found himself in a semiprivate room with a different roommate and closed
doors. Fortunately, team nursing prevailed here, with one staff nurse assigned to
a few patients. Still, the care was more fragmented, being dispensed as it was by
various members of the team, including practical nurses and aides.

Not surprisingly, Albert had eventually drawn comfort from the CCU's closely monitored environment. Now, transferred to a regular ward, he experienced a return of his previous feeling of fragility. He felt abandoned by Gottstine and her personnel, who, between drips and beeps, had tried to cheer him up. What would happen if he had another heart attack while recovering here? Now the skillful CCU nurses and physicians were far away. Could they arrive in time to save him? Anticipating this feeling of vulnerability, CCU nurses routinely checked on their former patients for several days to make sure they were recovering. The next day, Albert appeared quite pale and felt weaker. An examination by the CCU nurse detected a brief return of the previous arrhythmia. Albert was promptly returned to a Phase 2 room in the CCU and his digitalis dose adjusted. While he wandered around the premises, he came to witness another patient's cardiac arrest and resuscitation efforts, a traumatic experience that once more made him anxious. Could this happen to him? Was there still a chance that he would die at Mercy?[148]

Albert remained at the CCU until December 1 before being transferred once more to the medical floor. This meant still another room and a different roommate. His near obsession with the danger of experiencing a further arrhythmia made him fixate on his monitor rather than search for a friendly face. Both the ward's clinical specialist and the CCU nurse tried to teach him how to adjust to a convalescent state. However, although he was now ambulatory, Albert seemed to be looking inward, concentrating intently on the rhythms of his heart, and rarely socializing with other patients. Because of this behavior, he was brought to the attention of Mercy's Social Service Department, headed by a therapist, Richard Scarfetta, and assisted by a nurse, Jane Voss. Their goal was to understand the problems created by illness and disability for both patients and families, arranging referrals to community, medical, and social resources, including health-related agencies, following discharge. This assistance included the provision of home care nursing or space in a convalescent or nursing home facility.[149]

Albert was not well prepared for this transition to life in a medical ward. He still felt hurt and vulnerable, a man with a damaged heart, a weak body, and a tattered self-image. He worried intensely about a return of his previous arrhythmia, especially since he had been told that this could happen if he got upset or worried. In addition, there were the usual questions and anxieties about carrying out any type of physical activity. Although the CCU nurse hurriedly proceeded with some basic education about the contours of cardiac rehabilitation, Albert failed to express his anxieties fully. A booklet about postinfarction care and return to work further lowered his spirits. He vowed to retire after discharge, taking it easy and seeking closer ties with his remaining family members. During his last days at Mercy before going home, he found himself even without a roommate in the semiprivate ward room where he was convalescing.[150]

By now, Albert wanted badly to go home. Preparations were made to discharge him on December 3. The cardiology consultant recommended limited activity for the next two weeks while the patient continued taking his nitroglycerin tablets. Other medications were the long-term aspirin Ecotrin, digitalis (Lanoxin), a diuretic (Lasix), and potassium chloride. He was also told to use nitropaste every six hours. Although it must have felt like an eternity, Albert's total hospital stay had been only 15 days instead of the 39 days experienced by Joseph O'H. in 1954. Such shorter stays—now routine given the cost of hospitalization—forced many cardiac patients to transfer to a nursing home for convalescence or be cared for at home by family members and visiting nurses. One of his sisters arrived from Cleveland to take him to her home during the Christmas holiday. Albert was also to be followed in Mercy's outpatient department and referred to a psychiatrist for his presumed depression.

Two eventful weeks of fragmented care in different rooms, with diverse nursing and house staff personnel, were coming to an end. In contrast to his parents, he was still alive. In Albert's view, all that specialized high-tech care had been successful, but unlike Joseph, he failed to experience his recovery as a rebirth. Perhaps part of this response was attributable to his personality, not his medical care, but, according to Albert, his physicians and nurses had frequently forgotten that the wires placed on his skin were actually linked to a human being, not a heart-lung machine. Looking to the future with apprehension, Albert regretted the lack of a closer relationship with his caregivers, both at Mercy and with his private physician. However, under the circumstances, personal contacts with caregivers and other patients in the CCU were nearly impossible to achieve except perhaps with Gottstine, the supervisor, herself a remnant of the old Mercy nursing staff of the 1950s. Perhaps the real healing would begin in Cleveland during Christmas.[151]

"Moving forward under God"

By the mid-1970s, as Albert F. continued his slow recovery, the traditional mission of the Church and its ministry to the sick continued to be called into question. In an address given at the third annual Catholic Health Assembly, Pellegrino, now chairman of the board of the Yale-New Haven Medical Center, returned to a discussion of the true Catholic identity of hospitals. Most dangerous was the impact of President Lyndon B. Johnson's Great Society and its governmental concern for society's poor, virtually eliminating the traditional role of charity. The very existence of Catholic hospitals was further threatened by a confluence of powerful forces, including the growing membership crisis within the religious congregations, the intrusions of governmental and third-party agencies, and community influences on policy, as well as the complexities of hospital management and the rising costs of operations. These societal influences tended to secularize religious institutions, which were forced to focus on and respond to such political and financial challenges. "We can no longer assume that hospitals that are canonical Catholic are de facto Catholic or even totally Christian," Pellegrino said.[152] Hospitals like Mercy hired a new layer of professional managers primarily interested in the bottom line to guide them through the rapids of fiscal solvency. In her 1975 report, Mercy's Sister M. Annunciata acknowledged the growing uncertainties fueled by inflation and the implementation of certain mandated government programs.[153]

Meanwhile, the authorities at Mercy Hospital, prodded by the local bishop, decided in 1975 to create a formal pastoral program with Father Krupa at the helm, together with one additional priest and three Sisters. All members were to be trained for three months in clinical psychology and had to possess adequate interviewing skills. Awareness of the spiritual needs of hospital patients became an official policy, with members of the team frequently visiting those in need, their interviews to be written up and subjected to critical analysis by the group.[154] Like other Catholic health care facilities, Mercy had to comply with the revised ethical code developed by the National Conference of Bishops. Given the internal ambiguities of this document and the fact that bishops could make their own interpretations, the rules caused confusion. Creation of a "conscience clause" in 1973 as an amendment to the Public Health Service Act gave institutions and individuals the right to refuse participation in procedures and therapies at odds with their religious or moral values, providing a basis for subsequent ethical decision making, including the option to cease what were termed *extraordinary means* in treating the terminally ill.[155]

In 1976, the hospital's board of directors appointed Sister Sheila M. Walsh, also a registered nurse, as the new administrator of Mercy, replacing Sister. M. Annunciata, who became mother superior general of the Sisters of Mercy in the Buffalo diocese. Walsh was keen about issues of nurse and patient autonomy, advocating the concept of team care and supporting the rise of paramedical workers. Under the banner of "independence through interdependence," the national organization of Sisters of Mercy began a process of organizing multiunit hospital corporations, with eight of the nine "provinces" sponsoring hospitals, for a total of 125 institutions throughout the country. This strategy seemed necessary to counteract the influence of the for-profit hospital chains gradually emerging on the American health care scene. Such corporate restructuring and business emphasis were obviously at odds with the Sisters' congregational organization and original vow of poverty, but the twin issues of efficiency and quality care, so frequently stressed throughout the century, were once more perceived as the essential engines of survival and growth. Above all, the Sisters of Mercy wanted to retain influence and control over their institutions to fulfill their apostolic mission.[156]

At Mercy Hospital in Buffalo, meanwhile, construction of Phase II began as originally envisioned, with four floors added to the McAuley Building. By 1979, the institution had become the fifth largest hospital in Erie County and the second largest employer in South Buffalo. Patient care, notably for the elderly, made up a high proportion of its admissions. Moreover, Mercy's Emergency Room—now a major provider of primary care as the number of general practitioners dwindled—

was now one of the busiest in the county, with more than 40,000 visits recorded in 1978. The obstetric unit registered the county's largest number of births—2,751. In the jargon of the times, however, these were "loss leaders"—services insufficiently reimbursed and definitely unprofitable but still considered a function of the pronatalist and charitable orientation governing Catholic hospitals.[157] As Sister M. Annunciata insisted, "our goal is to be a true community hospital."[158]

At this point, however, South Buffalo residents represented less than a third of the patient population. By 1978, more than half of the admissions came from the adjacent southern suburbs. Consolidating its reputation for up-to-date coronary care, Mercy also continued to feature the only hospital-based mobile CCU in the city. Shorter stays meant that more hospital beds became available, to the extent that, in the early 1980s, some could not be filled, a first in the hospital's history. To be sure, the Sisters had retained their traditional frugality. Ever prudent, they were discriminating and economical buyers of hospital supplies. Since they avoided all waste, the costs of patient care at Mercy remained lower than at other comparable community hospitals in the Buffalo area.

Another critical issue disturbing the traditional hospital atmosphere at Mercy was the unionization of the growing variety of health care personnel. Such organizational efforts initially received Church support but were subsequently opposed by Catholic hospitals, especially after Congress passed legislation in 1974 extending coverage of the Labor/Management Relations Act to all nonsupervisory employees working in voluntary, nonprofit health care institutions and granting them the right to unionize.[159] Hospitals wanted to remain competitive in an era of cost cutting. Labor costs, a major budgetary item of all hospitals, had been steadily rising in the early 1970s, threatening further increases in expenditures and forcing the substitution of professional nurses by trained assistants, especially licensed practical nurses. However, Church leaders continued to advocate the rights of workers to fair wages and working conditions. Mercy participated in subsequent efforts to counter the threat of unionization, explaining that unions placed employees and management in an adversarial relationship, a threat to their carefully nurtured apostolic mission. The Sisters explained that allegiance to a union and its agenda would clash with the values and mission of Catholic hospitals and reduce their quality of care.[160]

In Buffalo, the right to strike was viewed by the Sisters of Mercy as abolishing an individual's power to select his own relationship with an employer. These problems continued to affect most Catholic hospitals during the ensuing decade, as hospital employees demanded a greater voice in setting hospital policies and making staffing arrangements. In time, however, pressures to unionize certain staff groups, including the nurses and many technical service personnel, proved irresistible, leading to strife, strikes, and layoffs and disrupting the hitherto congenial hospital atmosphere. During their rounds in the CCU, protesting nurses wore black ribbons or pins proclaiming "no justice," further raising the anxiety level of

already worried patients. To compound the problems, radical changes in the regulation and financing of health care, a malpractice crisis in New York State after
1985, and the patients' rights movement contributed to a deterioration of the traditional relationship between caregivers and their patients.[161]

Under the leadership of Sister M. Annunciata, who eventually became president and chief executive officer of the Mercy Health System of Western New
York, the South Buffalo hospital continued to promote, at least rhetorically, the
values of compassion, hospitality, and commitment to medical excellence. As Sister Sheila declared, "this is our life ministry of presence and service. We must be
thoroughly prepared to maintain our civil and corporate rights, not simply to survive and operate hospitals, but rather to maintain witness to the sanctity of life
and our reverence of it."[162] Yet the spiritual influence of the dwindling cadre of
Mercy Sisters was waning. Religious status with its potential for social control, was
no longer the sole determinant of relationships. Administrative and programmatic
decisions became more pragmatic, following "safe" directions already implemented elsewhere. Parochialism remained the rule. Although the owners and administrators of a multi-million-dollar hospital business, the Sisters had a critical
advantage. They could play the political game with no personal axe to grind since
their vows precluded any personal benefit or gain. Their fiduciary role covering
the marginalized and poor, the vulnerable and voiceless, gave the Sisters of Mercy
a potent moral platform from which to deal with the complexities of the American health care system. But how successful were they?[163]

Although they had proven to be fast learners, no broad vision beyond their
traditional charitable philosophy guided the Sisters of Mercy as they faced the
forces unleashed during the 1960s and 1970s, among America's most turbulent
decades in health care delivery. The nuns displayed tenacity and vitality in the face
of multiple societal pressures, admirable qualities derived from their religious and
nursing training.[164] Riding the new waves of antiauthoritarianism and laicization
in the Catholic Church, these Sisters had salvaged their power through collective
decision making, including the participation of prominent community leaders on
their board of directors. Operating throughout the 1970s with an iron fist hidden
in a velvet glove, the Mercy Sisters remained in charge of key administrative and
management positions, including nursing services, the laboratory, pharmacy, and
radiology departments, as well as the business office and medical records. Final
approvals were still sought at the top of the pyramid—Sister M. Annunciata at
the Mercy Order's mother house—while the remaining Sisters held the reins of
administrative power on the General Council and individual hospital boards, as
well as on planning committees.

However, the growing complexities of running a not-for-profit hospital in
America now required a broad spectrum of outside expertise in finance, insurance, management, and law. In the final analysis, what may have made the difference at Mercy was a small but devoted group of house and attending physi-

cians, especially O'Brien, Malloney, and Prezio. These men employed the tools of education—rounds, seminars, conferences—to improve the quality of medical care at Mercy, placing this community hospital at the level of larger, university-affiliated, and state-of-the-art institutions in downtown Buffalo. Moreover, Mercy's educators built bridges to other institutions and geographical areas, thus transcending the provincialism of South Buffalo and creating a mecca for specialty training, especially in cardiology. In the trade-off, however, Mercy Hospital lost part of its intimate, familiar, even "motherly" environment.[165]

Still, the Sisters of Mercy tried to hold the hospital to its traditional apostolic mission. For the Sisters, compassion for patients and devotion to God remained the key values. Most Sisters had been trained as nurses and, later, as X-ray technicians and physical therapists. Their dedication and commitment to their cause was the glue needed to hold the hospital together.[166] Increasingly, the dwindling numbers of Sisters gave way to lay caregivers and growing layers of administrators who were carefully screened to ascertain their agreement with the hospital's traditional apostolic mission.[167] Loyalty to this cause continued to be greatly valued in a society increasingly contemptuous of such behavior. Many of the new employees were enrolled in national leadership development programs, and their institutional performances were closely monitored. Periodic "mission effectiveness" sessions were held at the hospital to examine and discuss the desired values.

In time, the Sisters of Mercy came to realize that administrative, business, and technical skills had to take their rightful place next to moral qualities. Their systematic efforts to educate employees about the basic tenets of Mercy's caring philosophy had become a constant struggle. Fragmentation and subspecialization of the caregivers and the increasingly technological character of their interventions became formidable barriers to focusing on the patient's spiritual needs. Yet, bent on ignoring the corporate structures and the culture of consumerism forced upon her institution by the evolution of the American medical marketplace, Sister M. Annunciata continued to insist that "Mercy Hospital exists for the purpose of serving God by providing Christ-like care of the highest quality to the patients we serve regardless of race, color, religion, or financial status. Our dedication to preserving life and the dignity of man constantly calls upon each of us to provide the best we can offer, the highest level of ethics and professional standards."[168] Given the resilience and spiritual tenacity of the remaining Sisters of Mercy, the struggle endures.

NOTES

1. Mercy Hospital, *Mercy's Fifty Years*, Buffalo, NY, privately printed, 1954, p. 66.
2. To protect confidentiality, the patient's name and other identifying details have been altered. Information was obtained from clinical charts and personal interviews with family members in November 1994 and May 1996.

3. Mercy Hospital had been recently certified by the Joint Commission on Accreditation of the AHA. The first list of fully accredited hospitals in the United States and Canada, based on criteria of proper administrative structures and efficient management, was issued in April 1954.

4. Personal interview with Sr. Sheila M. Walsh, May 1996. For details see W. C. Mc-Cready, "The Irish neighborhood. A contribution to American urban life," in *America and Ireland, 1776–1976, The American Identity and the Irish Connection*, ed. D. N. Doyle and O. D. Edwards, Westport, CT, Greenwood Press, 1980, pp. 247–59.

5. Personal interview with "Joseph's" surviving wife, November 1994.

6. James B. Herrick published a paper titled "Clinical features of sudden obstruction of the coronary arteries" in *JAMA* 59 (Dec. 7, 1912): 2015–20. His aim was to assist clinicians in reaching a diagnosis during the patient's lifetime instead of at the autopsy table. For an overview see W. B. Fye, "Acute myocardial infarction: A historical summary," in *Acute Myocardial Infarction*, ed. B. J. Gersh and S. H. Rahimtoola, New York, Elsevier, 1991, pp. 3–13.

7. *Mercevents* 4 (December 1958): 8. In the opinion of CHA officials, the Emergency Room together with the admitting desk and the cashier's office were three critical hospital areas where prospective patients and staff members could come into conflict. To help the encounter run smoothly, the CHA produced a series of publications under the titles *Making Friends with Your Hospital Public* and *Making Friends Through Public Relations*.

8. See Andrew Greeley, *That Most Distressful Nation: The Taming of the American Irish*, Chicago, Quadrangle Books, 1972, p. 109. For a discussion of cultural differences in sickness behavior see I. K. Zola, "Pathways to the doctor—from person to doctor," *Soc Sci Med* 7 (1973): 677–89.

9. J. P. Boland, "Religious aspects of sisters' hospitals," *Hosp Progr* 2 (1923): 285. See also Aaron I. Abell, *American Catholicism and Social Actions: A Search for Social Justice, 1865–1950*, Garden City, NY, Hanover House, 1960.

10. Sr. J. of the Cross, "The Catholicity of the Catholic hospital," *Hosp Progr* 31 (October 1950): 300–02.

11. *Mercy's Fifty Years*, p. 42.

12. "Western New York State Heart Group boasts 81 Erie members," *Erie County Med Bull* 27 (January 1950): 20.

13. For an overview see P. R. Fleming, *A Short History of Cardiology*, Amsterdam, Rodopi, 1997. A critical study of the shifting contours of this specialty in Britain is C. Lawrence, "Moderns and ancients: The new cardiology in Britain 1880–1930," in *The Emergence of Modern Cardiology*, ed. W. F. Bynum, C. Lawrence, and V. Nutton, London, Wellcome Institute for the History of Medicine, 1985, pp. 1–33. For the United States consult J. D. Howell, "Hearts and minds: The invention and transformation of American cardiology," in *Grand Rounds. One Hundred Years of Internal Medicine*, ed. R. C. Maulitz and D. E. Long, Philadelphia, Univ. of Pennsylvania Press, 1988, pp. 243–75.

14. "Chamber told area's growth potential is second to none in the US," *Buffalo Evening News* (Jan. 27, 1954), p. 35.

15. Editorial, "The G. P.—physician of the whole patient," *Hosp Progr* 31 (August 1950): 225.

16. "An analysis of the medical profession in Erie County," *Erie County Med Bull* 30 (May 1953): 8.

17. Concerns expressed by the Erie County chapter of the American Academy of General Practice; see *Erie County Med Bull* 27 (January 1950): 12 and (February 1950): 12–15. Also see "GP chapter on the march," Ibid. 27 (May 1950): 9, 20.

18. Mercy Hospital, Monthly report from the Medical Record Committee, April 1954, Hospital Archives.

19. Mercy Hospital, Minutes, Executive Committee meeting, April 6, 1954, Hospital Archives.

20. Personal interview with surviving family members, November 1994.

21. Greeley, *The Taming of the American Irish*, p. 128.

22. In a 1953 census, Erie County actually listed nine cardiologists. At this point, the training of physicians such as O'Brien was subsidized by the federal government following the passage of the National Heart Act of 1948. See W. Bruce Fye, *American Cardiology: The History of a Specialty and Its College*, Baltimore, Johns Hopkins Univ. Press, 1996, p. 9.

23. USDHEW, *Vital Statistics of the United States, 1954*, "Mortality data," Washington, DC, USGPO, 1956, vol. 2, p. 444.

24. Iwao M. Moriyama et al., *Cardiovascular Diseases in the United States*, Cambridge, MA, Harvard Univ. Press, 1971, pp. 49–118.

25. For details see "Addition planned for nurses' home at Mercy Hospital," *Buffalo Evening News* (Jan. 21, 1954), p. 44, and (Mar. 18, 1954), p. 30.

26. The original hospital standardization program was conducted yearly by the American College of Surgeons until the AHA decided in 1950 to operate its own program. For details see J. S. Roberts et al., "A history of the Joint Commission on Accreditation of Hospitals," *JAMA* 258 (Aug. 21, 1987): 936–49, and C. H. Patterson, "Joint Commission on Accreditation of Healthcare Organizations," *Infect Control Hosp Epidemiol* 16 (1995): 36–42.

27. Appointed by Pope Pius IX 10 years earlier, Timon had already created an impressive parochial network of institutions, including churches and orphanages, schools, and hospitals. For details see Sr. M. Gerald Pierce, *Unto All His Mercy: The First Hundred Years of the Sisters of Mercy in the Diocese of Buffalo, 1858–1958*, Buffalo, NY, Savage Lithography Co., 1959, and A. Doyle, "Nursing by religious orders in the US, part II, 1841–70," *Am J Nurs* 29 (August 1929): 959–69.

28. For an overview see E. Kolmer, "Catholic women religious and women's history, a survey of the literature," in *The American Catholic Religious Life*, ed. J. M. White, New York, Garland, 1988, pp. 127–39. See also Thomas Donahue, *History of the Catholic Church in Western New York*, Buffalo, NY, 1904.

29. For information about the Sisters' service to poor and uneducated Irish Catholics see E. A. Ryan, "The Sisters of Mercy: An important chapter in church history," *Theol Stud* 18 (June 1957): 253–70. More information is available in Sr. M. Eulalia Herron, *The Sisters of Mercy in the United States, 1848–1928*, New York, Macmillan, 1929, and in Elinor T. Dehey, *Religious Orders of Women in the US*, Hammond, IN, W. B. Conker, 1930.

30. For details see Kathleen Healy, ed., *Sisters of Mercy: Spirituality in America, 1843–1900*, New York, Paulist Press, 1992. See also Sr. M. Beata Bauman, *A Way of Mercy: Catherine McAuley's Contributions to Nursing*, New York, Vantage Press, 1958.

31. Kathleen Healy, *Frances Warde: American Founder of the Sisters of Mercy*, New York, Seabury Press, 1973. For a general history of Buffalo see Mark Goldman, *High Hopes: The Rise and Decline of Buffalo*, Albany, State Univ. of New York Press, 1983.

32. The Tifft St. story is recounted in detail by Sister Gerard, *Unto All His Mercy*, pp. 169–76. Also consult Bernadette McCauley, "Who Shall Take Care of Our Sick? Roman Catholic Sisterhoods and Their Hospitals, New York City, 1850–1929," Ph.D. diss., Columbia Univ., 1992. A summary of McAuley's views appears in "Sublime anomalies: Women religious and Roman Catholic Hospitals in New York City, 1850–1920," *J Hist Med* 52 (1997): 289–309.

33. *Report of the Mercy Hospital, Tifft Street, Buffalo, NY, for the Year ending Dec. 31, 1905*, Buffalo, NY, privately printed, 1905, Hospital Archives. For earlier Buffalo institutions see J. Richardson, "A tale of two nineteenth-century hospitals: Buffalo Hospital of the Sisters of Charity and Buffalo General Hospital," in *Medical History in Buffalo, 1846–1996: Collected Essays*, ed. L. Sentz, Buffalo, State Univ. of New York Press, 1996, pp. 47–60.

34. See the brochure *Mercy Hospital Building Campaign $500,000*, Hospital Archives.

35. "Organize 'tank-corps' in Mercy Hospital drive," *South Buffalo News* (Nov. 15, 1923), p. 8.

36. *Mercy Hospital Building Campaign*, Buffalo, NY, 1924, Hospital Archives.

37. See Sister Gerard, *Unto All His Mercy*, pp. 316–39, and the pamphlet *Mercy Hospital, 25th Anniversary, 1904–1929*, Buffalo, NY, Baker Jones, 1929, Hospital Archives. Details about nursing are presented in Sr. Mary Immaculata, "Weak points in the nursing service of Catholic hospitals," *Hosp Progr* 6 (February 1925): 54–56.

38. Information concerning this campaign can be found in the *Buffalo Courier Express* (May 7, 1948), p. 103–04. In the newspaper, the vicar general of the Buffalo diocese, the Rev. John J. Nash, is quoted as saying that the campaign was "unique in the history of Buffalo in that Protestants and Catholics will go forth together on a common errand of mercy."

39. At this time, almost 70% of the Catholic hospitals reporting construction projects did not request Hill-Burton funding. See the editorial "Does new epoch call for new planning?" *Hosp Progr* 31 (January 1950): 1. For a discussion of community–hospital relations see P. R. Hawley, "Medicine as a social instrument: The hospital and the community," *N Engl J Med* 244 (Feb. 15, 1951): 256–59.

40. "Mercy Spreads Her Wings," Building Fund Drive and Inaugural Program, Hospital Archives.

41. "Handicapped aided in new therapy unit," *Buffalo Courier Express* (Jan. 15, 1950), p. B6 4–5. In 1948, the hospital also created a two-year School of X Ray Technology.

42. H. Jeghers and J. O'Brien, "An experiment in making the hospital a graduate medical center," *JAMA* 158 (May 28, 1955): 243–52. Clinical research was another goal. See A. E. Maffly and C. K. Howan, "A community hospital can do research," *Mod Hosp* 82 (February 1954): 87–89.

43. In 1952 the House of Delegates of the State Medical Society of New York had approved a resolution recommending the establishment of general practice departments in voluntary hospitals. This was reaffirmed in May 1954. See "House of Delegates transacts enormous volume of business," *Erie County Med Bull* 31 (June 1954): 7–8.

44. The arrangement stipulated that some of the academics would make monthly visits to Buffalo, while one Mercy intern per month was authorized to join the university program in Washington. Similar arrangements were completed with newly established Kenmore Mercy Hospital in Buffalo and St. Jerome Hospital in Batavia. See "Georgetown professor to inaugurate affiliation program at Mercy Hospital," *Erie County Med Bull* 28 (July 1951): 22.

45. "Mercy is unique here in rehabilitation," *Buffalo Courier Express* (Jan. 25, 1953), p. 8C 1–3.

46. "The apostolate of the Catholic hospital," *Hosp Progr* 32 (October 1951): 299.

47. The first convention of the CHA was also held in Milwaukee on June 24–26 and attended by 200 sisters, lay nurses, and physicians representing 43 Catholic hospitals from 12 states. Father Moulinier was elected the first president of the new organization and became its dominant personality in the following decade. "The chronological development of the Catholic Hospital in the US and Canada," *Hosp Progr* 21 (April 1940): 122–33.

48. C. J. Kauffman, "The push for standardization: The origin of the Catholic Hospital Association, 1914–1920," *Health Progr* 71 (January–February 1990): 57–65, and C. J. Kauffman, "The leadership of Father Moulinier—the CHA comes of age, 1921–1928," *Health Progr* 71 (March 1990): 41–48. For details, see his *Ministry and Meaning: A Religious History of Catholic Health Care in the United States*, New York, Crossroad, 1995.

49. C. J. Kauffman, "Years of transition—internal developments under Fr. Schwitalla, 1928–1947," *Health Progr* 71 (April 1990): 33–37.

50. For an overview of changes in American nursing see Barbara Melosh, "*The Physician's Hand: Work Culture and Conflict in American Nursing*," Philadelphia, Temple Univ. Press, 1982, pp. 159–205.

51. Personal interview with Mary Ann Gottstine, May 1996.

52. Mercy Hospital's Nursing School, 1954, Hospital Archives.

53. *Mercy's Fifty Years*, p. 66.

54. Personal interview with Sr. M. Annunciata Kelliher, November 1994.

55. A. M. Mater and H. L. Jaffe, "Treatment of acute coronary occlusion," *NY State J Med* 55 (July–December 1955): 3239–46.

56. D. Schechter, "As doctor sees nurse—and the same to you, sir," *Mod Hosp* 81 (October 1953): 61–65.

57. For a critique see Jo Ann Ashley, *Hospitals, Paternalism, and the Role of the Nurse*, New York, Teachers College Press, 1976.

58. *Mercy's Fifty Years*, p. 60.

59. Gottstine interview, May 1996.

60. Ibid.

61. *Mercevents* 1 (April 1955): 3.

62. Personal interview with Dr. Joseph Prezio, November 1995.

63. For a historical view see J. D. Howell, "Early perceptions of the electrocardiogram: From arrhythmia to infarction," *Bull Hist Med* 58 (1984): 83–98. See also J. Burnett, "The origins of the electrocardiograph as a clinical instrument," in *The Emergence of Modern Cardiology*, pp. 53–76.

64. S. Schnur, "The current dispute concerning anticoagulants in acute myocardial infarction," *JAMA* 156 (Nov. 20, 1954): 1127–30.

65. While Catholic hospitals in the early 1950s comprised 27% of the 875 institutions with approved internships, only 13% of these hospitals received a full complement of house officers, with 31% attracting no interns at all. See M. R. Kneifl and K. Pohlen, "The Catholic Hospital: Health care facts," *Hosp Progr* 32 (June 1951): 196–200.

66. R. L. Coser, "Authority and decision-making in a hospital," *Am Sociol Rev* 23 (1958): 56–63.

67. R .G. Hutchins, "Most nurses choose marriage," *Mod Hosp* 82 (April 1954): 69.

68. Sister Annunciata interview, November 1994.

69. Personal interview with Father Krupa, November 1995.

70. *Mercy's Fifty Years*, pp. 19–20.

71. See Andrew M. Greeley, *Religion as Poetry*, New Brunswick, NJ, Transaction, 1994.

72. W. T. Mulloy, "Catholic Association stresses apostolic duty," *Mod Hosp* 79 (July 1952): 150.

73. J. Flanagan, "Personnel problems: A Catholic approach," *Hosp Progr* 31 (March 1950): 66–67, and "See no relief in hospital costs," *Erie County Med Bull* 31 (January 1954): 30.

74. H. B. Burchell, "Acute myocardial infarction, a discussion of certain controversial issues," *Calif Med* 80 (April 1954): 281–87.

75. S. A. Levine and B. Lown, "Armchair treatment of acute coronary thrombosis," *JAMA* 148 (1952): 1365, and A. M. Mitchell et al., "The armchair treatment of acute myocardial infarction," *Am J Nurs* 53 (June 1953): 674–76. For a controlled, comparative study of bed rest and chair rest see J.R. Beckwith et al., "The management of myocardial infarction with particular reference to the chair treatment," *Ann Intern Med* 41 (July–December 1954): 1189–95.

76. Personal interview with Sr. M. Victorine Collins, November 1994.

77. T. J. Radtke, "The rosary is good medicine," *Hosp Progr* 32 (March 1951): 66–67.

78. The New York Heart Association was a leading organization involved in this problem. See Editorial, "Can the cardiac work," *NY State J Med* 55 (Apr. 15, 1955): 1123, 1125.

79. Again, the patient's name and other identifying details have been changed to protect confidentiality. Some details of his hospitalization were obtained through a personal interview in May 1996.

80. Fye called the CCU concept "a new heart care paradigm." See *American Cardiology*, p. 250.

81. USDHEW, "Mortality," in *Vital Statistics of the United States, 1974*, Rockville, MD, PHS, 1976, p. 624.

82. W. J. Walker, "Coronary mortality: What is going on?" *JAMA* 227 (Mar. 4, 1974): 1045–46. See also F. J. Stone, "Epidemiological factors related to heart disease," *World Rev Nutri Diet* 12 (1970): 1–42.

83. For details see Fye, *American Cardiology*, pp. 249–94.

84. Death rates were highest for the Northeast and Middle Atlantic region of the United States. See W. B. Kannel et al., "Epidemiology of coronary heart disease," *Geriatrics* 17 (1962): 675–90, and S. Pell and C. A. D'Alonzo, "Immediate mortality and five-year survival of employed men with a first myocardial infarction," *N Engl J Med* 270 (Apr. 30, 1964): 913–22.

85. See K. L. White and M. A. Ibrahim, "The distribution of cardiovascular disease in the community," *Ann Intern Med* 58 (1963): 627–36.

86. Buffalo had a Comprehensive Planning Council made up of local health care providers and state officials. See "Hospital must prove need to expand," *Buffalo Courier Express* (Feb. 19, 1973), p. 8.

87. H. W. Day, "History of coronary care units," *Am J Cardiol* 30 (September 1972): 405–07. See also by the same author "An intensive coronary care area," *Dis Chest* 44 (1963): 423–27. See also B. Lown et al., "The coronary care unit: New perspectives and directions," *JAMA* 199 (Jan. 16, 1967): 188–98, which describes the model unit at the Peter Bent Brigham Hospital in Boston.

88. For an analysis see H. Waitzkin, "A Marxian interpretation of the growth and development of coronary care technology," *Am J Pub Health* 69 (December 1979): 1260–68.

89. J. Fairman, "Watchful vigilance: Nursing care, technology, and the development of intensive care units," *Nurs Res* 41 (January–February 1992): 56–60.

90. V. Dormer, "Progressive patient care," *Nurs Mirror* 108 (1959): II–IV.

91. See, for example, the editorial by C. A. Sanders, "The coronary-care unit: necessity or luxury?" *N Engl J Med* 288 (Jan. 11, 1973): 101–02. The editorial referred to an article in the same issue by B. S. Bloom and O. L. Peterson, "End results, cost, and productivity of coronary care units," 72–78. Responding to a series of letters, the authors raised the issue of whether it was "ethical to use scarce resources on unproved treatment when the same funds could be used to provide proved treatment or prevention." *N Engl J Med* 288 (Apr. 5, 1973): 740.

92. D. J. Rothman, "The hospital as caretaker: The almshouse past and the intensive care future," *Trans Stud Col Phys Phil* 12 (1990): 163.

93. Ibid., 162.

94. Up to this point, the institution had been run by the religious administrator reporting to the mother superior of the Mercy congregation, together with the directors of nursing and medical education.

95. "Supplies ride the rails at Buffalo-Mercy Hospital," *Mod Hosp* 116 (March 1971): 93–97.

96. For developments in Catholic nursing see K. M. Straub and K. S. Parker, eds., *Continuity in Patient Care: The Role of Nursing*, Washington, DC, Catholic Univ. of America Press, 1966.

97. In December 1968, at a testimonial dinner in her honor, Sister M. Sacred Heart was characterized as having "never lost sight of the fact that patients at hospitals are human beings, not merely numbers on a chart." *Buffalo Evening News* (Dec. 6, 1968), n.p., Hospital Archives.

98. Sr. M. Annunciata had worked as a trained nurse at Mercy Hospital and was appointed assistant director of the Nursing Service in 1966. Without any other administrative experience, she was suddenly thrust into her new supervisory position at a critical time when the new building project needed to be promoted and funding for it secured. She admitted that, at day's end, she would take out her frustrations by playing tennis against a wall in the hospital's subbasement. Interview, November 1994.

99. S. M. Blaes, "Reimbursement problems of Catholic hospitals," *Hosp Progr* 56 (1975): 46–50, 54.

100. E. F. Rosinski, "The community hospital as a center for training and education," *JAMA* 206 (Nov. 25, 1968): 1955–57.

101. John J. O'Brien to Sr. M. Annunciata, Feb. 14, 1975, Hospital Archives.

102. See album of newspaper clippings, Mercy Hospital Library.

103. K. Meyer, "The social movement for change within the Catholic Church," in *Religion and the Social Order: Vatican II and U.S. Catholicism*, ed. H. R. Ebaugh, Greenwich, CT, Jai Press, 1991, vol. 2, pp. 187–201.

104. Yet, there was a strong need among people involved in the most intimate ministries to recapture a sense of sacredness and dignity of service. "Without the desire to serve, there remains a cold theologian, a heartless doctor and scientist and a merciless nurse and technician—practicing a trade. Professionalism is a state of intellectual and moral proficiency which one must earn." J. J. Flanagan, "Patient care," *Hosp Progr* 43 (June 1962): 73–74.

105. M. A. Neal, "American sisters: Organizational and value changes," in *Religion and the Social Order*, vol. 2, pp. 105–21. See also S. B. Armiger, "Mutual expectations of laymen and religious," *Hosp Progr* 47 (April 1966): 75–77, 109–10.

106. J. J. Flanagan, "What is the Catholic hospital apostolate?" *Hosp Progr* 47 (March 1966): 49–51. See also Philip Gleason, *Keeping the Faith: American Catholicism Past and Present*, Notre Dame, IN, Univ. of Notre Dame Press, 1987.

107. Sr. M. Victorine interview, November 1994.

108. See *Mercevents* 17 (January 1974): 4–5. See also K. D. O'Rourke, "Is your health facility Catholic?" *Hosp Progr* 55 (April 1974): 40–44, 66, and W. D. Kenney and C. P. Ceronsky, "Developing Christian values in a Catholic health facility," *Hosp Progr* 55 (October 1974): 32, 36–37.

109. Sr. M. Victorine interview, November 1994.

110. T. F. O'Meara, "Christian ministry and health service," *Hosp Progr* 54 (January 1973): 89–94.

111. C. A. Hangartner, "Implications for nursing education from Vatican II," *Hosp Progr* 47 (October 1966): 63–66, 78.

112. Sr. M. Annunciata, "Philosophy of Mercy Hospital," *Mercevents* 13 (July–August 1970): 2.

113. P. C. Reinert, "The role of religion in management," *Hosp Progr* 48 (September 1967): 59.

114. L. Hoban, "What is the future of the Catholic hospital?" *Hosp Progr* 48 (July 1967): 64–71, 98. See also M. Ewen, "Removing the veil: The liberated American nun," in *Women of Spirit*, ed. R. Ruether and E. McLaughlin, New York, Simon & Schuster, 1979, pp. 255–78.

115. E. D. Pellegrino, "What makes a hospital Catholic?" *Hosp Progr* 47 (November 1966): 67–70.

116. "In every act and service, the Catholic hospital must see its patients as children of God, as heirs to the infirmities of the body—not to be judged but served. . . . Even the benefits of the Christian theology of disease and suffering are too infrequently available. Perfunctory contact with overbusy chaplains will not suffice. . . . To fail in charity is to defect from the prime purpose for the separate existence of the Catholic hospital." Pellegrino, "What makes a hospital Catholic," 70.

117. F. M. Taylor, "A new generation of Catholic hospitals," *Hosp Progr* 47 (June 1966): 80–84.

118. L. Hoban, "Problems facing Catholic hospitals," *Hosp Progr* 48 (July 1967): 64–71, 98.

119. See executive director's report in "1969 CHA convention report," *Hosp Progr* 50 (August 1969): 75. For background information on health policy see D. M. Fox, "The consequences of consensus: American health policy in the twentieth century," *Milbank Q* 64 (1986): 76–99.

120. "We no longer have a self-enclosed Catholic subculture in this country. Religious are no longer confined to cloister. Catholic hospitals are no longer isolated from other related institutions, organizations, and agencies." "1969 CHA convention report," 75.

121. In another address to the CHA in 1969, Edward V. Ellis, associate dean at Penn State University, discussed the challenge faced by many Catholic hospitals located in deteriorating inner city neighborhoods (St. Elsewhere). He suggested that these institutions should be agents of social change by becoming involved with their residents and attempt to meet their needs and expectations. See his article "Changing neighborhoods: The challenge to stay," *Hosp Progr* 51 (January 1970): 39–43.

122. J. Tortorici, "The Catholic hospital: Catalyst in the health crisis," *Hosp Progr* 54 (July 1973): 42–46.

123. "Guidelines on the responsibilities, functions, and selection criteria for boards of trustees" *Hosp Progress* 51 (February 1970): 35–46. See also National Association of Catholic Chaplains, *The Apostolate to the Sick: A Guide for the Catholic Chaplains in Health Care Facilities*, St. Louis, CHA, 1967.

124. "Interview with Sr. M. Maurita," *Hosp Progr* 51 (August 1970): 24–28, and P. Scharper, "The health apostolate: some spiritual dimensions," *Hosp Progr* 52 (September 1971): 72–75.

125. Richard A. McCormick, *Health and Medicine in the Catholic Tradition*, New York, Crossroad, 1984, pp. 8–14, and J. F. Whealon, "Questions and answers on the ethical and religious directives for Catholic hospitals," *Hosp Progr* 52 (October 1971): 70–75.

126. J. M. Comey, "The documents of Vatican II and the Catholic Hospital," *Hosp Progr* 51 (June 1971): 49–51, 56. Also see Sr. M. Maurita, "Strengths and weaknesses of the Catholic health care system," *Hosp Progr* 54 (April 1973): 55–60.

127. McCormick, *Health and Medicine*, pp. 105–23. For a response to Father McCormick's publication see E. F. Diamond, "A physician views the directives, *Hosp Progr*

54 (February 1973): 70–72 and M. B. Dish and W. C. Hunt, "A dialogue on the directives," *Hosp Progr* 54 (March 1973): 46–52.

128. W. J. Burghardt, "Towards a theology of the health apostolate," *Hosp Progr* 52 (September 1971): 66–71.

129. About 30–50% of the patients in CCUs had confirmed myocardial infarction. R. E. Collins, "Guidelines for a small hospital CCU," *Hospitals* 46 (Sept. 1, 1970): 72–74, 188.

130. Gottstine interview, May 1996.

131. L. E. Meltzer and J. R. Kitchell, "The development and status of coronary care," in *Textbook of Coronary Care*, ed. Meltzer and A. J. Dunning, Philadelphia, Charles Press, 1972, pp. 3–25.

132. For a brief summary see R. Mulcahy, "Intensive coronary care: Current status and future prospects," *Cardiovasc Clin* 2 (1971): 87–101. See also J. Willis Hurst et al., eds., *The Heart, Arteries, and Veins*, 3rd ed., New York, McGraw-Hill, 1974, pp. 985–1161.

133. M. Z. Davis, "Socioemotional component of coronary care," *Am J Nurs* 72 (April 1972): 705–09. For a personal account see T. M. Schorr, "The vigil," *Am J Nurs* 75 (February 1975): 235.

134. For an insightful patient experience on entering a CCU see F. Storlie, "Double entendre in a CCU," *Am J Nurs* 74 (April 1974): 666–68, and the literary account in Arnold J. Mandell, *Coming of Middle Age: A Journey*, New York, Summit, 1977.

135. For details see S. L. Roberts, "The patient's adaptation to the coronary care unit," *Nurs Forum* 9 (1970): 57–63.

136. M. Fennal, "Becoming a CCU nurse," *Am J Nurs* 73 (September 1973): 1540–43, and D. J. Rowlands, "Coronary care I. The coronary care unit: Its organization and the nurse," *Nurs Times* 70 (Jan. 3, 1974): 10–13.

137. M. Ferrigan, "New nursing horizon: Cardiac nurse specialist," *Int Nurs Rev* 13 (April 1966): 19–20. For new teaching techniques see M. M. Wiener et al., "Nurse training goes modern," *Hospitals* 45 (Oct. 1, 1971): 74–80.

138. M. Manthey et al., "Primary nursing," *Nurs Forum* IX (1970): 65–84, and J. Fairman, "Watchful vigilance: Nursing care, technology, and the development of intensive care units," *Nurs Res* 41 (1992): 56–60.

139. A study of the qualifications exhibited by coronary care nurses in Western New York is E. R. Kellberg, "Coronary care nurse profile," *Nurs Res* 21 (1972): 30–37. See also A. H. Powell et al., "The cardiac clinical nurse specialist; teaching ideas that work," *Nurs Clin North Am* 8 (December 1973): 723–33.

140. D. Judge, "The new nurse: A sense of duty and destiny," *Mod Healthcare* 2 (October 1974): 21–27, and M. Manthey et al., "Primary nursing, *Nurs Forum* 9 (1970): 65–83. See also M. K. Aydelotte, "Issues of professional nursing: The need for clinical excellence," *Nurs Forum* 7 (1968): 72–86.

141. Eventually, Mercy Hospital surrendered to the prevailing market forces, opening a stress laboratory in 1975 and, soon thereafter, its own cardiac catheterization laboratory. See H. B. Burchell, "Important events in cardiology 1940–1982: A retrospective view," *JAMA* 249 (Mar. 4, 1983): 1197–1200, and J. D. Howell, "The changing face of twentieth-century American cardiology," *Ann Intern Med* 105 (1986): 772–82.

142. Harvey Feigenbaum, *Echocardiography*, Philadelphia, Lea & Febiger, 1972.

143. For details see N. H. Cassem and T. P. Hackett, "Sources of tension for the CCU nurse," *Am J Nurs* 72 (August 1972): 1426–30, and by the same authors "Stress on the nurse and therapist in the intensive-care unit and the coronary-care unit," *Heart Lung* 4 (1975): 252–59.

144. In spite of the fact that this ceremony was now authorized as a routine sacrament,

it frequently increased the patient's anxiety. See T. J. Toohey, "The challenge of the new rite of anointing," *Hosp Progr* 55 (May 1974): 60–63, 88.

145. T. Theorell and P. O. Wester, "The significance of psychological events in a coronary care unit," *Acta Med Scand* 193 (1973): 207–10, and J. J. Lynch et al., "The effects of human contact on cardiac arrhythmia in coronary care patients," *J Nerv Ment Dis* 158 (1974): 88–99. See also G. E. Burch, "Hospital routine and the heart patient," *Am Heart J* 88 (November 1974): 674–75.

146. F. Storlie, "A patient named Mara," *Am J Nurs* 43 (May 1973): 822–23. For another narrative about heart attacks see Max Lerner, *Wrestling with the Angel, a Memoir of My Triumph Over Illness*, New York, Norton, 1990, pp. 120–28.

147. E. A. Reid and E. M. Feeley, "Roommates: To have or have not," *Am J Nurs* 73 (January 1973): 104–07.

148. See R. M. Sezekalla, "Stress reactions of CCU patients to resuscitation procedures on other patients," *Nurs Res* 22 (January–February 1973): 65–69.

149. "Social services, helping care for the 'whole person,' " *Mercevents* 17 (July–August 1974): 4–5.

150. Recent studies have confirmed the deleterious influence of loneliness and isolation before and after heart attacks, emphasizing that love and caring are important factors in survival and rehabilitation. See Norman Cousins, *The Healing Heart*, New York, Avon Books, 1984.

151. For a discussion of patient stories see A. H. Hawkins, "A change of heart: The paradigm of regeneration in medical and religious narrative," *Perspect Biol Med* 33 (1990): 547–59.

152. E. D. Pellegrino, "The Catholic hospital: options for survival," *Hosp Progr* 56 (February 1975): 42. See also C. J. Kauffman, "Preserving a Catholic presence in the U.S. healthcare system," *Health Progr* 71 (August 1990): 35–46.

153. "We cannot allow ourselves to be affected by the uncertainty around us. We have to continue to do our planning, to make our changes, to improve Mercy wherever and whenever we can." Sr. M. Annunciata "A view for 1975," *Mercy Hospital, Buffalo, NY, Annual Report*, 1975.

154. The Mercy group sponsored a clinical pastoral education program to priests, ministers, religious individuals, and lay persons seeking certification as chaplains. See R. E. Wheelock, "CHSLP pastoral care model," *Hosp Progr* 56 (January 1975): 48–52.

155. For details see Orville N. Griese, *Catholic Identity in Health Care: Principles and Practice*, Braintree, MA, Pope John Center, 1987, pp. 461–504. A recent discussion of the Catholic position is M. V. Angrosino, "The Catholic Church and U.S. health care reform," *Med Anthrop Q* 10 (1996): 3–19.

156. This topic is treated in greater detail in Geraldine M. Redican, "Catholic Hospital Systems: History, Development and Policy Implications," Masters in Public Affairs thesis, Univ. of Texas, Austin, May 1981. The slogan comes from an unpublished CHA paper, quoted on p. 104. See also the panel discussion at the symposium "The future model of the Catholic hospital," *Hosp Progr* 55 (October 1974): 42–60.

157. This was especially true for the Emergency Room, increasingly the destination for those without health insurance and physicians. The quotation "When a hospital has empty beds, Medicare and Medicaid patients are better than cold sheets" is attributed to W. Walker, director of Management Information Systems, Catholic Health Association, St. Louis, in November 1980. See Redican, "Catholic Hospital Systems," p. 69.

158. "Mercy Hospital: Deep roots and a strong spirit," *Buffalo Evening News—The Magazine* (Sept. 23, 1979), pp. 4–7. See also R. L. O'Brien and M. J. Haller, "Investor-

owned or non-profit? Issues and implications for academic and ethical values in a Catholic teaching hospital," *N Engl J Med* 313 (July 18, 1985): 198–201.

159. For details see J. D. Miller and S. M. Shortell, "Hospital unionization: A study of the trends," *Hospitals* 43 (1969): 67–73.

160. See S. Kochery, "The non-profit hospital and the union," *Buffalo Law Rev* 9 (1960): 255–73.

161. For a recent example of a nurses' strike see J. Daniel, "Sisters, can you spare a dime?" *The Nation* (July 10, 1995): 54–58.

162. Mercy Hospital, Annual Report for 1973, Hospital Archives.

163. Mercy Hospital was cited in 1983 for noncompliance with the provisions of the Hill-Burton program to provide $200,000 worth of free care for 20 years to poor patients. Instead, the hospital attempted to collect some of its bills from individuals eligible for this program. Moreover, as part of its charitable obligations, Mercy wrote off free care dispensed to sick priests and nuns. See *Buffalo Evening News* (June 30, 1983), p. B 5. On Hill-Burton see H. Perlstadt, "The development of the Hill-Burton legislation: Interests, issues, and compromises," *J Health Soc Policy* 6 (1995): 77–96.

164. "We must constantly ask ourselves: what makes us different?" Sr. Sheila, May 1996. See also E. D. Pellegrino, "Catholic hospitals: Survival without moral compromise," *Health Progr* 66 (May 1985): 42–49.

165. Prezio interview, November 1995. See also the transcript of John J. O' Brien, "History of the Mercy Hospital, Buffalo, NY affiliation with Georgetown University Medical School, Washington, DC, 1951 through 1968," a paper delivered at Mercy Hospital's 25th annual Research Symposium, June 13, 1991, Hospital Archives.

166. Sr. M. Annunciata interview, November 1994.

167. For an excellent discussion see Helen R. Fuchs Ebaugh, *Women in the Vanishing Cloister*, New Brunswick, NJ, Rutgers Univ. Press, vol. 2, pp. 78–93. Also see Kevin D. O'Rourke, *Reasons for Hope: Laity in Catholic Health Care Facilities*, St. Louis, CHA, 1983.

168. Sr. M. Annunciata, "Respect for life," *Mercy Hospital, Buffalo, Annual Report, 1975*. For further discussion of the Catholic hospitals' struggle to retain their religious identity see Sr. Jean K. deBlois, "The Catholic Hospital: An Analysis and Critique of the Theological Rationale for Its Identity and Continued Existence," Ph.D. diss., Catholic Univ. of America, 1987, and Philip S. Keane, *Health Care Reform: A Catholic View*, New York, Paulist Press, 1993.

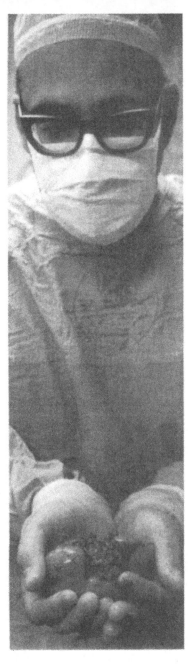

11

HOSPITALS AS BIOMEDICAL SHOWCASES

Academic Health Centers and Organ Transplantation

Transplantation became a very large miracle, perhaps the least anticipated and potentially the most important one in the history of medicine.
Thomas E. Starzl, 1992[1]

Searching for a donor

On September 23, 1984, two women were admitted to the Kidney Transplantation Unit of the University of California at San Francisco (UCSF). Faith T., a 29-year-old clinical dietitian from nearby Fremont, and Nancy P., a 31-year-old nurse from San Jose, were both long-standing diabetics suffering from end-stage renal disease (ESRD), and had been kept alive for the past year by frequent dialysis treatments. Their choice of hospital was easy. In both instances, physicians and dialysis nurses had strongly recommended UCSF, a world leader in renal transplantation and conveniently located nearby. Working in the health-care field, both Faith and Nancy knew about the institution's famous surgeons and state-of-the-art technology. Both suffered from complications of their disease, including high blood pressure and diabetic retinopathy, for which they had already received laser treatments. In early 1984, Nancy had suffered from uremic pericarditis, which was treated with a pericardial window. Unlike Faith, she kept a diary about these experiences and remembered having a very "rocky" dialysis. The periodic sessions left her exhausted, but she remained hopeful: "You have to look at the positive things; that's kind of what I do in life," Nancy recalled.[2]

In 1972, Congress had taken the unprecedented step of extending Medicare coverage to all persons under the age of 65 who suffered from ESRD. Part of a mandated amendment to the Social Security Act, this legislation eliminated all financial obstacles, allowing physicians and surgeons to focus entirely on medical eligibility criteria. Before long, government intervention had created a new service industry, with dialysis and transplantation centers mushrooming nationwide.[3] The shift from family-assisted home care to hospital and clinic dialysis centers dramatically expanded such care. By the end of 1982, 92% of patients on hemodialysis were being treated in a dialysis facility. Only 8% were treated at home, more than half of these by continuous ambulatory peritoneal dialysis. The ESRD program, covering about 5,000 patients at a cost of about $135 million in the early 1970s, rapidly grew by 1981 to 64,000 patients at a cost of $1.4 billion.[4] The legislation also mandated that patients such as Faith and Nancy be better informed about other care options, including transplantation.

Transplantation attracted not only persons with significant organ breakdown who definitely needed replacements, but also a larger number of individuals with partial organ failures who were unwilling to face lifelong medical management. Being relatively young and facing potentially long lives punctuated by dialysis several times a week, both Faith and Nancy had begun to seriously consider the option of renal transplantation in early 1984. One of Faith's older sisters had already died of complications from diabetes in her early thirties. Two decades earlier, juvenile-onset diabetics had not been considered ideal candidates for transplantation because of their fragile vascular state and uncertain metabolic control.

Since its inception in 1964, however, the Transplantation Unit at UCSF had been quite influential in changing this perception among physicians and patients.[5] Still, prospective organ recipients naturally posed the question: would a transplant really work for me? Would it save my life or merely extend my suffering? During their frequent dialysis sessions, Faith and Nancy had encountered nurses who strongly advocated the transplantation procedure, but they also met patients who had submitted to surgery, only to experience the agony of an organ rejection. What should they do? Perhaps the safer course was to continue dialysis. Eventually, both convinced themselves that a kidney transplant, especially if the organ came from a living donor, would offer a good opportunity to return to a more normal life. In 1984, patients with living related grafts had a 92% chance of success during the first year, with 71% retaining a functioning transplanted organ after five years, and about 50% after a decade.[6] Those odds warranted the gamble of surgery. One could always hope that future scientific breakthroughs would provide better drugs to arrest organ rejection.

By the early 1980s, kidney transplants had clearly made the transition from experimental procedure for critically ill individuals to accepted therapy for an expanding number of secondary medical conditions that impaired kidney function, including diabetes. Technical innovations, better immunological screening, and the advent of new immunosuppressants had contributed to this success. However, the specter of organ rejection still created uncertainties. Despite the promises of cyclosporin A, viewed as the new miracle drug in cadaveric transplantation, surgeons still preferred, if possible, living donors related to the recipients. Given the increasing shortage of organs, a new group of biologically unrelated donors—emotionally linked spouses or friends—rapidly joined the pool of donors, provided that their motives were equally "altruistic."[7] Thus, since the early 1960s, organ transplantation had raised a number of ethical, legal, and social issues.[8]

Organ procurement, whether from living related or unrelated and cadaver donors, presented unique problems. Among these was the protection of the health and rights of both recipients and donors.[9] Moral guidelines negotiated by philosophers and the courts were based on the concept of "encouraged voluntarism," whereby rational adults could make arrangements to donate organs voluntarily while alive or after death.[10] Legally sanctioned living wills and donor cards facilitated donation following passage of the Uniform Anatomical Gift Act in 1968.[11] In the case of cadaver organs, advanced patient directories or permission from the next of kin were necessary. Yet potential donors often stopped breathing before death, and their organs were thus permanently damaged by lack of oxygen and failed circulation.[12]

The advent of intensive care units since the late 1950s, however, had created technologies that sustained life in irreversible coma cases in which the brain was completely nonfunctional in a viable organ system.[13] Following recommendations of the Harvard Medical School Ad Hoc Committee to Examine the Definition of Brain Death in 1968, a consensus formed around criteria for what was termed *brain death*, employing clinical and electroencephalographic signs. The legality of such a definition facilitated the procurement of viable cadaver organs for transplantation, especially from accident victims, in whom the heartbeat and circulation were artificially maintained to ensure whole body perfusion prior to organ extraction.[14] But how should the scarce resources of transplantation be distributed?[15] In 1983, a private firm, United Network Organ Sharing (UNOS), became an important source of information for over 130 kidney transplant centers. However, UCSF was not among them, preferring instead to follow its own supply pathways.

Because of the lack of a centralized network of procurement and distribution, kidneys were still sought by individual hospitals and a number of independent organ procurement agencies. In the case of much more scarce hearts and livers, appeals for donors proliferated in the media, and even legislators found themselves involved in such quests. Unlike kidneys, these other organ transplants were still considered experimental, and their cost was not covered by many health insurance companies or the federal government. The questions Who shall live?, Who shall pay?, and Who shall decide? were of paramount concern to ethicists, policy makers, insurers, and the public.[16] As the gap between demand and supply widened in the late 1970s, the question of organ donations for profit was raised.[17] Since we live in a capitalist system, in which everything has its price, why should human organs be exempted? Robin Cook's novel *Coma*, subsequently made into a popular film, raised the specter of illegal organ harvesting by unscrupulous surgeons. Harmful to the medical profession, images of ghouls and cannibals entered the public imagination, a veritable replay of the grave-robbing exploits of yesteryear. In 1983, a would-be kidney broker, International Kidney Exchange, located in Reston, Virginia, asked 7,500 hospitals around the country whether they were interested in buying or selling human kidneys through the company. The organs offered—at a price of $5,000 each—were to be harvested from commissioned donors in the United States and abroad. Although the plan was roundly denounced as immoral and unethical, the specter of a commercial market in human organs remained.[18]

In addition to moral and legal questions, transplant surgeons raised technical issues as well.[19] How viable would these purchased organs be? How well could such potential donors be screened? At UCSF, Juliet Melzer adamantly opposed the sale of organs by living donors in the United States. She preferred healthy, motivated volunteers to give of their free will. Indeed, only altruism could provide proper donor gratification.[20] But could it be that the surgeons' resistance to a trade in organs was also a protective strategy to avoid exposure of the existing commercialization of transplantation surgery itself, including the high costs of procedures and the high income of practitioners?

Indeed, Faith and Nancy needed to ask: who would pay for their kidney transplant? Organ transplantation was viewed as expensive and labor intensive, but the money taboo operating in American medicine traditionally inhibited the intrusion of financial considerations in the choice of particular forms of health care. After surgery, those who had received transplants needed close postoperative monitoring and lifelong treatment with immunosuppressants, another source of medical expenses. Should cost be the deciding factor when evaluating therapy options?[21] One of the salient arguments in the debate centered on the question of whether transplantation was indeed the most cost-effective solution. An average year of dialysis, including physicians' fees, cost about $18,000 per patient, while the kidney transplant cost $37,000 during the first year. If it was successful, however—and the clinical statistics were steadily improving—expenses would decrease thereafter to about $4,000 per year for continuous immunosuppression.[22]

Surgeons repeatedly argued that, in the long term, transplants would cost the

Medicare program much less than lifelong dialysis, an argument that ignored the mortality rates of both procedures and the need for repeated transplants following rejection. More important, eligibility continued to broaden as an increasingly old population began to be afflicted by chronic renal failure secondary to other diseases, especially diabetes.[23] As the results continued to improve, increasing numbers of patients were placed on waiting lists. By 1983, an estimated 70,000 patients were eligible for ESRD benefits, but only 5,358 had received transplants in 1982. The number of patients operated on after age 65 increased 700%, while the number of diabetic patients like Faith and Nancy who qualified for transplants increased 800%.

In a cost-conscious era like the early 1980s, proponents of transplantation argued that it saved lives, alleviated unnecessary suffering, and improved the quality of life of those who submitted to surgery. One of UCSF's surgeons, Oscar Salvatierra, Jr., stressed that America was a compassionate and humanitarian society where nobody could put a dollar figure on life and quality of life. Health was one of our most cherished possessions, and citizens should not be shortchanged when a new technology became available.[24] But did ability to pay enter into the decision making? Who should get a transplant? American women, minorities, and the poor were transplanted at lower rates than more affluent and resourceful citizens.[25] To complicate matters in the early 1980s, a significant number of foreign patients, especially those from the Middle East and South America, came to the United States to receive transplants. In fact, in the Washington, DC, area they comprised nearly 35% of those being grafted. Many of the patients were wealthy and politically well connected; others were sponsored and financed by their own governments. Rumblings about a "green screen," based on the ability to pay in U.S. currency, were heard across the land. A few visitors from abroad came with their own donors in tow, listed as "relatives" (many were poor, coerced, or paid off to volunteer an organ), who had already undergone tissue typing in their country of origin.[26] Given the ethical, political, and economic problems created by such additional demands, discussions concerning the possibility of establishing quotas for foreign visitors ensued. Fortunately, the proliferation of transplantation centers around the world during the 1980s lessened the demand from foreigners.

Fortunately for Faith and Nancy, Medicare paid in 1984 for all medical expenses during the entire month in which the transplant took place and extended this coverage to include two additional months prior to the procedure if hospitalization for preparations became necessary. This eligibility ended 36 months after surgery unless rejection had occurred and dialysis or another transplant was contemplated. Posttransplant services for successful patients included periodic outpatient examinations to monitor for rejection or recurrence of kidney disease. The costs of postoperative therapy, however, were covered for only 60 days, raising the issue of who would pay for the permanent aftercare, especially following the advent of cyclosporin, a very effective but expensive drug. At this point,

Medicare would not pay for the drugs even though surgeons strenuously argued that they increased the success of the transplantation. Thus, in the early 1980s, surgeons were often forced to submit patients to a means test before performing a transplant to determine if the patient could receive the improved but more expensive drug therapy. Poor patients could not always depend on public fundraising campaigns to pay for cyclosporin and keep them alive, but this was not a concern for Faith and Nancy, who had stable, well-paying jobs to go back to if their transplants were successful.

With financial considerations resolved, both women started their search for a live organ donor, beginning with their own families. In 1982, approximately 31% of the 5,358 transplants performed in the United States involved living related donors. Once the subject was raised, Faith and Nancy found very supportive relatives, including healthy siblings willing to allow themselves to be tested for tissue compatibility and, if necessary, to donate a kidney. Faith came from a close-knit Irish family, and while initially hesitant to ask anybody to make such a generous sacrifice, all her siblings were screened after she popped the question. However, family members were concerned enough about the implications of such an organ donation to seek psychological counseling. In the end, the best match was Faith's sister Megan, who promptly agreed to donate one of her kidneys. "Whatever fears they [siblings] must have had about being a potential donor were probably balanced by the fear of losing another family member," recalled Faith.[27]

Nancy later remarked on the awkwardness of asking somebody to donate an organ and the unexpected responses to that request. In her case, both parents and two sisters volunteered immediately to be typed and crossmatched, while her brothers at first refused to submit to such tests. In the end, and probably under considerable family pressure, Nancy's brothers Dan and Jim also agreed to be checked. All the relatives came to San Francisco to be tested in March 1984, and Dan turned out to be the ideal candidate. In California, the Golden State Transplant Services not only matched organs to potential recipients, based on tissue type and blood group, but also prepared waiting lists for liver and heart organs based on medical urgency and distance from the transplant centers. If not placed regionally, some organs were exported to other countries because of the lack of a national registry and logistical problems there. Dan, a busy contractor, expressed the wish to postpone the operation until later in the year. His wife, one of Nancy's best friends from high school, continued to be opposed, fearful that Dan could die during the surgery. Thus, by her own admission, Nancy spent a long, frustrating summer on dialysis because Dan had been unwilling to call UCSF to schedule his appointment for the preliminary surgical workup. Finally, in mid-September, he came to San Francisco after his sister's transplant operation had already been scheduled.

Both experiences reflected gift-exchange issues common to all organ transplantation. As described by philosophers and health professionals, this "gift of life" was embedded in profound emotional and symbolic contexts, leading to the creation of special relationships between organ donors and recipients. Often, relatives of potential recipients were reluctant to comply but considered such requests as compelling family obligations. Others feared disapproval and felt guilty about their ambivalence. Ethicists wondered whether the donors' autonomy was being compromised by their filial duty. The higher number of live female donors and those holding less important jobs suggested that organ donation was often viewed as a natural extension of domestic female obligations.[28] For males like Nancy's brother Dan, on the other hand, the gift of an organ assumed greater importance, since he considered himself a busy and irreplaceable family provider. Finally, there were "black sheep" donors, individuals whose past transgressions made them subject to family disapproval and who consented to the donation as a way to make amends, a form of sacrifice and redemption. On the positive side, many prospective donors were enthusiastic and considered this an act of great altruism, often based on their moral or religious views—a chance to do something worthwhile.

Under the circumstances, transplant practitioners encountered a host of ethical problems in their role as gatekeepers, evaluating the prospective candidates' physical and psychological eligibility for organ donation.[29] Frequently remaining silent about specific reservations, the surgeons simply determined the donors' "total compatibility," a euphemism that disguised potential social and psychological disagreements as medical excuses. Donors who decided to give up an organ spontaneously, even before receiving all the information necessary to give informed consent, were just as troubling as those who hesitated. To further complicate matters, some transplant surgeons may also have felt that the removal of a kidney from a healthy donor constituted a violation of their ethos to do no harm, and they preferred to graft organs obtained only from cadavers. After all, patients such as Faith and Nancy were surviving on dialysis, and their lives were not immediately threatened, unlike individuals with failing hearts and livers. The desire for a better quality of life needed to be balanced with the risks of general anesthesia and major surgery awaiting their siblings.[30]

A third candidate for renal transplantation, Patricia B., a 39-year-old kindergarten teacher from Northern California, was to join Faith and Nancy's pilgrimage to UCSF. She had a history of hypertension after her second pregnancy, with progressive renal failure that had recently required dialysis three times a week. A newcomer to these treatments, Patty had tolerated dialysis poorly, developing severe nausea, vomiting, and a migraine type of headache each time she was subjected to the procedure. The option of a kidney transplant was discussed with her by a physician, and as in the cases of Faith and Nancy, Patty's own Irish family stood firmly behind her when she broached the question of a family donor. "Geographically as well as emotionally, we're a close family. But we never talked about a transplant because they didn't want to say: oh, you are probably going to need one soon," remembered Patty.[31]

After the standard tests, Patty's fraternal twin sister, Kathleen, was found to be the ideal donor. Patty remembered feeling quite guilty about accepting a kidney from a sister. "How do I accept such a big thing?" she mused, a reflection of the indebtedness typically felt by many organ recipients. When she discussed this guilty feeling with her dialysis technician at Kaiser Permanente, the nurse replied that Kathleen, the donor, was a "lucky" individual for having the once-in-a-lifetime opportunity to provide another person with a lifesaving gift. But, as was common with transplant patients, Patty was still left with the psychological and moral burden of indebtedness without opportunities for reciprocity. While clearly an act of self-sacrifice and love among family members, this "tyranny of the gift" caused transplant surgeons to downplay these human dynamics by attempting to reframe organ donation as merely a problem of biology and supply.[32]

Patty also raised the issues of autonomy and control. The uncertainties surrounding her current renal status, together with the complications of dialysis and the possibility of organ rejection, weighed heavily on her. As for others, hospitalization was for Patty a threatening experience, representing a loss of control and the specter of dehumanization. Would the surgeons and nurses focus exclusively on her physical condition?[33] Within the context of a modern American value system that stressed autonomy and self-sufficiency, submission to an assigned sick role was difficult to accept. "I guess the whole thing [transplantation] is one of not being in control. When you are sick and you need an organ, you don't have control."[34]

From teaching hospitals to academic health centers

When the three potential organ recipients came to San Francisco for their transplantation surgery, the UCSF hospitals and clinics operated under the direction of Chief Executive Officer William B. Kerr. The facilities included a general acute-care teaching complex—Moffitt Hospital—with 560 beds, a neuropsychiatric institute with 70 beds, and an ambulatory care center with 20 major clinics and faculty practices together receiving about 200,000 patient visits per year. UCSF's hospitals were well known throughout the world. Recent surveys revealed that only 63% of all hospital patients resided in San Francisco and the greater Bay Area. The rest came from other parts of California, the continental United States, and abroad.[35]

As early as 1900, American medical leaders had stressed the importance of the hospital in medical education and research.[36] Referring to the success of the Johns Hopkins Hospital since the opening of its medical school, professor of pathology William H. Welch remarked in 1907 that "the most valuable asset of a medical school is the possession of an endowed, good general hospital [whose] main purpose is to serve the interests of medical education while serving the best interests of the patients."[37] Welch went on to recommend that such an institution be supplied with clinical and pathological laboratories to carry out the modern scientific activities of diagnosis and treatment. The educator Abraham Flexner also adhered to the Hopkins model in his 1910 report on the state of medical schools in the United States and Canada, recommending that students receive practical training in hospital wards, dispensaries, and clinical laboratories. Unfortunately, few contemporary American hospitals were willing or even capable of assuming such educational and investigative roles. Most were private voluntary organizations or charitable municipal hospitals lacking the necessary facilities and determined to control their own staff appointments. The issue of academic control, however, was paramount for ensuring adequate clinical teaching.[38]

That same year, however, a series of affiliations between medical schools and hospitals in Boston, New York, and St. Louis provided the necessary momentum for further arrangements and the construction of new academic institutions. Whether private or public, many hospitals began to recognize the benefits of acquiring the services of a prestigious, full-time medical staff appointed by the universities, together with the provision of expensive laboratory equipment needed to conduct diagnostic and therapeutic activities based on the latest scientific knowledge.[39] The universities benefited equally from such associations with hospitals, especially the public ones caring for charity patients, since they provided the faculty and students with extended clinical facilities and the necessary teaching material to pursue research and training. To accommodate the needs of their academic partners, many of these teaching hospitals improved and expanded their facilities through generous philanthropic donations, some—like those of the Rockefeller Foundation—earmarked for such educational purposes.[40]

This marriage of convenience, however, did not survive without tensions. As suggested by Flexner's blueprints, university hospitals not only served the needs of medical education, but rapidly became leaders in training interns and residents in the various specialties and subspecialties. Drawbacks for the hospitals included not only the loss of control over their medical staffs, but complete surrender of their institutional objectives to the needs and goals of their academic partners. Not only were routines disrupted by the steady influx of medical students and house staff, but patient selection was increasingly dictated by the research and teaching interests of a rapidly expanding faculty, especially after the Second World War.[41]

Growing medical specialization fostered teaching hospital admissions based on referrals at the expense of community-based general care. Many of the selected patients were research subjects in a number of controlled clinical trials carried out under the supervision of research teams. Funding was a key factor in this development. Federal resources provided under the Hill-Burton Act in the late 1940s, and then research and training grants from the National Institutes of Health in the 1950s and 1960s, provided capital for the construction and renovation of teaching hospitals.[42] This modernization demanded the acquisition of new equipment—

especially complex technology—and additional staffing with specialized personnel. During those two decades, the growth rate of institutional budgets averaged 15–18% per year, while the nation's gross national product expanded by only 5–9%.

When Henry K. Beecher published his influential article on the ethics of clinical research in 1966, he acknowledged the increasing use of patients as experimental subjects since World War II. Beecher explained that this activity had taken place primarily in government, university, and private hospitals, citing a 17-fold increase in annual research expenditures between 1945 and 1965 at the Massachusetts General Hospital and a 624-fold increase at the National Institutes of Health. Indeed, according to Beecher, university hospitals—viewed as the intellectual backbones of the American health care system—were now populated by a new generation of able and entrepreneurial full-time academics trained and supported by federal grants. Relevance was defined by particular lines of investigation and superior grantsmanship. Since their professional identity, prestige, and income were closely linked to their investigative activities at the bench and the bedside, deans, departmental chairs, and professors needed expanded bureaucratic structures to organize their activities.[43]

Such concentration limited involvement with broader social and economic issues. Warnings were issued in the 1960s that this growing indifference to the needs of the American people would have dire consequences and deprive medicine of the support it required. "The medical school must descend from Mt. Olympus and come to grips with the social problems of medicine and face the public and its representatives," declared one leader. A clarion call to become involved in current issues of medical care needed to be reflected in the medical curriculum, with the addition of courses in sociology, economics, and history. Medical school graduates were ill prepared to understand the political and social forces that defined the medical profession and guided its future. "Medicine must help to shape its own destiny. The option will be removed if it ignores its social responsibility. A sound relationship based on mutual understanding between teaching hospital and medical school can only serve to strengthen the work of both."[44]

Driven by the advances of biomedicine and by efforts to market the new knowledge at the bedside, university hospitals in the mid-1960s expanded the scope of their specialized diagnostic and therapeutic facilities through a mixture of federal and private funding. Although construction funds dwindled, capitation and research grants continued to flow, increasingly supplemented in the 1970s by generous reimbursements for care rendered to Medicare and Medicaid patients, as well as payments from private insurance companies. Instead of looking beyond their institutional walls to communities, university hospitals now increased even more the range and complexity of their health care facilities through the creation of specialized services. Units were opened for the management of cancer, coronary and intensive care, cardiac catheterization, trauma and microvascular surgery, diagnostic imaging, neonatal nurseries, neurosurgery, and organ transplantation. Less ill patients were shunted to ambulatory facilities. Instead of becoming involved in the solution of community social problems, university hospitals retained their position as flagships of prestigious academic medical centers located in the most important urban centers of America.[45]

Meanwhile, in the quest to conduct more biomedical research, medical education and graduate training in hospitals had taken a back seat. If they were not too busy in their laboratories, faculty members traveled extensively, presenting or discussing papers at meetings, screening grant applications at national panels, or consulting with pharmaceutical companies or other medical centers. Battered by bloated basic science curricula, medical students, mostly guided by residents, were now increasingly exposed to a selected population of patients suffering from esoteric and degenerative diseases, who were aggressively treated and often prevented from dying with the help of sophisticated medical technologies. Thus, future physicians learned to value and eventually to implement this narrow hospital-centered paradigm that promised professional prestige and more than adequate income.[46]

The house staff, in turn, traditionally employed as cheap labor, saw their specialty training period extended by several years. Because of the complexity and severity of illnesses being treated in academic hospitals, this work demanded greater knowledge and responsibility. Men and women in training, moreover, were selected on the basis of their academic skills, not their caring qualities. Faced with the intensity of the institutional routines and peer competition, all they wanted was to survive their ordeal. Instead of the expected rewards, hostility toward patients and strategies to avoid their demands became widespread among harried and dehumanized residents and interns.[47] Stress, frustration, and cynicism frequently boiled over, leading to protests and eventually legislation to curb some of the most grueling working schedules.[48]

By the late 1970s academic medical centers began to experience problems that seemed to threaten their hitherto spectacular development.[49] No longer desirable, capitation payments linked to increases in student enrollment became extinct. Federal research grants, diminished by inflation, were more narrowly directed, more competitive, and aimed at securing clinical applications, thus allowing less cost shifting to educational activities and causing a loss of institutional overhead. Since the academic centers had turned to clinical income as a compensatory device to expand and finance their operations, increasing indifference to the cost implications of their unique mission was troubling.[50] In spite of such difficulties, university hospitals still retained their dominant position as showcases of American biomedical achievement, especially in the area of what experts called the "technologies of failure" such as coronary bypass surgery and organ transplantation. As Faith, Nancy, and Patty expected, the goal was to cure or intervene in irreversible disease processes, thus prolonging life. In the latter instance, the exclusive emphasis on the biomedical aspects of disease required dying patients to undergo "multispecialty preterminal consultations."[51]

In 1983, Medicare was altered by the passage of legislation critical to all hospitals, but especially those affiliated with academic centers. Instead of relying on the hospitals to inform them of the costs of medical procedures, the federal government now established fixed payment rates for these services. Henceforth a number of "diagnosis-related groups" (DRGs), with their individual price tags for the care of specific medical conditions, were to guide reimbursement.[52] Teaching institutions such as UCSF now became vulnerable to competitive bidding that would fail to compensate Moffitt Hospital for its unique patient case mix and severity of illness, both dictated in part by academic research and educational programs. Moreover, all payers, government and commercial carriers alike, initiated programs to limit hospitalization through prior authorization, admission procedures, and concurrent review. These measures were all designed to cut costs by reducing the length of stay. In turn, prospective payment services were expected to force university hospitals to monitor physician performance, thereby reducing their scholarly activities, including research. To offset some of these financial strictures, university hospitals were expected to identify a number of profitable "product lines," among them organ transplantation.[53]

California's state assembly passed legislation in June 1982 to curtail the costs of the state's Medi-Cal (Medicaid) program, legislation that had an immediate negative impact on UCSF's hospital operations. The Reagan administration had begun shifting resources from social programs to the military, including a reduction of federal matching funds for Medicaid. Faced with a severe budget deficit and soaring expenditures, California enacted a law that allowed for selective contracting with hospitals for inpatient care to be provided to qualified recipients. The basis for awarding such contracts was no longer the traditional cost-based and fee-for-service system, but a competitive one designed to foster a price war between the various qualified institutions.[54]

As of January 1, 1983, California had also transferred the financial and administrative responsibility for medically indigent adults to its counties, thus forcing the larger ones to run their own programs and provide inpatient and outpatient services through county-owned facilities.[55] These measures resulted in an unprecedented loss of patient volume at UCSF, since prior to the county transfer, medically indigent adults still made up 7% of the Medical Center's outpatients and 5% of Moffitt's inpatients. To compensate for these losses, UCSF negotiated with the County of San Francisco to provide limited tertiary care services not currently available at San Francisco General Hospital. In spite of this stopgap measure, however, Moffitt Hospital's occupancy rate went from 77.6% the previous year to 69.5%.

The new state legislation also substantially reduced the benefits for the remaining Medi-Cal population, including restrictions on outpatient services and elective procedures. Moreover, in spite of bidding for inpatient care, UCSF was denied a Medi-Cal contract effective February 1983 and forced to transfer patients to other facilities. In early 1983, the monthly census fell by at least 10% in 14 of the 26 clinical services. Patient days declined by more than 10%. To survive and prosper in a contracting environment, UCSF and other centers were urged to develop cooperative contracting strategies and prepare for substantial price concessions.

Finally, the 1983–1984 report of the UCSF Hospitals and Clinics admitted that the institution was currently facing the most fundamental changes in health care delivery since the inception of Medicare and Medicaid. In the past, academic centers had competed successfully on the basis of the broad array of specialized services offered, the quality of care provided, and the state-of-the-art technology of their physical facilities. Escalating expenses and fees—used by hospitals to plug the deficits they were incurring for treating the uninsured poor—had been paid routinely by the government and the private health insurance sector, with the additional costs passed on in the form of premium hikes to employers and employees. However, the new reimbursement schemes adopted by Medicare, Medi-Cal, Blue Cross, and commercial insurance carriers focused on price competition, profoundly altering a way of life that had been structured by the federal government's entry into health care finance. At the same time, academic centers such as UCSF were also challenged by growing health maintenance organizations and new provider networks as business and industry refused to go along with further increases in health insurance premiums that would allow university hospitals to continue their cost shifting of underreimbursed or uncompensated care. For the fiscal year 1984–1985, therefore, UCSF prepared itself to face the necessity of living within a relatively fixed income. Other voluntary hospitals were not so lucky, and a wave of mergers and closings ensued.[56]

Speaking to UCSF's board of overseers in October 1983, one noted health economist concurred that the love affair between the American public and medicine, born after World War II, was over. During the previous decades, expenditures for health care had increased eightfold, medical personnel had doubled, and hospitals had been transformed into a $140-billion-a-year industry. Fed by federal pipelines and clever cost shifting, medical schools and academic health centers had flourished, financing research to expand the frontiers of knowledge, fostering further technological innovations, and producing too many new graduates. Although UCSF's hospitals, with an affluent community base and a small indigent population, were part of a leading American institution, they nevertheless seemed destined to join other members of this threatened species, namely, the municipal and community hospitals, in their fight for survival. With shrinking operating funds and long-term financial underpinnings in jeopardy, academic centers such as UCSF were urged to rethink their academic and assistential mission.[57]

As our trio of prospective kidney recipients and their potential donors pondered the personal issues of organ transplantation in 1984, alarming reports about the impending sale of McLean Hospital, one of Harvard's teaching institutions, to a for-profit corporation exposed the increasing economic woes afflicting academic hospitals. Limited reimbursement from Medicare and Medicaid had been combined with a freeze on rates. At the same time, labor and equipment costs continued to rise, affecting especially the oldest teaching institutions in need of greater capital improvements. The purchase offer from the Hospital Corporation of America was eventually rejected, based primarily on what one academic committee represented as a set of values whereby "the operation of hospitals, and particularly teaching hospitals, should not be influenced by the motivation for profit."[58] A year later, a financial analysis questioned whether teaching hospitals would become an endangered species if efforts to curb their budgets continued. The traditional practice of shifting the cost of educational programs to income derived from patients and their insurers seemed to be in jeopardy.[59]

Quest for excellence: Moffitt Hospital and UCSF

Once admitted to UCSF's Moffitt Hospital, the mood of incoming patients such as Faith, Nancy, and Patty fluctuated between fear and optimism. The Kidney Transplantation Unit, located on the 14th floor, housed 16–20 patients, distributed among four wards with four beds each and two additional semiprivate rooms. The entire floor, shared with the Obstetrics/Gynecology and Urology services, had only four public toilets and three shower/baths for close to 60 patients. When she reached the floor, Nancy's first impression was decidedly negative: "When I first went in, I thought, well, it's kind of old." After completing some formalities, she was led to a four-bed arrangement: "In a ward? I haven't seen these for a while, and oh, there is not even a bathroom in the room." Patty was less shocked since she had already visited the antiquated facilities two weeks earlier when her sister was being tested. "Oh my goodness, there are four to a room!" she remembered thinking. "Oh, there isn't even a bathroom for those four. It is in the hallway! I was amazed because I've been in hospitals with double and private rooms. Gee, this is really old!" The paradox of coming to the leading transplantation service in the world and seeing it housed in crowded, spartan facilities reminiscent of pre–World War II institutions did not fail to impress the newcomers unfavorably.

Since its inception in 1864, the University of California (UC) Medical Center had played a leading role in California medicine. Despite its modest proprietary beginnings, forged in the rough-and-tumble of San Francisco's gold rush with greedy adventurers, tubercular and scorbutic miners, and syphilitic prostitutes, the Toland Medical College had created an excellent teaching center that attracted a cadre of gifted students. Some of its French-trained surgeons, including Hugh H. Toland (1806–1880) himself, brought to their enterprise the tenets of the Paris clinical school: less emphasis on theoretical facts, textbook learning, and memorization and more on bedside observation.[60] If Toland had established his school in part to legitimize his own professional status, tarnished by petty local disputes, rivalries, and greed, his progressive educational plans were meant to transform students into active observers of the sick through a linkage with the newly created San Francisco City and County Hospital. The subsequent climb toward academic legitimacy included an affiliation with the University of California in 1873. A move in 1898 from its original location in North Beach brought the school to its current site on the lower slope of Mount Sutro, located in the windswept Sunset district of San Francisco south of Golden Gate Park.[61]

The next 20 years witnessed the birth of scientific medicine at the new Parnassus Avenue address, an era in American medicine strongly influenced by German laboratory medicine. No longer in close proximity to San Francisco's municipal hospital, the school sought to establish its own clinical facilities following the successful model of Johns Hopkins and other leading universities. To make room for such an urgently needed hospital, the Medical Department in 1906 finally shifted the departments of anatomy, physiology, and pathology to the Berkeley campus under the deanship of Arnold D'Ancona (1860–1928).[62] Years later, the UC Medical Department sought to consolidate its position in San Francisco by establishing additional clinical affiliations with the San Francisco General Hospital and Presidio Hospital. Meanwhile, Dean Herbert C. Moffitt (1867–1951) laid plans to build a new hospital at the west end of the Parnassus site, precisely when suggestions were made to move the entire medical campus across the Bay to Berkeley. Although delayed by the onset of World War I, the new pavilion-type 225-bed University of California Hospital finally opened in 1917.[63]

In the 1930s, the Medical Department finally consolidated its precarious toehold on Sutro hill and began an extended period of educational reform under the leadership of deans Robert Langley Porter (1870–1965) and Francis E. Smyth (1895–1972). During this time, the UC Hospital was already too small to serve the educational and service needs of the institution. Larger medical school enrollments and a broader range of specialized services demanded a second acute-care facility. Planning for an additional 450-bed hospital was aided by a $2 million bond issue approved in 1940 by Governor Earl Warren. Moreover, all medical school departments were to be reunited at one location in San Francisco. World War II delayed these projects. However, in 1947 the Berkeley faculty made another effort to extract the Medical Center from San Francisco, a proposal soundly defeated by the San Francisco faculty. That same year, an Office of Architects and Engineers became responsible for developing a master plan that included the new hospital. In 1949, the university regents officially designated the campus as the UC Medical Center, San Francisco.

By the early 1950s, then, the medical center's consolidation finally seemed underway. To furnish enough space on the Parnassus site for the returning basic sciences departments, construction of a Medical Sciences Building to house classrooms and research and teaching laboratories began. The new university hospital, named after the former dean, was to be linked functionally to these facilities at every floor. This arrangement epitomized the new bench-to-bedside creed that sought to apply the newest discoveries of biomedical research to the clinical management of patients. For better or worse, the decision to allocate funds for the construction of this hospital definitively committed the University of California to a separate branch on the San Francisco site.

Designed by Timothy and Milton Pflueger, the cross-shaped, 485-bed high-rise Moffitt Hospital, with its steel frame and concrete exterior—designed to withstand a nuclear attack—slowly took shape amid construction delays. Each of the original 12 floors was devoted to a particular medical specialty. The original patient units were small, not exceeding 30 beds, arranged in typical pre–World War II style with four- and six-bed wards. At the time of its official opening on March 18, 1955, Moffitt Hospital was already deemed obsolete by experts in hospital design. At its dedication, the hospital was nevertheless hailed as "the nucleus of one of the world's foremost medical teaching facilities . . . an integration of the medical school's basic science with their related clinical departments."[64]

By June 14, 1955, 240 patients on gurneys and in wheelchairs were moved from the old University Hospital to the new facility. Surgery occupied an entire floor with a sweeping 10-room operating pavilion, wired for closed-circuit broadcasting and television reception. One floor housed the beds and laboratories of the Cancer Research Institute, another the X-ray facilities, including 22 cubicles placed around a darkroom. The lead-lined rooms shielded the facility from the radioactivity used in the treatments for cancer. Finally, four floors were assigned to the College of Pharmacy and three to the School of Dentistry; the Nursing School received only one. The inaugural brochure had mentioned that "a feature that will bring joy to patients admitted early in May will be a two-way communication system between nurses and patients."[65] Moffitt's four-bed patient rooms were air conditioned and provided with oxygen and vacuum outlets built into the walls.

In the meantime, construction of the 13th floor continued. Completed in June 1957, it housed the new Cardiovascular Research Institute. This entity was to comprise 26 laboratories and research areas together with four units containing a total of 16 beds. A diverse group of medical investigators under the direction of the newly appointed physiologist Julius H. Comroe, Jr., began its interdisciplinary work on cardiac, pulmonary, and vascular diseases. Then, after more than half a century of separation, the basic science departments of anatomy, physiology, and biochemistry returned to the Parnassus campus from Berkeley. A 14-story addition to the Medical Science Building, completed a year earlier, provided additional space for teaching, research, and a medical library. A year later, the Cardiovascular Research Institute with its 22 separate research laboratories opened its facilities in Moffitt Hospital, a joint venture between the university and the National

Institutes of Health. Other units followed in quick succession: an International Center for Medical Research and Training (1960) and a Hormone Research Laboratory (1967).

The year 1958 also represented another milestone: the campus became a separate administrative and academic unit in the UC system with its own provost, who was promoted to chancellor in 1964. Perhaps even more important, 1958 signaled the beginning of UCSF's most extraordinary phase: the expansion of biomedical research, which in less than two decades placed the institution on par with top academic medical centers in the United States and abroad. Upon its final completion in 1965, Moffitt Hospital was considered the largest and most costly (over $24 million) modern teaching hospital in the western United States. UCSF had become a regional center expected to provide specialized, high-quality care. Among Moffitt Hospital's jewels were the Neurological Center, including the Brain Tumor Research Center, Orthopedic Surgery, a national leader in hip and knee replacements; the Intensive Care Nursery featuring treatment of hyaline membrane disease; and specialized pediatric services in cancer, diabetes, heart disease, gastroenterology, and immunology. Finally, there was the Transplantation Service, one of the largest in the world. But further modernization was already an urgent priority; inadequate size and design promised functional obsolescence, and the facilities were no longer in compliance with contemporary state health and safety codes. An official report indicated that the hospital was "almost totally lacking in proper patient amenities,"[66] a judgment that preceded by nearly 20 years the comments made by Nancy and Patty on their arrival. A capital improvement program suggested additional modern facilities for another 200 beds.

Responding to perceived academic and health service needs, UCSF's long-range plans by 1965 included the purchase of several city blocks extending to the southern edge of Golden Gate Park, with conversion of some residences into additional offices and clinics. In response, neighborhood opposition grew. Academic centers nationwide, many located in decaying urban neighborhoods, were increasingly condemned for employing deceptively expedient methods in procuring real estate to remodel and expand facilities without considering their impact on adjacent neighborhoods and infrastructure. Like other American academic health centers, UCSF had not directly served the needs of its immediate community. Moreover, many professional and clerical staff members lived elsewhere, commuting daily to the academic ghetto in private cars and special buses.

The early 1970s introduced new elements into the planning process. The old UC Hospital was found to be seismically unsafe and slated for closure, even demolition. Unfortunately, the original 1898 campus had been laid out on the fog-shrouded north slope of Mount Sutro, comprising three separate low-rise buildings arranged in U-shaped fashion, with their axes perpendicular to Parnassus Avenue. Subsequent additions had contributed to an unbroken wall of buildings, further extended in the 1950s by the Medical Sciences Unit and Moffitt Hospital. With the construction of the new outpatient facility on the other side of the street, however, high-rise buildings now crowded both sides of the Parnassus shelf, making it not only a very congested artery, but also a wind tunnel for the cold westerly breezes blowing from the ocean.

The planned closing of the old UC Hospital demanded that Moffit be re-modelled and that an additional wing be constructed.[67] As they pondered the ex-pansion and remodeling projects, the local architects working with UCSF plan-ners considered environmental concerns and trends in urban aesthetics. They tried to soften and humanize the impact of this Manhattan-style high-rise complex, starkly visible for miles on its rocky perch. At the same time, they supported a philosophy of openness and tried to foster the campus–community cooperation lacking during prior projects.[68] Thus, the UCSF plans for the further expansion took shape amid public hearings and environmental impact studies. However, fear-ing a further deterioration of the residential areas surrounding UCSF, adjacent neighborhood organizations expressed strong opposition. Their new determina-tion to protect the real estate value and residential quality of the neighborhoods confronted the space-hungry university and threatened its efforts to retain a pre-eminent position in biomedical research and specialized medical care. In the face of bitter resistance from community activists, as well as city and state officials, the UC Board of Regents was forced in October 1976 to approve a compromise Long Range Development Plan (LRDP). The university agreed to limit its campus boundaries, a restriction that would both slow down the Moffitt expansion and further crowd the campus.[69]

In 1972, the State of California had passed a Health Sciences Bond Issue and earmarked $28.4 million for the remodeling project. Following the 1976 agree-ment, Chancellor Francis A. Sooy (1915–1986) announced the modernization and extension program, including the construction of a 15-floor hospital wing to be functionally integrated with the existing facilities at Moffit.[70] In the end, Moffitt's modernization program was hailed as a critical phase in the development of UCSF's Medical Center. In view of the momentous scientific and technological developments over the past two decades, the hospital had to redesign its space to accommodate new diagnostic and treatment facilities. Patient and caregiver com-plaints about the poor conditions for care and recovery in the existing patient rooms and nursing units prompted extensive remodeling. A new emergency room, waiting rooms, and supply areas were also added.[71]

Given a shortage of public funds, private money was sought to complete the project. The new 15-floor hospital wing, named the Joseph M. Long Hospital in honor of its donor, was officially dedicated on October 1, 1983. More than 15 years of planning and construction had created a general acute-care teaching hos-pital complex totaling 560 beds, together with an ambulatory care facility. At the opening ceremony, Chancellor Julius Krevans reiterated the ideal that "the uni-versity teaching hospital shares with other hospitals a concern for the patient who is in the hospital today." In his speech, Roger Boles, chief of the clinical staff, was more accurate in his assessment of UCSF's mission: the provision of highly specialized, technologically intensive "cutting edge" tertiary care based on up-to-date scientific knowledge. "We strive," said Boles, "to bring to our patients the most modern and sophisticated advances in medicine and surgery from our research laboratories and similar facilities around the world."[72]

Renal transplantation:
Scientific, clinical, and professional contours

Even before admission to Moffitt Hospital, new patients such as Faith, Nancy, and Patty were already paired with members of UCSF's Transplantation Service. Talking to the surgeons was deemed critically important. Further information for the patients was provided in the outpatient clinic by a clinical coordinator, Gloria Horns, in spite of the fact that at this time, most incoming patients were sick and tired from dialysis and therefore not in the best frame of mind to listen. Horns herself had designed some educational materials for the patients and their families, and the staff used preoperative dialysis sessions at various Bay Area centers to teach patients about transplantation. The aim was to ensure that all candidates would feel somewhat comfortable with their impending surgery.[73]

The intent of these educational efforts was to minimize patient bewilderment and anxiety about their therapeutic choice. As in other areas of medicine, uninformed patients could easily be deceived about the validity of unproven therapeutic claims. To avoid this, a Kidney Transplant Dialysis Association had been established, made up of transplant and dialysis patients and their families. Started in New England but now national in scope, this all-volunteer group was dedicated to helping other kidney disease patients cope with the potential psychological, financial, and social problems linked to their condition. The organization placed special emphasis on individual contact between patients, helping prospective transplant candidates to overcome some of their fears and anxieties. A patient manual describing the medical, financial, and emotional aspects of kidney disease and its management was an important step in the educational process.[74]

The modern era of transplantation had begun in the 1950s with a transfer of nonregenerating vital organs.[75] While this was a period of scientific and technical successes, its also created a number of new moral and social problems. The first experimental kidney transplant was performed in 1951 by David Hume in Boston, using a cadaver donor. For the next four years, both Hume and another surgeon, Joseph Murray, continued this procedure, but most patients died shortly after surgery.[76] On December 23, 1954, however, Murray and nephrologist John Merrill successfully carried out the world's first living donor transplant using a kidney from the patient's identical twin. Given this perfect tissue match, the operation, which took place in Boston at the Peter Bent Brigham Hospital, was successful.[77]

Because of tissue rejection, early kidney transplants from live donors were generally restricted to twins or close relatives, but still the issue of immunosuppression had to be considered. The first attempts to halt the immunological destruction of transplanted organ were made out in Paris and Boston between 1959 and 1962, involving total body radiation. In 1959, Murray transplanted a kidney from a fraternal twin recipient who had been exposed to such radiation, but several additional transplant patients died, mostly of secondary infection. Working with transplants from blood relatives, Jean Hamburger, in Paris in 1960, used a combination of radiation and steroids to treat the recipients successfully.[78]

Further success and a return to the option of using unmatched cadaver organs was made possible by the use of the new immunosuppressant drug azathioprine (Imuran), introduced in 1961. Imuran inhibits the metabolism and multiplication of cells, especially lymphocytes. At this point, Rene Küss introduced the concept of "cocktail" or multiple-agent therapy to delay rejection, using a combination of 6-mercaptopurine and Imuran. Joint Imuran and prednisone treatments followed a year later. With the use of live, related donors and combined immunosuppression, the practice of transplantation was to advance rapidly. However, it would still be fair to characterize kidney transplantation in the early 1960s as experimental, carried out by a small group of surgeons.[79]

In March 1962, another pioneer, Dr. Thomas E. Starzl, performed the first human kidney transplant at the University of Colorado Medical Center, again with an identical twin as the donor. By November of that year, he had successfully employed a combination of radiation and a cocktail of Imuran and prednisone to delay rejection in patients receiving homografts from living, related family members. Starzl's approach was considered a major breakthrough, although pessimism persisted about the long-term function and survival of the grafted kidneys, especially during the early weeks after a successful transplant before the body adapted to the graft.

The immunological processes responsible for rejection continued to be viewed as powerful and relentless, a subject of much discussion and speculation during the ensuing decades.[80] *Time* magazine's cover story on May 3, 1963, about surgical advances since World War II included the practices of organ transplantation, informing the public about its gradual ascent as a subspecialty. Starzl published an influential paper in October 1963 recommending that transplantation become another routine clinical service. Murray proposed the creation of a worldwide kidney transplant registry to be based in Boston. Amid professional euphoria and increased public expectations, the "gold rush" in kidney transplantation began around the mid-1960s, with 25 new programs created in the United States.[81]

Not surprisingly, this period of great optimism in the transplantation field led to the founding in 1964 of a journal, *Transplantation*, another indicator of professional development. Although heavily dependent on the availability of live donors, the number of procedures rose sharply. Improvements in dialysis allowed better preparation of patients for transplantation. Another major contribution to clinical transplantation was the use of antilymphoblast globulin (ALG) to prevent tissue rejection, introduced by the transplant surgeon John Najarian from UCSF. From the beginning, the use of family donors (25% of all transplants) created a biological advantage over cadaver allografts. Since cadaver kidneys were usually removed from donors who had died from cardiac arrest, they were exposed to a critical period of ischemia (lack of blood circulation) that could render them unsuitable. Better methods of retrieval and preservation were necessary. Working on this problem, Najarian's UCSF colleague, Folkert O. Belzer, achieved a dramatic improvement in cadaver kidney transplants after recognizing the presence of an agonal vasospasm in the main renal artery and main intrarenal branches mediated by the release of catecholamines from the adrenal glands. Pretreatment of potential kidney donors with a bilateral adrenalectomy before their deaths eliminated this problem. It appeared that cadaver transplants could now be performed electively instead of on an emergency basis.[82]

Moreover, Belzer discovered a method of rapidly freezing and thawing organs that caused unstable lipoproteins to precipitate in the plasma. The removal of these lipoproteins enhanced the preservation of organs through plasma perfusion. In August 1967, Belzer tested his new preservation method in a clinical situation, transplanting a cadaver kidney 17 hours after obtaining the organ. Following this landmark case, hypothermic perfusion became a reality. Using a portable machine, Belzer's team made the rounds of local hospitals in pursuit of donated cadaver kidneys. In the absence of regional or national organ banks or networks, procurement became highly competitive, with transplant surgeons or their representatives battling each other at the bedside of potential donors. In the meantime, publicity surrounding spectacular heart transplants reached an early peak, sensitizing the public to the possibilities of organ replacement.[83]

Later, during the 1970s, the fledgling field of renal transplantation went through a period of consolidation, with some improvements observed in data collection and tissue typing, as well as better sharing of information about organ procurement among institutions. At this point, there were three requirements for a standard academic transplantation program. First, centers needed to integrate surgical and medical disciplines, with a need for clinical subspecialties such as nephrology and immunology and the availability of complex diagnostic and therapeutic facilities. Second, they had to sponsor an active research program focused on organ preservation issues, the testing of histocompatibility, and the physiopathology of organ rejection. Here an alliance of basic scientists, surgeons, and internists was critical. The third requirement was a census of transplanted patients for clinical research and teaching purposes. Not surprisingly, all three conditions could best be met in academic medical centers.

Transplant surgeons decided to establish their own professional society with support from the "big shooters," leaders in the burgeoning field, including Thomas Starzl, Mel Williams, and Folkert Belzer. The first regular annual meeting took place in Chicago on May 23, 1975.[84] The new American Society of Transplant Surgeons (ASTS) had 180 charter members, who elected Starzl as their first president. Instead of openly becoming a political lobbying organization for transplantation issues, the membership depicted ASTS as a scientific group organized to support research and educate the public about issues surrounding transplantation. The Society also established a new journal to publish the results of investigations conducted by members. An educational committee coordinated the Society's input into a national educational campaign, a professional strategy that soon allowed ASTS to become involved with various federal agencies and congressional committees.[85]

The Society also attempted to provide guidelines for clinical investigation. Researchers were told to follow closely the principles established in the Belmont Report, a document prepared by the National Commission for the Protection of Human Subjects of Biomedical and Behavioral Research in July 1974.[86] The new policies protected patients' rights and insisted on informed consent, forcing researchers to disclose the potential risks and benefits of their clinical studies. Selection of subjects for randomized trials was also suggested as a final step toward drug certification. Not surprisingly, a basic clash of ideologies and objectives between independent clinical researchers and the new federally mandated Institutional Review Boards ensued. Starzl and other transplant surgeons resented what they characterized as the creation of a bureaucratic, governmental watchdog capable of questioning their clinical decisions and interfering with patient selection. Insistence on randomized trials as instruments of discovery had, in Starzl's words, become "trialomania."[87]

Soon, as other organs became transplantable, the ASTS broadened its scope. To make transplantation a prestigious surgical subspecialty independent of the American Board of Medical Specialists, ASTS's early leadership concerned itself with professional credentials and the requirements of formal education and training. This was particularly important during the presidency in 1977–1978 of John Najarian, who, after leaving UCSF, had established a training program at the University of Minnesota. Najarian called for the development of more such programs and the accreditation of transplant fellowships. He also invited basic scientists in genetics and immunology to address Society members, a move that cemented the cooperation between basic scientists, nephrologists, and surgeons. Over the next decades, Najarian's measures ensured the successful development of the field, characterized by very high incomes and professional power.[88]

Physicians and ethicists, meanwhile, debated the question of dialysis versus transplantation. Which procedure provided the best chance for survival? With the introduction of reliable vascular access through the creation of a radiocephalic arteriovenous fistula in the arm, as well as the less commonly employed method of peritoneal washings, maintenance hemodialysis had become available in the 1960s. Nevertheless, as better-preserved cadaver organs, adequate tissue matching, and less toxic drugs to prevent rejection appeared, transplantation became the preferred method of managing ESRD. It was argued that dialysis was merely a temporary bandage; by contrast, transplantation was hailed as a permanent "cure." The former condemned patients to fluctuating levels of activity and well-being, disrupted jobs and living routines, and required frequent trips to a dialysis center.

Transplantation was, hopefully, a single surgical event, followed by sustained, almost total recovery and less cumbersome lifelong monitoring. Despite more favorable survival statistics, however, the hazards of prolonged immunosuppression still posed significant risks, as did the appearance of new diseases in the transplanted population, including cancers, especially lymphomas (32 times more prevalent in transplant patients than in the general population), especially the reticulum-cell sarcoma variety. Other complications included redistribution of body fat, stretching and thinning of abdominal skin, cataracts, bone decalcification, peripheral neuropathy, and diabetes. Moreover, transplant patients were more susceptible to bacterial and viral infections such as hepatitis B that assumed epidemic proportions at transplant centers worldwide during the 1960s, with many deaths also reported among the health-care personnel who treated transplant patients.[89] Noncompliance with the antisuppressant regimen spelled disaster and prompt organ rejection. As soon as physicians learned more about the long-term effects of transplantation, debates concerning the quality of life for the postoperative patient began in earnest. Some transplanted patients found themselves caught between two risky alternatives, although there was always the option of returning to dialysis. In spite of the risks, 38,650 kidney transplants were performed between 1973 and 1982. Indeed, by the end of 1982, about 16,000 people already lived with functioning grafts.

But who should receive transplants? Initially, lack of standard patient selection protocols hampered this decision. What was the true incidence of renal failure in a community? Based on patient enrollments reported to the End-Stage Renal Disease Medical Information System, those suffering from terminal renal failure constituted about 100 per 1,000,000 population, with about 25% of those suffering from diabetes. In the United States alone, nearly 82,000 patients were enrolled in this program by 1983. As of December 31, 1982, there were 65,765 dialysis patients, of whom 6,700 held places on a transplant waiting list. Criteria for all potential recipients included an age range between 10 and 55 (for Medicare benefits), clinical stability of their renal condition, and lack of a secondary medical condition. Donors, in turn, were screened for age between 2 and 65 years, general health prior to terminal hospitalization, absence of infection and cancer, circumstances of death, and renal status before death.

After the issue of potential organ availability was settled for patients such as Faith, Nancy, and Patty, the next step was to ascertain whether the donor's organ was genetically compatible with the recipient to minimize bodily rejection. Tissue matching had been instituted in 1964, creating a new cottage industry for clinical tissue typing based on the new field of histocompatibility. Questions were raised about the quality of the antigen match and the clinical outcome. How could the antigens in donor cells be detected? One way was to examine circulating lymphocytes in the blood of both donors and recipients. The tests employed to determine tissue adequacy included blood type and human leukocyte antigen (HLA) tissue type compatibility. The Nobel Prize winner Sir Peter Medawar (1915–1987) had confidently predicted in the 1960s that the next advance in transplantation would be an antirejection therapy based on antilymphocyte serum (ALS). An antibody test was developed using serum of the prospective recipient mixed with white blood cells from the planned donor. This crossmatch between donor cells and recipient serum had led in 1966 to a marked decrease in hyperacute organ rejection. Still, lack of correlation between clinical outcomes and the quality of matching in unrelated cases persisted.[90]

A crossmatch ensured the absence of antibodies to the donor organ. This test was repeated several times during preparation of the living related donor, including 48 hours before the transplant. Another procedure was the mixed lymphocyte culture (MLC), whereby blood samples from the living donor and the recipient were mixed to determine tissue compatibility. Finally, surgeons employed donor-specific blood transfusions (DST) for patients scheduled to receive a living donor transplant. The procedure consisted of small transfusions with donor blood at two to three specific intervals to test the suspected histocompatibility. If, two weeks after a blood transfusion, the potential recipient developed antibodies, the planned transplant was canceled. Transplanting only those patients who did not make antibodies to their relative's blood greatly improved the chance of success.

Transplantation surgery consisted of placing the graft—living or cadaveric—in the right pelvis rather than in the usual kidney location in the back. The existing kidneys, therefore, remained undisturbed. The donor organ was connected to the internal or external iliac artery and vein, with the ureter connected to the bladder. If there were no complications, the actual operation took approximately two to four hours. During the immediate postoperative period, frequent tests were required to monitor the early function of the transplanted kidney. These included daily blood samples, renal scans or sonograms, and perhaps kidney biopsies if early rejection was suspected. Renal scans allowed physicians to assess the blood flow and function of the transplanted kidney and to determine whether slow functioning was the result of acute tubular necrosis or urinary retention in the bladder. This procedure was usually performed the day after surgery, after the Foley catheter was removed, or if rejection was suspected. The renal sonogram demonstrated whether parts of the transplanted kidney were blocked or if any fluid had collected around the organ. In addition, it was often necessary to examine tissue obtained from a biopsy specimen of the transplanted organ, especially if the recipient's original disease had begun to recur in the transplant or if rejection was suspected in spite of steroid treatment. Organ rejection was an expected but feared side effect of transplantation, and most people who received a new kidney experienced a small degree of tissue rejection, generally within the first month following surgery.

By the early 1980s, this rejection was controlled by some form of global immunosuppression, except in isografts between genetically identical persons such as identical twins. The purpose of any such regimen was to prevent graft rejection with a minimum of side effects. From the early period on, Imuran (azathioprine) and prednisone had been the mainstay of immunosuppression, but these drugs also decreased the white blood cell count, exposing patients to a variety of opportunistic infections as well as the development of lymphatic cancers. Doctors still frequently employed antilymphoblast globulin (ALG), a purified antilymphocyte antibody obtained from horse serum, which could be sensitized through the injection of human lymphocytes obtained from the thoracic duct. At first, ALG was injected intramuscularly at the time of transplantation, but this method caused severe pain and swelling, prompting a change to intravenous injections. ALG could not be given on a long-term basis because of the transplant recipient's reaction to horse protein and its connection to a higher incidence of viral infections and cancer formation. It was therefore often administered as a component of the triple-drug cocktail with reduced dosages of prednisone and Imuran.[91]

After 1980, the experimental use of another immunosuppressant, cyclosporin, suggested greater potential for increased transplant activity. In several studies, cyclosporin seemed to prolong allograft survival.[92] In fact, its routine use after 1984 precipitated a veritable transplantation boom in America and around the world. This drug also allowed a reduction in the administration of prednisone and thus drastically decreased the incidence of infectious complications. Transplantation advocates argued that even with its high cost—$ 4,000 to $6,000 per year— it paid for itself within the first year after surgery through shorter hospital stays and lower rates of postoperative organ rejection. Among cyclosporin's drawbacks were its toxic effect on kidneys—more pronounced in transplant recipients—a possibly higher incidence of lymphoma and Kaposi's sarcoma, and neurological complications such as tremors and convulsions.[93]

As UCSF transplant surgeon Oscar Salvatierra indicated in 1984, the true goal of transplantation was "alleviation of suffering and the giving and prolongation of meaningful life." If patients were to be rehabilitated, however, "transplantation is not the cure, it is just the start."[94] As Faith, Nancy, and Patty considered surgery, postoperative management of immunologically deficient transplant patients was still fraught with great uncertainties. Nearly all patients developed infections, especially in the lungs, and many suffered from peptic ulcers. Those who rejected their grafts did so in the early weeks following transplantation, and had to return to dialysis before another donor could be found and a second transplant scheduled. Although acute and irreversible rejection decreased significantly due to the new immunosuppressive strategies, the chances of chronic graft failure after three months opened the possibility of additional transplants. Much was at stake for our UCSF trio as they got ready for their transplants.

World class: Transplantation at UCSF

At UCSF, the first kidney transplant was performed on January 8, 1964, employing an organ from a living identical twin.[95] The operation was carried out by Najarian, then a young surgeon and former graduate and house staff member of the medical school recruited a year earlier to lead the surgical research laboratories. Before this time, the University of California at Los Angeles had been the only other center on the West Coast doing such procedures. During the same year, Belzer joined Najarian at UCSF, and the two collaborated in setting up an independent transplantation service. In 1965, Najarian established the precedent at UCSF of accepting all patients seeking renal transplants, including high-risk and juvenile-onset diabetics such as Faith and Nancy.[96]

Both Najarian and Belzer were pioneers in the burgeoning field of clinical transplantation. In 1967, Najarian left for Minnesota and was replaced by Belzer and Samuel Kountz, a Stanford graduate; the two became codirectors of the Transplantation Service. Under Kountz, UCSF became in 1969 the site for the first clinical study to evaluate postoperative renal hemodynamics. At the time of Kountz's departure in late 1972 to assume the surgery chair at the State University of New York Downstate Medical Center in Brooklyn, the Service had already transplanted over 400 kidneys. Two years earlier, Kountz, son of a black Mississippi sharecropper, had been the principal advocate for the inclusion of an End Stage Renal Disease category in the evolving Medicare program. Kountz's political involvement challenged future surgeons and patients concerning ethnic and social diversity among transplantation patients. At UCSF, a steering committee was created including surgeons, a psychiatrist, and a chaplain to examine the philosophical, ethical, and social issues associated with organ transplantation. In mid-1972, Oscar Salvatierra, Jr., a graduate of the University of Southern California trained as a surgeon and urologist, became a postdoctoral fellow in the Transplantation Service. Salvatierra, whose father was of Spanish descent and whose mother had immigrated from Mexico, was attracted by Kountz's ability to combine the rigors of transplant surgery with political activism.

Working together, Belzer—now in charge—and Salvatierra demonstrated the dangers of prolonged high-dose immunosuppressive therapy. They showed that lower drug doses markedly improved a patient's postoperative course and decreased the risk of infection without jeopardizing kidney graft survival. In fact, massive doses only seemed to delay rather than prevent organ rejection. Belzer and Salvatierra also published a valuable article in *Transplant Proceedings* about the organization of an effective cadaver renal transplantation program.[97] Aware of the important medical dimensions of transplantation, UCSF became the first West Coast institution to initiate a partnership between transplant surgeons and nephrologists. It was based on the premise that transplantation created a host of new medical conditions in need of long-term monitoring by a kidney specialist. The approach was novel, with only four or five other internists nationally working in transplantation services at that time. Recruited by the Department of Medicine with a joint appointment in Surgery, nephrologist William J. Amend joined the team in 1974. A Cornell medical graduate who interned at UCSF between 1967 and 1969, Amend had been quite impressed by Kountz—"a role model with a sparkling personality"—during his stay in San Francisco. After a postdoctoral fellowship in Boston with John Merrill, also a nephrologist, who worked with surgeons Joseph Murray and David Hume, Amend arrived just as Belzer left San Francisco to become the chair of the Department of Surgery at the University of Wisconsin in Madison.[98]

In the same year, Dr. Paul Ebert, a pediatric cardiac surgeon from Cornell, succeeded Dr. J. Engelbert Dunphy as chairman of the Department of Surgery after a 10-year tenure in which UCSF's Transplantation Service had attained worldwide recognition. Ebert selected Salvatierra as the new director of the Service, and he and Amend forged a unique professional partnership characterized by Salvatierra as the new "template for clinical transplantation programs."[99] Inevitably, surgeons were to remain the glamour figures of the Service, while the "humble role of a nephrologist"—Amend's words—required a readiness "to pick up the mud."[100] Internists helped surgeons with clinical protocol and techniques, but more important, they bonded with patients. Their daily presence in the clinic and ward contrasted with the inaccessibility of the surgeons, who spent most of their time in the operating rooms, leading to frequent personal exchanges, critical for gaining patients' confidence and promoting compliance with the postoperative drug regimen. Amend's success in defining the medical role led to the appointment of another nephrologist, Flavio Vincenti, who joined the Service a year later.

During the 1970s, Ebert's hands-off stewardship of the Department of Surgery had important consequences for transplantation at UCSF. Service chiefs such as Salvatierra acquired significant autonomy and implemented their own agendas. Salvatierra was determined to build a nationally prominent program focused on the optimal delivery of transplantation technology. Another surgeon, Nicolas Feduska, soon joined the team. According to Robert Derzon, UCSF director of hospitals and clinics from 1970 until 1977, Moffitt Hospital in 1977 was spending about as much annually for essential services to ESRD patients as for all ambulatory care. Salvatierra not only proved to be an able surgeon, proud of the hospital's growing number of annual transplants, but his partnership with the nephrologists promised better care and improved results for the patients. The presumed cost effectiveness of this approach for ESRD patients was stressed repeatedly in reports and journal articles.[101] Detecting a wider spectrum of need, the Service began to include young children, the elderly, and those suffering from diabetes as candidates for surgery. In 1978, the Service celebrated its first 1,000 kidney transplants. In the tradition of his predecessors, especially Kountz, Salvatierra seldom turned down patients, and transplants were made available to wealthy foreigners and poor migrants, as well as underserved blacks and Latinos.[102]

From the early 1980s on, UCSF's Transplantation Service grew even more rapidly, with a doubling of referrals and an expanding number of procedures.[103] The presence of immunologist Marvin R. Garovay, recruited in 1981 from the Peter Bent Brigham Hospital in Boston to conduct modern histocompatibility testing, increased the interaction between transplant surgeons and a number of medical specialties. Involved in immunogenetics, Garovay was given the task of reducing sensitization by performing multiple donor-specific blood transfusions. Another newcomer was Juliet S. Melzer, a graduate of Northwestern University, who combined her surgical training, including transplantation, with laboratory experience in cellular immunology. Recruited in 1983 by Salvatierra, Melzer displayed an unusual mix of talent and training and was expected to infuse more research into the Service. By contrast, Salvatierra characterized himself as a "patient person," emphasizing care over research. Indeed, some of his colleagues viewed the donor-specific blood transfusions he pioneered as a useful clinical application of basic immunological information, not as the result of original experimental research.[104] Melzer admitted that she was glad to be working in such a prestigious transplantation program. Unfortunately, her original assignment, which called for devoting time to both basic science and surgery, proved impossible. From the start, she became totally immersed in the busy life of a surgeon, covering for Salvatierra and Feduska, who by then were traveling extensively around the country presenting their impressive results.

Salvatierra's Transplantation Service was quite active, doing more than 190 operations per year with only three full-time surgeons. By 1983, the count was up to 197 kidney transplants, and a year later there were 218. At the 9th International Congress of the International Society of Urology in 1983, Salvatierra, Amend, and their colleagues presented their experience with 1,800 renal transplants. "The idea of numbers was always discussed," recalled Melzer.[105] Salvatierra justified his near obsession with high numbers of transplants as a critical factor for the public acceptance and professional growth of the field. Clinical decision making required a large number of cases, and those successful statistics meant something to colleagues, politicians, and the public at large. Aided by an extensive computerized system, the UCSF Service built the best U.S. database on kidney transplantation, recording over 500 endpoints for their surgical results. Whether driven by economics, politics, or professional status, this concentration on case numbers remained another signature of UCSF's Transplantation Service.

With adequate administrative and academic support, the Transplantation Service became one of UCSF's crown jewels, as well as an important source of income for the hospital, since it was also a major client of the Radiology and Laboratory Medicine departments. Indeed, the Service reported a gain of 3.3% in patient days from fiscal year 1981–1982 to 1982–1983. With Ebert's blessing, all surgical fees obtained from organ procurement were diverted to a separate fund designed to promote the activities of the transplantation program, including research, education, and subsidies for patients with special problems. Frequently demanding more hospital beds and threatening to resign and take his patients elsewhere, Salvatierra built the largest kidney transplantation program in the world.

Organ transplantation occurred primarily in university hospitals because of its complexity, the ready availability of patients to be operated on, and the logistics of organ procurement. In contrast to surgery in private practice, transplantation was financially lucrative for academic medical centers. University hospitals had lost income following the implementation of the ESRD program, which had made dialysis widely available in private clinics and hospitals around the country. For its part, UCSF's Transplantation Service had become a pivotal part of the Surgery Department, its clinical activities fully reimbursable by the federal government. However, Salvatierra questioned whether the service was getting enough back for its substantial contributions to the financial health of the academic center. In the early 1980s research and education seemed to be lagging, and institutional support was flagging. Since Belzer's departure in 1974, no new research transplantation fellows had worked in the Service. First-year medical residents came through the Service to study problems of hypertension, renal failure, diabetes, nutrition, immunosuppression, and infectious disease, but the rotation was not very popular. Students frequently carped about preachy surgical attending physicians and lack of autonomy. Friction between the departments of Medicine and Surgery concerning coverage by the house staff occurred. During the early 1980s, fifth-year surgical residents assigned to the Service complained about their lack of responsibility. The gripe was that transplant surgeons gave residents little opportunity for hands-on training. First- and second-year residents were essentially limited to holding retractors.

As on other floors at Moffitt Hospital, the physical facilities for the Transplantation Service were inadequate, outdated, and crowded. Transplanted patients and their living donors were scattered all over the hospital, and there was rarely enough operating room time available for scheduled transplantation surgery. The Service's outpatient clinic, with small offices for surgeons and nephrologists, was located on the 8th floor; the inpatient service was on the 14th. For a time, any overflow—the so-called floating patients—went to the 10th-floor medical wards, outfitted with semiprivate rooms and their own bathrooms. "How come we didn't go to Long Hospital?" was the most frequently asked question after October 1983, posed by many patients familiar with the new facilities. In vivid contrast with the spartan facilities at Moffitt, Long Hospital had single and double rooms with bathrooms for privacy and comfort.

In late June 1983, three months before the arrival of Faith, Nancy, and Patty at the unit, UCSF's Transplant Service marked its 2,000th transplant, becoming the first center in the world to reach this number. Salvatierra and Feduska performed the milestone surgery. Nearly 40% of the procedures involved living and related donors. Because of the tremendous need for kidney donors, UCSF maintained an ongoing educational and referral program to encourage donations. The Service continued to be recognized for its pioneering work, including the development of a system to preserve cadaver kidneys for up to 72 hours, although most were transplanted within 48. This system, now used worldwide, involved placing the cadaver kidneys in portable preservation equipment, where their viability could be carefully maintained. Surgeons of the Service personally traveled to other hospitals to recover cadaver kidneys. Such trips not only involved institutions in the Bay Area, but also demanded flights throughout Northern California, extending as far south as San Luis Obispo and even Las Vegas.

Some hospitals had their own organ procurement programs. Professional education consisted of orienting hospital personnel and developing a commitment to cadaveric kidney retrieval. At UCSF and elsewhere, active staff surveillance identified and reported potential donors soon enough to make retrieval possible. Participants included nephrologists, neurologists, and neurosurgeons, Emergency Room physicians, nursing supervisors, unit managers, nurses, chaplains, and even social workers. The key role was played by a transplant coordinator in charge of hospital surveillance and notification procedures. Available around the clock, this person also reviewed medical records to identify potential donors.

In 1984, Ebert's decade in the Department of Surgery came to an end when he accepted the directorship of the American College of Surgeons. With his departure, a period of administrative tranquility and laissez-faire in the department ended.[106] Despite cuts in Medicare and Medi-Cal, however, the Transplantation Service continued to operate in the black and attracted an ever larger number of patients.[107] When in San Francisco, Salvatierra remained active in surgery—"always in the trenches," by his own description. When he was not busy performing surgery, his political agenda of passionately promoting the benefits of transplantation for needy patients took him to Sacramento and Washington for heavy lobbying with state and federal officials and legislators. Politics were very important to him as part of his activist identity. A decorated combat surgeon in Vietnam, Salvatierra had championed veterans' health issues, studied diabetes among Native Americans, and promoted minority access to care in California. Such multiple activities propelled him into leadership positions and membership in a variety of organizations, from the National Kidney Foundation to the presidency of the American Society of Transplant Surgeons.

In early 1983, Salvatierra and two other transplant surgeons met with representatives of Congress and the executive branch to discuss the need for a national system of organ procurement and distribution. His multiple contacts with Congressman Albert Gore, Jr., of Tennessee regarding this and other transplantation issues eventually led to the formulation of legislation to regulate the donation of human organs. Hearings were held between July and October 1983 before the Subcommittee on Health and the Environment, chaired by Rep. Henry A. Waxman of California. Among those who testified were Belzer, Salvatierra, and Starzl. However, after both the House of Representatives and the Senate had passed by wide margins their respective versions of a bill, Committee on Labor and Human Resources Chairman Orrin Hatch delayed convening the required conference committee to reconcile the legislation. The entire effort appeared to be in jeopardy, apparently a victim of political maneuvering to stymie Gore's senatorial ambitions. Here again, Salvatierra's behind-the-scenes efforts, including a letter to President Ronald Reagan, helped break the congressional deadlock and ensure passage of the National Organ Transplantation Act of 1984, a crowning tribute to Salvatierra's political efforts.[108]

"Rebirth" at Moffitt Hospital

In 1984, the Kidney Transplant Unit on Moffitt's 14th floor was a busy place. Waiting lists were long. With only 16 beds officially assigned to it, the medical and nursing staff had developed a priority system. They assigned available beds to transplant candidates and frequently sent donors to be worked up and even hospitalized for their nephrectomies in other surgical units. Transfers to the 11th floor, a primary medical service, were also common. To avoid boarding patients in other units, nurse-coordinators sometimes placed male and female patients in the same ward, a measure socially and psychologically uncomfortable for patients, families, and caregivers.[109] As in other departments at Moffitt, the unit was a classic example of the type of hospital space carved out of existing areas originally earmarked for interdisciplinary research, teaching, and patient care. Scheduled for remodeling, this was in 1984 the last user-unfriendly floor remaining in the building.

After their arrival, patients were generally seen by the inpatient coordinator-educator, Susan Hopper, a specialized transplantation nurse responsible for processing all newcomers. Susan had been hired in 1978 when the Kidney Transplant Unit got busier and the need arose to process and educate increasing numbers of pre- and postoperative patients. She also coordinated preoperative blood transfusions, attended educational sessions at neighborhood or community clubs, and for a time helped with organ procurement. Another clinical specialist, Peggy Devney, came in 1980 to assist in the education of ward nurses and patients. The service also had two social workers and a staff psychiatry liaison, Dr. Roger M. Lauer, together with an occupational and physical therapist. Lauer screened prospective donors and recipients for psychiatric histories, substance abuse problems, and episodes of noncompliance with the medical regimen.

Placed in the same four-bed ward, Faith and Nancy talked freely about their illnesses. The atmosphere in the unit seemed friendly, with physicians and nurses getting along with humor and efficiency. A day after her arrival, however, Faith became frightened by her high blood sugar level and the specter of losing control over her carefully managed diabetic condition. Teary-eyed, she walked around talking and spending time with her sister and donor, Megan. Diabetics presented particular challenges to medical and behavioral management. Stress and the effects of surgery changed insulin requirements, while medical attending physicians differed in their criteria of what constituted proper control of the disease. Moreover, not all diabetics were sufficiently disciplined in controlling their disease. Nancy was equally apprehensive, and both patients soon required an insulin drip. Yet, as Nancy recalled later, once she had met her new roommate, "I never had a second thought about being by myself."[110]

On September 25, orderlies wheeled both Faith and Nancy into the operating room to receive their new kidneys. Faith's surgeon was Juliet Melzer; Feduska performed the nephrectomy on her sister, Megan. After two attempts at perfusion following placement of the organ in the abdomen, the donor kidney had to be recooled, but the patient sustained only minimal blood loss and returned to the recovery room in good condition. For Nancy, the surgical roles were reversed, with Feduska installing the new kidney obtained by Melzer from Nancy's brother Dan. Nancy also survived her surgery in good condition. Renal scans obtained on the first postoperative day showed good uptake and excretion for both patients. No rejection was detected, and renal functions began to improve. The first two days after surgery were monotonous, with frequent interruptions from the nursing staff monitoring vital signs. Surrounded by machines and fitted with nasogastric tubes and Foley catheters, Faith and Nancy lay immobile and anxious, hoping that their grafts would be successful. Both were now placed on the immunosuppressant regimen of Imuran and prednisone. Then Patty received her kidney. Here again Feduska was the primary surgeon, while Salvatierra operated on the donor, her sister Kathleen. Her kidney had two urethers, complicating the surgery, but both procedures were uneventful. Back in the hospital room, the bonding continued. Recalled Nancy: "After we got back after our surgery, in the first days, we were glad we were all together because every night we would lay awake. It was like a great slumber party. We would lay awake at night all talking and we really got to know each other, sharing our feelings, we got real close. We'd have breakfast in the morning and we kind of shared all our visitors. It was real fun."[111]

Hospitalization, of course, demanded periods of privacy and isolation followed by socializing. The early postoperative period was punctuated by grogginess and immobility, better handled in seclusion, but with four patients in the same room at different stages of recovery, this period was short-lived. Patients talked to each other, sharing common experiences that facilitated kinship. Within days of Faith's and Nancy's surgeries, the clubby atmosphere fostered by the now archaic ward arrangement had a strongly positive effect, recognized by the staff and the patients themselves. As soon as they became ambulatory, patients even strolled the hallways. On the downside, however, once patients were relieved of their catheters about a week after surgery, they spent most of their time standing in lines for the three available toilets, intent on producing hourly urine specimens during the day that were required for the second postoperative week. At night, this process had to be repeated every two hours.

All three women spent their entire hospitalization period in a four-bed room. According to Faith, "I would have felt very lonely, isolated and scared in a private room," adding, however, that "there are definitely disease states where I can imagine myself wanting privacy, but this [kidney transplantation] was not one of them."[112] Occupying the fourth bed was Arlene W., a woman in her mid-50's who had her transplant the same day as Patty. From the first postoperative day, Arlene had a hard time. Clinical manifestations of rejection set in early, and a biopsy of her new kidney was obtained. Placed again on dialysis, she remained in bed most of the time, nauseated and vomiting, only to have her transplanted kidney removed. In spite of her condition, Arlene was included in the room activities. Not only did Faith, Nancy, and Patty come from large families, but their personalities and jobs allowed them to bond easily. Arlene, by contrast, seemed more private and retiring, seldom receiving visitors, but she came to enjoy her roommates' frequent guests.

At UCSF's Transplantation Unit, nursing was critical, especially because of occasional staff shortages and the high volume of patients. In the 1980s nursing was poised for a quantum leap toward professional autonomy. Feminist perspectives and the concept of civil rights had coalesced with notions of individual autonomy and self-fulfillment.[113] Nurses in American hospitals everywhere now played a greater and better-defined role. As so-called clinical specialists, they performed a multiplicity of tasks, from hands-on care to teaching other nurses, as well as educating the patients. However, there remained unresolved issues concerning the traditional conception of nursing as a womanly service, as well as the more prosaic question of whether there were still enough jobs available for those entering the field.[114] Old hierarchical disputes with medicine and its practitioners were being revisited, with the traditional "game" between them in jeopardy. Instead, hospitals widely adopted a team concept, creating a collective of caregivers involving not only doctors and nurses but also a series of technicians and assistants.[115]

Kidney transplantation fit well into a mechanical model of medicine, in which attention focused primarily on the recovery of physiological functions. Delivery of "compulsive" nursing care in the early 1980s included strict attention to the details of fluid intake and output. Nurses were urged to discard traditional caregiving rituals and ground their practices in the logical application of scientific knowledge.[116] Under the circumstances, the nursing staff provided technical information and support, relying on the patients themselves to seek out family members and friends for their emotional needs, a normal sequence of events in modern, increasingly impersonal patient–caregiver relationships. Given the complexity of transplant management, the nurses were part of a comprehensive care system that demanded a great deal of patient compliance.

The model of nursing care employed at Moffitt broke down the pre- and postoperative periods, assigning different teams of competent nurses to each phase and forcing patients to take the initiative in learning more about their posttransplant management. An earlier horizontal model of care and education, in which one nurse was assigned to each new patient from preadmission screening until posttransplant discharge, was abandoned. This method had allowed caregivers to familiarize themselves with the whole hospitalization process of their assigned patients, thus serving the nurturing needs of both nurses and patients. But by the time Faith, Patty, and Nancy entered the unit, the feeling was that no single nurse needed to bear total responsibility for a particular patient. The older method contributed to caregiver burnout and hampered scheduling flexibility. If a particular caregiver was unavailable, the system broke down and patients felt insecure.

A guiding philosophy in the early 1980s, therefore, was to ensure that patients quickly learned to manage their own care in the hospital through the employment of support groups instead of dependence on particular caregivers. The intense teaching sessions usually started after removal of the Foley catheters. At first, Faith seemed somewhat hostile to the postoperative instruction provided by the nurses, comparing it to homework in grade school. With her master's degree in nutrition and her sophisticated diabetes management skills, Faith was proud of her knowledge of renal disease.

From the outset, however, Faith, Nancy, and Patty came to appreciate the specialized nursing staff on Moffitt's transplantation ward. Lower doses of immunosuppressants had lessened anxiety about infection. Nurses no longer wore protective gear, a fact that reassured patients who might otherwise have become frightened by the isolation routines and garb. To ease patient discomfort, the clinical coordinators became involved in every aspect of care, including dialysis, preparations for transplant surgery, the multiple donor-specific blood transfusions, and postoperative monitoring. They also adopted the role of patient advocates in their relationships with the surgeons, a legal metaphor created within the new patients' rights movement.[117] Regular nurses tried hard to overcome the difficulties caused by Moffitt's antiquated space configuration and its impact on patients by their steady presence and displays of good humor.

Living in close quarters, patients such as Faith, Nancy, and Patty not only learned together but also checked on each other during their recovery phase. From the beginning, most organ recipients developed a love-hate relationship with their surgeons. For some, surgeons were intimidating demigods who had provided the "gift of life." To communicate their gratitude, some patients attempted to ingratiate themselves with their "saviors," even behaving obsequiously, trying to develop a spiritual, almost mystical attachment.[118] Others frequently complained that the surgeons "floated in and out," that they did "their magic and then disappeared" because they spent so much time in the operating room, not a surprise in a service performing on average nearly four kidney transplants per week. For their part, transplant surgeons feared that technical mistakes would harm their charges. As Starzl remarked, "the transplanted patient is a delicate piece of fragile glass."[119] In general, the transplant surgeons got caught up in the momentum of their unending string of surgeries, worried about the lack of donors but immensely gratified by their accomplishments and often embarrassed at being placed on pedestals. Surgeons—those working at UCSF seemed an exception—also easily found themselves giving primacy to medical education and research rather than to patient care.

By contrast, nephrologists such as Amend and Vincenti frequently visited the wards, making regular morning rounds with the surgeons, nurses, house staff, and medical students and chatting with individual patients. Then there were afternoon sessions without patient visits, restricted to the caregiving team composed of a surgeon, nephrologist, resident, clinical coordinator, and head nurse, who freely discussed the latest clinical developments of the newly operated patients or those experiencing postoperative complications.[120] Endowed with a good sense of humor, Amend and Vincenti were cast in a far less threatening role than the cranky, sleep-deprived house staff members and thus were rewarded with a warmer reception from the patients.[121] The presence of these nephrologists satisfied the need for physicians to "be there" on the wards for their recovering patients. Amend was especially effective in diffusing anxiety, patiently explaining the ups and downs of the postoperative period. In all, the UCSF team of attending physicians exemplified a fortuitous blend of the traditional decisive activist approach exhibited by surgeons and the slower, more methodical and thoughtful medical approach.

By October 1, Faith was doing better, with a renal scan showing good uptake and excretion. She was no longer suffering bladder spasms, and her Foley catheter was to be removed the following day. What would happen next? Here the efforts of an empathetic nephrologist such as Amend were critical. Kindness and humor were supplemented by Amend's penchant for employing index cards on which he wrote down and drew pictures of all the pertinent information for recovering patients. This included rudiments of renal pathophysiology, decision tree analysis, and treatments. Each patient thus obtained a personalized and dated statement from Amend, a memento many were proud to keep.[122]

One of Faith's critical observations about hospital life at Moffitt concerned trust. In her view, modern American patients were usually well educated in health matters. When hospitalized, however, ideally they needed to stop trying to second-guess the medical and nursing staff and assume that good care would be forthcoming in a professional manner. This was particularly difficult for Faith, given her unfortunate prior experiences at another university hospital and her own compulsive diabetes management. In truth, some diabetics were notorious "control freaks," poised to wrest this function from the transplant nurses as soon as possible. Concerned about daily fluctuations in her blood sugar, Faith very much wanted to resume command of her body. In her steroid-induced euphoria, she insisted on relinquishing control only if the caregivers promised to do as good a job as she expected from herself. Faith's repeated threats to administer her own insulin from syringes stuffed into her handbag elicited opposition from the caregivers. Following careful negotiations with the residents and nurses, she finally surrendered after reaching an agreement—she still remained skeptical—for joint management.[123]

Given the high level of stress experienced by both caregivers and patients in such an intense, busy ward, Dr. Lauer, the staff psychiatrist, headed off potential trouble by making daily rounds early in the morning accompanied by a social worker. As in other parts of the institution, some patients strongly resented hospital routines and their loss of freedom. Lauer tried, in most instances, to change staff expectations rather than patient behavior. His goal, however, was to emphasize the patients' need to organize their new posttransplant lives according to carefully designed management plans. A new lifestyle, necessary to ensure the long-term viability of the graft, demanded increased responsibility and self-care from each transplanted patient.[124] This typical American self-care approach was challenged in the early 1980s by the influx of Saudi Arabian and Latino patients, who preferred to shift the educational responsibilities to spouses and relatives.[125]

At the onset of transplantation, the expectations were minimal. However, once the new organ—the ticket to a better life—seemed to be fairly well established, expectations soared. Ambulatory patients were eager to regain previous levels of activity, although they knew they would never get back to the "blind normal." Poised at the threshold of such a life, many had grandiose expectations. Doctors and nurses were seen as the agents enabling such a miracle, but the patients' own sense of the critical role they were to play in making the transplant a permanent condition suggested the need for a total remake of their lives.[126] In an almost religious sense, transplant patients viewed their hospital experience as a rebirth and hoped for a permanent deliverance from the hated dialysis sessions and other crippling limitations.

By early October, however, Patty had already complained of intense pain around the incision area and could not get relief from medications. Nursing notes from October 7 revealed that Patty had discussed with her roommates her feelings about the surgery and the outcome of her transplant. On the ward, a creeping uncertainty began to replace the early postoperative euphoria. Like many other patients before them, Patty, Faith, and Nancy felt an acute sense of mortality, daring to live just one day at a time. As one observer commented, patients at this stage of their recovery felt as though they were sitting on a powder keg, which was ready to explode and thwart their dreams of a better life.[127]

While Faith and Nancy redoubled their efforts to cheer up Patty, her wall chart displaying her laboratory results suggested a decline in renal function. In full view of staff and patients, the graphs were posted next to the door of each hospital room, containing the daily laboratory results of bodily functions. This system, employed worldwide since the 1960s and endorsed by the American College of Surgeons, provided easy reference for nurses and surgeons monitoring the progress of their postoperative patients. Moreover, the data were quite useful for house staff and attending physicians during rounds in reaching therapeutic decisions. The message from caregivers was that everything concerning patient management was out in the open, and that medical information was being shared and could play a role in patient education.

At Moffitt, however, nurses posted daily the new laboratory values for all to see in a climate of apprehension and often fear. Far from being reassured, some patients became excessively focused on, even obsessed with, the numbers. Patty later remembered the daily practice of "going up to the wall chart with a knot in the stomach." Patients with higher creatinine values got more staff attention and support from other patients. Patty explained that she "felt for the people who were not progressing as successfully as I was for the first two weeks. I thought it was kind of a downer to go out and see this [information] in public."[128] This angst about numbers prompted further educational efforts by the nurses designed to play down the importance of such laboratory results and help patients get on with their lives. Again, Patty: "In a way it was nice—other people knew and were trying to help, and support. But I don't know that I would have wanted everybody saying 'Oh, I'm so sorry for you.' That's what bothered me."[129] Some postoperative patients even became jealous because their roommates were faring better.

In an effort to counteract severe anxiety, Lauer led weekly sessions of a transplantation support group, open to all patients in need of further reassurance. Meeting every Thursday afternoon, this gathering was also attended by nurses, social workers, and a chaplain. Postoperative outpatients and potential transplant candidates frequently joined in. As in other patient groups, the freewheeling discussions were aimed at creating patient solidarity and bonding with staff members. On the ward, meanwhile, patients were encouraged to talk to each other about their frustrations and feelings regarding their temporary loss of control following surgery.

On October 8, Patty expressed further frustration with the comprehensive patient teaching program. Lacking advanced medical knowledge, she was somewhat concerned that all this information, including that concerning the side effects of drugs such as prednisone, was being provided after the fact. For many patients, compliance with the new array of immunosuppressants, so critical for the survival of the graft, could easily be jeopardized if the information was not furnished in a timely manner. In response, Peggy Devney had developed a new approach to the problem by installing bulk medication containers at the bedside. The rationale was that patients should be further encouraged to take an active role in learning their home care routines—including the ingestion of pills—if the medication was readily available. Not to be forgotten in this educational process was the patient's family, no longer an obstacle but now considered a vital partner in future care.[130]

On October 11, Patty became quite upset. She had started running a high fever and realistically feared that this represented the onset of organ rejection. The house staff ordered blood and urine cultures, a chest X-ray, and a renal scan. By the next day, Patty openly acknowledged her resentment of the fact that her clinical course was less favorable than that of Faith and Nancy. Feeling abandoned, and with the prospect of returning to dialysis too painful to contemplate, Patty could not hide her deep disappointment and even withdrew temporarily from her friendly roommates.[131] Was the celebrated "rebirth" in jeopardy?

Two weeks after surgery, the side effects of prednisone, depression, and weight gain experienced by most patients were another common stress point in the postoperative process requiring careful monitoring and frequent reassurance.[132] Physicians and nurses, both at UCSF and at other transplantation centers, continued to stress strict postoperative compliance with the dietary and especially the immunosuppressive regimen, insisting that some of the negative effects were transitory. Obviously, the success of the transplant hinged on strict adherence to the established protocol. However, the educational program resonated better with patients who were already quite independent, health-conscious, and disciplined. Sometimes family members were forced to assume this educational burden, especially if the patients were children.[133] Not surprisingly, frustrated patients, including Faith, Patty, and Nancy, began raising quality-of-life issues that had meaning well beyond hospitalization.

Making transplantation routine

On October 13, Nancy P. was discharged from Moffitt Hospital after an uneventful recovery. At that time, the average hospital stay for a transplant patient receiving a kidney from a living donor at UCSF was 15–18 days; for a cadaver transplant it was 24 days, more than double that of Najarian's unit at the University of Minnesota. At UCSF, however, patients continued to be thoroughly indoctrinated in their postoperative routines while they were still in the hospital. Patty appeared teary, lethargic, and depressed to her friends, seemingly resigned to the possibility of losing her new kidney. As the surgeons explained, another graft was always an option. She now exhibited renewed pitting edema below her knees, a form of fluid retention believed to be secondary to an incipient rejection of her new kidney. Concerned, the attending physicians obtained a renal biopsy. With Nancy gone, Patty was now comforted by Faith and the quieter Arlene.

Faith T. was discharged the next day, feeling very well and now able to regulate her blood sugar. "I almost didn't want to go home. [The hospital] can be a lonely place, but these people took my loneliness away, at a real level," she commented. Faith also stressed the importance of the humor displayed by caregivers such as Amend and her new roommates, which was "probably a better healer than many medications."[134] On the same day, however, a bitterly disappointed Patty was forced to submit once more to dialysis, with its attendant nausea and headaches. The renal biopsy showed signs of an acute but minimal tissue rejection, with marked medullary congestion and focal tubular necrosis. Although both the nurses and Patty's husband remained very supportive, Patty continued to be anxious and depressed. Fortunately, a week later, Patty's rejection process stopped, and her kidney functions seemed to stabilize. A brief visit from Faith and Nancy, who were now being followed by the nephrologists in the outpatient clinic, also decidedly lifted her flagging spirits. They all walked the halls together and performed their required postoperative exercises.

Finally, on October 24, Patty B. was also discharged. Her pain was now seemingly under control, and her previous mental depression had lifted. Her blood pressure, however, remained high. Reflecting on her hospitalization, Patty recalled that although the four-bed ward looked antiquated, even primitive, because of its lack of bathroom facilities, "when I was there it was great. The [arrangement of] four in a room was probably really helpful to all of us. I suppose I would have had more questions and concerns and maybe reservations if I didn't have that group of people to communicate with who were going through the same thing I was going through."[135] Patty's journey was over.

After a long delay, meanwhile, both houses of Congress unanimously passed the National Organ Transplant Act, and President Reagan signed the legislation on October 19, 1984, just as the three patients were recovering from their transplants in Moffitt Hospital. The new law established a national registry for all organ transplants and made the purchase and sale of organs for transplantation purposes illegal. The ASTS, under Salvatierra's presidency, and the International Transplantation Society had strongly supported the bill in the face of opposition from the AMA and the American College of Surgeons, which considered the proposals an unnecessary intrusion into private medical practice. Members of the executive branch, including Reagan, had branded it another example of undesirable governmental intrusion. This landmark act also addressed problems related to organ procurement, establishing a national Organ Procurement and Transplantation Network (OPTN) with already organized local and regional procurement agencies.[136] The arrangement also suggested the establishment of a national standard for all potential recipients. Eventually, the first network contract was awarded in 1986 to the nonprofit United Network for Organ Sharing (UNOS), and a plan for its operation was approved on October 1, 1987. While the financial issue of posttransplant therapy remained unsolved, this legislation created a task force charged with evaluating all reimbursement problems, including coverage of outpatient cyclosporin therapy and payments for nonrenal organ transplantation. As Starzl saw it, "transplantation was being woven into the fabric of American society and of conventional medical care."[137]

After 1984, renal transplantation became an even more established therapy, but issues of organ procurement and allocation, as well as cost effectiveness, still pose ethical and economic dilemmas.[138] The concept of brain death continues to challenge entrenched cultural views about human vitality and viability. The public continues to fear that efforts to expand the pool of available organs could translate into less than energetic therapeutic measures to put off death, thus increasing the potential for organ harvest. At the same time, the experimental nature of lifelong immunosuppression continues to present problems. Many experts argue that kidney transplantations never fully restore health since they merely substitute the side effects of the drugs for the symptoms of chronic kidney failure, thus setting up a lifelong battle against organ rejection and infection. Some have described renal transplantation, when successful, as merely giving the patient a "holiday from dialysis," although organ recipients hope that the procedure will allow them to retire permanently from such treatments.

Subsequent technological improvements, including the routine employment of cyclosporin, have created a faster rate of turnover, cutting hospital stays to 5 or 6 days for transplants from living donors and 12 days for cadaver donors, about a third of the previous length. Moreover, by capping the costs of specific organ transplants, the advent of Medicare's Diagnosis Related Groups has further shortened the hospital stay.[139] Even nursing care, comprising about 30–40% of total hospital expenditures, was reigned in as part of federal efforts to "bring rationality into the provision of health care services."[140] According to Gloria Horns and Peggy Devney, by the 1990s discharge plans were being made even before the patient received the transplanted kidney. While more economical, however, shorter hospitalizations carry a considerable human price. Given such a brief institutional sojourn, both patient education and in-house socialization have taken a back seat. Suggestions are now being made for the organization of hospital-based, supervised convalescent facilities instead of allowing discharged transplant patients to linger in nearby hotels and motels for which insurance companies will not pay.[141]

From a demographic perspective, renal transplantation is bound up with America's changing disease patterns. Like other developed countries, the nation had experienced an epidemiological transition from acute to chronic disease since the early twentieth century, followed by an impressive extension of life expectancy responsible for increasing the number of its older citizens. But what are the ends of medicine? Our hubris and our refusal to accept limits have extended to the aging process and mortality. Should life-prolonging treatment be provided to everyone, regardless of cost?

This imperative to deny death has likewise fueled the growth of the organ transplantation field, leading to what one critic has coined an effort to "slash and suture our way to eternal life."[142] Although the government retains a limited responsibility for health care, it has committed itself at the federal and state levels to pay for a number of health care schemes—including organ transplantation—broadly defined as entitlement programs designed for special groups in American society. These potentially open-ended claims on public resources characterize the field of transplantation. As Najarian asked in the 1970s, "Should society devote its economic and manpower resources, required hospital space and technology, for the treatment of a relatively small number of patients?"[143]

Provided with new technologies and drugs, transplantation in the 1990s has become increasingly routine, involving multiple organs as well as retransplants. Health has really never been a social good in American society, but has become instead the responsibility of individuals. With human organs now considered another form of merchandise, the altruistic gift relationship that lent earlier transplantation a moral quality is quickly vanishing. Since cultural taboos continue to hamper the availability of transplantable organs, consumers have created a commercial market of international scope, threatening the personhood of many poor Third World inhabitants—especially in India and among Chinese political prisoners—a development that has prompted the creation of a task force on transplantation and bodily integrity.[144]

In the end, kidney and organ transplantation in general can be seen as another paradigm mirroring the dilemmas of the fragmented American health care system. Among them is the link between employment and the right to health care, which creates inequality of access and forces specific individuals to make emotional and highly public appeals for resources and services. This is especially dramatic in the case of organ donations. Caregivers, for their part, have entered into increasingly bureaucratic and financial relationships with profit-making health-care businesses, jeopardizing their traditional professional ethos and commitment to service. Until recently, however, health care decisions, including transplantation, remained insulated from economic considerations, since a rationing system based on the ability to pay would seem to threaten Americans' autonomy, freedom of choice, and belief in limitless medical progress. Nobody has questioned the phenomenon of multiple kidney retransplants, particularly in an expanding population of diabetics, that threatens to escalate costs dramatically.[145]

Another important issue is the lack of both national and regional planning in transplantation, since the American hospital system remains largely decentralized. Pleas for regional cooperation have been voiced since the 1930s. Such measures are believed to contain medical costs by avoiding the duplication of facilities, equipment, and personnel. For the most part, individual or merged institutions continue to value pluralism and competition. While the issue of organ procurement eventually forced the creation of regional networks, top transplant programs such as UCSF's continue their independent efforts to secure such organs.

While federal capitation payments forced American university hospitals to cut costs, a 1984 comparison of UCSF's Moffitt Hospital with several European counterparts in Leuven, Berlin, Leiden, and London also revealed the persistence of institutional differences similar to those disclosed in 1929 for general hospitals. The expectation of this study was that perhaps in the United States, "as university hospitals move into a price-competitive era, they may come to resemble their European counterparts,"[146] an assumption that somewhat naively disregarded American cultural traditions that cannot be altered by economics alone. Not surprisingly, the conclusions of the report highlighted the tendency of American medicine to serve a population of unscreened, self-referred, and insured patients who were acutely ill, many requiring intensive care, whereas the Europeans admitted only a select population. Patients admitted to Moffitt were quickly subjected to a barrage of expensive, technologically sophisticated diagnostic tests and therapies, with the assistance of numerous physicians, nurses, house staff, and technicians, before being discharged to complete their recovery elsewhere. The process was accomplished with significant input from the often assertive American patients and their families, who influenced clinical decisions and demanded aggressive interventions, even in potentially terminal illnesses. Compared to the annual budget of similar European hospitals, that of UCSF's Moffitt was substantially higher. Items not represented abroad included the staff's fringe benefits for health insurance and the $1.5 million spent annually for malpractice insurance premiums.

By 1988, the final remodeling phase of Moffitt Hospital forced the transfer of the Transplantation Service to the ninth floor of the adjacent Long Hospital, where it remains today. Here semiprivate and private rooms look out toward Golden Gate Park or Mount Sutro. This modern facility provides far greater privacy, access to private bathrooms, and amenities such as television, which had been demanded by many patients. At the same time, however, the single rooms require individual nursing care and supervision, a barrier to further efficiency, and significantly inhibit efforts to socialize.[147] In fact, social workers must spend more time with individual patients, who now have fewer people to talk to than they had in shared facilities. As Faith characterized her experiences with roommates a decade earlier, "I don't know if words would ever be sufficient to be able to describe the absence of isolation that occurred when I went through this experience."[148] Moreover, these spatial arrangements affect the posttransplantation educational program. Now the patients need to be gathered together for the group teaching sessions. Another important factor is the gradual shortening of the hospital stay, which also hampers the establishment of relationships with caregivers.

Institutional socialization and the personal connections that now seem so unimportant have migrated to outpatient clinics, since patients discharged early must return there initially three times a week following surgery. In retrospect, Patty B. commented in 1994 that "just coming for my clinic visits is always a high . . . because I know that I've got a second chance at life. It's just a very special type of thing. And UCSF plays into that. My whole experience here was kind of a miraculous journey."[149]

To this day, Faith, Nancy, and Patty remain good friends, and each of them, in her own way, continues to be an example to many persons who are trying to gather the courage to choose a renal transplant, especially from a living donor.[150] In her capacity as a clinical dietitian, Faith encourages such people with her descriptions of the positive experience and support she received while hospitalized with Patty and Nancy. For her, the stay at UCSF "was unquestionably the most positive medical experience of my entire life."[151] Mutual understanding concerning the immanence of time and hope for a better future were the fruits of hospital life on that small, antiquated ward. In his recent autobiography, Starzl acknowledged the central role patients have played in organ transplantation, enduring the endless experimental diagnostic tests and therapeutic procedures. "Ultimately they, in their suffering, were the ones who made all triumphs of medicine possible," he acknowledged, adding that the patients "gave meaning to what we did or tried to do."[152]

NOTES

1. Thomas E. Starzl, *The Puzzle People: Memoirs of a Transplant Surgeon*, Pittsburgh, Univ. of Pittsburgh Press, 1992, p. 3.

2. Personal interviews with Faith T. and Nancy P., January 1994. The patients were selected after a meeting with Juliet S. Melzer and William J. Amend, Jr., October 1993.

3. For details see David J. Rothman, *Beginnings Count: The Technological Imperative in American Health Care*, New York, Oxford Univ. Press, 1997, pp. 88–109, and Renee C. Fox and Judith P. Swazey, *The Courage to Fail: A Social View of Organ Transplants and Dialysis*, 2nd ed., Chicago, Univ. of Chicago Press, 1978.

4. R. J. Rubin, "Epidemiology of end stage renal disease and implications for public policy," *Publ Health Rep* 99 (September–October 1984): 492–98, and R. W. Schmidt et al., "The dilemmas of patient treatment for end-stage renal disease," *Am J Kidney Dis* 3 (1983): 37–47.

5. N. J. Feduska, et al., "Dramatic improvement in the success rate for renal transplants in diabetic recipients with donor-specific transfusions," *Transplantation* 38 (December 1984): 704–08.

6. Statistics provided by R. Duca, chief administrative officer for the Surgery Department, UCSF's Transplant Service, 1994.

7. J. M. Prottas, "Encouraging altruism: Public attitudes and the marketing of organ donation," *Milbank Q* 61 (1983): 278–306, and C. H. Fellner and S. H. Schwartz, "Altruism in disrepute: Medical versus public attitudes toward the living organ donor," *N Engl J Med* 284 (1971): 582–85.

8. J. Murray, "Moral and ethical reflections on human organ transplantation," *Linacre Q* 31 (1964): 54–56, and David Lamb, *Organ Transplants and Ethics*, London, Routledge, 1990, pp. 7–23. For an excellent summary of the issues see R. C. Fox et al., "Social and ethical problems in the treatment of end-stage renal disease patients," in *Controversies in Nephrology and Hypertension*, ed. R. G. Narins, New York, Churchill Livingstone, 1984, pp. 45–70.

9. For background see Richard M. Titmus, *The Gift Relationship*, London, Allen & Unwin, 1971.

10. A. L. Caplan, "Organ transplants: The costs of success," *Hastings Center Rep* 13 (1983): 23–32.

11. For details see A. M. Sadler et al., "Transplantation: A case for consent," *N Engl J Med* 280 (Apr. 17, 1969): 862–67.

12. A. L. Caplan, "Ethical and policy issues in the procurement of cadaver organs," *N Engl J Med* 311 (Oct. 11, 1984): 981–83.

13. For a historical perspective see E. H. Ackerknecht, "Death in the history of medicine," *Bull Hist Med* 42 (1968): 19–23.

14. "A definition of irreversible coma: Report of the Ad Hoc Committee of the Harvard Medical School to Examine the Definition of Brain Death," *JAMA* 205 (Aug. 5, 1968): 337–40. See D. Wikler and A. Weisbard, "Appropriate confusion over 'brain death,' " *JAMA* 261 (Apr. 21, 1989): 2246, and David Lamb, *Death, Brain Death, and Ethics*, London, Croom Helm, 1985.

15. J. K. Iglehart, "Transplantation: The problem of limited resources," *N Engl J Med* 309 (July 14, 1983), 123–28.

16. R. A. Rettig, "The politics of organ transplantation: A parable of our time," in *Organ Transplantation Policy, Issues and Prospects*, ed. J. F. Blumstein and F. A. Sloan, Durham, NC, Duke Univ. Press, 1989, pp. 191–227.

17. C. B. Carpenter et al., " 'Free market' approach to organ donation," *N Engl J Med* 310 (Feb. 9, 1984): 395–96, and K. J. Bart et al., "Increasing the supply of cadaveric kidneys for transplantation," *Transplantation* 31 (May 1981): 383–87.

18. G. J. Annas, "Life, liberty, and the pursuit of organ sales," *Hastings Center Rep* 14 (1984): 22–23.

19. D. A. Ogden, "Consequences of renal donation in man," *Am J Kidney Dis* 2 (March 1983): 501–11.

20. Personal interview with Juliet S. Melzer, October 1993. Se also M. Hoffman, "Is altruism part of human nature?" *J Person Soc Psychol* 40 (1981): 121–37.

21. R. W. Evans, "The socioeconomics of organ transplantation," *Transplant Proc* 17 (1985), suppl. 4, 129–36.

22. In fact, later figures showed that Medicare spent on average $32,000 per year for each patient on dialysis, while a renal transplant cost "only" $56,000 the first year and about $6,000 yearly thereafter for three years, when eligibility for this reimbursement ended. The figures are taken from N. G. Levinsky and R. A. Rettig, "The Medicare end-stage renal disease program: A report from the Institute of Medicine," *N Engl J Med* 324 (Apr. 18, 1991): 1144–45, and quoted in Renee C. Fox and Judith P. Swazey, *Spare Parts: Organ Replacement in American Society*, New York, Oxford Univ. Press, 1992, p. 75.

23. R. A. Rettig, "The politics of health cost containment: End-stage renal disease," *Bull NY Acad Med* 56 (January–February 1980): 115–37, and more recently P. M. McNeill, *The Ethics and Politics of Human Experimentation*, Cambridge, Cambridge Univ. Press, 1993.

24. See O. Salvatierra, Jr., "The role of organ transplantation in modern medicine," *Heart Transplant* 4 (1985), 3: 285–89.

25. C. M. Kjellstrand, "Age, sex, and race inequality in renal transplantation," *Arch Intern Med* 148 (June 1988): 1305–09.

26. Melzer interview, April 1994.

27. Faith T. interview, January 1994. For an overview see Roy Y. Calne, *A Gift of Life: Observations on Organ Transplantation*, New York, Basic Books, 1970. A poignant story concerning the issues of transplanted organs can be found in Richard Selzer, "Whither thou goest," in *Imagine a Woman and Other Tales*, New York, Random House, 1990, pp. 3–28.

28. For a different view of the decision-making process see C. H. Fellner and J. R. Marshall, "Twelve kidney donors, *JAMA* 206 (Dec. 16, 1968): 2703–07, and by the same authors, "Kidney donors revisited," *Am J Psychiatry* 134 (1977): 711–14.

29. See Fox and Swazey, *The Courage to Fail*, pp. 5–39.

30. For details see Roberta G. Simmons, Susan Klein Marine, and Richard L. Simmons, *Gift of Life: The Effect of Organ Transplantation on Individual, Family, and Societal Dynamics*, (1977) reprint, New Brunswick, NJ, Transaction Books, 1987, pp. 153–97.

31. Personal interview with Patricia B., January 1994.

32. Fox and Swazey, *Spare Parts*, pp. 31–72. See also T. Parsons et al., "The 'gift of life' and its reciprocation," *Social Res* 39 (1972): 367–415. The classic anthropological study is Marcel Mauss, *The Gift: Forms and Foundations of Exchange in Archaic Societies*, trans. I. Cunnison, Glencoe, IL, Free Press, 1954.

33. A. J. Krakowski, "Hospital encroachment on the patient—dehumanizing effects of progress," *Public Health Rev* 10 (1982): 11–25.

34. Patricia B. interview, January 1994.

35. "UCSF: Mission and Goals," 1983, Archives and Special Collections, UCSF Library and Center for Knowledge Management (hereafter UCSF Archives).

36. An editorial entitled "Medical schools and hospitals" declared that "indeed, to a large extent, the hospital with its wards, its outpatient departments, its operating rooms, its dead-house and its laboratories, is the medical school," *JAMA* 35 (Aug. 25, 1900): 501.

37. W. H. Welch, "The relation of the hospital to medical education and research," *JAMA* 49 (Aug. 17, 1907): 531–34.

38. "A hospital under complete educational control is as necessary to a medical school as is the laboratory of chemistry or pathology." H. S. Pritchett, "Introduction," in Abraham Flexner, *Medical Education in the United States and Canada* (1910), reprint, New York, Arno Press, 1972, p. ix.

39. For background see W. B. Fye, "The origin of the full-time faculty system," *JAMA* 265 (Mar. 27, 1991): 1555–62.

40. Kenneth M. Ludmerer, *Learning to Heal*, New York, Basic Books, 1985, pp. 219–33.

41. W. Bauer, "The responsibility of the university hospital in the synthesis of medicine, science, and learning," *N Engl J Med* 265 (Dec. 28, 1961): 1292–98.

42. On Hill-Burton see H. Perlstadt, "The development of the Hill-Burton legislation: Interests, issues, and compromises," *J Health Soc Policy* 6 (1995): 77–96.

43. See, for example, H. Beecher, "Ethics and clinical research," *N Engl J Med* 274 (Jun. 16, 1966): 1354–60, and D. J. Rothman, "Ethics and human experimentation: Henry Beecher revisited," *N Engl J Med* 317 (Nov. 5, 1987): 1195–99.

44. J. H. Knowles, "Medical school, teaching hospital, and social responsibility, medicine's clarion call," in *The Teaching Hospital: Evolution and Contemporary Issues*, ed. J. H. Knowles, Cambridge, MA, Harvard Univ. Press, 1966, pp. 143 and 145. Knowles was director of the Massachusetts General Hospital, Harvard professor, and president of the Rockefeller Foundation. See also his "The balanced biology of the teaching hospital," *N Engl J Med* 269 (Aug. 22, 1963): 401–06 and 450–55.

45. As one author observed, "the designation 'hospital' apparently is no longer appropriate and is being replaced, wherever possible, by the term 'medical center' which is far more prestigious." M. B. Rosenblatt, "The medical center or the hospital," *Bull NY Acad Med* 47 (July 1971): 731.

46. A useful discussion concerning this paradigm and its possible substitution for another is S. A. Schroeder, "Expanding the site of clinical education: Moving beyond the hospital walls," *J Gen Intern Med* 3 (1988): 5–14.

47. See Terry Mizrahi, "Coping with patients: Subcultural adjustments to the conditions of work among internists-in-training," *Social Probl* 32 (1984): 154–66, and her book *Getting Rid of Patients*, New Brunswick, NJ, Rutgers Univ. Press, 1986. The legislation to curb the 120-hour week was adopted by New York State in 1989, in part as a result of the Libby Zion case. See Natalie Robins, *The Girl Who Died Twice: The Libby Zion Case and the Hidden Hazards of Hospitals*, New York, Delacorte Press, 1995.

48. M. J. Asken and D. C. Rahan, "Resident performance and sleep deprivation: A review," *J. Med Educ* 58 (1983): 382–88, G. W. Small, "House officer stress syndrome," *Psychosomatics* 22 (1981): 860–69, and J. H. Pfiffering, "Coping with residency distress," *Resident Staff Phys* 29 (1983): 105–11.

49. D. E. Rogers and R. J. Blendon, "The academic medical center: A stressed American institution," *N Engl J Med* 298 (Apr. 27, 1978): 940–50, J. K. Iglehart, "Moment of truth for the teaching hospital," *N Engl J Med* 307 (July 8, 1982): 132–36, and R. H. Ebert and S. S. Brown, "Academic health centers," *N Engl J Med* 308 (May 19, 1983): 1200–07.

50. For discussion of the issues see A. S. Relman, "Who will pay for medical education in our teaching hospitals?," *Science* 226 (Oct. 5, 1984): 20–23. See also Association of American Medical Colleges, *A Description of Teaching Hospital Characteristics*, Washington, DC, AMMC, 1982.

51. M. Fulop, "The teaching hospital's modern deathbed ritual," *N Engl J Med* 312 (Jan. 10, 1985): 125–26.

52. M. G. Goldfarb and R. S. Coffey, "Change in the Medicare case-mix index in the 1980s and the effect of the prospective system," *Health Serv Res* 27 (August 1992): 385–415, and L. Hughey Holt, "DRGs (Diagnostic Related Groups): The doctor's dilemma," *Perspect Biol Med* 29 (Winter 1986): 219–26.

53. J. K. Iglehart," Medicare begins prospective payment of hospitals," *N Engl J Med* 308 (Jun. 9, 1983): 1428–32, and S. S. Bergen, Jr., and A. C. Roth, "Prospective payment and the university hospital," *N Engl J Med* 310 (Feb. 1, 1984): 316–18.

54. E. P. Melia et al., "Competition in the health-care marketplace: A beginning in California," *N Engl J Med* 308 (Mar. 31, 1983): 788–92, and J. Hadley, "Medicaid reimbursement of teaching hospitals," *J Health Polit Policy Law* 7 (Winter 1983): 911–26.

55. C. J. Schramm, "The teaching hospital and the future role of state government," *N Engl J Med* 308 (Jan. 6, 1983): 41–45.

56. A. Sager, "Why urban voluntary hospitals close," *Health Serv Res* 18 (Fall 1983): 451–75.

57. E. Ginzberg, "The love affair is over," *UCSF Mag* 7 (1984): 42–47.

58. B. J. Culliton, "University hospitals for sale," *Science* 223 (Mar. 2, 1984): 909–11.

59. W. J. Schwartz et al., "Is the teaching hospital an endangered species?" *N Engl J Med* 313 (July 18, 1985): 157–62.

60. For information on Toland see F. T. Gardner, "The little acorn: Hugh Huger Toland, 1806–1880," *Bull Hist Med* 24 (1950): 61–69.

61. For information on the Toland Medical College consult "Editor's table," school an-

nouncements, and Toland's 1864 introductory lecture, in *Pacific Med J* 7 (September–October 1864): 296, 315–25, 373–75.

62. It still is unclear whether the desire for an academic hospital in San Francisco was related to the shortage of clinical facilities after the devastating 1906 earthquake. Most information regarding the early history of the UC Medical Department is available in the UC Archives at Berkeley. The History of Health Sciences Department at UCSF has a brief historical chronology (unpublished) composed by Günter B. Risse and Nancy Rockafellar. The information will soon be available on an Internet Website.

63. Documents concerning UC Hospital's physical plant, UCSF Archives, AR 87–40, folder 8.

64. Gov. Earl Warren, quoted in *SF Examiner* (May 12, 1996), p. A10.

65. Moffitt Hospital Administrative Records, 1954–1976, UCSF Archives, AR 82–2, folder 6.

66. Moffitt's Modernization Project, Legislative Analysts' Review, February 1974, UCSF Archives, AR 85–15, folder 14.

67. Hospital Modernization at UCSF, August–October 1973, UCSF Archives, AR 82–3, folder 27, and dn-2, 5:1.

68. Most existing campuses were deemed "hard-edged," composed of defined, static, and isolated structures, whereas the new architectural trends dictated "soft-edged," multiuse complexes scattered among free spaces and capable of allowing future expansion and easy remodeling. Ibid.

69. J. Kilgore Robinson, "A plan for the '80s," *UCSF J* (1982): 1–2. See also Inner Sunset Action Committee vs. Matthews, the Regents et al., UCSF Archives, AR 82–3, folder 29.

70. When asked by UC President Hitch what would happen if the funds were not forthcoming, Chancellor Sooy replied that "I'll have the greatest free-form sculpture you've ever seen," in *Conversations with Francis Adrian Sooy*, UCSF Campus Oral History Project, p. 35, also in UCSF Archives.

71. Personal interview with Marilyn Flood, July 1994.

72. "A university teaching hospital is different," *UCSF Mag* 6 (1983): 6–7. For materials related to Long Hospital's dedication see Hospital administration folder, UCSF Archives, AR 86–25.

73. Personal interview with Gloria B. Horns, transplant coordinator, May 1994.

74. Ibid

75. For extensive background consult Francis D. Moore, *Transplant: The Give and Take of Tissue Transplantation*, rev. ed., New York, Simon & Schuster, 1972. Another useful synthesis is J. B. Saunders, "A conceptual history of transplantation," in *Transplantation*, ed. J. S. Najarian and R. L. Simmons, Philadelphia, Lea & Febiger, 1972, pp. 3–25.

76. J. E. Murray, "Remembrances of the early days of renal transplantation," *Transplant Proc* 13 (1981): 9–15. For background about renal diseases see S. J. Peitzman, "From dropsy to Bright's disease to end-stage renal disease," *Milbank Q* 67, Suppl. 1 (1989): 16–32.

77. Both provided brief recollections of their achievement: J. E. Murray, "Remembrances of the early days of renal transplantation," *Transplant Proc* 13 (March 1981): 9–15, and "Discovery: Reflections on the first successful kidney transplantation," *World J Surg* 6 (1982): 372–76. More recently, Murray wrote "Human organ transplantation: Background and consequences," *Science* 256 (1992): 1411–15. See also J. P. Merrill, "The development of human kidney transplantation—personal recollections," *Pharos* 47 (1984): 22–24.

78. J. P. Merrill, "A historical perspective of renal transplantation," *Proc Clin Dial Transplant Forum* 9 (1979): 221–25.

79. D. Hamilton, "Kidney transplantation: A history," in *Kidney Transplantation: Principles and Practice*, ed. P. J. Morris, 3rd ed., Philadelphia, Saunders, 1988, pp. 1–13. Morris also published a brief overview: "Kidney transplantation, 1960–1990," *Adv Nephrol* 20 (1991): 3–17.

80. See C. G. Groth, "Landmarks in clinical renal transplantation," *Surg Gynecol Obstet* 134 (1972): 323–28, and for details see Leslie Brent, *A History of Transplantation Immunology*, San Diego, Academic Press, 1997.

81. T. E. Starzl, "The development of clinical renal transplantation," *Am J Kidney Dis* 16 (1990): 548–56.

82. Personal interview with Nancy L. Asher, director of the Transplantation Program, September 1993.

83. F. O. Belzer and O. Salvatierra, "Renal transplantation: Organ procurement, preservation, and surgical management," in *The Kidney*, ed. B. M. Brenner and F. C. Rector, Philadelphia, Saunders, 1976, vol. 2, pp. 1796–1818.

84. F. K. Merkel and O. Salvatierra, "Founding of the Society," in *History of the American Society of Transplant Surgeons*, ed. O. Salvatierra and C. T. Lum, Minneapolis, Stanton Pub. for American Society of Transplant Surgeons, 1994, pp. 1–24.

85. G. M. Williams, "Those early years," in Salvatierra and Lum, *History*, pp. 43–45.

86. National Commission for the Protection of Human Subjects of Biomedical and Behavioral Research, *The Belmont Report: Ethical Principles and Guidelines for the Protection of Human Subjects of Research*, Washington, DC, USGPO, 1978.

87. Starzl, *The Puzzle People*, p. 241. For a contemporary view see J. F. Childress, "Who shall live when not all can live?," *Soundings* 53 (1970): 339–55.

88. J. Cerilli, "The first ten years," in Salvatierra and Lum, *History*, pp. 357–59.

89. H. Balner and R. L. Marquet, "Transplantation biology—past and present: Reappraisal of 'breakthroughs' since 1955," *Transplant Proc* 13 (March 1981): 13–18.

90. Moore, *Transplant*, pp. 166–99.

91. F. O. Belzer, "Immunosuppressive agents—a personal historical perspective," *Transplant Proc* 20 (June 1988): 3–7.

92. B. D. Kahan, "Cosmas and Damian in the 20th century?" *N Engl J Med* 305 (July 30, 1981): 280–81, and M. E. DeBakey, "Cyclosporin A: A new era in organ transplantation," *Comprehensive Ther* 10 (1984): 7–15.

93. D. J. Cohen et al., "Cyclosporin: A new immunosuppressive agent for organ transplantation," *Ann Intern Med* 101 (November 1984): 667–82.

94. Personal interview with William J. Amend, Jr., April 1994.

95. A brief history of the service can be found in N. L. Asher and A. S. Peele, "Transplantation at the University of California, San Francisco," *The Chimera* (ASTS) 4 (November 1992), No. 3: 1, 11–13.

96. J. S. Najarian et al., "Ten year experience with renal transplantation in juvenile onset diabetes," *Ann Surg* 190 (1979): 487.

97. F. O. Belzer and O. Salvatierra, "The organization of an effective cadaver renal transplantation program," *Transplant Proc* 6 (1974): 93–97.

98. Amend interview, April 1994. More information was provided by Oscar Salvatierra in an unpublished 1994 testimonial to Amend.

99. Personal interview with Oscar Salvatierra, June 1994.

100. Amend interview, April 1994.

101. O. Salvatierra et al., "Analysis of costs and outcomes of renal transplantation at one center," *JAMA* 241 (Apr. 6, 1979): 1469–73.

102. See, for example, O. Salvatierra, "Demographic and transplantation trends among minority groups," *Transplant Proc* 21 (1989): 391–96, and N. J. Feduska et al., "Cadaver

kidney transplantation provided from one center within a large geographical region," *Trans Am Soc Artif Intern Organs* 24 (1978): 270–77. More recently see C. M. Kjellstrand, "Age, sex and race inequality in renal transplantation," *Arch Intern Med* 148 (1988): 1305–09.

103. O. Salvatierra et al., "1500 renal transplants at one center: Evolution of a strategy for optimal success, " *Am J Surg* 142 (July 1981): 14–20.

104. O. Salvatierra et al., "Update of the University of California at San Francisco experience with donor-specific blood transfusions," *Transplant Proc* 14 (1982): 363–66, and N. J. Feduska et al., "Donor-specific transfusions prior to renal transplantation in diabetic recipients," *Transplant Proc* 17 (1985): 1066–68.

105. Melzer interview, April 1994.

106. For more details see the forthcoming collection of oral history interviews featuring UCSF surgeons in the post–World War II years conducted via the UCSF Campus Oral History Program, UCSF Archives.

107. Personal interview with Rudi Schmid, former dean of the Medical School, April 1994.

108. Salvatierra interviews, August 1993 and June 1994; *Congressional Record*, 98th Cong., 1st sess., 1984. In a letter to Chancellor Krevans dated February 27, 1986, Gore referred to Salvatierra as "the driving force behind the passage and enforcement of the National Organ Transplantation Act." Personal communication with Salvatierra.

109. Renal Transplant Center, 1975–1979, UCSF Archives, AR 83–2, folder 16.

110. Personal interview with Nancy P., January 1994.

111. Ibid.

112. Faith T. interview, January 1994.

113. S. R. Leighow, "Backrubs vs. Bach," *Nurs Hist Rev* 4 (1996): 3–17.

114. Susan Reverby, "A caring dilemma: Womanhood and nursing in historical perspective," *Nurs Res* 36 (1987): 5–11, and by the same author *Ordered to Care: The Dilemma of American Nursing, 1850–1945*, New York, Cambridge Univ. Press, 1987.

115. P. A. Prescott and S. A. Bowen, "Physician–nurse relationships," *Ann Intern Med* 103 (1985): 127–33. For an update see L. I. Stein et al., "The doctor–nurse game revisited," *N Engl J Med* 322 (Feb. 22, 1990): 546–49. See also S. Bunting and J. Campbell, "Feminism and nursing: Historical perspectives," *Adv Nurs Sci* 12 (1990): 11–24.

116. See, for example, M. M. Jackson, "From ritual to reason—with a rational approach for the future: An epidemiological perspective," *Am J Infect Control* 12 (1984): 213–20.

117. G. R. Winslow, "From loyalty to advocacy: A new metaphor for nursing," *Hastings Center Rep* 14 (June 1984): 32–40.

118. Toward the end of her hospitalization even Faith, who had quarreled with her caregivers, finally made peace with Melzer, with whom she had feuded for weeks, offering her a stuffed animal.

119. Starzl, *The Puzzle People*, p. 141.

120. I attended two of these rounds in April 1984 at the invitation of Melzer and Amend. See A. Arluke, "Roundsmanship: Inherent control on a medical ward," *Soc Sci Med* 14A (1980): 297–302.

121. R. C. Friedman et al., "Psychological problems associated with sleep deprivation in interns," *J Med Ed* 48 (1973): 436–41.

122. Amend interview, April 1994.

123. A useful overview of the issues is J. J. Mathews, "The communication process in clinical settings," *Soc Sci Med* 17 (1983): 1371–78.

124. For an informative analysis of these relationships see Cecilia M. Roberts, *Doctor and Patient in the Teaching Hospital: A Tale of Two Life-Worlds*, Lexington, MA, Lexington Books, 1977.

125. Personal interview with Peggy Devney, April 1994.

126. Personal interview with Roger M. Lauer, psychiatric consultant to the Transplantation Service, June 1994. This issue is discussed in Anne Hunsaker Hawkins, *Reconstructing Illness: Studies in Pathography*, West Lafayette, IN, Purdue Univ. Press, 1993, pp. 31–60.

127. M. Chambers, "Psychological aspects of renal transplantation," *Int J Psychiatry Med* 12 (1982–83): 232.

128. Patricia B. interview, January 1994.

129. Ibid.

130. M. A. Brandt, "Consider the patient part of a family," *Nurs Forum* 21 (1984): 19–23.

131. M. Chambers, "Psychological aspects of renal transplantation," *Int J Psych Med* 12 (1982): 229–36.

132. S. H. Basch, "Damaged self-esteem and depression in organ transplantation" *Transplant Proc* 5 (1973): 1125–27.

133. Devney interview, April 1994, and another with Pastora Blessing, August 1994.

134. Faith T. interview, January 1994.

135. Patricia B. interview, January 1994.

136. A. C. Novello and D. N. Sundwall, "Current organ transplantation legislation: An update," *Transplant Proc* 17 (1985): 1585–91.

137. Starzl, *The Puzzle People*, p. 280. For another recent history of organ transplantation see Calvin Stiller, *Lifegifts: The Real Story of Transplants*, Toronto, Stoddart, 1990.

138. For details see John Kilner, *Ethical Criteria in Patient Selection: Who Lives? Who Dies?* New Haven, Yale Univ. Press, 1990.

139. R. B. Fetter, "Diagnosis-related groups: The product of the hospital," *Clin Res* 32 (1984): 336–40, and J. E. Wennberg et al., "Will payment based on diagnosis-related groups control hospital costs?" *N Engl J Med* 311 (Aug. 2, 1984): 295–300.

140. E. J. Halloran and M. Kiley, "The nurses' role and length of stay," *Med Care* 23 (September 1985): 1122–26.

141. Devney and Horns interviews, April and May 1994, respectively.

142. R. C. Fox, "Afterthoughts: Continuing reflections on organ transplantation," in *Organ Transplantation: Meanings and Realities*, ed. S. J. Youngner, R. C. Fox, and L. J. O'Connell, Madison, Univ. of Wisconsin Press, 1996, pp. 252–72.

143. R. J. Howard and J. S. Najarian, "Organ transplantation—medical perspective," in *Encyclopedia of Bioethics*, ed. W. T. Reich, New York, Free Press, 1978, vol. 3, p. 1165. For an update consult C. R. Stiller, "Organ and tissue transplants—medical overview," in ibid., rev. ed., New York, Macmillan, 1995, vol. 4, pp. 1871–82.

144. D. J. Rothman, "The international organ traffic," *NY Rev Books* 45 (Mar. 26, 1998): 14–17. See also Andrew Schneider and Mary P. Flaherty, *The Challenge of a Miracle: Selling the Gift*, Pittsburgh, Pittsburgh Press, 1985, and more recently Margaret J. Radin, *Contested Commodities*, Cambridge, MA, Harvard Univ. Press, 1996.

145. P. A. Ubel et al., "Rationing failure: The ethical lessons of the retransplantation of scarce vital organs," *JAMA* 270 (Nov. 24, 1993): 2469–74.

146. S. A. Schroeder, "A comparison of Western European and U.S. university hospitals," *JAMA* 252 (July 13, 1984): 240.

147. A. Seelye, "Hospital ward layout and nurse staffing," *J Adv Nurs* 7 (1982): 195–201.

148. Faith T. interview, January 1994.

149. Patricia B. interview, January 1994.

150. A. Spital and R. Spital, "The living kidney donor, alive and well," *Arch Intern Med* 146 (October 1986): 1993–96.

151. Faith T. interview, January 1994.

152. Starzl, *The Puzzle People*, p. 339.

12

CARING FOR THE
INCURABLE

AIDS at San Francisco
General Hospital

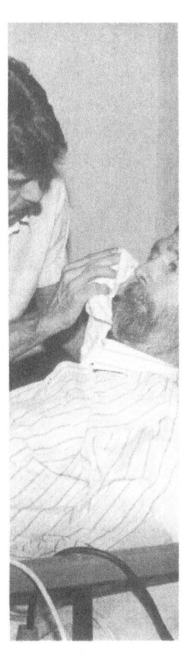

I became a patient here on 5 B last Saturday. I was overjoyed to become a part of this spirited community. This is a haven. I am lucky. I am on a spiritual high and determined to keep my optimism and humor till the end. With these marvelous healers all about me, it should be easy.

J. S. Selby[1]

An early AIDS portrait: "Warren"

By early 1984, while Faith, Patty, and Nancy were receiving dialysis treatments, the San Francisco gay community was in turmoil. For about three years, a growing number of its members had been coming down with what appeared to be a new disease with severe and protean clinical manifestations. Doctors called it *AIDS*, an acronym for the medical term *acquired immune deficiency syndrome*. This scientific label described a progressive loss of immunity responsible for a host of infections and cancers ending in death. Since the 1960s a favorite destination for hippies and gays, San Francisco was turning into a graveyard for many of its vibrant young newcomers. Victims of some still poorly understood disorder that robbed them of their inner defenses, some gay men were wilting and shrinking.

They became pale caricatures of themselves in a crowd of men who loved to show off their sculpted bodies.

As the number of AIDS cases mounted, the region's most widely read gay newspaper printed its first obituary in March 1983. This section quickly became a regular feature, scanned by apprehensive readers who wanted to keep track of acquaintances and personalities in the community. In sharp contrast to San Francisco's leading newspapers, which artfully concealed the cause of death, the *Bay Area Reporter* began publishing brief but vivid biographical sketches written by friends and family members openly disclosing AIDS as the reason for the demise. Rather than creating a panic, the writers intended to "out" the deceased in terms of this new disease as part of summing up and validating the lives of those they loved. Instead of being banished once more to their closets with formal obituaries, the dead were often sketched in intimate terms, their lives portrayed as meaningful and symbolic of a stigmatized community determined to overcome another crisis.[2] AIDS indeed challenged a set of widely assumed American expectations: a long life, pursuit of happiness, control of infectious diseases, and the invisibility of death. One eyewitness lamented that "we ought not to have to worry about dying, for God's sake. Instead, our worries should concern simple things—whether to buy Skip or Jiffy. Thanks to AIDS our choices are no longer simple. We no longer have control over what we are expected to deal with."[3]

Such obituaries commonly recalled the courage and strength as well as the *joie de vivre* and humor displayed by those who had fallen victim to AIDS. As the new disease assumed epidemic proportions, many young gay males were grudgingly coming to terms with the clinical uncertainties and lack of effective treatments. As anxious readers glancing at these announcements wondered whether it soon would be their turn to fall ill, the stories—like the AIDS quilt—testified that those who were dying did so with dignity and class. In fact, to further stress the nobility of their suffering and death, military metaphors represented AIDS patients as engaging in heroic "battles" with the disease. They were often portrayed as faithful foot soldiers felled in the service of their cause, at war with a scourge that threatened the very survival of the gay community.[4] "They did the best they could," insisted one writer. "They may not have achieved immortality but what the hell, they tried. It is as fitting an epitaph as any."[5]

Among them was Warren J., a writer, performer, and book illustrator, who also worked as a volunteer at the Harvey Milk Archive. Originally from Oak Ridge, Tennessee, the 34-year-old man played the piano, danced and acted, designed and sketched. He had graduated from the University of North Carolina with a degree in theater arts. Like many young gay men Warren came from a traditional family, although his parents were now divorced. His father had remarried and worked as a nuclear engineer at the Oak Ridge power plant, while his mother remained a homemaker. In 1975, at a conference in Florida, Warren had met Kelly H., and they began a 10-year relationship during which they often lived together, especially after moving to San Francisco in the early 1980s. In a sense, they were both latecomers to a city that for almost two decades had welcomed an expanding gay population emptying the closets of America.[6]

Indeed, by 1980, the city was seen as the gay capital of the country, if not the world, home to about 100,000 mostly young gay males—nearly one out of every five city adults—spreading out in all directions from the heart of the Castro district in Eureka Valley that they now claimed as their own. In an unprecedented migration, more than half had moved to San Francisco during the 1970s, lured by its history of tolerance for a broad spectrum of lifestyles and behaviors. By the late 1970s, the gay community had diligently re-created the institutions of small-town America, sponsoring more than 150 civic and religious organizations, publishing nine newspapers, and supporting three Democratic political clubs. At the time of Warren's arrival, gays wielded great political and economic power, although the wrenching events surrounding Harvey Milk's assassination in 1978 and the manslaughter conviction of his murderer that ended in a riot had widened traditional divisions.[7]

Warren's new home town, the Castro, was Oz, a refuge for the persecuted tribe and a symbol of gay liberation. The new shock troops of urban renewal had assisted San Francisco's transition from a manufacturing city to one with an economic base in the financial and service industries. Originally a decaying working-class neighborhood populated by Irish and German immigrants, Eureka Valley had lured newcomers because of its affordable housing. Soon gentrified, the restored, colorful Victorian houses on the slopes of Twin Peaks were populated by mostly single white men. As Warren explored the area's numerous bars, restaurants, stores, and book shops, he became aware that the Castro was now an exclusive gay turf and an overwhelmingly male enclave in a city of distinct, ethnically diverse neighborhoods. The prevailing dress code was a combination of cowboy and lumberjack attire, with plaid shirts, blue jeans, hiking boots, leather vests, and tweed or bomber jackets. With their short hair and sunglasses, "Castro clones" wearing such outfits erotically showed off their fit bodies as they cruised the strip.[8]

A critical component of the new gay identity being forged was sexual liberation. While gay sexual mores had a long tradition, the self-contained nature of the San Francisco gay community tended to amplify their impact. The explosive celebration of newly won freedoms expressed itself spasmodically in parades and all-night parties. Recreational drug use was common. The result was a high level of sexual activity and experimentation taking place in "meat palaces" such as bars, bath houses, and sex clubs mostly scattered in the "Valley of the Kings," the old warehouse district south of Market Street. In this carnival atmosphere, close to half of the sexually active males admitted to or boasted contact with at least 500 partners, while close to a third claimed to have had over a 1,000. Many believed that diseases such as gonorrhea and syphilis—rampant, according to San Francisco's Health Department—were necessary admission fees for pleasure. "Besides, what did it matter if we got sick?" declared one of them. "Penicillin fixed everything."[9]

Following his arrival in San Francisco, Warren also tasted the fast-track world of sex and drugs before settling down with one partner, his friend Kelly. In late 1981 and early 1982, however, he frequently became ill. At first he experienced recurrent minor symptoms such as swollen lymph nodes, night sweats, bouts of abdominal cramps and diarrhea, followed by weight loss. Like other sexually active gay males in San Francisco, he was not overly alarmed. In the late 1970s, the incidence of sexually transmitted diseases in San Francisco, including hepatitis B and bowel conditions such as giardiasis and amebiasis, was increasing, and it was starting to concern private physicians and public health officials, including medical detective Selma Dritz.[10] In 1980, Dritz noted the dramatic rise in these conditions in all major metropolitan centers of the country with a significant gay population and called for public education to create greater awareness of the problem among caregivers and citizens. Paradoxically, such a proposal had the potential to stigmatize further the new gay communities. According to Dritz, the proper solution was to involve them directly in the endeavor.[11]

Like other young gay men in San Francisco with similar complaints and no health insurance, Warren sought medical care at the Haight-Ashbury Free Clinic, making his first visit on August 8, 1982. Going to a clinic was a fact of life for many liberated gay males, fostering a sense of camaraderie and solidarity. Following a radiological examination of his gastrointestinal tract, which was reported as normal, the attending physicians made a tentative diagnosis of irritable bowel syndrome. To guard against a possible infection, Warren was given sulfa drugs, followed by a course of another medication for possible parasitic infection—giardiasis—now commonly referred to as "gay bowel disease."[12] But by December 1983, his general condition had deteriorated enough to warrant hospitalization at the City and County of San Francisco General Hospital (SFGH), where he was admitted with a diagnosis of AIDS.

During his extended stay at SFGH's new 5 B ward, Warren spoke often about his reactions to AIDS. Like other gay men suffering from this fatal illness, Warren complained that he had failed to leave a legacy. Dying young before he had accomplished something meaningful concerned him. Lacking a religious framework that could endow his suffering with meaning and purpose, he turned to education. The story of his encounter with this senseless and cruel disease would give Warren's brief life the significance he craved. "He was convinced that he had not made a mark in the world," recalled Kelly.[13] Soon, Warren's mind was made up. His experiences with AIDS would help others who had contracted the disease. He went on to assist the hospital staff in confronting issues surrounding AIDS care and dying and also spent considerable time on the telephone, reassuring other members of the gay community. As the illness took its toll, however,

Warren was unable to document his own story and became receptive to the idea that his life and struggle with AIDS be written by a friend. Bearing witness to the impact of AIDS on his life would be part of the chronicle of this epidemic.[14]

At this time, half of the deaths from AIDS still occurred at home, where relatives and friends gathered for "life" or "farewell" parties. Under those circumstances, most recalled the salient experiences of their brief lives, especially the move to San Francisco from faraway places in the Northeast, Midwest, and South. This was what Warren had wanted, but in spite of his own wishes, he died at the hospital in April 1984. Following his death, a friend wrote a play about Warren's and his peers' experiences as AIDS patients, based on a series of interviews she had conducted with patients and caregivers at SFGH. The play, Warren's legacy and validation of his courage and compassion, was first produced at the Seven Stages theater in Atlanta in August 1984, then moved for the next two years to Los Angeles and Iowa. Not surprisingly, the setting for *Warren* was the so-called AIDS ward at SFGH.[15]

San Francisco General Hospital: Tradition and evolution

Warren's destination, San Francisco's "General," had a history stretching back to the early days of California's fabled gold rush.[16] On July 18, 1857, the first establishment began admitting patients in an old schoolhouse located in North Beach at the corner of Stockton and Francisco Streets.[17] In 1864, Hugh Toland, president of the nearby proprietary medical college that would become UCSF, offered to run the 150-bed hospital. Following protracted negotiations, Toland and his faculty received permission a year later to use the facilities for clinical instruction. Not surprisingly, the move generated public opposition. People feared that physicians would experiment on patients and that inexperienced students would cause harm. This small facility nonetheless became so overcrowded in the 1860s that the authorities decided to build a new hospital. As with other contemporary institutions such as Johns Hopkins and Eppendorf, its design followed the pavilion plan, with separate wards linked by a covered walkway. The new 400-bed establishment, located south of the city's center near Potrero Hill, opened on August 27, 1872. Although fears of human experimentation were periodically voiced, a new agreement was reached in 1873 with the former Toland Medical College, now the Medical Department of the University of California, to have the institution also serve as a clinical facility for the training of medical students.

By 1896 the all-wood building had become inadequate, even dangerous, given the growing demand for care.[18] Wrote John Williamson, the director of the facilities: "for a quarter of a century they have served as a refuge for every known form of disease. They are saturated with filth and impregnated with germs. They are a menace to the health of the community in which they are located. They are a disgrace to civilization and an ulcer upon the municipality."[19] Following the 1906 earthquake, as bubonic plague broke out in the obsolete hospital, plans for a replacement site oscillated between the Laguna Honda Almshouse tract and the original Potrero location. Property owners in the Mission district, hoping to turn the old site into a park, favored the distant setting at Laguna Honda. Patient demand, however, came from the central population centers of the city closer to the Potrero site. The ground was higher, and the area was sunnier and warmer than the windswept west. The original site having been chosen, the old, rat-infested building was officially condemned in September 1907 and burned down a few months later.[20]

Seven years later, the new SFGH had risen from the ashes of the old and was officially dedicated on May 1, 1915. Built for approximately $3.5 million, which had been raised through municipal bonds, the 700-bed, steel-frame hospital complex consisted of 10 main buildings on the pavilion plan, although by now that building style had become nearly obsolete elsewhere in the country.[21] Each four-story building was linked by a system of underground tunnels. The entire nine-acre area was enclosed by an iron grill fence and lighted at night by about 40 ornamental electroliers.[22] Less than a decade later, however, these splendid facilities were again hopelessly overcrowded, and long waiting lists greeted those who wished to enter. Most inmates were chronically ill indigents who remained in the institution for long periods of time.[23] In the 1930s, efforts were made to transfer them to the city's almshouse and use the facilities for particular populations with specific diseases and social needs.[24] Further expansions and the creation of ambulatory clinics helped to improve conditions until the end of World War II.

Like most municipal hospitals, SFGH began to decline during the 1950s as the middle class migrated to the suburbs. Uninsured patients from private institutions were dumped there. The ensuing erosion of the city's tax base contributed to the fiscal deterioration of municipal government, causing cutbacks in medical services. Political interference jeopardized the professional autonomy of SFGH's administration. In spite of repeated calls for reform, the hospital was also hampered by antiquated governance and Byzantine purchasing requirements. As a large institution housing patients supported by public and charitable funds, SFGH had developed a productive relationship with the two local medical schools, UCSF and Stanford, acquiring an academic medical staff and a capable house staff. Given San Francisco's municipal conditions, however, there was concern that funds provided by medical schools for teaching students and residents were actually being spent in patient care. With the support of the presidents of UC and Stanford University, as well as hospital officials and members of the city's Public Health Department, demands to modernize medical care were made to the local authorities. However, the San Francisco Board of Supervisors rejected a three-year plan to reallocate funds.

In 1959, Stanford University ended its long relationship with SFGH when it moved all its operations south to an area near Palo Alto. Even UCSF threatened to sever its own affiliation. The impending crisis prompted a new agreement between the City and County of San Francisco and the UC Medical School. As part of this affiliation, the university would provide medical supervision and instruction at the General, while the city continued to furnish the necessary nursing and support services. As Ellis D. Sox, director of San Francisco's Public Health Department, reported, the newly forged partnership guaranteed that SFGH patients would receive the best possible medical care at the least possible expense to the taxpayer.[25]

Beginning in 1960, SFGH embarked on a vigorous program to change its image and its mission. Instead of a typical county institution caring for all types of patients, half of them afflicted with chronic diseases, the hospital was to become an active medical center providing acute medical and surgical care to medically indigent residents of the city.[26] At one level, this required substantial patient transfers to other facilities and the organization of home care programs for the chronically ill. More important, the hospital expanded its medical and nursing staffs, developed more ambulatory facilities, and created adequate clinical and laboratory facilities. The last were gradually provided under contracts with UCSF, including programs such as intensive care, a premature baby clinic, and neurosurgery. However, the passage of Medicare legislation in 1965 threatened the continued viability of SFGH, like that of urban public hospitals throughout the country, losing many of the qualifying elderly patients to private institutions. On the other hand, by providing reimbursement schemes for health care services to the elderly, disabled, and needy, the federal government in the mid-1960s further accelerated the transformation of SFGH into a modern community hospital serving the acute medical needs of all sectors of the city.[27]

Given SFGH's obsolete and decaying physical facilities, a fateful decision was made in 1965 to build a new Medical Center at the heart of the hospital complex. Supported by city and university authorities and financed by a state bond issue, plans continued despite the strong objections of the San Francisco Medical Society, whose members feared the increased competition. As Medicare patients exited the institution, they were replaced by injury and drug victims requiring emergency care. By 1972, a new Trauma Service came into existence as new techniques, including ventilators and intravenous fluids, became lifesaving procedures available for patient management around the clock.[28] While SFGH struggled to modernize in the early 1970s, lack of municipal funds to hire the necessary specialized staff prompted strikes by nurses and house staff, forcing the Joint Commission on Accreditation of Hospitals to place the institution on probation. A string of assertive nursing directors were particularly active, concerned about the quality of hospital care and thus forging new roles for the nurses in clinical decision making.[29] SFGH was hampered by its divided city, state, federal, and university governance and financing schemes. Facing significant budgetary shortfalls, the hospital continued to drift amid calls from health planners to stop the new construction and close the entire complex as high vacancy rates developed in nearby private San Francisco institutions.[30]

In spite of setbacks and delays, SFGH's new 584-bed Medical Center was officially dedicated on July 19, 1976. An outstanding design feature of the building was the "stacking" of all emergency and critical-care departments and the linkage of these ward units by high-speed elevators and conveyor systems.[31] Soon this modern facility attracted Medicare and Medi-Cal patients who had previously gone to other institutions. However, the federal revenue could not offset the devastating budget cuts in 1978, following the statewide approval of Proposition 13 limiting California property taxes. Mass resignations of nurses and other layoffs followed, and accreditation was suspended. SFGH fought hard to survive. In the end, the institution succeeded because of its modern facilities, university-affiliated medical staff, and outstanding nursing, all providing state-of-the-art care in the increasingly competitive hospital marketplace.

By the early 1980s, as Warren and his friends cruised the Castro, public hospitals across the country were in critical condition. In California, nearly half of the county institutions had closed since 1964.[32] Although San Francisco was "overbedded," SFGH provided services to the working poor, the unemployed who failed to qualify for welfare, and the vast number of underinsured, undocumented immigrants who were ineligible for public assistance.[33] Public hospitals such as SFGH were being flooded with charity patients, fruits of President Reagan's economic recession and the steady decline in private insurance coverage.[34] Members of the city's Board of Supervisors continued to grumble about the hospital's $20 million annual budget, but they and the citizens were well aware that they were getting a bargain. A major reason was the hospital's long-standing affiliation with UCSF. Financial and technical university support linked SFGH to cutting-edge basic and clinical research. In addition to developing a first-rate trauma center, the university had obtained private and public grants for research laboratories at this public hospital. These included the Gladstone Institute for Cardiovascular Disease, the Rosalind Russell Arthritis Institute, the Gallo Institute for studies on alcoholism, and the Lung Biology Center.[35]

At the same time, contract services allowed UCSF to maintain its powerful clinical and teaching presence in the hospital. In return for excellent opportunities for teaching medical students, interns, and residents—there were 185 in 1983—the university continued to provide clinical services. In that year 175 full-time UCSF faculty members were based at General, supplemented by 350 volunteer clinical attending physicians. Training programs enabled SFGH to staff its wards and clinics at lower salaries than those paid by other institutions contracting with full-time specialists. Although viewed as clinical material, patients received excellent medical care—paid for by both Medicare and Medi-Cal—that employed sophisticated but costly technology.[36]

Fixed payment rates for health care services under Medicare in 1983 and California's new Medicaid regulations offering competitive contracts to hospitals also affected SFGH, accentuating the two-tier health care system prevailing in the United States.[37] This new contract, and the transfer of the medically indigent from state to county facilities in that same year, swelled the hospital's population. At the same time, the institution became the destination for a number of Medi-Cal and even paying patients referred for specialized care under contracts with UCSF. This connection was to include Warren—suffering from the new scourge known as AIDS.[38] Indeed, the newly established clinic devoted to the treatment of AIDS patients was to be cited as a shining example of positive relationships between SFGH and UCSF and their caregivers.[39] As a result of these important academic linkages, SFGH became widely known as the best public hospital in the country.[40]

Framing AIDS in the early 1980s: Lifestyle, cancer, or infection?

While Warren's symptoms brought him into contact with a primary care facility, other gay men sought out local dermatologists to treat their multiple purple-brown skin spots, diagnosed as Kaposi's sarcoma (KS), a rare form of cancer. This condition had previously been observed only in older men or individuals taking immunosuppressive drugs. The rapidly growing lesions were starkly visible on the arms, legs, and chest and disfigured the handsome faces of youthful sufferers. Early in 1981, Marcus Conant, a UCSF clinical professor of dermatology, began seeing several cases of KS in young men, as did colleagues in Los Angeles and New York. Similar experiences were recorded by Paul Volberding, a young UCSF oncologist, who came to SFGH in July. The lesions spread quite rapidly, and the condition seemed fatal. KS had first been reported by an Austrian dermatologist, Moritz Kaposi, in 1872, based on the study of five patients seen between 1868 and 1871. Kaposi believed that the disease was lethal within two or three years, and that the tumors could affect internal organs as well as the skin.[41] Until the 1950s, only about 600 cases of KS had been reported in the world literature. However, the true incidence and prevalence of the disease remained a puzzle, with only biopsy-confirmed skin lesions usually recorded. A link to homosexuality was never probed. In any event, fears about the social and legal consequences of publicly admitting such a sexual preference would have made it almost impossible to ascertain such a link.[42]

In the developed world KS had already been linked in the 1970s to immunosuppression in cases of organ transplantation, especially kidney implants such as those sought by Faith, Nancy, and Patty. However, discontinuance of such drug-induced states often reversed the development of the tumors. To assess the new situation, a KS workshop took place at UCSF on September 15, 1981, to evaluate these patients and attempt to treat them with chemotherapy.[43] In early December, at the annual meeting of the American Academy of Dermatology held at the Moscone Center in San Francisco, Conant and others distributed the first pamphlet about this new and more aggressive variety of the disease.[44] In rapid succession over the next few months, about 80 cases were reported nationally and the homosexual linkage was made explicit, fueling fears that a veritable epidemic of "gay cancer" was in the making.[45]

At the same time and in the same urban centers, physicians, some of them specializing in infectious diseases, encountered other young men suffering from fever, weight loss, and respiratory symptoms. Many were diagnosed as having a pneumonia caused by *Pneumocystis carinii*, a usually nonvirulent protozoan, discovered in 1910.[46] More recently, however, this organism had been found to cause virulent pneumonia in individuals suffering from leukemia, usually children, who had been medically immunosuppressed in the course of treatment. More important, some of these patients with pneumonia, all of them gay, also suffered from KS and other opportunistic infections such as candidiasis, herpes zoster virus, and cytomegalovirus disease.[47] The so-called gay bowel syndrome, in turn, encompassed a variety of conditions ranging from parasitic infestations to herpes and other sexually transmitted ailments. Included in the etiologic mix was the widespread use of recreational drugs among most patients afflicted by these conditions. The most prominent were legally sold nitrates that enhanced orgasm when inhaled, popularly known as *poppers*.[48] At this point, both cancers and infections were associated with the immunologic effects of an unknown process or condition seemingly connected to the gay lifestyle.[49]

Historically, the construction of a new disease model is a complex process, with many participants, including physicians, scientists, nurses, epidemiologists, and politicians, as well as the patients and the public at large. Often the initial framing is clinical, involving the sick, those around them, and the medical professionals being consulted. The traditional goals are to collect information on the various complaints and to recognize physical manifestations capable of being linked to existing clinical conditions, biological understandings, and social judgments. Next, physicians attempt to find categorical relationships between the new information and the previously known medical conditions. In this instance, cancers such as KS and opportunistic infections were related to a state of lowered cellular immunity.[50] While the total inventory of signs and symptoms remained blurred, a consensus had been created among caregivers to label the new condition. This action was critical for the disease to achieve nosological status and social validation. Giving a name to the new condition also summoned needed diagnostic and therapeutic services, facilitated scientific research, and allowed standard collection of data for epidemiological purposes. References to a *gay plague* and—early in 1982—*gay-related immunodeficiency* (GRID) were common responses.[51] In March 1983, the acronym AIDS was used to describe the central dysfunction perceived to be responsible for the broad spectrum of disease manifestations, a scientific framing of the disorder based on clinical laboratory studies.[52]

The fact that AIDS patients were male, gay, and sexually active immediately suggested that the new syndrome was another sexually transmitted disease like gonorrhea and syphilis, a fact that linked AIDS to the moral stigma attached to them. At this time, homosexuality was no longer considered a psychiatric condition. As the gay liberation movement proclaimed sexuality as a key attribute of their members' newly constructed identity, it also suggested that gays were susceptible to a particular constellation of diseases, just as ethnic groups could suffer from their own specific ailments. From a medical point of view, then, being gay meant that certain conditions like the cancers and bowel infections could be legitimately characterized as *gay bowel* and *gay cancer* diseases associated with lifestyle and perhaps even as an altered physical constitution that was responsible for the immunological failure.[53]

While scientists studied the characteristics and causes of this presumed immunological exhaustion as well as a possible retroviral etiology, a parallel epidemiological framework placed the available clinical observations within the context of environment and society. Why was this disease appearing now? Where was it coming from? Had a nasty bug been introduced into the United States or was it the result of a random mutation of existing microorganisms? What role did demographic and social factors such as gay life play? Here again, definitions of risk groups and behaviors were informed by existing biases concerning the gay lifestyle.[54] Sexual activity was much more visible and socially acceptable in the gay community than in the larger society, but its vaunted frequency was probably exaggerated by many gay men.

Gradually, over the following year, a complex web of causality was established linking lifestyle, homosexuality, anal sex, drug use, and previous venereal disease as being cumulatively responsible for AIDS. In June 1982, an article about opportunistic infections and immune deficiency in homosexual men appeared, bringing all these factors together.[55] Identified among other infectious agents were *Pneumocystis carinii*, *Cryptococcus neoformans*, and *Candida albicans*. Medical authors wondered whether the immune deficiency was initiated by the host's response to an infectious agent or was simply the consequence of the gay lifestyle, which gradually damaged and eventually destroyed the human immune system.[56]

All these scientific, clinical, and epidemiological constructions of AIDS were linked to cultural and social frameworks that sought to provide meaning for the new phenomena.[57] Since clinical researchers concentrated their studies on the gay men who had first come to their attention, part of this scaffolding was based on the notion that homosexual promiscuity and drug abuse were to blame.[58] Indeed, the epidemiological data confirmed that gay males who had engaged in more frequent sexual encounters were at greater risk. Hypothetical linkages between the perceived amorality of anonymous sex and the new disease tended to further discredit AIDS sufferers, already shunned because of their homosexuality.[59] On the positive side, such stigmatization ultimately helped to rally the gay community around AIDS sufferers, creating greater awareness about the health implications of being gay and sexually active.[60] As popular perception of the existence of AIDS increased, weird notions concerning its origins and routes of transmission emerged, based in part on contradictory scientific information distorted and sensationalized by the media. Were evangelical Christians right when they postulated that AIDS was God's punishment for what they viewed as a perversion? Some members of the gay community resorted to paranoia, believing in a government plot, a form of germ warfare designed by the Reagan administration to suppress the gay lifestyle. Was this a conspiracy involving the FBI or the CIA? A widespread rumor believed by Warren and his friends was that AIDS had resulted from a faulty laboratory experiment in genetic engineering, leading to the creation of an artificial and nefarious superbug that, like the Andromeda strain, had accidentally escaped or been deliberately allowed to escape from its flask to doom a particular sector of humankind.[61]

From the start, the new disease entity was also enmeshed in a variety of political frameworks. In formulating policies, different levels of government, foundations, health professional groups, and community organizations rapidly focused on AIDS sufferers as potential dangers to public health.[62] In assigning blame for the appearance of AIDS, history seemed to repeat itself in San Francisco. During the 1900 bubonic plague in the city, the authorities had focused on its stigmatized Chinese inhabitants, holding them responsible for introducing and spreading the epidemic. Linkages with promiscuity, poor hygiene, and drug abuse were established. Constitutional weakness and filthy living habits were held to be responsible for the appearance of the scourge, leading to the quarantine of the entire ethnic neighborhood, Chinatown.[63]

Based on the early evidence, the American response focused narrowly on the homosexual connection, even though AIDS was already perceived to be overwhelmingly heterosexual in most other regions of the world, especially in Africa. The early assumption was that this epidemic was another temporary mystery, like Legionnaire's disease, soon to be resolved and thus contained. The first formal move made by the public health authorities was in July 1981, when the Centers for Disease Control (CDC) sounded the alarm over the emergence of KS in its monthly bulletin.[64] But how could AIDS sufferers be monitored and controlled?

Local and state governments responded by activating existing public health protocols and bureaucracies. Traditional epidemiological data collection and enforcement procedures such as compulsory contact tracing and segregation were suggested. However, many procedures were now at odds with recently hard-won civil libertarian standards of privacy and due process. In March 1982, epidemiologists at the CDC announced that over 50 of the reported cases in New York and Los Angeles were temporally related and proved that these persons had had sex with each other.[65] Fearing contagion, an alarmist minority of the general public demanded the complete isolation of those diagnosed with the disease, raising the specter of new quarantines and forceful removal of the sick to isolation hospitals, some of them to be located on islands.[66]

As these debates began, further research on the scourge was called for. Aided by a $50,000 grant awarded by the American Cancer Society to conduct clinical studies, a KS clinic opened at UCSF in January 1982 under the joint directorship of Conant and Volberding.[67] Given the unusual aspects of this cancer and its association with lymphadenopathies and rare pulmonary and intestinal infections, these men were joined by epidemiologists Selma Dritz and Andrew Wallace, as well as by virologist Jay Levy and consultants in immunology, pulmonary diseases, and gastroenterology.

Although faced with a mounting toll of sick and dying comrades, San Francisco's gay community first reacted to the AIDS epidemic with denial and incredulity. However, public education regarding AIDS, including the known risk factors for contraction and spread, was of paramount importance. Based on the available scientific, clinical, and epidemiological information, physicians recommended safe sex practices. In another first, Conant and others decided to establish a private KS Education and Research Foundation in May 1982 to plan educational programs for those most at risk of contracting the disease.

Meanwhile, UCSF's KS clinic focused on early clinical evaluation and diagnosis. Caring for this cancerous disease became an organizing principle for the interaction of dermatologists and oncologists. A division of labor ensued whereby patients already evaluated at the KS Clinic were sent to the newly opened oncology facility at SFGH for treatment, including, if necessary, hospitalization. Located on the fifth floor of the hospital's new building and managed by Volberding with the help of a nurse, Gayling Gee, this outpatient clinic on Ward 5 B opened on July 1, 1982, as another branch of the hospital's Department of Medicine under the leadership of Dr. Merle Sande. With no examining table—the ward was being used as a dormitory for house staff—Volberding was forced to check the patients on beds occupied at night by those on call. Most patients were white, middle-class males, well-educated and employed, who had private health insurance, a fact that greatly facilitated the subsequent creation of health care services for them. SFGH was the only institution in Northern California to treat AIDS openly.[68]

At the same time, Conant's KS Foundation began offering a referral service for those in need of medical advice. A call-back system operated by community volunteers sought to follow up and monitor these individuals, a precursor to San Francisco's efficient AIDS case management program.[69] As the number of cases mounted in 1983, Volberding was named director of a new SFGH Division of AIDS Activities, which included members from other clinical divisions, including infectious diseases, pulmonary medicine, oncology, and general medicine. The division was to have its own administrative infrastructure within the hospital's Department of Medicine, and it was designed to coordinate all medical activities, ensure responsibility for patient flow within the institution, and test new drugs.[70] Moreover, Volberding became responsible for teaching house staff and students about the clinical aspects of AIDS. At the clinic, meanwhile, he was joined by Dr. Constance Wofsy, an emergency physician, who was the acting chief of the hospital's Infectious Disease Unit. Wofsy went to work at 5 B half a day a week, seeing those who exhibited symptoms of infection such as swollen lymph nodes and respiratory difficulties.[71]

Flooded with patients, Volberding requested financial assistance from the city. He and Wofsy projected another load of at least 40 cases of KS during the 1982–1983 fiscal year. Responding to the increasing health threat, the city government approved $40,000 in July for converting another facility at the hospital into an AIDS clinic scheduled to open in January 1983. Other funding sources came from UCSF and the community. The specter of a growing number of very sick patients being admitted to the wards suggested the need to establish an outpatient facility that could provide the necessary medical and social services, thus minimizing the use of inpatient care. At this time, blood banks also began to discourage gay men at risk from donating blood.[72]

By September 1982, it seemed clear that AIDS was a sexually transmitted, blood-borne disease spread in a manner almost identical to that of hepatitis B. At the same time, a new study published in a leading medical journal postulated that multiple factors rather than a novel virus induced AIDS in gay males. One was sexual promiscuity and the exchange of bodily fluids, repeatedly exposing healthy men to semen, which was believed to possess immunosuppressive effects. Another was cytomegalovirus, which could reactivate the widespread Epstein-Barr virus responsible for infectious mononucleosis and lymphomas. As a means of prevention, the authors recommended restricting some forms of sexual activity and employing condoms.[73]

Fear of contagion gripped hospital staff and other patients. By the end of the year, Volberding was finally evicted from 5 B after a pregnant female resident expressed fear about sleeping in beds used to examine AIDS patients. In response, formal AIDS infection control guidelines were instituted. Early in March 1983, an Infection Control Task Force chaired by Sande and composed of physicians, nurses, administrators, lawyers, and ethicists was appointed to deal with the issues of risk to health personnel posed by AIDS at both hospitals and clinics.[74] Based on the available information, blood and enteric precautions were implemented, including placement of puncture-proof containers for needle disposal in each hospital room.[75] At this point, no health worker had become ill from treating AIDS patients, yet a period of great anxiety and high stress began for all caregivers until the low infectivity of the disease became clinically apparent and an antibody test to detect its presence was made available in 1984.

Warren, meanwhile, experienced several recurrences of his flu-like symptoms. He pondered the use of homeopathy or vitamins as the solution.[76] In November 1982, he again consulted with the Haight-Ashbury Clinic after developing a papular, pruritic rash, considered by caregivers to be allergic and treated with Benadryl. Two months later, across town, the first AIDS outpatient clinic in Ward 86 opened at a corner of the SFGH complex. Its 3,500 square feet of space were far away from the new medical center, located on the top floor of an old red brick pavilion building with a Spanish-tiled roof trimmed with copper gargoyles. At this time, the floor still functioned in part as an alcohol detoxification clinic and hosted an exercise class. After years of neglect, the unattractive interior included elevators splattered with graffiti. The outpatient clinic was initially staffed by two physicians, Volberding and Wofsy, and functioned three and a half days a week as both a referral clinic and a treatment facility for primary and specialized care. Concerned about infection, janitors wore makeshift space suits when they cleaned the building.

The promise of clinical research also set Ward 86 apart from many others at SFGH. Researchers offered patients access to drugs still unavailable on the market. With a grant from the Schering pharmaceutical firm, Volberding conducted trials on his patients suffering from KS with recombinant alpha interferon, a natural antiviral protein believed to possess antineoplastic properties. As in earlier times, the promise of a cure using this and other drugs motivated many AIDS sufferers to overcome their fears and prejudices about coming to a public hospital.[77]

On Wednesday afternoons, Volberding and Wofsy held informational sessions for patients on topics linked to their disease, including social and legal issues. Soon the number of patient visits increased to about 200 per month. The clinic quickly outgrew its assigned space and added the other half of the floor. A gay physician, Donald Abrams, joined Ward 86 in July 1983. Together with Volberding and Wofsy, head nurse Gee, and nurse practitioners J. B. Molaghan and Garry Carr, they formed a small but congenial family. All shared one big office space with little partitions in the partially renovated ward. Chipped paint graced the walls; the floors were aged linoleum, and dim light fixtures hung by wires from the ceiling. "It was something from the Addams Family," commented Abrams.[78] Despite the relatively poor quarters, most of his 200 lymphadenopathy patients were willing to travel across the city to be seen at SFGH. "It was more important who was seeing them than where they were being seen," Abrams recalled.[79]

Who "owns" AIDS in San Francisco? Planning Ward 5 B

Because of the distance between the clinic and SFGH's main facilities, Ward 86 secured a group of multidisciplinary consultants and began providing its own laboratory services in a public, decentralized institution supported by a variety of financial sources. This unusual situation brought together a group of young physicians—inexperienced upstarts in the eyes of their senior colleagues—many of them dissatisfied with the medical status quo in the rest of the hospital. Senior hospital attending physicians had devoted their professional lives to a spectrum of traditional diseases. Many now hesitated to get involved in what appeared to be a confusing new syndrome. As Volberding was fond of saying, there was no gray hair anywhere around this disease. Why would anyone want to devote his or her energy to such a bizarre syndrome erupting among what some depicted as the "gay fringe"? The multidimensional clinical character of AIDS made the physicians who treated it the renegades of traditional medical specialties, just as their gay charges were outcasts of society. Forced together, they created their own family.

Given the range of opportunistic infections in people with AIDS, clinical research and treatment required from the start cooperation among a diverse team of medical specialists. The situation demanded flexibility and innovation from professionals not usually trained to work together. As Conant observed, "one of the things that medicine does well is communicate vertically; one of the things it does poorly is communicate horizontally."[80] But the challenges of this new disease engaged the attention and curiosity of all physicians drawn to the clinic. Although Volberding freely admitted his ignorance and fear, an incredible excitement seized those caregivers whom fate had brought together to witness the birth of a clinical entity.

In 1983, the patients of UCSF's KS clinic were shifted to SFGH's Ward 86 for treatment, a move attributed in part by gays to a lack of enthusiasm for housing large numbers of stigmatized AIDS patients at Moffitt Hospital. Moreover, the academic medical center was keenly interested in preserving its tertiary care referrals and pursuing already established and well-funded lines of scientific research. Volberding was happy to receive these patients at the General. "They were part of my career now," he later recalled.[81] In a search for new clues, detailed questionnaires were prepared for the patients to document the particularities of their lives prior to their illness. Sande, in turn, was more keenly aware of the ongoing competition between the medical services at Moffitt Hospital and SFGH and was eager to improve the latter's clinical programs: "We saw AIDS and we grabbed it" as an opportunity to build another center of excellence within the city's public hospital, he later recalled.[82] While the university remained actively involved in the clinical and scientific framing of AIDS, it was excused from organizing more specific clinical services at its crowded Parnassus campus.

Ward 86, operating without a rigid appointment schedule, had prospective patients present themselves at the front desk to determine what was bureaucratically termed *intake eligibility*. Because of the influx of former UCSF patients and others previously seen by private practitioners, Ward 86 created its own administrative system. Name, place of residence, and insurance status had to be ascertained, and the staff processed all laboratory procedures. At this time, Abrams still had a number of reservations about the clinic. Earlier, he had strongly objected to the rundown physical plant. In fact, he and Volberding personally repainted the elevator. Like others, Abrams also felt that "having all the AIDS patients segregated on one unit was discrimination and homophobia." Soon, however, he had to admit that "it seemed to work pretty well . . . . It provided a target for the gay community to make contributions . . . ultimately obviously a wise decision and it has served as a model."[83]

The whole operation at Ward 86 was closely linked to UCSF by direct phone lines and personnel. Still, being confined to SFGH felt like a loss of status to some caregivers and an insult to their patients. Abrams, who initially saw these patients at the UCSF clinic, was quite upset with the change of location. "My patients were very sophisticated, intelligent people that had a high socioeconomic status." The thought of "herding them all over to San Francisco General to be treated in that place which is not particularly wonderful" was "a terrible affront." "The thought of having them wait for X rays, sitting next to people that are chained and shackled and wearing orange prison uniforms was very bad."[84] Indeed, some of them refused to leave the university clinic.

In May 1983, Volberding, still a junior clinician, obtained a three-year $1.2 million grant from the National Cancer Institute to support and expand research on AIDS. This award, one of several made to medical centers around the country, was designed to help fund research currently being carried out by investigators located at various San Francisco locations.[85] To the surprise of their superiors, the rapidly expanding family of young Turks successfully organized clinical services and, like Volberding, also proved their mettle in the struggle for federal research funds awarded for biomedical projects. As scientific medicine became involved with AIDS, information obtained from individual patients helped researchers to formulate hypotheses about the biological mechanisms of disease, design laboratory projects, and carry out epidemiological surveys. Although science initially lagged behind, some laboratory science fields, particularly virology and immunology, became respected partners on the road to knowledge essential to interpreting the growing clinical experience of AIDS.[86]

However, physicians could not deal with the immune system alone; they had to treat the whole patient. Scientific knowledge had to be applied within the context of every human life. The paradox of AIDS was this: while medical science struggled to contribute to a better understanding of the disease, the medical art, full of uncertainties and doubts and frequently derided as a bastion of subjectivity, was to experience a renaissance. Moreover, the traditional patient/physician dyad was replaced by a much broader relationship. Doctors or nurses were not the only healers, but were joined in that art by counselors, relatives, friends, and other patients. Indeed, AIDS and caring for its victims had become the "property" of many constituencies and caregiving groups in San Francisco.[87]

For Volberding, patients above all needed to be made comfortable. His own background in oncology had taught him the critical importance of psychosocial care. Thus, from its very beginning, Ward 86 utilized a number of counselors in patient management. A clinical psychologist, Paul Dague, suggested the inclusion of Shanti volunteers to provide emotional support for patients. Established in 1974 by psychologist Charles Garfield, the Shanti Project was originally located in Berkeley, serving as a bereavement counseling group for terminal cancer patients in the Bay Area. In 1981, however, one of the Shanti volunteers, the psychologist Jim Geary, created an AIDS support group in San Francisco. After assuming the directorship in 1982, Geary obtained city grants for the Project and its volunteers and offered its services to Ward 86. The idea was to provide peer counseling from individuals trained in sympathetic listening, role playing, massage, and small group interaction. In each instance, the permanent staff matched the counselors with individual patients. A psychiatry resident, James Dilley, provided additional counseling, and he later managed to obtain a half-time city-funded position to continue working with both the staff and inpatients.[88]

The health risks inherent in treating AIDS patients also created tensions among health care professionals torn between altruism and self-interest. As persons and professionals, physicians had to confront their own values, emotions, and prejudices while facing the terror generated by KS eruptions, multiple infections, and gradual bodily wasting. Discussions concerning the social obligation of health professionals to treat dangerously ill and terminal patients ensued.[89] Was there a social contract, even a professional oath? Stories circulated about practitioners fleeing contagion during past plague and cholera epidemics. Could history become a justification for physicians to refuse care? At first, AIDS was assumed to behave like any other cancer, but the multiple opportunistic infections, blood transmission, and high mortality generated considerable fear among caregivers of contracting the disease. "For the next year and a half we lived in real dread," recalled Volberding.[90] Periodically, they would all believe themselves afflicted with AIDS. Wofsy, the infectious disease expert, wore gloves when palpating for lymph nodes in armpits and the groin. Yet nobody was supposed to admit to fear. Many of the medical residents were especially afraid of the AIDS patients, and for some time the issue threatened recruitment to UCSF's residency training programs. House staff members feared not only for themselves, but also for their spouses, partners, and children.[91]

The SFGH authorities were equally alarmed. An increasing number of very sick AIDS patients flooded the hospital's inpatient facilities. The institution seemed in danger of being converted into an AIDS hospital. At this point, Sande prepared to curb the population of AIDS patients to about a third of the available teaching beds, a traditional measure designed to place house staff needs ahead of those of patients. Anxiety and homophobia greeted sufferers on admission to various wards. Most persons with AIDS were isolated in private rooms located at the end of a unit. Frightened nurses, garbed in caps and gowns, made no pretense about their dislike for these patients. Some febrile, shivering patients were forced to get up at night and change their own soaked bedsheets. Dragging their intravenous stands along, they often had to fetch their own food trays left outside their rooms by apprehensive members of the Dietary Department.[92] Patients' complaints fell on deaf ears or were channeled to SFGH's complex administrative bureaucracy, with predictable results.[93]

As the situation became more serious, straight and gay caregivers at SFGH started lobbying for the establishment of a separate facility where AIDS patients could be spared the discriminatory, often uncaring treatment they were receiving. In March 1983, the idea of consolidating the inpatients with AIDS to improve their care found some supporters among the other staff. At this point, nearly half of the people afflicted with the disease in the Bay Area were coming to SFGH's clinics and wards for evaluation and treatment, making this hospital the repository of more patients with the disease than any other institution in the country. Volberding and Wofsy approached Sande with the idea of creating a separate inpatient facility devoted to AIDS patients. The rationale was similar to that responsible for creating the outpatient clinic. At this point, AIDS seemed to be a new and lethal disease caused by an unknown but presumably infectious agent. An isolated wing thus made sense for both the patients and their potential caregivers. Like all SFGH units, the new section would be headed by a nurse.[94]

After approval from the hospital administration, Clifford Morrison, a nurse, was selected to design and organize this new ward, known as the Medical Special Care Unit. Morrison had begun as a Shanti volunteer and then worked at SFGH's psychiatric facilities. Because of his link to the gay community and his friendship with the hospital's director of nursing, he was an ideal candidate for the project. Within weeks, however, Morrison realized the monumental hurdles confronting the hospital, physicians, nurses, and AIDS patients before proper care could be provided. At first, the gay community opposed the creation of a separate unit, since this meant giving in to the popular hysteria demanding the removal and isolation of all AIDS victims based on traditional quarantine schemes. In fact, such plans were quickly denounced as a blueprint for a new "leper colony" designed to protect the rest of SFGH's hospital population.[95]

For Morrison, however, it began to make sense to have a small model unit capable of pulling together all the institutional resources presently devoted to AIDS. Ward 5 B, the original oncology facility with its 12 beds, was located in a corner of the new hospital building and could be easily isolated as a respiratory intensive care unit. Here all patients would occupy private rooms, more for their own comfort than for segregation purposes. To avoid any sense of quarantine, medical staff would encourage open visitation. For Morrison, Ward 5 B was definitely modeled after other oncology units, but with a new focus: a more complex disease requiring a sophisticated staff to administer intensive drug therapies and provide psychological support. Since the hospital administration was under considerable pressure to demonstrate its commitment to the care of AIDS patients, Morrison's plan for the separate ward was approved in April 1983.[96]

With only three months left before the planned opening, Morrison quickly organized his unit with support from gay community organizations and health professionals willing to staff it. An essential qualification was that AIDS patients would be treated with dignity. Morrison decided to implement the primary care concept, which meant that the unit would have a nursing rather than a medical focus, emphasizing the education of patients and their own involvement in care. He was emphatic about this unorthodox approach; it did not imply special treatment for one particular group of hospital patients but just plain quality care. The decision to have separate rooms for each patient not only conformed to infection control policies, but also acknowledged the perception that at advanced stages of illness the patients needed some privacy. The only structural change was the installation of sinks with foot pedals and soap dispensers to allow the staff to wash their hands frequently in compliance with institutional isolation rules.[97]

Morrison's call for volunteers to staff the new unit met with a very favorable response, and he ended up interviewing about 35 individuals for the initial 12 positions. Applicants were asked basic questions about their philosophy of health care and nursing, their views on terminal care, death, and dying, and their attitudes toward gay men and drug users. In his interviews with prospective staff members, Morrison discussed the latest epidemiological information available on AIDS, as well as the perceived risk factors and infection control measures. Those selected came from varied backgrounds, but all had considerable clinical experience, including exposure to cancer patients or intensive care, perhaps working in a hospice or mental ward. More than half were either gay men or lesbians. In addition, three Shanti counselors were to provide services seven days a week, with a backup psychiatrist on call for patients with acute breakdowns or suicidal conditions.[98]

The final pool of volunteer nurses hired by Morrison represented some of the best San Francisco could offer. Since the mid-1960s, staff nurses in the Bay Area had struggled to improve their working conditions and salaries. Through collective bargaining, unionized nurses had finally increased their political power at SFGH in the face of weak administrative leadership, thus laying the groundwork for nursing's stronger voice in patient management and staff assignments. Many nurses were social activists who had elected to work at this hospital because they liked caring for the disenfranchised, downtrodden, and newly arrived immigrants. Many naturally gravitated to AIDS patients as another stigmatized minority. Others, like Diane Jones, who became one of the night nurses, were recommended by the AIDS patients themselves scattered in the various hospital wards.[99]

In planning their work at Ward 5 B, nurses decided to work in teams that included physicians, social workers, nutritionists, and mental health staff. In doing so, the nurses eliminated two concerns still afflicting their profession: their progressive removal from the bedside and their traditional bondage to medicine. In a display of the egalitarian culture pervading San Francisco's gay community, Morrison even refused to assume the title *head nurse*—which implied a hierarchical decision-making structure—opting instead for the democratic label *nursing coordinator*. In doing so, he signaled his decision to establish a novel consensus-building arrangement that would also ensure professional autonomy for the nurses and allow for more flexible control over staffing schedules.[100]

As planned, the 12-room inpatient unit received its first patients on July 26, 1983, as Warren and his friends were performing a Shakespearean play in Golden Gate Park. Morrison himself processed all admissions. Only the most acutely ill patients were brought to Ward 5 B, with less sick patients being distributed to other units. Given the nature of this disease, family members and friends were allowed to stay in the room with the patient, an arrangement that helped lift morale and foster effective counseling essential in managing young patients afflicted with a fatal illness. Provided with ample windows, these rooms were arranged around a U-shaped corridor encircling workstations, a conference room, and storage facilities. The yellow and orange rooms and hallways of the newly redecorated ward were cheerful. The place gave an impression of festivity and airiness. There were flowers and house plants everywhere.[101]

Morrison's apprehension that the gay community would condemn the ward as another warehouse for the sick and dying proved unfounded. Within its first four months of operation, the AIDS ward had over 100 admissions. Ironically for a city hospital frequented by the poor, always on the brink of financial insolvency and in danger of losing its accreditation, well-heeled, respectable gay men now clamored to be admitted. Indeed, shifting from its initial Cinderella status, the ward started to add luster to a hospital with the usual image problems of any charitable city and county institution. The professional volunteer staff quickly developed a keen sense of camaraderie, and the unit exuded optimism. The idea that AIDS was just a temporary crisis requiring a decisive but short-term response persisted among caregivers and patients. The gay community was being severely tested but expressed its readiness for the challenge: "I've never in my life been so proud to be gay as I am now," admitted Morrison. "Gay people have been stereotyped as being weak, but we're dealing with it. We're strong, we're handling it."[102] Patients seemed to agree. "I want everyone to know how fantastic and wonderful the care is here. People should know that this is a place where they will be healed. The staff does its best for you."[103]

Gay pride: Patients' rights and responsibilities

By now, many local practitioners had substantially increased their understanding of AIDS' symptoms, modes of transmission, and risk factors.[104] The causative agent remained a mystery, and there was no diagnostic test that could detect the disease. At the national level, the Department of Health and Human Services made AIDS its first research priority. The search was definitely on for an infectious agent, probably a virus, believed to be transmitted through blood and blood products and known to attack the T_4 cells of the immune system. Researchers at the Pasteur Institute in Paris claimed to have discovered such an agent, but American scientists continued their efforts to verify these findings. Homosexual promiscuity was still considered a major factor in the etiology of the disease. Volberding reported encouraging results from his interferon trials in the treatment of KS, but the response rate was comparable to that of treatment with conventional chemotherapy.[105]

The diagnosis and treatment of AIDS was, therefore, still very much in a state of flux when the new ward was being assembled. Warren, for example, remained in diagnostic limbo for many months before he was admitted to Ward 5 B. When he went to the Haight-Ashbury Free Clinic in April 1983 and again in May, complaining of cramps and diarrhea, the practitioners there tested him for bacterial and parasitic bowel infections, finding nothing. Still, they prescribed a seven-day course of Flagyl. Despite his worries, there was no talk yet about his having AIDS.

This slowness to come to a diagnosis of AIDS derived not just from the medical community's still incomplete understanding of the disease, but also from a lack of education about the disease in the gay community. Neither the San Francisco Health Department nor the city's gay organizations had mounted effective educational efforts directed at the stigmatized community, although the issue of transmission through bodily fluids seemed scientifically proven. In May 1983, the Harvey Milk Club distributed a pamphlet on the subject, and the *Bay Area Reporter* eventually printed a "manifesto" warning that AIDS could be sexually transmitted. Not surprisingly, this information elicited critical responses from community leaders who denied its accuracy. By June, the CDC in Atlanta had reported 1,641 cases of AIDS nationally—71% in homosexual men, 17% in nonhomosexual intravenous drug users, 5% in Haitians irrespective of sexuality, and 1% in hemophiliacs. That month, newspapers and magazines carried a record number of articles about the new plague.

Still, many gay men found it difficult to face the possibility that the spread of AIDS might be curtailed by changing their sexual practices. They found themselves in the dilemma of being asked to reexamine their feelings about sex and human relationships in the name of some hypothetical collective responsibility, without a clear notion of whether this sacrifice would affect them personally or their immediate friends.[106] A possible decision by the city's health authorities to close San Francisco's bath houses was labeled "genocidal." As one observer remarked, sex for gay men was a badge of self-esteem and aggressiveness, as well as the foundation of a social identity, a liberating behavior for a stigmatized sector of American society. Living in a culture with a heightened sense of sexuality among

the young, it was difficult for gay men to curb such practices unilaterally, particularly since the general population remained adversarial or even hostile. Without
cohesive family networks to counsel them, many young men pursued their own
agendas, regardless of the consequences.[107]

Later that summer, Warren and Kelly performed together in Shakespeare's
play *The Tempest* in Golden Gate Park. Warren started this engagement with a
lot of energy but seemed to tire quite easily. This was especially apparent in the
performance of somersaults during the show. After performing them he appeared
disoriented, and had a hard time standing up and keeping his balance. Diarrhea,
further weight loss, and night sweats weakened him. Although both he and Kelly
suspected AIDS as the cause of Warren's symptoms, physicians at the Haight-
Ashbury Clinic remained skeptical. Most gay men still associated AIDS with the
appearance of KS, a visually obvious illness. Each morning, they nervously inspected their faces and panicked at the sight of every emerging spot or pimple.
Moreover, every cold, every swollen lymph gland, and every bout of diarrhea
caused alarm.

Perhaps Warren's illness could be labeled an *AIDS-related complex (ARC)*,
representing a cluster of symptoms and conditions that could eventually lead to
AIDS. Nevertheless, Warren remained in a frustrating nosological limbo. There
was nothing definite in spite of several radiological studies of his upper and lower
gastrointestinal tract. Lacking alternatives for a second opinion because of his financial status, Warren remained anxious and concerned. As one caregiver at
SFGH's new Ward 5 B, Allison M., remarked, "To feel horrible and not have a
validation for it is a terrible way to live."[108] Following another visit by Warren on
July 11, physicians at the neighborhood clinic finally referred him to the Gas-
troenterology Clinic at SFGH for further studies of his chronic diarrhea. A new
workup included a sigmoidoscopy and a negative rectal biopsy, but the attending
physicians, suspecting AIDS, also tested him immunologically with a PPD tuberculin skin test, which was positive. A brief visit to SFGH's Emergency Room for
chest congestion later that month finally led to a referral to the AIDS outpatient
facility at Ward 86. Here Warren was first seen by Wofsy on August 1, 1983.[109]

Patient assignments to individual physicians were based on a preliminary
screening conducted by nurse practitioners. When Warren first came to the clinic,
a division of labor had been established whereby Volberding continued to plan
research programs and care for malignancies such as KS and lymphomas. Wofsy,
an infectious disease specialist, would treat patients with opportunistic infections,
and Abrams would deal with all those individuals affected by other AIDS-related
conditions, including the lymphadenopathy syndrome now defined by the term
ARC. Those attending Warren at the clinic immediately suspected that he had
AIDS since all of his symptoms fit the pattern of illness that was plaguing many
young men in San Francisco. Stool cultures for *Cryptosporidium*, however, were
negative. Although he feared that he probably had AIDS, Warren remained in de-

nial since nobody had officially diagnosed him. He continued to experience diarrhea and fatigue despite antibiotic treatments and better nutritional management.[110]

By September, news reports of a workshop on retroviruses at the Cold Spring Harbor Laboratory suggested that the cause of AIDS was indeed a virus isolated from some of the victims of the disease. At this point, the number of cases officially reported had already risen to 2,259, with pneumocystis pneumonia being the most common opportunistic infection in more than half of them. According to statistics compiled by the San Francisco Health Department, more than 87% of the reported cases in 1983 were white males. The CDC was still fighting the perception that AIDS might be spread through casual contact, but the public was becoming increasingly nervous. In San Francisco, the Stonewall Gay Democratic Club held a panel discussion on gay male sex after AIDS. It featured the issues of the baths, promiscuity, monogamy, and celibacy within the context of individual and community responsibilities in the current health crisis.[111]

In early December, Warren and Kelly joined San Francisco's ACT Company to perform in Charles Dickens' *A Christmas Carol*, but merely a week into the run, Warren could no longer climb the two flights of stairs built on the stage. At this point, he consulted a homeopathic physician in Marin County, who, believing that the symptoms reflected allergies, took him off most food articles except rice cakes and raw fish, prescribing some herbal remedies and vitamins. Discouraged, Warren made plans to return to Tennessee and stay with his parents. However, when Kelly brought Warren to SFGH's AIDS clinic for a regularly scheduled appointment on December 12, Warren's condition had seriously deteriorated, especially over the previous weekend. A nonproductive cough had joined the night sweats and profuse diarrhea. His temperature was below normal (96°F), and his blood pressure was low. The examining physicians decided to admit him to Ward 5 B, the inpatient facility, to run further tests and possibly develop a treatment plan. His attending physician was Dan Wlodarcyzk, and his current intern was Mark Smith. By this time, more than 100 patients had already been treated in this unit, most of them for acute pneumonia. Although a majority left the hospital improved—the mortality rate was less than 5%—these patients were now returning for treatment of a second and much more serious bout of pneumonia. After his arrival in the ward, Warren was placed in room 17 B, considered to have the best view in the entire unit. By his own admission, the panorama of hills surrounding San Francisco reminded him somewhat of his native Tennessee.[112]

For Warren it was a relief to know for certain that he had AIDS. Filled with frustration and fear, he had fought off for more than a year and a half the various infections that could now be reinterpreted as early manifestations the disease. The diagnosis also accomplished another goal: it qualified Warren for Medi-Cal benefits to pay for his hospital care. Unfortunately, the attending physicians discovered that the state refused to pay for any experimental drugs prescribed for his treatment. Now, placed under a cooling blanket to reduce the high fever and night sweats, Warren paradoxically seemed at peace with himself. He had been planning to return to Tennessee to visit his parents at Christmas but was now forced to break the news to them that he was not coming because he was quite sick with AIDS. After the initial shock, his family members were quite supportive in spite of tensions lingering from the summer of 1983, when he had revealed to them that he was gay. At that time, Warren had returned to his hometown in the belief that his mother was dying. When he "came out" to his parents, his father was quoted as saying that he did not comprehend this but would stand by him because he was his loving son. Given the advanced state of his mother's emphysema, Warren felt guilty about returning to San Francisco after a few weeks to be with his lover and other friends.[113]

While hospitalized on Ward 5 B, Warren received care from rotating teams of house physicians, although Wofsy, Volberding, and Abrams continued to function as attending physicians, teachers, and consultants. The house physicians reviewed cases with the nurses at conferences on Tuesday afternoons. Diane Jones, one of the night-shift nurses, characterized this as "fish-bowl medicine."[114] As in other municipal teaching hospitals, day-to-day medical care remained in the hands of the house staff. Many residents, however, were still afraid of AIDS patients. The multiple diseases on display on the ward appeared to be overwhelming, and contagion still seemed a good possibility. "Part of me was holding back," admitted one medical resident, "but I lost my fear after treating them as people with a problem."[115]

Following bronchoscopy on December 19, Warren's respiratory symptoms were diagnosed as pneumocystis pneumonia. Doctors immediately ordered intravenous trimethoprim-sulfa (Septra) and painful intramuscular injections of pentamidine for three weeks, both routine treatments for opportunistic infections. A lumbar puncture on December 22 added meningitis to the previous diagnoses. Warren's gastrointestinal condition was finally determined to be cryptosporidiosis, for which he received intravenous amphotericin B, the highly nephrotoxic drug dubbed "amphoterrible," that also caused a horrible taste in the mouth. Finally, Warren was also placed on alpha-interferon, the drug Volberding used in his KS studies to boost the immune system.[116]

Given the rudimentary knowledge about AIDS, all caregivers, both nurses and physicians, learned from newspapers, the patients, and each other. As Abrams recalled, nurses quickly became experts in the care of AIDS patients and had to educate the transient house staff on a need-to-know basis. "The docs don't have much input and really can't take much credit for the success of 5 B," remarked one nurse.[117] Following Warren's admission, the nursing notes described him as extremely intelligent and informed, cooperative, quiet, witty, and insightful. Like others before him, he demanded detailed information about his condition and the nature of all prescribed treatments. This strategy allowed patients like Warren to gain some semblance of control over what appeared to be a complex and unpredictable disease. In fact, some patients compulsively monitored the latest news and treatments—some even subscribed to medical journals—and appeared at times embarrassingly better informed about the latest studies than their caregivers. Such a diffusion of medical knowledge turned the traditional Aesculapian authority of the physician on its head, placing new demands on the behavior of health professionals. In shaping a much more collaborative model of care, medical dogmatism gave way to a measure of humility and collegiality.[118]

After a week in Ward 5 B, however, the usually soft-spoken Warren became angry and discouraged with the house staff. Their behavior, he thought, was patronizing, and many ignored Warren's demands for respect and attention as a full-fledged partner in treatment. Most of Warren's frustration centered on the conflicting opinions he received. Physicians had determined that he was suffering from three opportunistic infections at once, and they all needed to be treated separately. How could this be? Had they been present all along? At the same time, sulfa drugs made him quite nauseous, while amphotericin contributed to profuse night sweats and renal damage. Like many other patients and nurses, he began seriously to question his medical regimen.[119]

Warren's skepticism reflected profound changes in contemporary attitudes and expectations. Since the 1960s, a wave of individualism and questioning of authority in America had begun spilling over into the health care sector, fueling demands for patient autonomy and freedom of choice. An expansion of the notion of personhood combined with demands for civil rights.[120] By pressing for a share in the medical decision-making process, the sick challenged the status of the physician as the undeniable authority regarding health matters. This movement was an attempt to demystify medicine as part of a broader movement that distrusted experts, demanding truth telling and informed consent. As the so-called New Age became more mainstream, signs of what was being portrayed as a "revolt of the patient" could be observed everywhere, but especially in California.[121] Such a partnership was sought in the face of a dominant view of medical care as a commodity in a consumer market, an approach particularly entrenched in America, as exemplified by the story of Paula during the Depression.[122] Subsequently, private and government insurance programs had transformed care into an entitlement. Hospitals, for their part, were still hierarchically organized and therefore categorized as "human rights wastelands."[123]

Such individualism and demand for patient autonomy were closely linked to a social movement of the 1960s identified as the "Age of Aquarius" or the "counterculture" that promoted a philosophy of life linking a person's physical and emotional realms in a quest for a new spirituality. With their focus on holistic health and their challenges to authority, Aquarians demanded that medicine no longer focus only on physical ills, but also take into account individual needs, concerns, and suffering. The desired goal was no less than a restoration of the personhood of the patient, and biomedicine was criticized for being excessively reductionist, sexist, and racist. Many persons—including Warren—subscribed to the traditional notion of a natural healing force: the mind (or soul), a powerful "healer within," responsible for the efficacy of positive emotions on bodily phenomena. This new patient activism and empowerment were strongly reflected on Ward 5 B, where patients, together with caregivers, became prominently involved in the medical decision-making process. To implement such partnerships, people with AIDS demanded additional health information and psychological support to understand the meaning and implications of medical diagnosis, treatment, and prognosis. In their despair, many also began experimenting with alternative treatments.[124]

Working with AIDS patients at SFGH, psychiatrist Dilley tried to determine the behavioral characteristics that put certain young men at greater risk of contracting the disease. Persons suffering from AIDS in San Francisco were in a special bind. As noted earlier, gay pride and power had been highest in the city just prior to the epidemic. Stigmatized by mainstream society and without roots in their adopted communities, some of these men often also felt lonely and guilty about their status and sexual freedom, searching in vain for validation in a largely hostile world outside of their own neighborhoods.

Some wondered whether a negative self-image could actually impair the immune system and cause the dreaded disease. Among those hospitalized at SFGH, many openly expressed their internalized homophobia and shame in the form of self-doubt, guilt, and even self-hatred. Could homosexual sex be, after all, unnatural? Were they really allowing themselves to be infected despite knowing the risks? Falling ill with AIDS was often rationalized as a deserved punishment. Under such circumstances, why should they merit hospital care? Perhaps psychological factors such as previous bouts of depression created the necessary susceptibility for an infectious agent to cause AIDS. If this was true, preventive counseling could be important.[125]

These feelings, especially the erosion of self-esteem exacerbated by hospitalization, were precisely those that Warren and others would try to prevent through their example and writings. After three years, fear of AIDS alone could no longer sustain its powerful deterrent quality. To be sure, there were signs that a majority of the gay community was attempting to adjust to the epidemic threat. Changes in behavior did occur, particularly abstinence and safer sex through the use of condoms, less anal sex, and reduced exchanges of bodily fluids. Many, however, persisted in practicing what was now dubbed "unsafe" sex, some of it in the bath houses and sex clubs. Finally, there was the irony of AIDS, gradually dissolving those perfect male bodies, wrecking the self-image of physical beauty and fitness prevalent in the gay community. One volunteer characterized the relentless clinical march of AIDS as saying good-bye to body functions one at a time. In a culture obsessed by youth, many AIDS sufferers gradually realized that their most treasured possession, their own bodies, were relentlessly wasting away and had to be given up.

Patients cope with sickness in many different ways. Some become silent, depressed, and withdrawn. Others express a great deal of interest, even fascination, in the details of their disease. At Ward 5 B, many of the AIDS patients had a hard time knowing how to control and where to direct their anger and resentment, at times blaming themselves for having contracted the scourge. Some transferred their rage to people around them, including friends, relatives, and hospital staff who could be blamed for inflicting even more pain. In his first weeks on Ward 5 B, Warren attempted to control his emotions by demanding that Kelly leave him alone and by insisting on dealing with the hospital-paid caregivers in an impersonal, often critical manner. "If people didn't go through these things, they would not be human," noted Allison M., the head nurse, "they'd be robots."[126]

The art of nursing: Life on Ward 5 B

Since the days of Florence Nightingale, nursing had changed significantly in both philosophy and outlook. Nurses were now also educators, researchers, and administrators, skilled in the management of special diseases.[127] Despite their growing professionalization, they were still viewed as humanizers. At its core, the nursing role remained one of personal contact, communication, and empathy that created therapeutic relationships and promoted healing.[128] "Caring is the heart of nursing," insisted one contemporary nursing leader.[129] Just as some physicians insisted on practicing the art rather than the science of medicine, nurses employed their communication skills, feelings, and intuition to make contact with the sick. Perhaps staffing patterns, as well as the scope and pace of technological interventions previously noted in organ transplantation, conspired against such emotional involvement elsewhere, but SFGH's Ward 5 B offered unique opportunities.[130]

In the face of AIDS, medicine appeared impotent, capable only of palliating symptoms, which placed nursing at the center of patient care. Moreover, the hospitalized AIDS patients usually lacked traditional personal support systems. Most were considered outcasts by their families, while some of their acquaintances and friends either stayed away out of fear of contagion or were ill themselves. The loneliness could be devastating, and the need for companionship was acute. The burden of understanding patients' perspectives and integrating a new terminal illness into nurses' experience represented a rebirth of the caring role, which on other hospital wards was frequently displaced in the name of institutional rationality and efficiency. According to Morrison's blueprints, the patient–nurse relationship on 5 B was to be multidimensional as well as task-oriented, in contrast with more specialized models. "Caregiving is heart work," commented a Shanti volunteer.[131] Indeed, the "new" caring was described as the art of total involvement, a return to the historical roots of nursing. Previous stereotypes of nursing as a nurturing, womanly occupation had obviously survived, although a considerable number of the nurses were now male. Most patients on the AIDS ward established an emotional relationship with someone on the staff. As one patient remarked, "I know how the pioneers must have felt fearing what was ahead of them," adding that "my bed is like a covered wagon and we are all on a wagon train helping each other in a time of need."[132]

Most of the multidisciplinary emotional support team assembled on Ward 5 B was composed of nurses, social workers, Shanti counselors, chaplains, volunteers, and community members, who all wanted to work closely with AIDS patients. The nurse–patient ratio was higher than in other SFGH wards, and the technological assistance was state of the art. The nurses worked 12-hour shifts to take care of a dozen very sick patients.[133] Traditional hospital rituals designed to express sympathy and concern, such as greeting of patients, laying on of hands, and taking the pulse acquired even greater poignancy. "That's one of the things that is amazing about that ward," remembered Kelly. "People make relationships."[134] A key caring role was reserved for the gay community. As Morrison remarked, "I think that 5 B has become the property of the community. The community feels very proud of it."[135] Indeed, gay health workers acted in many ways as community representatives while discharging their caregiving responsibilities. The gayness of the nurses, who were frequently afflicted by self-doubt, now provided patients with a powerful sense of identity and connection. Another male nurse, George J., declared that "one of the great strengths of this ward is the support that comes from a community that feels itself under attack by this disease. The community is galvanized."[136] As care providers, they showed solidarity during this time of trouble. "There is a strength in us being together and supporting each other. People can sit down at that conference room—nurses, doctors, patients—and talk about the issues that come up—sexuality, lifestyle, treatment, homophobia—we discuss it," recalled Morrison.[137]

Under such circumstances, the traditional professional distance was easily eliminated. On selected occasions, both patients and caregivers even admitted their homosexuality to each other—an event of great emotional significance, especially for some volunteer staff members hitherto undecided about their own sexual orientation. The laying on of hands, an ancient healing art relegated to fringe practitioners, experienced an important rebirth at this time, practiced by the nurses, friends, and therapists. Massage, a traditional technique, played an important role in fostering relationships with patients. Taught by Irene S., a therapist with hospice experience, touch therapy seemed to ease the feelings of fear and isolation most patients experienced. "Our hands are a direct extension of our hearts, of how we feel," commented Irene. "A touch says I love you, I care for you, and you are worthy of that love and care."[138] Another caregiver explained that a loving touch provided much needed relief for patients who were constantly prodded, poked, and hurt in the course of treatments.[139] Many of the relationships forged on 5 B survived the patients' discharge, and it was not uncommon for caregivers to receive visits and be asked out on dates by their former charges.[140]

This unique hospital setting prompted a number of reflections about the contemporary philosophy of nursing. Staff members made distinctions about the nature of their work. In the modern secularized world, some were no longer motivated by pity and redemptive zeal. While the Christian framework still provided this rationale of compassion as an agenda for personal salvation, the approach of most nurses on 5 B sprang from notions of secular humanism, holism, and individual autonomy. The staff related to the patients as human beings and even as friends. We nurse "not out of charity but human understanding" was the clarion call on the ward.[141] As fellow humans, the sick and their families needed to be treated with respect. The one-on-one interaction was a display of shared humanity. Yet the human experience of suffering and the caring response to it inevitably returned to earlier religious constructions. Some caregivers continued to employ Christian thought and imagery. On a tour of Mexico, one nurse, George J., became fascinated by the vivid statues of a suffering Christ, Mary, and the saints: "As I was kneeling it came to me that I care for people who look like that. At all times in history there are people who are going through that. I feel interested in that human experience. I am fearful of it and drawn to love it."[142]

Nurses also performed the traditional menial tasks of body care and hygiene, together with the specific and often highly technical interventions required by modern therapeutics. For nurses, hitherto steeped in bureaucratic work, the intimacy created by touching, bathing, and cleaning sick bodies was inspirational. Because of the exhausting physical duties and emotional involvement, however, the heavy workload necessitated furloughs to prevent burnout. For most, this caregiving was based on reciprocity. Being members of the gay community, they feared falling ill with the same disease afflicting their present charges. Statements such as "What comes around goes around" and "I know that I would want to be treated decently if I came down with AIDS" were common.[143]

At the center of this nursing was genuine engagement with patients, frequent talks, empathy, and reassurance. While day chores allowed less time for conversation, night nursing, freed of certain routines, provided opportunities for lengthy and intimate encounters.[144] "Nursing on that ward is like performing an act of devotion," commented Allison M., adding that it was always absorbing and encompassing, "almost like a vigil." The intensity of the personal relationships with patients was reflected in the statement of another staff member, who admitted, "I think healing is always based on love. That is the energy I use when I am working with healing someone. It's my own love, and it's the love for the world at large." This remark aptly reflected the healing function of nursing, usually lost among the bureaucratic routines and technical interventions typical elsewhere.[145]

When asked about her activities during Warren's hospitalization, Elissa C., one of the nurses on 5 B, replied: "I believe that a sick person needs an advocate who understands and tries to get the patients what they need, help them, inform them, help them process and deal with their feelings."[146] Such patient advocacy was not uncommon elsewhere in the hospital but was perhaps much more potent on a ward housing individuals traumatized by social stigma as well as a deadly disease. Restoring self-respect and empowering patients to assume as much control as possible over their bodies were lofty goals, sometimes difficult to accomplish since many patients were acculturated to remain passive in medical matters. Not surprisingly, the nurses played important roles in providing medical information, holding discussions with patients concerning code status and quality-of-life issues.

According to a patient handout produced by the ward nurses, patient education and advocacy were critical.[147] The ward had a small conference room where everybody, patients and caregivers, came together, forming bonds of friendship and intimacy. Reflecting some of the radical democratic values governing gay culture, patients and their families went together to the health professionals' AIDS update meetings, read the medical literature about the disease and its treatments, and freely debated the information with caregivers. Weekly staff conferences involving physicians and nurses transmitted new information and promoted the ongoing educational process associated with a new disease. Besides helping patients understand their opportunistic infections, the nurses explained organ system involvement, the origin of multiple symptoms, the meaning of laboratory tests, and the potential benefits and drawbacks of treatments. Some procedures, including lumbar and bone marrow punctures, bronchoscopies, and brain biopsies, were frightening. "God," groaned one patient, "they'll never be able to call us sissies again."[148] Caregivers spoke also about precautions to be taken after discharge. Unfortunately, not enough was known at this time about the evolution of AIDS to provide patients with clear options. Many effects of therapy remained uncertain, with patients basically just "buying time" by keeping the multiple opportunistic infections at bay. Frequent tests monitored white blood cell counts and hematocrits in patients taking amphotericin. Indeed, the bloodletting carried out daily by phlebotomists to meet the requirements of laboratory medicine bore striking similarities to the traditional therapeutic venesections of yesteryear based on humoral premises.

Angry with some of the doctors over their behavior toward him, Warren connected on a personal level with many nurses on 5B, especially Allison M. and two night nurses, Charles C. and Diane Jones. Charles, who was also gay, already had considerable experience caring for AIDS patients, and he was quite willing to listen to newcomers such as Warren, who were often angry and frightened about their new diagnosis, which was tantamount to a death sentence. Charles encouraged Warren to resume his drawing, aware that the young man wanted to fill the rest of his life with art. Sharing experiences within a similar cultural and gender background facilitated the establishment of personal relationships between nurses and patients. In addition, the shared experiences of already discharged patients made them a valuable emotional resource for patients confined to the ward, and the former often returned to console others after their outpatient clinic visits on Mondays and Thursdays. "You always hear a lot of laughter when patients come back after they are discharged to say hello," commented Morrison.[149]

Under Morrison, 5 B quickly became SFGH's most unconventional unit. Community support took many forms, including the daily delivery of newspapers, as well as donated pastries and toiletries. The patients, not the hospital, were empowered to designate the significant others who would have resident privileges, reflecting a local culture that sought to redefine the parameters of the American family. Family and friends flocked to the ward, in part to bring good will and cheer to the patients, but also curious to learn more about this new disease. In the beginning, visitors donned gowns and masks, since AIDS sufferers were presumably contagious and needed to be kept in isolation, but these rules changed when it became apparent that the sickness could not be transmitted through casual contact. To respect the privacy of all patients, the ward's locator board carried only the patients' first name and last initial. During the first three weeks on 5B, Warren often hosted groups of 9 or 10 friends in his room. He was blessed with an expressive face, a keen sense of humor, and a flair for the dramatic, and his theatrical presence in the ward remained etched in the memories of his friends and caregivers. Laughter followed him everywhere. Inevitably, as hospitalization dragged on, fewer visitors came. On the ward, meanwhile, ambulatory patients pushed their intravenous feeders around in the hallways, talking to each other. As in Moffitt's Kidney Transplant Unit, patients helped each other fight their illness, their boredom, and their pain. In the rooms, one could hear bursts of laughter over the steady hiss of respirators, and the steady humming of the refrigerated blankets that kept the pneumocystis-bred fevers below 103°F.

According to one account, Ward 5 B was the most entertaining unit at SFGH. Here the celebration of gay freedom and liberation from discrimination continued unabated. An air of festivity permeated an otherwise harrowing experience of gloom and doom. The upbeat party atmosphere was created with music booming from radios and television sets, while patients and visitors mingled in the halls, telling jokes. At holiday time, gay volunteer groups handed out presents, served gourmet dinners, and offered massages. A group called the Godfather Fund threw a party and distributed slippers, teddy bears, and shaving utensils to the patients. Entertainment, such as performances by Sharon McKnight, the popular cabaret singer, wearing her black and white feather boa, enlivened hospital life for the men on "death row" sipping what could very well be their last glasses of champagne. In the tradition of gay "camp" humor a number of baptisms, weddings, and bon voyage parties routinely took place on the ward. But the starker reality of AIDS never departed: at the first baptism, everybody took extraordinary precautions in compliance with the infection-control protocol. "I got kids at home," remembered one volunteer. All participants wore masks and gowns as they plunged the patient into a bathtub full of water in the presence of a minister.[150]

Although in intensive treatment for pneumonia and meningitis, Warren was strong enough to receive visitors. Indeed, his father, mother, and stepmother came to San Francisco at around Christmas 1983. Since they were sick—his father suffered from diabetes and his mother had severe emphysema—they visited only briefly. Warren had a number of good talks with his father, Wiley, when both his mother, Florence, and stepmother, Helen, were away. Florence appeared to be used to hospital routines and remained somewhat aloof, while Warren's father tried harder to understand what was going on. Sad but open and accepting of the people around his son, Wiley provided support and was appreciative of the help provided to his son by the hospital staff. Warren's friend, Rebecca R., also came to the ward daily for several weeks, conducting interviews with caregivers that would form the core of her theatrical production. The first Christmas on Ward 5 B—also known as "the island in a sea of selfishness"—featured a big dinner to which the entire hospital staff, community leaders, patients, and their families were invited. Tables brimmed with traditional holiday food, including turkey, ham, stuffing, and gravy, as well as salads and desserts. A custom-decorated Christmas tree and sacks of wrapped presents provided a traditional holiday atmosphere. A steady stream of visitors arrived bearing gifts, including boxes of Godiva chocolate and what one volunteer characterized as "small versions of Walgreens,"—the drugstore—including soaps, razors, toothbrushes, and shampoo.[151]

Besides the official staff, 5 B was constantly populated by other volunteers, some of them just visitors, others bringing in more food. Zany Rita Rocket, a travel agent, served Sunday brunches to patients and their visitors and tap danced in the hallway. Another volunteer, in her quest to stimulate lagging appetites and sagging spirits, brought marijuana-laced brownies to grateful patients. One volunteer was identified as the "bath queen"; others were very proficient at giving massages. Still others simply delivered blood samples or wheeled the patients around. Many volunteers were relatives of AIDS patients who had died; a few eventually became patients themselves on 5 B.

Kelly had many good memories of the ward and the people who worked there. He said there was "a wonderful feeling to the ward; it was one of the first hospital situations in which I felt the staff was committed to creating a community." Previously, all of Kelly's experiences with hospitals had left him feeling dehumanized, but the staff of 5B "treated the patient as a whole person, not as parts of a chart."[152] Still, he strongly doubted that life was being prolonged by the drug treatments the patients received there. Perhaps the opposite was true. "The medical community is not used to having to deal with those diseases and a lot of the drugs employed are highly toxic . . . if anything, I think there is a tendency to shorten people's lives in the hospital."[153]

Managing death and dying

Contemporary experience suggested that AIDS becoming increasingly synonymous with death. A week after his admission, Warren got to see a Shanti
counselor summoned by Kelly. Often called in by the ward's social worker, the
volunteers—most of them gay and some of them AIDS sufferers themselves—
circulated freely from room to room, offering their services. "Every day I walk
into somebody's room uninvited and let them know who I am and that I am available to them," recalled Jan, one volunteer.[154] Shanti trained its counselors to engage individual patients and create a human bond, especially with those who were
lonely or receptive to discussing issues surrounding their illness and impending
death. One counselor remembered writing a will for one of his patients. Shanti's
approach was to look at the whole patient and determine all perceived physical
and emotional needs. Just listening to the dying could be a healing experience.
Responses and words were not based on formulas but were left to the intuition
of the caregiver. As one of them recalled, these encounters were sometimes very
intense but helpful.[155]

Although AIDS reintroduced the reality of death to public consciousness,
American culture largely ignored it, even denied it. Everyday routines and social
encounters allowed for little contact with the dying and the dead. Moreover, the
rhythm and intensity of the typical technologically driven hospital life prevented
opportunities for listening and talking. But neither death nor talk of death could
be avoided on Ward 5 B, which, in contrast with the life-giving transplantation
unit at Moffit, appeared to be a "recruitment center for the morgue," even a "death
house."[156] Because of their young age and stigmatized status, AIDS patients frequently expressed doubts about the meaning of their lives. Slow death in an institution could be a lonely fate, especially if in the final analysis feelings of unful-
fillment and futility arose. Moreover, patients like Warren faced the reality of
waning control over a body ravaged by disease. Some were absolutely terrified
about the future. When and how would they lose final control over their bodies?
Would it be very painful?

Dying concerned all patients hospitalized on 5 B. Our cultural assumption is
that all hospitalizations will be for the better, that lives, if not saved, can at least
be prudently prolonged. Yet Ward 5 B seemed different. Here modern medicine
revealed a limited ability to stem the course of opportunistic infections consum-
ing the patients. Caregivers could only promise to make the dying process more
comfortable through the generous use of pain killers like morphine. For practitioners who considered themselves capable of battling disease with success, death
was the ultimate enemy, to be fought off at any price. Thus, AIDS patients expressed recurrent fears about being caught in the middle of this war, adding physi-
cian-induced suffering to their dying. In spite of such perceptions, Morrison and
his staff worked hard to create a supportive environment that acknowledged the

shifting expectations of those who were in danger of losing their lives. The quid pro quo was that patients taught the staff the reality of dying, while the staff, in turn, responded by teaching patients the reality of love and understanding. "I think we have created a nice place to die here in the hospital," observed George, one of the nurses.[157]

To be sure, persons die the way they live, exhibiting a great variety of responses that reflect our society's pronounced individualism. Some remain fearful and anxious; others come to terms with their fate and make peace with themselves or those around them. In the AIDS ward, some patients wanted to be left alone, refusing nourishment and medication, while others desperately sought company and hoped to prolong their lives. As one observer declared, "we come to the conclusion that the most important thing about dying is to have control over how we go about the business of doing it."[158] In any event, it seemed important for caregivers to be there as needed and hold vigils with their patients, following traditions that probably went back in time to the dawn of humankind. One female intern sat up with Warren all night, listening to his stories and learning a great deal about dying. This was an important albeit exhausting bonding experience for everyone, nowadays practiced especially in cancer wards and intensive care units.

For many, the question arose as to whether AIDS' clinical manifestations and moral implications denied its sufferers a good death. But could dying become a form of healing, a reconciliation with oneself and one's life? Within days of receiving his AIDS diagnosis, Warren talked extensively with Kelly about funeral arrangements. Hoping to stay in control even beyond his death, Warren planned another theatrical performance. Since he had been involved in filming dances, he demanded to be laid out in his white unitard, his face covered with white makeup. After cremation, Warren's ashes were to be dispersed on a farm in Nashville owned by the person he had previously danced with.

Death and dying on Ward 5 B also brought home the importance of code status, especially in the event of unexpected neurological complications and mental impairment. On admission, patients were requested to sign a directive expressing their wishes with regard to possible resuscitation efforts in the event of an emergency. As in other hospitals, American patients had the right to make informed decisions about the scope and length of their care and, moreover, to make judgments concerning their quality of life in relation to complications arising from their diseases and treatments.[159] Given the high death rate in the AIDS ward during its first year, these concerns were quite realistic, although the long-term evolution of AIDS was still unknown. The modern deathbed ritual of multiple subspecialty consultations was largely omitted. "We can make death comfortable," explained Morrison. "They'll fight and fight and fight. And then it comes to the point that they'll say I just can't take it anymore, and then, they'll die."[160]

Some of the patients and caregivers had problems with the so-called death and dying industry spawned by health practitioners, psychologists, and bioethicists in the 1970s. The most often quoted book on this topic was Elizabeth Kübler Ross' *On Death and Dying* (1969) in which the author postulated that the process of human dying involves five progressive stages ending with acceptance.[161] While useful for unravelling some of the attitudes towards death imbedded in a complex of cultural beliefs and practices, Kübler Ross' scenario possessed no empirical validation and no claim on universality. Actual management of dying patients based on such a model could be problematic. In the experience of caregivers on 5 B, not every dying patient accepted his fate peacefully. Death continued to be an unpredictable human event, something less easy to control than the books described. Lack of a consensus about the "right" way to die hobbled both patients and their caregivers. Some patients even felt guilty: "I am not dying according to plan" was a frequent comment. Frustrated, some AIDS sufferers improvised unique mixtures of previous religious and military death myths, variously stressing acceptance and afterlife or the heroism and liberation of this final rite of passage.[162] In a sense, 5 B patients perceived themselves as death row inmates, except that they did not know the manner of their demise. Nurses, in turn, felt that there was an excessive fear of dying. "We all have these ideas of what death is but how it takes place and the reality is invariably very different, especially with this disease," observed Allison M.[163]

For some caregivers, the intensity of their ministry began to take its toll. The long hours, the frustration of witnessing the hopelessness and suffering of the patients, the futility and high toxicity of medical treatments, coupled with administrative snafus, all fostered burnout or compassion fatigue. To be sure, many of the nurses had come from other units such as oncology, where similar situations prevailed, although the patients were mostly older. Efforts to deal with helplessness and grief drained them emotionally. "You die with every patient that touches you as a person," remembered Diane Jones.[164] Eventually, angry and depressed, some caregivers had to end their intense emotional involvement to continue functioning. Like soldiers fighting in the trenches, they showed clear signs of the traumatic stress syndrome commonly known as battle fatigue. A protective detachment became necessary as nurses and counselors accepted the reality of death and the constant turnover of patients. Some were forced to take brief leaves of absence to regain control over their own lives and repair family relationships. But "you really never got away," remembered Diane. The nightmare went on endlessly. To help themselves, the caregivers created their own support group, meeting regularly with Dilley, the psychiatrist, to share their feelings and reduce stress.[165]

According to Kelly, Warren failed to share fully the Shanti death preparation strategy designed for him during his final months at SFGH. With his combative spirit, he still had hope that he could beat his illness. A Pollyanna at heart, Warren never felt sorry for himself. According to Kelly, he treated his counselor as a new audience for his stories, thereby avoiding the "heavy stuff." Ken, the counselor, insisted that his function was merely to validate a patient's suffering. "Volunteer counselors are trained to be with someone, not to have an agenda of their own . . . they are trained to reflect what the client is feeling and whatever he is feeling is right. We don't judge."[166] Warren's narratives became a strategy for coping with AIDS, to reaffirm his identity, and to revisit some of the highlights of his young career. The volunteer apparently was delighted to interact with a patient still full of life and exhibiting so many interests. "It was wonderful to sit in his room and hang out with him," Ken later recalled.[167]

While Warren and others continued to deny the imminence of death and to express optimism, hoping perhaps to lick the disease and leave the hospital, the Shanti counselors tried more realistically to prepare patients for their long-term prognosis by moving them along the continuum outlined by Kübler Ross. While other sick individuals in the ward said their goodbyes and died, Warren gallantly continued to struggle for life, even after the complications of the disease had robbed him of most of his faculties. As another staff member remarked, the young men on 5 B were less fearful of actually dying than of losing their lives, lives full of plans and dreams, now reluctantly to be abandoned. Under such dramatic circumstances, Ward 5 B became the target for radical Christian groups who sought to convert some of the dying patients. Preying on their fears, clergymen sought to manipulate the sick and attempt moral recovery. Under the guise of delivering toothbrushes, toothpaste, and other personal items, one team of SOS (Save our Souls) missionaries invaded a particular room, prepared to give "witness" to its inmate. On another occasion, a zealous volunteer chaplain tried a similar proselytizing ploy, but to no avail. Many were summarily ejected from the premises, although they claimed to have received a summons from individuals requesting to be saved. A special Catholic gay organization, Dignity's Ministry to People with AIDS, was authorized by SFGH's coordinator of chaplains to assist those in need. Like other hospital patients, those requesting pastoral care were provided with a clergyman of their choice.[168]

After losing his job and giving up his apartment, Kelly spent many nights in the hospital, and the staff of 5 B became like a family to him and Warren, supporting both of them. In early January 1984, complications from the drug treatment forced physicians to stop Warren's amphotericin B treatments. His family had a history of kidney stones, and Warren passed such a stone, followed by profuse bleeding. He remained at SFGH for most of the next month. As his respiratory difficulties subsided, the sulfa drugs were stopped. With his blood condition and renal function improved, amphotericin was resumed. Vertigo and extreme fatigue remained, and pain management continued. On February 17, Warren received a Hickman catheter to facilitate self-administration of intravenous amphotericin B to control his cryptococcal meningitis. As his opportunistic infections lessened under aggressive therapy, he became well enough to check himself out of the hospital into a Shanti residence on February 20, 1984. More than a year earlier, the Shanti Project had begun opening a number of hospice-type care centers in private houses. Home, however, was not always the expected place of solace and intimacy, but an equally contested space shattering notions of greater comfort and familiar support.[169] There Warren remained under the supervision of a visiting nurse and planned to make follow-up visits to the outpatient clinic for blood examinations to monitor the side effects of his drug treatment. He also had a tube put in his chest for further aerosol treatments with pentaminine to keep the pneumocystis pneumonia in check. A follow-up examination three days after entering the hospice disclosed some clinical improvement. Warren appeared alert, his lungs were clear, and he was told to return to the clinic in one week to monitor his blood status while continuing to take the amphotericin. Had he conquered the infections through sheer courage and determination?[170]

Upbeat, Warren's renewed goal was to draw and write about his experiences. Friends provided him with a word processor but to no avail. The side effects of his drug therapy kept him "zonked out" most of the day, making him depressed and despondent. On March 8, another visit to Ward 86 found him gaunt and wasted but free of neurological, respiratory, and gastrointestinal symptoms. The intravenous amphotericin regimen, however, had induced a precipitous drop in Warren's hematocrit, suggesting bone marrow failure or another infection. On March 14, therefore, Warren was brought back to the clinic for a blood transfusion. During this time, Shanti also provided a therapist who tried to assist his healing by employing an alternative treatment: visualization. This method consisted of letting the patient tell stories about his life and find a common thread tying them together that might be responsible for the disease. Warren's plan was to complete two additional weeks of drug therapy before flying back home to Tennessee for a brief visit. He did not wish to return as an invalid, forcing his father and stepmother to care for him.[171]

Unfortunately, Warren's father, Wiley, was unable to find a practitioner in Knoxville willing to look after Warren—at the time few physicians dared to see AIDS patients—and the plan had to be dropped. The prospects of being hospitalized and possibly placed in total isolation far away from San Francisco were daunting. "He would have been treated as a leper," speculated Kelly. The question, however, turned out to be irrelevant. Within a week, Warren experienced a dramatic seizure and was taken by ambulance to SFGH's Emergency Room on March 20, where he had another attack without losing consciousness. He was then transferred to the hospital's Neurology Unit and readmitted to the AIDS ward the following day. Everyone, including Warren himself, had hoped that he could spend his last days at a hospice, but it became clear that, after the grand mal attack, he was too sick to be discharged.

Following his return to Ward 5 B, Warren appeared mentally clear, with normal speech, but complaining of headaches. A test was positive for the cryptococcal antigen, suggesting a recurrence of his previous meningitis.[172] Seizures continued during the first week of hospitalization, despite large doses of anticonvul-sive medication. Warren also had difficulty walking and experienced persistent headaches, nausea, and vomiting. The seizures were devastating, with Warren be-coming progressively aphasic before their onset. Nobody could predict when they would occur, and there seemed to be no way to prevent them. On March 28, the physicians discontinued Warren's amphotericin treatments because of his recur-rent leukopenia. Given the seriousness of his condition, Wofsy signed a "do not resuscitate" (DNR) order after obtaining permission from Warren's father. By March 31 Warren was confused, frequently climbing out of bed and in need of restraints. Suspecting herpes encephalitis, physicians ordered a computed tomog-raphy scan, but the results were inconclusive. A test for herpes, however, came back positive, and Warren was placed on the antiviral agent Acyclovir. As he strug-gled in Ward 5 B, San Francisco became increasingly embroiled in the bath house controversy. Under pressure from Mayor Diane Feinstein and members of the Board of Supervisors, Dr. Melvyn Silverman, director of the San Francisco De-partment of Public Health, promised to formulate guidelines banning sex activ-ity in bath houses. Gay community activists responded strongly, suggesting that such measures were "killing" the gay liberation movement.[173]

In early April, Warren's headaches became progressively more severe. The seizures were quite dramatic and frequent, in spite of higher doses of dilantin. In-creasingly, Warren needed more time to regain his speech and overcome his dis-orientation. A pattern developed in which he went for two days without seizures and then had a series of four or five epileptic fits followed by a long period of un-responsiveness. His progressively impaired mental status became a source of de-spair for both caregivers and friends. Gone were the smile, the pep, the optimistic stance. Even the Shanti counselor felt totally helpless and stopped his visits. A de-bate ensued among the caregivers about the wisdom of performing a brain biopsy, but the ward nurses, in their patient advocacy role, strongly opposed the proce-dure. In another vain attempt to control Warren's symptoms, the physicians once more increased the doses of dilantin and phenobarbital.

As Kelly remembered, Warren "just really shut down. I think the last two weeks he was just lying there waiting for his body to stop."[174] Warren had finally come to terms with the inevitable outcome and now seemed more at peace with his suffering and impending death. After all, he had for a time responded coura-geously to the challenges of a cruel disease, he told his friends. Perhaps Warren shared the feelings of another AIDS-infected gay man who had recently admitted that "in some ways I even look forward to death as a rest, a release from care. It will be nice not to have to worry about the future anymore—about happiness and success, about ambition and fulfillment. It will be nice not to have to try so hard to find 'meaning' in everything and to make every moment count."[175] As Warren was dying, Mayor Feinstein declared April 2–8 as AIDS Prevention Week in the city to stress the importance of disseminating all available information on the new disease. Six hundred new victims were expected to be diagnosed in the Bay Area before the end of the year.

Back at Ward 5 B, the attending intern wrote of a plan to discharge Warren to a Shanti residence on April 8 if no further seizures occurred. However, the patient's lingering lethargy and new complaints of headaches forced physicians to modify this plan by sending him temporarily to a hospice. This transfer was in turn cancelled because of Warren's deteriorating condition. By April 11 he was unresponsive and moribund, again with a spiking fever. At 7.30 AM on April, 13, 1984, Warren was found dead in his room. No autopsy was performed. His death certificate listed respiratory arrest, herpes zoster, encephalitis, and AIDS as the main causes. Other problems were chronic diarrhea caused by the parasitic protozoan cryptosporidium, cryptococcal meningitis, and other opportunistic infections.

Warren's body was cremated immediately. He thus joined San Francisco's "city of ghosts," another of those ethereal residents just floating around, never exhibited in death in funeral homes or buried in their own plot of land.[176] His funerary wishes were respected and his ashes taken to Nashville to be scattered on the grounds of his friend's farm. In the presence of his family and friends, congregated in the evening around a bonfire, Warren's ashes were blown with the help of a fan into filmed images of his dances projected against the dark sky, thus allowing the reflection and his ashes to mingle before returning to the ground. As the ceremony ended, a burst of fireworks exploded in a final salute to a man who wanted so much to leave a legacy to posterity. Warren's struggles with AIDS had demonstrated the power of the human spirit and the value of life.

The lessons of AIDS

Warren's experiences with the *San Francisco model* of AIDS care deserve further comment, particularly because Wards 86 and 5 B soon became internationally famous, attracting physicians, nurses, community leaders, politicians, and celebrities from all over the world. Their multidisciplinary approach for delivering care had been shaped in part by the unique epidemiological characteristics of the disease in the city, as well as by the personalities of those who chose to devote their attention to patients suffering from AIDS. In its early phase, Ward 5 B was perceived as a combination of modern hospital and hospice. Believing in the acute nature of the disease, the unit "patched up" patients and fought the broad panorama of infectious diseases resulting from impaired immunity. When these measures failed, caregivers provided for a dignified death. The military metaphors, traditionally *de rigueur* in medical discourse, were adopted by both caregivers and patients as they spoke of young men being felled by an invisible enemy. As in other hospital-based "skirmishes" and "trench warfare," conditions such as shell shock and battle fatigue soon afflicted perennially overworked staff members.

Many visualized Ward 5 B as operating like a MASH unit, where caregivers were confronted day and night with sick and dying individuals, engaged in a war that was bound to end soon.

The ward's primary role was nursing together with additional medical intervention. Given their limited expertise in the early 1980s, physicians mainly monitored clinical progress with the help of laboratory information and attempted to deal with the opportunistic infections using a conventional array of antibiotics and highly toxic chemotherapeutic agents. AIDS was difficult to diagnose, treat, and prognosticate. While deaths were frequent, possible cures were also expected and eagerly discussed. Insufficient statistics about the lethal nature of AIDS spawned renewed hope. Although it seemed unclear to contemporaries whether AIDS had already peaked, historical perspectives from previous epidemics offered reassurance and promised future relief. As one early sufferer declared, "eventually I think they'll find a cure whether it is ten months or ten years."[177]

By contemporary standards, Warren had remained in the hospital for an extensive period. His first 70-day hospitalization ended in February, but he was readmitted in March for another 23 days before his death. One Shanti volunteer recalled, "Warren wanted to die on the ward in 'his' room." He had lived in this healing space for so long that everybody readily identified it as "Warren's room." "Rooms are like mausoleums," remarked the volunteer. "They have memories of the people occupying them."[178] For Warren, 17 B was no longer a randomly assigned, impersonal hospital room, but an environment filled with his possessions, as well as recent memories of good times spent with friends and family. Within a year, however, the average stay in the AIDS ward went down sharply to 12 days. Thanks to prompt aerosol treatment, patients now easily survived a second and even a third bout of pneumocystis pneumonia and were then promptly discharged. Three years later, in 1987, AIDS patients remained in the hospital for only seven or eight days thanks to the improved outpatient facilities and options for home treatment. Life expectancy, meanwhile, remained about 18 months after the onset of the first symptoms.[179]

April 1984 turned out to be the crest of another demoralizing mortality wave for SFGH's Ward 5 B, with 15 deaths recorded during that month alone. A new statistical tool, the city's *AIDS Report*, inaugurated by Dr. Mervyn F. Silverman, by April 30 listed 41 new AIDS cases and a total of 19 AIDS deaths. To contemporaries of Warren in San Francisco, AIDS was seen as a subacute, frequently fatal disease predominantly affecting younger white males. Warren's age group (30–39) represented by far the most numerous contingent of AIDS cases (53%). Viewed by race and ethnicity, whites still accounted for 91% of all AIDS victims and most of them admitted to being gay, a critical statistic in understanding life and caregiving in SFGH's AIDS ward.[180] Meanwhile, the CDC reported the existence of almost 4,000 cases in the United States. The four "H's"—homosexuals, Haitians, hemophiliacs, and heroin addicts—emerged as the most likely spreaders of AIDS.

As the first anniversary of Ward 5 B neared, the original generation of AIDS patients was gradually dying. Warren was among the first cohort of persons diagnosed with the complications of this disease after their immune systems were irreversibly damaged. Even aggressive treatment of the multiple opportunistic infections seemed to provide little hope of success, especially following involvement of the central nervous system. On April 24, 11 days after Warren's death, Margaret Heckler, then secretary of health and human services, announced that virologist Robert Gallo and his collaborators at the National Institutes of Health had discovered the virus that causes AIDS, an event strongly disputed by French investigators who had already made a similar claim. A test to detect the HTLV-III virus—as this particular human T-cell leukemia virus was named—was to be available soon, and a vaccine was promised within 18–24 months. In its May 4 issue, the journal *Science* published Gallo's and French scientist Luc Montagnier's findings causally linking the new retrovirus to clinical AIDS.[181] This was the same month in which the film star Rock Hudson was also diagnosed with the disease, and a new era of a more sympathetic portrayal of AIDS patients by the media ensued.[182]

Like previous episodes of mass disease, AIDS exposed critical fault lines in the American health care system.[183] At one level, the myth of our perceived conquest of infectious diseases was shockingly pierced. Until AIDS occurred, the prevailing notion was that the microbe hunters had succeeded. Now professional arrogance seemed to paralyze medicine's response. At the outset, the disease was not taken seriously. Remembered Conant: "We believed that the challenge we faced in finding out what was causing Kaposi sarcoma was going to be very much like toxic shock syndrome, or Legionnaire's disease."[184] The likely scenario was familiar to everyone. Basic science would quickly identify the bacterium or virus, and then specific antibiotics or antiviral drugs would be tested, eventually neutralizing or slaying the invading culprit. Good epidemiological tracing, in turn, would reveal the pattern of transmission and provide the necessary clues for prevention. Such optimism, however, was partially dashed as physicians and scientists traveled a slow road to identifying the cause of AIDS.

On another front, traditional American hospital organizations seemed unable to cope with people suffering from AIDS. It soon became clear that special facilities devoted entirely to the diagnosis and care of this disease were desirable to enhance the quality of care and reduce its costs. From an efficiency standpoint, hospitals needed a substitute for ineffective and expensive treatment of AIDS patients in scattered intensive care and isolation units. From their very inception, SFGH's Wards 86 and 5 B operated on one level as acute, highly technical, interventionist care models for treating a complicated illness with a poor prognosis. At issue were a number of tenacious and recurrent opportunistic infections waxing and waning in the face of highly toxic drugs. New knowledge and skills were demanded from doctors.[185] As house officers, attending physicians, and visitors, a cadre of young physicians, many of them gay, learned this management in San Francisco's well-organized clinical showcase.

At another level, AIDS forced a reevaluation of the attitudes and behavior of caregivers. In spite of the risk of contagion, physicians were reminded of their professional responsibilities for treating the sick. In addition to providing drug therapy, they were forced to pay greater attention to the mental and emotional status of their patients and to review the limits of their technical intervention. "I think it [AIDS] has brought back the art of medicine into our medical education process," admitted Sande.[186] Greater sensitivity to quality-of-life issues was imperative, as were efforts—previously ignored or denied by modern medicine—to orchestrate a good death. AIDS forced the prevailing hospital culture to face the issue of dying, requiring caregivers to restructure their work.[187] These circumstances demanded out- and inpatient counseling, private rooms, support groups, referral services, and community outreach. For those professionals who really cared and shared their burdens with patients, the personal rewards could be great, but hospitals were also keenly aware of the risks involved in such total care. Efforts to avoid the burnout of hospital personnel, including counseling and rap sessions rarely considered before, eventually became institutionalized in hospitals throughout the United States.

"Everything one can come up with in medicine just first happened with AIDS," insisted Wofsy, including methods for tracking the development of new drugs, advanced medical directories, the confluence of medical and nursing functions, and a reformulation of the patient–physician relationship to allow for greater patient input.[188] The arrangements eventually became a model for the management of chronic care for other diseases. Services were shifted from the hospital ward to the clinic and from the clinic to homes or hospices.[189]

Because of the complex, multiorgan involvement in AIDS, the cost of care was high—double that of other infectious diseases—leading to attempts by hospital authorities to share this cost with federal, state, and local governments as well as private sponsors, including insurance companies, foundations, and community organizations. A typical course of the disease in the early 1980s usually meant that patients needed frequent clinic visits and multiple hospitalizations. In general, AIDS treatments were very expensive because of their intensity and duration.[190] Laboratory monitoring of the disease and drug therapies involved extensive bacteriological culturing and multiple biopsies. Infection control measures, social services, and counseling created additional costs. For physicians, specialization in AIDS was demanding and time-consuming, without the usual financial rewards, especially for those who treated hospital patients covered by Medi-Cal. The extensive involvement of dedicated volunteers became critical in providing the scope and level of care demanded by the clinical contours of AIDS.

At one level, the San Francisco model stressed a holistic approach, borrowed in part from oncology via those afflicted with KS, but also because patients belonged to a stigmatized sector of the population whose social and behavioral characteristics played a decisive role in organizing their care. By painting AIDS as a special disease, recalled Wofsy, caregivers made it clear that they intended to offer its victims a special level of effort. Traditional medical paternalism, steadily in retreat since the 1960s, gave way to a more cooperative relationship between caregivers and well-informed patients. Although always contested, the physician's authority was further challenged by AIDS, given the rudimentary knowledge of the disease and the uncertain outcome of medical treatment. Rather than making unilateral decisions, practitioners provided options and made recommendations. Such dialogue was facilitated by the nature of those who suffered from AIDS. "This sudden influx of highly articulate young questioning people," explained Wofsy, "was stunningly stimulating and held the physician to the kind of expectation that private patients hold their practitioners to."[191] Physicians such as Volberding, Abrams, and others put their personal lives on hold, becoming totally immersed in the unfolding epidemic as caregivers, researchers, administrators, patient advocates, and even political activists.

Because of their nursing and community involvement, AIDS units such as SFGH's Ward 5 B stimulated the emergent hospice movement. As early as December 1983, the Hospice of San Francisco had contracted with the city's Public Health Department to include AIDS patients among its terminally ill residents. Given the escalating expenses and shorter stays at hospitals, similar opportunities to become intimately involved with patients and provide loving care also shifted to other similar institutions such as the city-run Laguna Honda Hospice. However, given the chronic personnel shortages, where would one find the highly specialized and dedicated nurses who were necessary? More important, how could whole communities be mobilized successfully to combat other diseases? Morrison's comments in 1984 echoed those of Wofsy. Both were optimistic: "AIDS has changed health care so that it will never be the same again. Issues that have been problems for years came all of a sudden full blown to the surface. Whether people want to acknowledge it or not, health care will be better because of this." Morrison added that "it is a real shame that it took AIDS for us to do what we are doing. I hope it will catch on, not just for AIDS, but for everything. I really see that the way we are running 5 B is a very simple way to run nursing units in a hospital."[192]

San Francisco's multidisciplinary approach emphasized human care rather than technical medical assistance alone. It thus required novel ways to provide hospital care and utilize community services. Nursing's more prominent role in clinical decision making, its renewed devotion to social and psychological issues, set the tone. A return to both the art of medicine and the art of nursing reestablished a measure of human contact that had been gradually dissipating in the twentieth century as caregivers focused on and declared "war" on disease rather than being concerned with caring for sick persons.

Given society's strong denial of the reality of death, the absence of a paradigm for "good dying" led to a number of improvisations and new rituals. At Ward 5 B, patients such as Warren returned to teach their most important lesson: healing and dying are fundamental human experiences best achieved through intimacy, communication, and communal support. The early AIDS story in San Francisco exemplified a dramatic shift in the goals of medicine, prompting physicians once more to address human suffering and pain. Diagnostic and therapeutic strategies attempted to make sick persons comfortable and maximize their functions, not just to extend life for its own sake. This focus required a close working relationship between caregivers and patients to create options in harmony with their values and feelings. The therapeutic decisions taken by the caregivers of Ward 5 B were congruent with the long-term interests of the patients themselves, not just agendas prepared by physicians or insurance companies.

Warren's passage is our last patient journey through a hospital, undertaken within the complex medical and social context shaping life in San Francisco during the early 1980s. His final wish was granted. Through their personal accounts and stories of their pilgrimages, the dead live on in our world. They become examples, reminders of the collective struggle with AIDS. Warren's story of courage and empathy featured San Francisco's unique gay culture and its premier model of AIDS care. Like the portion of the AIDS quilt that honors his memory, Warren's story will remain part of the epidemic's early profile at a time when caring for AIDS patients was a novel experience intimately linked with dying and the limits of scientific knowledge. In San Francisco, the patients were all young males, and together with most caregivers, members of the local gay and lesbian community. Communication and bonding took place in an atmosphere of altruism and compassion seldom seen elsewhere in the 1980s. Parallels to earlier twentieth-century American hospitals as communal expressions of ethnic pride, identity, and responsibility are obvious.

Alexis, the seventh patient admitted to Ward 5 B after its opening in July 1983, put it best: "If we keep missing the point of this crisis, we will keep repeating mistakes. It's really going back to a very humanitarian approach. We've come out of the total scientific solution, and come up pretty empty-handed. Now we have to look beyond the statistics. We have to read between the lines. We have to look at the broader dimension of the human being. When we use the word 'humanitarian,' we are talking about a human being as opposed to an intelligent organism. That dimension is going to include the physical, the emotional, the intellectual, and the spiritual. There is no way to measure accurately three of those, and yet we are trying desperately to do that. It really bothers me to see this opportunity missed by humanity to help itself and to become a bit more patient with itself."[193]

With AIDS as experienced in Ward 5 B of SFGH during 1984, we have indeed come full circle from the early Christian shelters created in the Roman Empire nearly 2,000 years earlier. "Caregiving is one way for humans to learn about humanity," observed one Shanti counselor. "It is not only about simply doing for others. It's also about self-acceptance and honest intentions. The best caregivers are those who come to work not out of guilt or professional necessity, but because they have been touched by the soul of another human being."[194] With insights into AIDS' ability to threaten the integrity of patients' personhood, many caregivers in Ward 5 B achieved an intuitive understanding of their patients' suffering. Sharing meanings and values as well as socioeconomic status, both parties established a truly healing kinship, in spite of the therapeutic failures and frequent deaths. Here the hospital truly embodied the traditional *hospitalitas* or gift relationship between caregivers and patients. One nurse, Gary C., suggested the best epitaph for Ward 5 B: "Once upon a time there was a disease called AIDS and these rooms were filled with people who were loved by people with love."[195]

NOTES

1. From a letter dated December 18, 1984, and addressed to San Francisco's Mayor Dianne Feinstein. Book of testimonials, SFGH's Ward 5 A.

2. Mike Hippler, "Blue Thursday: A Community Confronts the AIDS Crisis," Gay and Lesbian Historical Society of Northern California, Box 90-12. See also R. A. Padgug and G. M. Oppenheimer, "Riding the tiger: AIDS and the gay community," in *AIDS: The Making of a Chronic Disease*, ed. E. Fee and D. M. Fox, Berkeley, Univ. of California Press, 1992, pp. 245–78.

3. M. Hippler, "AIDS, a personal exploration; the new gay ward at SFGH," *Bay Area Rep* 8 (Oct. 20, 1983): 16.

4. S. L. Montgomery, "Codes and combat in biomedical discourse," *Science as Culture* 2 (1991): 341–90. See also Anne Hunsaker Hawkins, *Reconstructing Illness: Studies in Pathography*, West Lafayette, IN, Purdue Univ. Press, 1993, pp. 61–77.

5. Hippler, "AIDS, a personal exploration," 223.

6. Personal interview with Kelly H., January 1994. For details on the historical development of the American gay community see Dennis Altman, *The Homosexualization of America, the Americanization of the Homosexual*, New York, St. Martin's Press, 1982, and George Chauncey, *Gay New York: Gender, Urban Culture and the Making of the Gay Male World, 1890–1940*, New York, Basic Books, 1994, especially pp. 1–29.

7. J. D'Emilio, "Gay politics and gay community: The San Francisco experience," *Socialist Rev* 11 (January–February 1981): 77–104, partially republished as "Gay politics and community in San Francisco since World War II," in *Hidden from History: Reclaiming the Gay and Lesbian Past*, ed. M. B. Duberman, M. Vicinus, and G. Chauncey, Jr., New York, New American Library, 1989, pp. 456–73. For background see John D'Emilio, *Sexual Politics, Sexual Communities: The Making of a Homosexual Minority in the US, 1940–1970*, Chicago, Univ. of Chicago Press, 1983, and Susan Stryker and Jim Buskirk, *Gay By the Bay*, San Francisco, Chronicle Books, 1996.

8. For a brief introduction to San Francisco's gay community see Frances FitzGerald, "The Castro-I" *The New Yorker* (July 21, 1986): 34–70. More details are provided in this author's *Cities on a Hill: A Journey Through Contemporary American Cultures*, New York, Simon & Schuster, 1986.

9. Hippler, "Blue Thursday," p. 218. For an analysis of the reactions to sexual freedom

see D. Altman, "Sex: The frontline of gay politics," *Socialist* Review 43 (September–October 1982): 3–17, and S. Epstein, "Moral contagion and the medicalizing of gay identity: AIDS in historical perspective," *Res Law, Deviance, Social Control* 9 (1988): 3–36.

10. W. Szmuness et al., "On the role of sexual behavior in the spread of hepatitis B infection," *Ann Intern Med* 83 (1975): 489–95. For details on hepatitis B see William Muraskin, *The War Against Hepatitis B: A History of the International Task Force on Hepatitis B Immunization*, Philadelphia, Univ. Pennsylvania Press, 1995.

11. S. Dritz, "Medical aspects of homosexuality," *N Engl J Med* 302 (Feb. 21, 1980): 463–64, and W. F. Owen, "Sexually transmitted diseases and traumatic problems in homosexual men," *Ann Intern Med* 92 (1980): 805–08. For background see B. Hansen, "American physicians' earliest writings about homosexuals, 1880–1900," *Milbank Q* 67 Suppl. 1 (1989): 92–108.

12. M. J. Schmerin et al., "Giardiasis: Association with homosexuality," *Ann Intern Med* 88 (1978): 801–03.

13. Kelly H. interview, January 1994. For a bibliography of AIDS narratives see T. F. Murphy and S. Poirier, eds., *Writing AIDS: Gay Literature, Language, and Analysis*, New York, Columbia Univ. Press, 1993.

14. Hawkins, *Reconstructing Illness*, p. 68.

15. Rebecca Ranson, *Warren*. I am indebted to the playwright for the opportunity of reading her script.

16. I employed a chronology prepared by Nancy Grey Osterud and her graduate students. Further information is contained in two unpublished papers prepared by them: "San Francisco General Hospital in Historical Perspective" (November 1990) and "The Changing Mission of San Francisco General Hospital" (July 1991). Hospital Archives. Courtesy of Moses Grossman.

17. See the editorial "Hospitals are one of the necessities of modern times," *Pacific Med Surg J* 5 (1862): 311–15.

18. Editorial, "San Francisco city and county hospital," *Occid Med Times* 4 (1890): 381–87, and "Hospital notes," *Calif Med J* 15 (1894): 225–28.

19. Editorial, "City and county hospital," *Pacific Med Surg J* 40 (1897): 96–97.

20. For details of the bubonic plague epidemic and the hospital see G. B. Risse, "The politics of fear: Bubonic plague in San Francisco, California, 1900," in *New Countries and Old Medicine*, ed. L. Bryder and D. Dow, Auckland, NZ, Pyramid Press, 1995, pp. 1–19, and "A long pull, a strong pull, and all together: San Francisco and bubonic plague, 1907–1908," *Bull Hist Med* 66 (1992): 260–86. See also L. Eloesser, "The City and County Hospital of San Francisco: Recollections of far away and long ago," *Am J Surg* 118 (October 1969): 493–97.

21. T. W. Huntington, "What the new hospital means to San Francisco," *Pacif Coast J Nurs* 11 (1915): 291–92.

22. R. G. Brodrick, "New San Francisco Hospital is finest of its kind," *The Modern Hospital* 5 (November 1915): 311–20. See also J. Irvine, "A brief history of the San Francisco General Hospital," *UCSF Alumni/Faculty Assoc Bull* 18 (1974): 2–6.

23. Haven Emerson and Anna C. Phillips, *Hospitals and Health Agencies of San Francisco, 1923: A Survey*, San Francisco, Community Chest, 1923, especially pp. 27–83.

24. Leontina Murphy, "Public Care for the Dependent Sick in San Francisco, 1847–1936," M.A. thesis, Univ. of California, Berkeley, 1938, pp. 124–54.

25. Osterud, "SFGH in historical perspective," p. 35.

26. F. W. Blaisdell, "The pre-Medicare role of city/county hospitals in education and health care," *J Trauma* 32 (February 1992): 217–28.

27. F. W. Blaisdell, "Development of the city/county (public) hospital," *Arch Surg* 129 (1994): 760–64.

28. San Francisco Department of Public Health, "San Francisco General Hospital," in *Annual Report 1971–1972*, pp. 35–40, and *Annual Report 1972–1973*, pp. 39–50.

29. For background see J. S. Roberts et al., "A history of the Joint Commission of Accreditation of Hospitals," *JAMA* 258 (Aug. 21, 1987): 936–40, and Joan I. Roberts and Thetis M. Group, *Feminism and Nursing: An Historical Perspective on Power, Status, and Political Activism in the Nursing Profession*, Westport, CT, Praeger, 1995.

30. N. M. Christensen, "City/county hospitals: An endangered species," *Arch Surg* 129 (1994): 903–07. For details see Richard E. Brown, *Public Medicine in Crisis: Public Hospitals in California*, Berkeley, Univ. of California Press, 1981.

31. "The San Francisco General Hospital Medical Center," *SFGH News*, commemorative issue, July 1976, and the keynote address by Francis J. Curry, "The beginning of a new era for SF General," *SFGH News* 5 (September 1976): 1–2.

32. E. R. Brown, "Public hospitals on the brink: Their problems and their options," *J Health Politics Policy Law* 7 (Winter 1983): 927–44, and J. K. Iglehart, "Federal policies and the poor," *N Engl J Med* 307 (Sep. 23, 1982): 836–40.

33. J. Feder and J. Hadley, "The economically unattractive patient: Who cares?" *Bull NY Acad Med* 61 (January–February 1985): 68–74.

34. J. Feder et al., "Falling through the cracks: Poverty, insurance coverage, and hospital care for the poor, 1980 and 1982," *Milbank M F Q* 62 (Fall 1984): 544–66, and K. Davis, "Reagan administration health policy," *J Public Health Policy* 2 (1981): 312–32.

35. L. Lingaas, "The 'General,' " *UCSF Mag* 6 (1983): 36–44.

36. J. Kadley, "Medicaid reimbursement of teaching hospitals," *J Health Politics, Policy Law* 7 (1983): 911–26.

37. H. Waitzkin, "Two-class medicine returns to the US: Impact of Medi-Cal reform," *Lancet* 2 (November 1984): 1144–46.

38. San Francisco Department of Public Health, *Annual Report 1982–1983*, pp. 11–12.

39. See UCSF's *Synapse* 28 (Mar. 1, 1984): 1, 3, and *SF Chronicle* (Feb. 23, 1984), p. 4. More information was obtained from personal discussions with former UCSF School of Medicine Dean Rudi Schmid.

40. Stuart H. Altman et al., eds. "Introduction," in *Competition and Compassion: Conflicting Roles for Public Hospitals*, Ann Arbor, Health Administration Press, 1989, pp. 1–13. For background information see Harry F. Dowling, *City Hospitals: The Care of the Underprivileged*, Cambridge, MA, Harvard Univ. Press, 1982.

41. L. H. Breimer, "Did Moritz Kaposi describe AIDS in 1872?" *Clio Med* 19 (1984): 156–58.

42. For a historical background of the possible origins of AIDS see Mirko D. Grmek, *History of AIDS: Emergence and Origin of a Modern Pandemic*, trans. R. C. Maulitz and J. Duffin, Princeton, NJ, Princeton University Press, 1990. Another recent contribution is Jaap Goudsmit, *Viral Sex: The Nature of AIDS*, New York, Oxford Univ. Press, 1997. Cases occurring before the current epidemic are considered in D. Huminer et al., "AIDS in the pre-AIDS era," *Rev Infect Dis* 9 (November–December 1987): 1102–08.

43. "Workshop on Kaposi's Sarcoma, sponsored by the NCI and the Task Force on KS and opportunistic infections of the CDC," *Cancer Treat Res* 66 (1982): 1387–90.

44. Marcus Conant, Leake Historical Lecture, UCSF, March 5, 1992. Transcript available at History of Health Sciences Dept., UCSF.

45. A. E. Friedman-Kien et al., "Disseminated Kaposi's sarcoma in homosexual men," *Ann Intern Med* 96 (1982): 693–700. A useful compilation of the early research articles

concerning AIDS is R. Kulstad, ed., *AIDS: Papers from Science, 1982–1985*, Washington, DC, American Association for the Advancement of Science, 1986.

46. An early study of this condition is H. Masur et al., "An outbreak of community-acquired *Pneumocystis carinii* pneumonia," *N Engl J Med* 305 (Dec. 10, 1981): 1431–38. Among these patients were several intravenous drug abusers. See also S. E. Follansbee et al., "An outbreak of *Pneumocystis carinii* pneumonia in homosexual men," *Ann Intern Med* 96 (1982): 705–13.

47. W. L. Drew et al., "Prevalence of cytomegalovirus infection in homosexual men," *J Infec Dis* 143 (February 1981): 188–92.

48. J. P. Vandenbroucke, "Amyl nitrate use by homosexuals," *Lancet* 1 (Feb. 27, 1982): 503.

49. D. T. Durack, "Opportunistic infections and Kaposi's sarcoma in homosexual men" (editorial), *N Engl J Med* 305 (Dec. 10, 1981): 1465–67. For a historical approach see G. B. Risse, "Epidemics before AIDS: A new research program," in *AIDS and the Historian*, ed. V. A. Harden and G. B. Risse, Washington, DC, DHHS, 1991, pp. 2–12, and C. E. Rosenberg, "What is an epidemic? AIDS in historical perspective," *Daedalus* 118 (1989): 1–17.

50. Editorial, "Immunocompromised homosexuals," *Lancet* 2 (December 1981): 1325–26. For a perspective see Arthur M. Silverstein, *A History of Immunology*, San Diego, Academic Press, 1989.

51. M. S. Gottlieb et al., "Gay-related immunodeficiency (GRID) syndrome: Clinical and autopsy observations," *Clin Res* 30 (1982): 349A.

52. V. Harden and D. Rodrigues, "Context for a new disease: Aspects of biomedical research policy in the US before AIDS," in *AIDS and Contemporary History*, ed. V. Berridge and P. Strong, Cambridge, Cambridge Univ. Press, 1993, pp. 182–202, and V. Harden, "Koch's postulates and the etiology of AIDS: An historical perspective," *Hist Philos Life Sci* 14 (1992): 249–69. For background see D. Nelkin, D. P. Willis, and S. V. Parris, eds., *A Disease of Society: Cultural Institutional Responses to AIDS*, Cambridge, Cambridge Univ. Press, 1991.

53. I am indebted to Christine Molnar for tracing the medical literature on sexually transmitted diseases prior to AIDS—especially papers produced by gay physicians—and for pointing out how it provided a language and framework for conceptualizing AIDS in its early stages.

54. G. M. Oppenheimer, "In the eye of the storm: The epidemiological construction of AIDS," in *AIDS: The Burdens of History*, ed. E. Fee and D. M. Fox, Berkeley, Univ. of California Press, 1988, pp. 267–300, and A. G. Fettner and W. A. Check, *The Truth About AIDS: Evolution of an Epidemic*, New York, Holt, Rinehart & Winston, 1984. See also J. W. Curran, "The CDC and the investigation of the epidemiology of AIDS," in *AIDS and the Public Debate*, ed. C. Hannaway et al., Amsterdam, IOS Press, 1995, pp. 19–29.

55. D. Mildvan et al., "Opportunistic infections and immune deficiency in homosexual men," *Ann Intern Med* 96 (June 1982): 700–04.

56. See also R. E. Stahl et al., "Immunological abnormalities in homosexual men; relationship to Kaposi's sarcoma," *Am J Med* 73 (August 1982): 171–78. For an overview see Peter Conrad and Joseph W. Schneider, *Deviance and Medicalization*, St. Louis, C.V. Mosby, 1980, pp. 172–213. With respect to an infectious agent see C. A. Ross, "Challenges in clinical virology (1958–1974): A personal viewpoint," *J Infect* 11 (1985): 7–14.

57. C. E. Rosenberg, "Disease and social order in America: Perceptions and expectations," in *AIDS: The Burdens of History*, pp. 12–32.

58. J. Fort, "Sex and drugs: The interaction of two disapproved behaviors," *Postgrad*

Med 58 (July 1975): 133–36. See also Dennis Altman, *AIDS in the Mind of America*, Garden City, NY, Anchor Press, 1986, pp. 30–57.

59. C. Warren, "Homosexuality and stigma," in *Homosexual Behavior*, ed. J. Marmor, New York, Basic Books, 1980, pp. 123–41.

60. Jeanne Kassler, *Gay Men's Health*, New York, Harper & Row, 1983, and D. Ostrow et al., eds., *Sexually Transmitted Diseases in Homosexual Men: Diagnosis, Treatment and Research*, New York, Plenum, 1983.

61. Kelly H. interview, January 1994.

62. More information is provided in Steven Epstein, *Impure Science: AIDS Activism and the Politics of Knowledge*, Berkeley, Univ. of California Press, 1996.

63. See C. McClain, "Of medicine, race, and American law: The bubonic plague outbreak of 1900," *Law Social Inquiry* 13 (1988): 447–573, and Risse, "Politics of fear," pp. 1–19.

64. CDC, "Kaposi sarcoma and pneumocystis pneumonia among homosexual men," *MMWR* 30 (1981): 305–07. For background information see Elizabeth W. Etheridge, *Sentinel for Health: A History of the Centers for Disease Control*, Berkeley, Univ. of California Press, 1992, pp. 321–40.

65. F. Lozada, S. Silverman, and M. Conant, "New outbreak of oral tumors, malignancies, and infectious diseases strike young male homosexuals," *CDA J* 10 (March 1982): 39–42.

66. D. F. Musto, "Quarantine and the problem of AIDS," in *AIDS: The Burdens of History*, pp. 67–85.

67. S. S. Hughes, "The Kaposi's Sarcoma Clinic at the University of California, San Francisco: An early response to the AIDS epidemic," *Bull Hist Med* 71 (1997): 651–88.

68. "History of the AIDS program," San Francisco General Hospital, Ward 84/86 Collection (hereafter SFGH Ward 84/86 Collection), Archives and Special Collections, UCSF Library and Center for Knowledge Management (hereafter UCSF Archives).

69. For details see Deborah Russell, "The San Francisco Model: Lessons from the First Decade of the AIDS Crisis," M.A. thesis, San Francisco State University, 1993 (UCSF Archives).

70. M. A. Sande, "The AIDS epidemic: Blueprint of a hospital's response," *Trans Am Clin Climat Assoc* 99 (1987): 185–95.

71. SFGH Ward 84/86 Collection, series III, UCSF Archives.

72. Ibid., series IV, "Contracts," and series V, "Budget and Finances."

73. J. Sonnabend et al., "Acquired immunodeficiency syndrome, opportunistic infections, and malignancies in male homosexuals," *JAMA* 249 (May 6, 1983): 2370–74.

74. For a historical review see A. Zuger and S. H. Miles, "Physicians, AIDS, and occupational risk," *JAMA* 258 (Oct. 9, 1987): 1924–28. See also A. R. Jonsen, M. Cooke, and B. A. Koenig, "AIDS and ethics," *Issues Science Technol* 2 (1986): 58–59.

75. J. E. Conte, Jr. et al., "The University of California at San Francisco Task Force on AIDS: Infection-control guidelines for patients with acquired immunodeficiency syndrome (AIDS)," *N Engl J Med* 309 (Sept. 22, 1983): 740–44.

76. A note chronicles a treatment with high doses of vitamins: C. S. M. Anderson, "I am recovering from AIDS," *Bay Area Rep* 8 (Oct. 6 1983): 14; for details see Irwin Stone, *The Healing Factor: Vitamin C Against Disease*, New York, Grosset & Dunlap, 1972.

77. P. Kondlapoodi, "Interferon in the treatment of Kaposi sarcoma," *N Engl J Med* 309 (Oct. 13, 1983): 923.

78. Interview with Donald I. Abrams in *The AIDS Epidemic in San Francisco: The Medical Response, 1981–1984*, Regional Oral History Office, Bancroft Library, Univ. of California, Berkeley, 1996, vol. II (hereafter, *AIDS in San Francisco*, ROHO).

79. Ibid. See also SFGH Ward 84/86 Collection, series II, UCSF Archives.

80. Conant, Lecture, UCSF, March 5, 1992.

81. Interview with Paul Volberding in *AIDS in San Francisco*, ROHO, 1995, vol. I.

82. Interview with Merle Sande in *AIDS in San Francisco*, ROHO, vol. IV (unpublished).

83. Abrams in *AIDS in San Francisco*, ROHO, vol. II.

84. Ibid.

85. Victoria A. Harden, "The NIH and biomedical research on AIDS," in *AIDS and the Public Debate*, pp. 30–46. For a history of the National Institutes of Health see Harden, *Inventing the NIH: Federal Biomedical Research Policy, 1887–1937*, Baltimore, Johns Hopkins Univ. Press, 1986.

86. A. J. Ammann et al., "Acquired immune dysfunction in homosexual men: Immunologic profiles," *Clin Immunol Immunopathol* 27 (June 1983): 315–25. For details, David Weatherall, *Science and the Quiet Art: Medical Research and Patient Care*, Oxford, Oxford Univ. Press, 1995.

87. Personal interview with Diane Jones, December 1993. See also A. R. Moss et al., "AIDS in the 'gay' areas of San Francisco," *Lancet* 1 (April 1983): 923–24.

88. Russell, "The San Francisco Model," p. 60.

89. S. H. Wanzer et al., "The physician's responsibility towards hopelessly ill patients," *N Engl J Med* 310 (Apr. 12, 1984): 955–59.

90. Ibid. See also D. M. Fox, "The politics of physicians' responsibility in epidemics: A note on history," *Hastings Center Rep* 18 (April–May 1988): 5–10, and J. O'Flaherty, "The AIDS patient: A historical perspective on the physician's obligation to treat," *Pharos* 54 (Summer 1991): 13–16.

91. Volberding, *AIDS in San Francisco*, ROHO, vol. I and R. Steinbrook et al., "Ethical dilemmas in caring for patients with acquired immunodeficiency syndrome," *Am Int Med* 103 (1985): 787–90. For an overview, see W. J. Curran, "Legal history of emergency medicine from medieval common law to the AIDS epidemic, *Am J Emerg Med* 15 (1997): 658–70.

92. Jones interview, December 1993.

93. J. A. Nicholas, "Burying a PWA brother and complaints about hospital care," *Bay Area Rep* 9 (Apr. 19, 1984): 30.

94. Volberding, *AIDS in San Francisco*, ROHO, vol. I.

95. Rebecca Ranson, AIDS interviews at Ward 5 B, San Francisco General Hospital, courtesy of the author (hereafter Ranson, SFGH interviews), chap. III.

96. Volberding, *AIDS in San Francisco*, ROHO, vol. I.

97. Jones interview, December 1993.

98. Ranson, SFGH interviews, chap. III.

99. Jones interview, December 1993.

100. Randy Shilts, *And the Band Played On: Politics, People and the AIDS Epidemic*, New York, St. Martin's Press, 1987, pp. 354–57.

101. A somewhat breezy account of SFGH and AIDS was published by the journalist Carol Pogash, *As Real as It Gets: The Life of a Hospital at the Center of the AIDS Epidemic*, New York, Birch Lane Press, 1992.

102. M. Hippler, "Learning about Ward 5 B at SF General," *Bay Area Rep* 8 (Nov. 3, 1983): 18.

103. M. Hippler, "Patrick Walker, patient on Ward 5 B," *Bay Area Rep* 8 (Nov. 17, 1983): 20.

104. M. S. Gottlieb et al., "The acquired immunodeficiency syndrome," *Ann Intern Med* 99 (1983): 208–20.

105. P. Volberding, "Therapy of Kaposi sarcoma in AIDS," *Semin Oncol* 11 (March 1984): 60–67. See also SFGH Ward 84/86 Collection, series IV, "Contracts," UCSF Archives.

106. F. FitzGerald, "The Castro-II," *The New Yorker* (July 28, 1986): 45–63. For a useful discussion concerning the pitfalls of AIDS education see W. Odets, "The fatal mistakes of AIDS education," *SF Bay Times* 15 (May 4, 1995): 3–7.

107. S. Seidman, "Transfiguring sexual identity: AIDS and the contemporary construction of homosexuality," *Social Text* 19/20 (Fall 1988): 187–206, and S. Kleinberg, "Life after death," *The New Republic* (Aug. 11, 1986): 30–33.

108. Rebecca Ranson, SFGH interviews, chap. VII.

109. Information obtained from Warren's clinical record at Ward 86.

110. Kelly H. interview, January 1994.

111. See announcement in *Bay Area Rep* 8 (Dec. 1, 1983): 13.

112. Ward 86 clinical information and Kelly H. interview, January 1994.

113. Ibid.

114. Jones interview, April 1994.

115. For an early view of the risk see G. N. Burrow, "Caring for AIDS patients: The physician's risk and responsibility," *Can Med Assoc J* 129 (1983): 1181, and later R. M. Wachter, "The impact of the acquired immunodeficiency syndrome in medical residency training," *N Engl J Med* 314 (Jan. 16, 1986): 177–80. See W. J. Friedlander, "On the obligation of physicians to treat AIDS: Is there a historical basis?," *Rev Infect Dis* 12 (1990): 191–203.

116. Jones interview, December 1993.

117. Ranson, SFGH interviews, chap. VI.

118. For a critique see T. Mizrahi, "Coping with patients: Subcultural adjustments to the condition of work among internists in training," *Social Probl* 32 (1984): 156–66.

119. Kelly H. interview, January 1994.

120. One of the most influential works on this subject is Paul Ramsey, *The Patient as Person*, New Haven, Yale Univ. Press, 1970.

121. J. S. Levin and J. Coreil, " 'New Age' healing in the US," *Soc Sci Med* 23 (1986): 889–97. For details see Marilyn Ferguson, *The Aquarian Conspiracy: Personal and Social Transformation in the 1980s*, Los Angeles, J. P. Tarcher, 1980.

122. For more details see M. Haug and B. Lavin, *Consumerism in Medicine: Challenging Physician Authority*, Beverly Hills, CA, Sage, 1983. Another example of this approach is Charles B. Inlander and Ed Weiner, *Take This Book to the Hospital with You, A Consumer Guide to Surviving Your Hospital Stay*, rev. ed., New York, Pantheon Books, 1991.

123. The issue is well articulated in G. J. Annas, "The hospital: A human rights wasteland," *Civil Lib Rev* 1 (1974): 15–35. See also W. J. Curran, "The patient's bill of rights becomes law," *N Engl J Med* 290 (Jan. 3, 1974): 32–33.

124. See L. Kopelman and J. Moskop, "The holistic health movement: A survey and critique," *J Med Philos* 6 (1981): 209–35, and J. J. Kronenfeld and C. Wasner, "The use of unorthodox therapies and marginal practitioners," *Soc Sci Med* 16 (1982): 1119–25.

125. R. Shilts, "Of course, nobody had planned on this," *SF Chronicle, This World* (Jan. 15, 1984): 17–18.

126. M. Hippler, "The nurses of ward 5 B," *Bay Area Rep* 8 (Dec. 1, 1983): 18.

127. For details, see P. Lister, "The art of nursing in a postmodern context." *J Adv Nurs* 25 (January 1997): 38–44.

128. For a moving example see N. T. Littlefield, "Therapeutic relationship: A brief encounter," *Am J Nurs* 82 (September 1982): 1395–99.

129. C. H. Jordan, "Caring and sharing: Spectrums of practice," *AORN J* 38 (December 1983): 1003.

130. For a valuable insight see Patricia E. Brenner, *The Primacy of Care: Stress and Coping in Health and Illness*, Menlo Park, CA, Addison-Wesley, 1989.

131. H. Salort, "I show up, I pay attention, and I care," in Charles Garfield, ed., *Sometimes My Heart Goes Numb: Love and Caregiving in a Time of AIDS*, San Francisco, Jossey-Bass, 1995, p. 63.

132. Hippler, "Blue Thursday," p. 197. See also M. Forstein, "The psychosocial impact of the acquired immunodeficiency syndrome," *Semin Oncol* 11 (1984): 77–82.

133. For another witness account see M. Hippler, "The new gay ward at San Francisco General," *Bay Area Rep* 8 (Oct. 20, 1983): 16–18.

134. Kelly H. interview, January 1994.

135. Ranson, SFGH interviews, chap. III.

136. Ibid., chap. VI.

137. Ibid., chap. III.

138. D. Chapin, "The healing touch," *SF Examiner/Chronicle*, "Image" section, Feb. 9, 1986, pp. 11–12, and P. Heidt, "Effect of therapeutic touch on anxiety level of hospitalized patients," *Nurs Res* 30 (1981): 32–37.

139. M. Salort, "I show up," p. 60.

140. Jones interview, December 1993.

141. Ibid.

142. Ranson, SFGH interviews, chap. VII.

143. Ibid.

144. For a personal account see D. Gregory, "My night on the AIDS ward," *Bay Area Rep* 8 (Oct. 27, 1983): 15–18.

145. Ranson, SFGH interviews, chap. VII.

146. Ibid.

147. "Philosophy for 5 A," a ward pamphlet (at SFGH Ward 5 A).

148. Kelly H. interview, January 1994.

149. Ranson, SFGH interviews, chap. III.

150. See Shilts, *The Band Played On*, pp. 394–96.

151. Jones interview, December 1993.

152. Kelly H. interview, January 1994.

153. Ibid.

154. Ranson, SFGH interviews, chap. VIII.

155. Ibid.

156. Ibid., chap. VII. 1740–42, and C. Seale et al., "A comparison of hospice and hospital care for people who die: Views of the surviving spouse," *Palliat Med* 11 (Mar 1997): 93–100.

157. Ranson, SFGH interviews, chap. VI. The issue of dying as a positive emotional experience for patients, families, and caregivers has been powerfully argued by Ira Byock, *Dying Well*, New York, Riverhead Books, 1997.

158. Gregory, "My night on the AIDS ward," 18. For a recent discussion see Sherwin B. Nuland, *How We Die: Reflections on Life's Final Chapter*, New York, A. A. Knopf, 1994. For a discussion of prayer in modern hospitals see T. F. Dagi, "Prayer, piety, and professional propriety: Limits on religious expression in hospitals," *J Clin Ethics* 6 (1995): 274–79.

159. S. Vinogradov et al., " If I have AIDS, then let me die now!" *Hastings Center Rep* 14 (February 1984): 24–26.

160. R. Shilts, "Life in ward 5 B," *SF Chronicle*, "This World" section, Jan. 15, 1984, p. 8, and J. M. Adams, "Life and death on ward 5 A," in *Washington Post*, "Health, Science and Society" section, Dec. 12, 1989, pp. 12–13 and 14–15.

161. The most often quoted work on this topic is Elizabeth Kübler Ross, *On Death and Dying*, New York, Macmillan, 1969. The author postulated that dying involves five successive stages: denial, anger, bargaining, depression, and acceptance. See also her more recent book, *AIDS: The Ultimate Challenge*, New York, Macmillan, 1987.

162. Hawkins, *Reconstructing Illness*, pp. 91–124, and M. Fulop, "The teaching hospital's modern deathbed ritual," *N Engl J Med* 312 (Jan. 10, 1985): 125–26.

163. Ranson, SFGH interviews, chap. VII. See also D. Field, "We didn't want him to die on his own—nurses' accounts of nursing dying patients," *J Adv Nurs* 9 (January 1984): 59–70.

164. Jones interview, SFGH, April 1994.

165. For a recent analysis see J. A. Macks and D. I. Abrams, "Burnout among HIV/AIDS health care providers: Helping the people on the frontlines," in *AIDS Clinical Review 1992*, ed. P. Volberding and M. A. Jacobson, New York, M. Dekker, 1992, pp. 281–99.

166. Ranson, SFGH interviews, chap. IX, and Jones interview, April 1994.

167. Ranson, SFGH interviews, chap. VII.

168. A. White, "Fundamentalists make hay out of AIDS dead and dying," *Bay Area Rep* 9 (Mar. 29, 1984): 5.

169. See W. Ruddick, "Transforming homes and hospitals," *Hastings Center Rep* 24 (1994): S11–S14, and R. L. Rubinstein, "Culture and disorder in the home care experience: The home as sickroom," in *The Homecare Experience*, ed. J. F. Gubrium and A. Sankar, Newbury Park, CA, Sage, 1990, pp. 37–57.

170. Clinical information and Kelly H. interview, January 1994.

171. Ibid.

172. C. B. Britton and J. R. Miller, "Neurologic complications in AIDS," *Neurol Clin* 2 (May 1984): 315–39, and D. Armstrong, "Central nervous system infections in the immunocompromised host," *Infection* 12, Suppl 1 (1984): S58–S64.

173. P. Lorch, editorial, "Killing the movement," *Bay Area Rep* 14 (Apr. 5, 1984): 6–7.

174. Kelly H. interview, January 1994. For a moving personal account of an elderly man dying of AIDS see H. Brodkey, "Dying: An update," *The New Yorker* (Feb. 7, 1994): 70–77.

175. M. Hippler, "Deaths in the family," *Bay Area Rep* 8 (Dec. 8, 1983): 15.

176. Garfield, *Sometimes My Heart Goes Numb*, p. 171.

177. M. Hippler, "Patrick Walker," *Bay Area Rep* 8 (Nov. 17, 1983): 20.

178. Ranson, SFGH interviews, chap. XI.

179. Jones interview, SFGH, April 1994.

180. City and County of San Francisco, *SFGH Quarterly AIDS Surveillance Report*. For SFGH, also consult San Francisco Department of Public Health Annual Reports and San Francisco Controller Reports.

181. The history of this discovery can be found in R. C. Gallo and L. Montagnier, "The chronology of AIDS research," *Nature* 326 (1987): 435–36, and Gallo's *Virus Hunting: AIDS, Cancer, and the Human Retrovirus: A Story of a Scientific Discovery*, New York, Basic Books, 1989.

182. T. E. Cook and D. C. Colby, "The mass-mediated epidemic: The politics of AIDS on the nightly network news," in *AIDS: The Making of a Chronic Disease*, ed. Fee and Fox, pp. 105–08.

183. D. M. Fox, "AIDS and the American health policy: The history and prospects of a crisis of authority," *Milbank Q* 64 (1986): 7–33.

184. Conant, Lecture, UCSF, March 5, 1992.

185. J. L. Gerberding, "The University of California at San Francisco Task Force on AIDS. Recommended infection-control policies for patients with human immunodeficiency virus infection: An update," *N Engl J Med* 315 (Dec. 11, 1986): 1562.

186. Sande in *AIDS in San Francisco*, ROHO, vol. IV. See also D. R. Gordon, "Clinical science and clinical expertise: Changing boundaries between art and science of medicine," in *Biomedicine Examined*, ed. M. Lock and D. R. Gordon, Dordrecht, Kluwer, 1988, pp. 257–95.

187. F. G. Miller and J. J. Fins, "A proposal to restructure hospital care for dying patients," *N Engl J Med* 334 (Jun. 27, 1996): 1740–42. For these authors, the dichotomy between care and curing is misleading. See also T. E. Quill, *Death and Dignity: Making Choices and Taking Charge*, New York, Norton, 1993.

188. Interview with Constance Wofsy, *AIDS in San Francisco*, ROHO, vol. III, 1997. See also D. J. Rothman and H. Edgar, "AIDS, activism and ethics," *Hosp Pract* 26 (1991): 135–42.

189. J. C. Robinson, "The changing boundaries of the American hospital," *Milbank Q* 72 (1994): 259–75, and R. A. Kane, "Expanding the home-care concept: Blurring distinctions among home care, institutional care, and other long-term care services," *Milbank Q* 73 (1995): 161–86.

190. For details see Peter S. Arno and Karyn L. Feiden, *Against the Odds: The Story of AIDS Drug Development, Politics and Profits*, New York, HarperCollins, 1992.

191. Wofsy in *AIDS in San Francisco*, ROHO, vol III.

192. Ranson, SFGH interviews, chap. III.

193. Ibid., chap. XII.

194. Warner, *Sometimes My Heart Goes Numb*, p. xxii.

195. Taped remarks made at the 10th anniversary of Ward 5 B. See also *San Francisco General Hospital Ward 86/Ward 5A Tenth Anniversary, 1983–1993*, SFGH Archives.

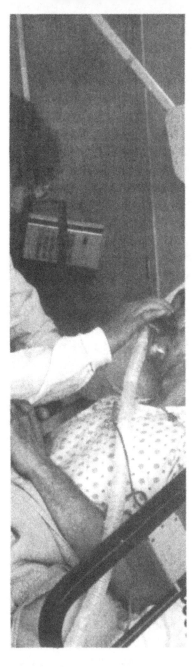

CONCLUSION

The Future of Hospitals as Healing Spaces

Wherever patient-focused care leads us in the years ahead, we must constantly remind ourselves why we began the journey in the first place—not in the service of some buzzword or faddish approach but to improve continuity and quality for patients.
J. Philip Lathrop, *The Health Care Forum*, 1992[1]

Evolution of hospitals: A profile

This historical review of hospitals has been episodic, a series of portraits, loosely arranged in chronological order but also strategically chosen to cover important themes and critical developments in the history of medicine and therapeutics. In each age and place, hospitals functioned as symbols of community solidarity, engaged in delivering culturally acceptable forms of social welfare and providing mechanisms for coping with suffering, illness, and death. As communities and cultures have changed over time, the roles and institutional boundaries of hospitals have changed with them.[2]

At the beginning, the hospital was a *house of mercy*, *refuge*, and *dying*, a place for seeking sanctuary. In Byzantium, the early guest houses represented a social coping mechanism in the face of famines, wars, epidemics, migrations and displacements, pilgrimages, and urbanization. Space in this communal shelter was provided for physical protection and spiritual comfort. The social welfare function was paramount, and the institution provided rest, food, clothing, care, and even medical consultations for the poor, displaced, and homeless. From the start, both church and secular authorities included hospitals within their public policies regarding epidemics, transforming them into tools for separation. A special variant, the *house of segregation*, was an instrument for isolation designed to control individuals considered threats to society such as lepers, plague victims, and the undeserving poor.

By the time of the Renaissance, as the modern state sought to protect and restore its working citizens as productive members of society, the hospital was transformed into a *house of rehabilitation*. If possible, deserving members serving in the armed forces needed to be mended and returned to active duty or retired as invalids. To serve their needs, governments created networks of military and naval hospitals. Henceforth, hospitals became tools for both physical and moral recovery. The former, secular goal led some institutions to accelerate the ongoing medicalization process by hiring more members of the medical profession for their caregiving staffs. After 1500, the original shelters splintered into hospitals, asylums, and prisons with somewhat overlapping functions. In Protestant Europe, hospitals also became enmeshed in new schemes of social control with more selective welfare functions. In Catholic countries, large shelters or general hospitals warehoused a broad spectrum of individuals, from the aged and chronically ill to lunatics and mendicants.

By the eighteenth century, state power focused on economics, science and health. The hospital became a *house of cure* through the mercantilist reforms of enlightened absolutism. Shelter, food, clothing, and moral revival still remained institutional goals, but medical and surgical treatments became paramount, perhaps lifesaving. Medicalized establishments increasingly restricted admissions to sick individuals, and in many places professionals assumed control of admissions and discharges. Hospitals also participated in the education of medical and later nursing professionals and contributed decisively to the creation of new knowledge about health and disease, especially medical theory and practice. Emphasis on systematic clinical observations, treatment and experimentation with drugs, and education transformed the hospital into a *house of teaching and research*. In Paris, the medical presence expanded further as physicians systematically dissected all inmates who died in the institution, allowing the hospital also to become a *house of dissection*. The result was a rapid development of pathological anatomy, clinicopathological correlation, and the rise of physical examination techniques.

A few decades later, further medicalization transformed the hospital into a *house of surgery*. Indeed, after 1850, the availability of general anesthesia and, later, antisepsis allowed for an expansion of surgical procedures, attracting a broader spectrum of patients—many of them belonging to the middle classes—and thus consolidating the hospital's reputation as a curative institution. Thanks to new advances in medical knowledge and technology, the early twentieth century witnessed the emergence of the hospital as a *house of science*. Equipped with clinical laboratories and X-ray facilities for diagnosis and treatment, hospital space was divided according to new medical specialties and equipment. Affiliated with academic institutions, many hospitals were transformed into centers of biomedical research and training. As acute, short-term facilities, they shed their convalescent and dying functions, which were transferred to nursing homes and hospices.

Hospitals have always mirrored the collective values of their sponsors, staffs, and patients. Seven hundred years ago, their humanitarian mission in Europe had been jeopardized by administrative greed and insensitivity toward the sick poor, leading to fierce competition for resources followed by waves of closings and consolidations lasting for several centuries. At the time, bloated institutional bureaucracies and callous caregivers discredited the hospitals' proverbial charity, which had been closely linked to Christianity. Today a similar phenomenon involving postmodern hospitals is currently unfolding worldwide, especially in the United States. The hospital has become a *house of high technology*, providing mostly intensive patient care with the aid of a wide array of powerful and complex diagnostic and therapeutic devices, from scanners to kidney stone crushers. The hospital still provides medicine's most acute and sophisticated interventions, but the bulk of health care delivery is moving out to clinics and patients' homes, leaving behind a costly surplus of hospital beds. Shifts toward primary care, health promotion, and disease prevention often bypass hospitals completely. In the United States, the widening gulf between ambulatory care locations and hospitals begins to resemble earlier British models that separated general practitioners and hospital consultants as part of an institutional rationing plan.[3]

Among hospitals, a veritable Darwinian struggle to survive has ensued. Between 1984 and 1993, 949 U.S. institutions closed. If current trends continue, more than a third of all existing American hospitals will either close or merge during the next decades. Demographics, epidemiology, and the current economic climate increasingly force hospitals—at a very high price—to provide only what they do best: highly technical, intensive care, ranging from neonatal nurseries to near-terminal geriatric lifesaving. From a technical point of view, new and less invasive diagnostic and therapeutic technologies can be provided in outpatient or day-care settings not requiring hospitalization. The result: patients with an ever narrower spectrum of diseases are admitted to hospitals. How, then, can hospitals survive financially while organizing their work in ways better suited to meet today's patients' needs?

While hospital functions continue to narrow, medical care at large is becoming more holistic in approach, moving toward the goal of a continuum of care that involves clinics and physicians' offices, convalescent facilities, hospices, and patients' homes. Under generous pre-1980s reimbursement systems, American health care was usually episodic and fragmented, afflicted with significant duplication of work while leaving important gaps in coverage. By contrast, organized and integrated transitions between health services and their institutions allow patients to move directly from ambulatory clinics or physicians' offices to hospitals, while the coordinated discharge from them to ambulatory clinics and home or hospice care creates an integrated plan of care. In many instances, hospitalization is now considered as a failure of the system. This level of organization involves all caregivers, but the multiple locations of the services can create communication problems between caregivers. It similarly presupposes the patients' cooperation and education in health matters, frequently achieved through reading materials but also through access to a telephone and electronic advice systems. Needless to say, this new approach involves a radical change in the American medical culture, prompting patients to move away from traditional, primary hospital-based care.[4]

Better living conditions and improved education, as well as preventive measures and better environmental control of certain infectious diseases, have led to birth control and extended life expectancy, creating an ongoing population shift toward an older society. Mature populations are more susceptible to a variety of chronic rather than acute diseases, an epidemiological change that leads to greater stress on long-term care issues rather than short-term interventions. Under such circumstances, patient functionality is best assessed and therapeutically managed in ambulatory settings rather than in expensive hospitals. Medicine's current emphasis on outcomes is driven by these demographic factors. Increasingly, health maintenance is the goal, with behavioral, lifestyle, social, environmental, and occupational issues becoming just as important as genetic predisposition and molecular interventions.

At the same time, aging patients mostly suffer from complex or multiple diseases, and hospitals continue to provide the intensive care necessary to neutralize the sudden breakdown of multiple organ systems or to stop the ravages of aggressive cancers. Here, however, a shifting ethic of terminal care now increasingly questions aggressive hospital treatment of the dying, tending to decrease the length and number of such heroic interventions. Patients wishing to retain control of their dying process increasingly transfer from hospitals to other institutions. Hospice care has become an increasingly popular alternative, perceived as allowing a "good" death, variously defined as involving freedom from pain, a peaceful environment, and personal dignity.[5]

Historically, hospitals have dealt openly with death and dying, with patients assembled in large wards routinely witnessing such events with a mixture of fear and comfort, as illustrated by the fate of Adolf of Cologne in Jerusalem's Hospital of St. John. Before the Enlightenment, dying in hospitals was considered a blessing for believers expecting salvation. Surrounded by prayerful caregivers and provided with the last sacraments, their redemption was complete. Following secularization, however, medicalized hospitals competing for charitable funds began shunning the fatally ill, viewing their management as a waste of their limited resources and their ultimate death as detrimental to an image built on low mortality statistics. Management concentrated on the purely physical manifestations of illness in keeping with the basic medical disease orientation. With recovery their avowed goal, hospitals made efforts to limit contact with the moribund and the dead, creating separate wards and morgues to house them.

In modern times, despite attempts to limit aggressive interventions and prolong life, hospital rituals still include specialized consultations at the deathbed.[6] Indeed, dying is frequently equated with treatment failure, and heroic efforts are made to prolong life at all costs. In the Western world, acute care hospitals remain dedicated to sustaining life through the employment of invasive technologies.[7] Only in very recent times has medicine come to terms with the futility of actively opposing death. With therapeutic options exhausted, some caregivers now aim to provide adequate pain control and a supportive environment that includes vigils by relatives.[8] In most hospitals, terminal care is still inadequate, especially concerning the relief of pain. The creation of separate palliative care units run by multidisciplinary teams of caregivers has begun to change the modern hospital's stubborn denial of death.[9] As Warren J.'s experience with AIDS at San Francisco General Hospital suggests, patients can be allowed to orchestrate their own dying in accordance with their individual social, spiritual, and cultural expectations.[10]

The new American spirituality

In the summer of 1997, the California Pacific Medical Center in San Francisco installed on its premises a labyrinth, a 36-foot-wide maze with its concentric paths leading to a rose-shaped center. Its designer considers the labyrinth as a symbolic path where—given the dwindling art of medicine—patients can learn to reconnect themselves with their former lives. Divided into four quadrants, the beige and cinnamon color design was painted on a fiberglass surface, allowing patients to enter from the sides and walk over a third of a mile before reaching the center. The labyrinth is based on designs discovered in the stone floors of French cathedrals, especially the Benedictine structures at Chartres. Its purpose is to provide an opportunity for meditation and relaxation for patients awaiting organ transplants, as well as for those recovering from other diseases. Many visitors, caregivers, and residents in of the hospital's neighborhood have extolled its presumed healing qualities.[11] Is this a symbol of a new commitment to the human side of medicine—part of developments already observed at the new AIDS ward of San Francisco General Hospital during the 1980s?

Healing is often accomplished by the sick themselves or may require the help of others. At the physical level, the process may include the end of pain and the restoration of bodily function. Those who consider themselves healed often experience a renewed sense of identity, security, and harmony with their family, community, and the world at large. Whether or not healing can take place in hospitals, however, is dependent on how well such institutions are able to foster a climate and a plan of action leading to recovery, one that takes account of both physical and spiritual needs. The hospital milieu is critical for mending body and soul. Environments and personnel conducive to healing include pleasant, comfortable surroundings, as well as skilled and sympathetic caregivers whose interventions are designed not only to counteract the effects of disease but also to address the emotional and spiritual needs of those who suffer within hospital walls.

Given their religious character, the early Christian shelters provided great spiritual solace but minimal physical comforts. The accent was on holism and communal life at the expense of individual privacy. Modern hospitals, by contrast, have reversed this emphasis and now focus primarily on individual physical rehabilitation in more fragmented and depersonalized environments. They have been aptly described as the "Land That Never Sleeps," with their sensory and work overload detrimental to rest and sleep while retaining the risks of earlier institutional cross-infection and caregivers' errors.[12] Regimentation, often inscribed in detailed regulations, also harkens back to earlier needs for confinement and segregation necessary to discipline a shelter full of strangers. To this day, people who travel into the strange world of hospitals continue to speak of a rather traumatic, intimidating transfer into an alien universe of sickness and strict rules. Often this removal constitutes a crisis of body, mind, and spirit.

Consumerism in medicine

Patients everywhere have become purchasers of health care services. The excessive commodification of health care now beginning to sweep the world has not been kind to hospitals or their clients. Both the rhetoric and the reality of consumerism in medicine display a number of basic contradictions and create paradoxes worth exploring historically. In the United States, the term *consumer* denotes a measure of familiarity with the product or service to be acquired or received, together with a dose of skepticism concerning its quality and thus the need for a guarantee of satisfaction and indemnity. The notion of the patient as a consumer suggests that hospital patients should be autonomous and informed partners in making care decisions and should exercise their right to authorize or refuse treatments. Such a participatory relationship was significantly strengthened following the appearance of AIDS in the early 1980s, as attested to by the practices followed at Ward 5 B of the San Francisco General Hospital. For most Americans, however, consumer choices in health care are difficult to make on the basis of the medical knowledge commonly available to them. Moreover, such options are now restricted by employers to a number of omnipotent insurance companies and their rigidly formulated service plans, which, in turn, are enforced by gate-keepers who no longer consider hospitalization as an entitlement. Consumer confidence in health care is declining.[13]

New managerial and financial imperatives

The American hospital industry of the 1990s has developed a patient-centered care scheme designed to achieve customer satisfaction by striving to make hospitals more pleasant, comfortable, and user friendly. In fact, the health care industry has characterized this approach as a "redesign of patient care so that hospital resources and personnel are organized around patients rather than around various specialized departments."[14] In recent years, architects have been persuaded to modify the interior of hospitals further, since the quality of institutional space remains an important factor in the outcome of medical care.[15] Ornate lobbies and plant-studded atriums greet newcomers. Single, well-furnished rooms with their own bathrooms, television sets, and video players have proliferated. To ensure privacy and provide a home-like ambiance, some institutions have even reconfigured entire wings into care suites, offering more privacy while allowing the sharing of lounging, library, and kitchen facilities. Gourmet meals and liberal visiting privileges further enhance the hospital experience. At its extreme, this approach involves the marketing of hotel-type services for privileged consumers longing for luxury by offering upscale floors or units resembling fine hotel suites equipped with antique furniture, Oriental rugs, and electronic communications, while throughout the country institutions caring for the poor are closing.[16]

To avoid excessive waits for caregiving personnel and to place services closer to the patient, the concept of a *focused* location has led to the creation of multiple nursing substations located in smaller *pods* or units caring for seven to nine patients. They are often monitored by individual bedside computer terminals that can access all pertinent clinical databases. Computers and pneumatic tubes also facilitate communication and transportation of specimens and lab results. All pods are surrounded by satellite pharmacies, laboratories, and radiological units, thus sparing patients frequent trips outside their immediate area except for surgery or other major procedures, as well as reducing the turnaround time for routine test reports and services.[17]

To achieve the goal of placing hospital patients in focused settings, the new care system seeks to provide—in the rhetoric of consumerism—*seamless* services, ostensibly to provide more *face time* devoted to interactions between patients and their primary caregivers. Former hospital routines, scheduling, coordinating, and documenting are now seen as too time-consuming. The solution, borrowed from other industry models, is to eliminate barriers between workers by training them to perform multiple tasks. This means dispensing with the usual parade of specialized caregivers, individuals performing narrow tasks such as phlebotomists, tray carriers, housekeepers, technicians, transporters, and clerks. In the hospital, this reorganization especially affects nursing, requiring reeducation and cross-training. In the managed care lingo, nursing skills must be shared, "leveraged" to other cross-trained ancillary workers.[18]

In many parts of the United States, therefore, nurses have resumed traditional tasks, including bed making and patient hygiene, that managers describe as "empowering" because they allow nurses a return to historically sanctioned domesticity and greater patient contact. Cross-trained, multidisciplinary caregiving teams (patient care associates composed of a nurse, practical aide, and technician) are now the norm. Nurses heading these teams are sometimes concerned about the quality of care offered by such untrained personnel and see the changes as part of a deprofessionalizing trend driven primarily by financial considerations. Although their jobs have been freed of many bureaucratic tasks, American nurses continue to have little time to share their humanity with patients because of their increased workloads, and burnout is frequent. Yet routine bedside caregiving remains one of the key opportunities for personal contact and for healing to begin.

The creation of multiple caregiving teams or panels has also diminished the physician's authority in hospitals.[19] Demoted to mere providers of medical services, physicians are subjected to the vagaries of hospital contracting, especially the rationing of specialist care. The new financial accountability in medicine has put an end to unfettered spending for medical procedures and therapies, including unnecessary diagnostic testing, surgery, and drugs that have accounted for significant rates of institutional mortality. Moreover, hospitals are experiencing a financially driven redefinition of what constitutes optimum scientific care leading to defined patient outcomes. The relentless American emphasis on cost and efficiency, as well as the transformation of the hospital into an intensive care institution, now also favors the development of a new practitioner: the *hospitalist*, a specialist devoted to and responsible for managing the care of hospitalized patients.[20]

Previous organizational schemes in hospitals—from Byzantium to the twentieth century—were based on a stable, hierarchical paradigm wherein rectors, directors, superintendents, or managers were entrusted to identify problems and take measures to correct them. Today's new management "science" has destabilized that hierarchy, calling for hospitals to diffuse expertise and encourage workers to be creative and cooperative. Because the problems encountered in complex organizations are no longer predictable, goes the logic, neither should be problem solving. Under these circumstances, periods of institutional chaos and disorganization are deemed necessary for truly creative work since order cannot be achieved in an incremental, linear, or predictive way. In today's hospitals, therefore, everything is in flux, including management layers and accounting systems, financial services and utilization rates, performance policies and staffing levels.[21]

Today, the mantra adopted by most American hospital managers is to reconstruct and streamline health care delivery. "Reengineering" has therefore become the constant in American hospital reform, attempting to reshape institutions for future success in their respective health care markets. To remain competitive, hospitals now periodically stage expensive "quality engineering" campaigns and often revise their strategic plans on a quarterly basis. But the result of these periodic "slash and burn" crusades—new waves of hiring, layoffs, and retraining of personnel, as well as new productivity formulas and across-the-board cuts—is often less a burst of creativity than an outbreak of anxiety about job security among the staff. These corporate decisions destroy loyalty and trust, and afflict even hospital administrators with stress and burnout, although some managers claim to find such a crisis environment exciting, even invigorating, if it helps hospitals to operate more efficiently. The ultimate goal of reengineering is, of course, to continue to shorten the patients' hospital stay and thus save money—what critics have characterized as "drive-through" hospitalization.[22] Even for patients enjoying luxurious accommodations, the experience is ever more fleeting.

Hospitals and the humanity of institutional care

Historically, the sick arriving in hospitals sought a semblance of balance and structure to reorganize and repair their damaged lives disrupted by suffering and disease. Institutional rituals and dedicated caregivers attempted to deal with the ambiguities of suffering and provide an environment suitable for such recovery.[23] In sharp contrast, the American reengineered house of crises offers a panorama of institutional flux. Patients suffer not only because their caregivers feel unsure about their places in the hospital hierarchy, but also because the order and stability so necessary to cope with the uncertainty of illness have been reengineered away, replaced by a climate of tension and stress.[24] Moreover, patients are torn between behaving as discriminating, informed consumers who should demand options available in the world of corporate medicine and their status as suffering, insecure human beings anxious to disclose feelings and complaints, trusting that their caregivers will show empathy and pledge to help them. Trust in people, not spreadsheets, remains an essential healing ingredient. Without it, neither physicians nor nurses can play their role as patients' advocates, thus compromising the healing process.[25]

For most of hospital history, religion was the bond that linked institutional mission, patronage, administration, staff, and patients. Today many hospital patients still turn to religion for solace and comfort.[26] Addressing the spiritual needs of patients is seen as complementary to conventional therapeutics and offers the potential for earlier recovery and discharge, two goals of managed care. Pastoral visits are thus promoted as cost-effective and are evaluated based on whether they can make a difference in patients' outcomes. In the intensely technical world of today's hospital, chaplains sometimes may be the only members of the care team willing to listen to their patients' feelings. In America, however, new schemes of pastoral care are replacing the traditional hospital ministry, considered too unfocused and open-ended. Visits from members of a pastoral team are now routinely scheduled by caregivers at what are considered critical junctures of the hospitalization process.

Like bodily processes, spiritual pathways are said by theorists of caregiving to have their own predictable order and cadence, and the chaplains must provide the guidance necessary to pull the patients through to the next step: "What it takes to heal is a journey, no one skips a stop on the trail."[27] Instead of being assigned by religious denomination, chaplains are chosen by medical specialty, including oncology, cardiology, trauma, and thoracic surgery. Moreover, they must be mobile, since their visits are arranged under diverse conditions and in various settings. In moments of anxiety and stress, chaplains are told to support and counsel patients by talking, praying, or holding hands. The encounter is not necessarily restricted to a discussion of the divine, but more often is an opportunity for patients to unburdened themselves of their fears. A "God does not heal alone" approach also encourages patients to become actively engaged in their recovery. Some are asked to employ meditation techniques to conquer their anxieties. In the eyes of its critics, the true goals of managed care's "sheep-dip" chaplaincy— herd 'em, dip 'em, and move 'em out—are financial and do not address the needs of many patients, who would like to control the pastoral visits without predetermined agendas and time constraints.[28]

In academic medical centers, patient passivity and emotional starvation are accentuated by a host of educational rituals, including frequent rounds involving attending physicians, house staff, consultants, medical students, and nursing coordinators. Being inspected and examined by retinues of residents and students—a common practice essential for clinical education since the mid-eighteenth century—accentuates patients' feelings of degradation and lack of privacy, particularly if these examinations are performed without attempts to secure prior consent or acknowledge human dignity.[29] Moreover, case presentations, grand rounds, and mortality and morbidity conferences all concentrate on the contours and peculiarities of disease states instead of referring to the sick person.[30] In spite of their depersonalizing effects, diagnostic rituals have therapeutical potential, but drugs and machines alone cannot accomplish this goal. Patients seek legitimation for their illnesses and look to those in authority for an eventual recovery.

Hospitals originally emerged as communal homes to shelter the needy and deal with their mortality, providing a human touch to those suffering within particular social and religious frameworks. Later, new medical agendas vigorously attempted to recover the health of inpatients and reintegrate them into their families and communities. As hospitals move into the twenty-first century to cater almost exclusively to short-term and intensive technological interventions, they need to devise new ways of making that care humane and responsive to patients' needs, fears, and hopes.[31] New management techniques and the commodification of medicine are forcing an American hospital system notorious for its bloated finances and decentralization to streamline services and correct notable inefficiencies. This may contribute to desirable institutional reforms, but business values can easily jeopardize the technical quality and humanitarianism inextricably linked to hospital services.[32] The logic of financial gain is already threatening to undermine the hospital's ability to function as a house of healing, prompting calls for a new institutional ethic that could guide caregivers in assisting a "wounded humanity."[33]

Ironically, the post-modern hospital may also be failing patients physically just as much as spiritually. Technical mishaps and adverse drug reactions increase with institutional complexity. A different threat is the presence of antibiotic-resistant germs responsible for a growing incidence of cross-infections reminiscent of yesteryear's hospitalism. At the same time, The American health care "product" has increasingly been placed on a starvation diet, sometimes depriving hospital patients of more expensive procedures—such as transplants—that could be lifesaving. To deliver it, less competent caregivers and patients become the guinea pigs and victims of countless managerial failures in fluctuating corporate structures and plans. Although designed to pamper consumers in more physically attractive surroundings, hospital "reengineering" in America may paradoxically fail to achieve true patient satisfaction and better outcomes.

Asked recently about health care in the next millenium, the current president of the American Hospital Association, Dick Davidson, tried to reassure the public, saying that "there will always be personal contact and caring. Everything we do is about human need. That's the constant over time."[34] Patient-centered care must be human-centered care, delivered in a supportive hospital environment that continues to provide the best and most appropriate care that medical science has to offer, without neglecting the emotional and spiritual aspects of illness. As traditional monuments to human empathy and benevolence, hospitals must remain houses of healing.[35]

NOTES

1. J. P. Lathrop, "The patient-focused hospital," *Healthcare Forum* 35 (May–June 1992): 78. Mr. Lathrop is vice-president of the Health Care Group at Booz, Allen & Hamilton, Inc., Chicago.

2. J. C. Robinson, "The changing boundaries of the American hospital," *Milbank Q* 72 (1994): 259–75.

3. E. Ginzberg, "Hospitals: From center to periphery," *Inquiry* 32 (Spring 1995): 11–13. See also Henry J. Aaron and William B. Schwartz, *The Painful Prescription: Rationing Hospital Care*, Washington, DC, Brookings Institution, 1984.

4. K. Lumsdon, "Crash course: Piecing together the continuum of care," *Hosp Health Networks* 68 (Nov. 20, 1994): 26–34. For background see C. Rosenberg, "Looking backward, thinking forward: The roots of hospital crisis," *Trans Stud Coll Phys Phila* 12 (June 1990): 127–50.

5. See, for example, Kenneth P. Cohen, *Hospice: Prescription for Terminal Care*, Germantown, MD, Aspen Systems Corp., 1979.

6. M. Fulop, "The teaching hospital's modern deathbed ritual," *N Engl J Med* 312 (Jan. 10, 1985): 125–26.

7. In the United States, attempts have been made to create new diagnostic groups for palliative care that would allow payment for end-of-life care in such hospitals. See C. K. Cassel and B. C. Vladeck, "ICD-9 code for palliative or terminal care," *N Engl J Med* 335 (Oct. 17, 1996): 1232–34.

8. J. H. Muller and B. A. Koenig, "On the boundary of life and death: The definitions of dying by medical residents," in *Biomedicine Examined*, ed. M. Lock and D. B. Gordon, Dordrecht, Kluwer, 1988 pp. 351–74.

9. F. G. Miller and J. J. Fins, "A proposal to restructure hospital care for dying patients," *N Engl J Med* 334 (Jun. 27, 1996): 1740–42, and C. Seale et al., "A comparison of hospice and hospital care for people who die: Views of the surviving spouse," *Palliat Med* 11 (March 1997): 93–100.

10. S. Payne et al., "Impact of witnessing death in hospice patients," *Soc Sci Med* 43 (December 1996): 1785–94.

11. See W. Carlsen, "Hospital following nontraditional path," *SF Chronicle* (June 6, 1997), p. A19.

12. L. L. Leape et al., "The nature of adverse events in hospitalized patients," *N Engl J Med* 324 (Feb. 7, 1991): 377–84, and for details, C. G. Mayhall, *Hospital Epidemiology and Infection Control*, Baltimore, Williams & Wilkins, 1996.

13. For more details see Marie Haug and Bebe Lavin, *Consumerism in Medicine: Challenging Physician Authority*, Beverly Hills, CA, Sage, 1983. Another example of this approach is Charles B. Inlander and Ed Weiner, *Take This Book to the Hospital with You, A Consumer Guide to Surviving Your Hospital Stay*, rev. ed., New York, Pantheon, 1991.

14. K. Lumsdon, "Putting patients first: Hospitals work to define patient-centered care," *Hospitals* 67 (Feb. 5, 1993): 14, and M. Kravitz et al., "Implementation of a new patient care role: Concept to reality," *J Nurs Admin* 27 (May 1997): 7–11.

15. For an overview see C. R. Horsburgh, Jr., "Healing by design," *N Engl J Med* 333 (Sep. 14, 1995): 735–40.

16. The conversion at Johns Hopkins Hospital cost $1 million, and the hospital now charges $725 per day for a room and $1,250 for a suite. See A. M. Nordhaus-Bike, "Deluxe in da hospital," *Hosp Health Networks* 70 (Apr. 5, 1996): 50–52. For a brief perspective see R. L. Martensen, "Hospital hotels and the care for the 'worthy rich,' " *JAMA* 275 (Jan. 24/31, 1996): 325

17. L. H. Avery, "Future unclear as nurses face workplace redesign and job redeployment," *AORN J* 60 (July 1994): 99–105, and P. Brider, "The move to patient-focused care," *Am J Nurs* 92 (1992): 26–33.

18. K. Lumsdon, "Will nursing ever be the same?," *Hosp Health Networks* 69 (Dec. 5, 1995): 31–35.

19. See Milton I. Roemer and Jay W. Friedman, *Doctors in Hospitals: Medical Staff Organization and Hospital Performance*, Baltimore, Johns Hopkins Univ. Press, 1971, pp. 29–48.

20. R. M. Wachter and L. Goldman, "The emerging role of 'hospitalists' in the American health care system," *N Engl J Med* 335 (Aug. 15, 1996): 514–16.

21. Based on the book by Michael Hammer and James Champy, *Reengineering the Corporation: A Manifesto for Business Revolution*, New York, Harper Business, 1993. See also Michael Hammer, *Beyond Reengineering: How the Process-Centered Organization Is Changing our Work and our Lives*, New York, Harper Business, 1996.

22. K. Lumsdon, "Mean Streets: Five lessons from the front lines of reengineering," *Hosp Health Networks* 69 (Oct. 5, 1995): 44–52, and J. L. Sherer, "Managing chaos," *Hosp Health Networks* 69 (Feb. 20, 1995): 22.

23. C. L. Bosk, "Occupational rituals in patient management," *N Engl J Med* 303 (Jul. 10, 1980): 71–76.

24. M. L. Lyon, "Order and healing: The concept of order and its importance in the conceptualization of healing," *Med Anthrop* 12 (1990): 249–68.

25. E. S. More, "Empathy as a hermeneutic practice," *Theoret Med* 17 (1996): 243–54, and D. E. Rogers, "On trust: A basic building block for healing doctor/patient interactions," *Pharos* (Spring 1994): 2–6. See also S. K. Toombs, *The Meaning of Illness: A Phenomenological Account of the Different Perspectives of Physician and Patient*, Boston, Kluwer, 1992.

26. For a Catholic perspective see Edmund D. Pellegrino and David C. Thomasma, *Helping and Healing: Religious Commitment in Health Care*, Washington, DC, Georgetown Univ. Press, 1997.

27. T. Hudson, "Measuring the results of faith," *Hosp Health Networks* 70 (Sept. 20, 1996): 24–28. The article is based on an interview with a Catholic priest.

28. See letter by G. S. Nash in *Hosp Health Networks* 71 (Jan. 20, 1997): 8.

29. For recent narratives from medical students about this problem see A. Brewster, "A student's view of a medical teaching exercise," *N Engl J Med* 329 (Dec. 23, 1993): 1971–72, and R. R. Sargeant, "A patient in the teaching hospital: Balancing privacy and education," *Pharos* 58 (Summer 1995): 29–34. An eloquent narrative by an elderly male patient being catheterized before an assembly of student nurses is provided by B. Farwell, "Health care in America: An intimate glimpse," *Ann Intern Med* 125 (1996): 1005–06.

30. A. Arluke, "Roundmanship: Inherent control on a medical teaching ward," *Soc Sci Med* 14 (1980): 297–302.

31. "No matter who provides the care, however, it will never be complete unless those responsible for it seek a far deeper understanding of the patient's social, economic, and ecological contexts than we do now. Becoming more aware of the psychological barriers to effective care is an essential part." J. P. Kassirer, editorial, "Is managed care here to stay?," *N Engl J Med* 336 (Apr. 3, 1997): 1014.

32. D. Mechanic, "Changing medical organization and the erosion of trust," *Milbank Q* 74 (1996): 171–89.

33. See R. T. De George, "The moral responsibility of the hospital," *J Med Philos* 7 (1982): 87–100, together with S. J. Reiser, "Hospitals as humane corporations," in *Integrity in Health Care Institutions: Humane Environments for Teaching, Inquiry, and Healing*, ed. R. E. Bulger and S. J. Reiser, Iowa City, Univ. of Iowa Press, 1990, pp. 121–29, and L. R. Churchill, " 'Damaged humanity': The call for a patient-centered medical ethic in the managed care era," *Theoret Med* 18 (1997): 113–26.

34. M. Grayson, "An interview with Dick Davidson," *Hosp Health Networks* 72 (Jul. 5, 1998): 16.

35. Wrote the oncologist Eric J. Cassel: "Observation of current hospital medicine suggests that its therapeutic power is largely rejected, untapped, undervalued, or merely neglected with resultant impoverishment of medical care," in *The Nature of Suffering and the Goals of Medicine*, New York, Oxford Univ. Press, 1991, p. 69.

INDEX

Abrams, Donald: and ARC patients 641; attending physician at San Francisco General Hospital, Ward 5 B 643; concern for patients 633, 635; involvement in AIDS care 662; in San Francisco General Hospital, Ward 86 633; *See also* acquired immunodeficiency syndrome; medicine, U.S. (20th c.), AIDS

academic medical centers, U.S. (20th c.): 576–82; educational rituals 684; evolution of 576–79; financing services of 577–81; Flexner report on 577; Harvard Medical School 347, 581–82; patients as experimental subjects in 578; Stanford University 624–25; training of house staff in 579. *See also* University of California, San Francisco

accidents: 12; and industrialization 468; riding 88, 91. *See also* trauma

accidents, automobile: 463–67, 488–92; American Motorist Association statistics 488; growing number of cars 489; legal and financial implications of 490–92, 499; medical care for victims of (*see* Madison General Hospital; S., Paula; trauma); national epidemic of 488–92; National Safety Council statistics of 489; pedestrians as victims 489. *See also* Madison, Wisconsin

acquired immunodeficiency syndrome (AIDS): 627–33, 658–64; AIDS-related complex (ARC) 641; CDC reports on 640, 642, 659; construction of 628–29; and cryptosporidiosis 643, 658; definition of 628–29; early understanding of cause 629–30; "gay bowel disease" 622, 628–29; and gay community 647–48; "gay related immunodeficiency" (GRID) 628; and infectious mononucleosis 632; Kaposi sarcoma or "gay cancer" (*see* Kaposi sarcoma); and lymphomas 632; neurological complications of 656–58; and opportunistic infections 628; patient experiences (*see* patients, AIDS); pneumocystis pneumonia 628, 643, 656; and public health 630–31, 640–41, 657; quilt 620; role of medicine in (*see* medicine, U.S. (20th c.), AIDS); scientific labeling of 619; and sexual promiscuity 629–31, 642; as sexually-transmitted disease 629; stigma associated with 645; viral origin of 639–40, 642, 660. *See also* nursing, U.S. (20th c.), AIDS; patients, AIDS

administration, hospital: 6–7; abuses in early Europe 218; in Ancien Régime institutions 294; authoritarianism in x; and character of institution 4; monastic standards for 6; power struggles with patrons 6; role of the Church in 5–8. *See also* organization, hospital

Adolf of Cologne: 134–38, 143–48; death in Jerusalem 134–35, 148; as inmate at Hospital of St. John, Jerusalem 145–46; pilgrimage to Holy Land 134–37 (*see also* Jerusalem); and Theoderic von Würzburg 134

Allgemeines Krankenhaus, Vienna (18th c.): 259–65, 267–71; administration of (see Frank, Johann P.; Quarin, Joseph); admission policies and routines 269–70; Brunonian medicine at (see Brown, John); clinical instruction in 276–78; description of 262–63; design competition for 262; dispensatory at 267; emergency room 267; Emperor Joseph II's sponsorship of 261–62; finances of 264–65, 268; hospital life in 268–73; institutional epidemics 266–67, 269–70, 275–76; lying-in facility 267; medical and surgical staffs 263, 267–68; mortality of caregivers 275–76; nurses at 263–64; opening notice 264; pathological museum 277–78; postmortem dissections 277–78; role of diet 267; salubrity (see hygiene, hospitals); surgery at 267; teaching cases 269, 275; transformation from almshouse 260–262; treatment of patients 268–73; trials with stimulants 271–73. See also Duschau, Johann; medicine, Vienna

almshouses: 81, 107, 183, 216, 266, 296, 502; General Hospital of Paris (Bicêtre and Salpêtrière Hospices) 294, 296; Grosses Armenhaus, Vienna 260, 261–62

Amend, William J.: nephrologist on transplantation team 596 (see also UCSF Transplantation Service); relationship with patients 603. See also transplantation, kidney; transplantation of organs

anesthesia: 12; and "calculus of suffering" 360; chloroform 363, 381–84; first amputation with ether 354–56 (see also Warren, John C.); hazards of ether administration 360; human experiments with 357; and Liston, Robert 359; at Madison General Hospital 492; publicity about first use of ether 357–59; use of "letheon" 352–361 (see also Morton, William)

antidotes (theriacs): 19; local antiseptics as 416; medical works about 96; Notker II's knowledge of 99–100; for plague poison 195; preparation of olio contraveneni 211. See also humoralism; therapeutics, medical

architecture, hospital: 6; Allgemeines Krankenhaus in Vienna 262–63; Asclepieion

temple 22–24, 34; Byzantine hostel 82–83, 123; Edinburgh Infirmary's Adams building 241–43; Eppendorf General Hospital 428–31; high-rise buildings 469–70, 473, 481; Hospital of St. John in Jerusalem 137; and hospitalism 266, 367–68, 403–06, 429–31, 469; hospitals as landmarks 5; interior design in modern U.S. hospitals 470, 483; 679, 681; Johns Hopkins Hospital 403–06; Madison General Hospital 479–80; Massachusetts General Hospital 346; Moffitt Hospital 582, 584–87; Necker Hospital 291; Roman valetudinarium 49–50; St. Gall infirmary and hostel 97–99; spatial organization 5–6

Aristides, Aelius: 15–20, 33–38; diagnosis of "consumption" 38; and Egyptian healing deities 15–17; and incubation 15–16, 32, 34–37; at Pergamon 16, 29,33–38; quoted by Osler, William 421; relationship with Asclepius 16, 36–7; in Rome 17–18, 20; and Sacred Tales (Hieroi Logoi) 16, 37; in Smyrna 15, 17, 20; symptoms of illness 17–18, 20, 35–38; treatments for 15–18, 20, 34–37. See also Asclepius, cult of; Greece, Ancient; medicine, Roman Empire

Asclepius (Esculapius): 15–17, 25–26; association with Imhotep and Sarapis 16–17 (see also religion); comparison with Christ 38; divine transformation of 20–21, 24, 79; Hygieia, daughter of 26, 50; linkage to Johns Hopkins Hospital 1028; as patron of Hippocratic physicians 25–26; as personal savior 36–38; portrayal by Aristophanes 31; provision of health advice 15–16, 34–37, 83–84; transformation into pan-Hellenic god 22. See also Aristides, Aelius; Asclepius, cult of; Asclepius, temple of; Greece, Ancient

Asclepius, cult of: 20–24, 28–33, 44, 50; Asclepiads (iatroi) 27–28; and Christianity 38, 79; development of 16–26, 33–34; expansion into Rome 22; faith, role of in 27, 31, 57–58; and Galen 33; function of dogs and snakes 22–23, 31; growing sophistication of 32–33; and healing ceremonies 28–34; incubation rites of 30–31,

34; medical cures of 32, 34–38; parallel developments in Egypt 16–17; rituals of 28–30, 33, 57–58; simultaneous rise of Hippocratic physicians 26–27; sufferer's role in cure 31, 36–37; testimonials of cures 23, 27, 20–30, 32–33; women as health seekers 28. *See also* Asclepius; Asclepius, temple of; Galen; Greece, Ancient; Roman Empire

Asclepius, temple of (Asclepieion): 24–28, 56–57; at the Athenian Acropolis 22, 24–25, 33; baths at 22–24, 34–35; at Cos 21, 29; description of typical complex 22–24, 28, 34; destruction of temples 38; endowments to 32–33, 37; at Epidaurus 21–25, 29–30, 32–34; festivals and athletic events at 33, 36; as forerunner to hospital 56–59; illnesses seen at 28; at Lambaesis 59; location of 22; at Pergamon 11, 15, 22–23, 29, 33–37; Piraeus 22; prayer at 28; priesthood of 29, 31; as refuge from persecution 28; in Roman Empire 24; as shelter 56–57; sociability at 58; spa-like atmosphere of 35; staff 33, 37; on Tiber Island in Rome 22, 208; visits from physicians to 27. *See also* Aristides, Aelius; Asclepius; Asclepius, cult of; Greece, Ancient; medicine, Roman Empire

Auenbrugger, Leopold: *Inventum Novum* 315; percussion method of 243, 325; physician- in-chief at Spanish Hospital 272. *See also* diagnosis, medical; medicine, Vienna

Austrian Empire (18th c): medical police in 260; cameralism in 259; enlightened despotism in 258–59; imperial capital of (*see* Vienna, Austria); reign of Joseph II 258–65; status of physicians and surgeons 277. *See also* Allgemeines Krankenhaus, Vienna; medicine, Vienna

B., Patty: 569–76, 599–607. *See also* UCSF Transplantation Service

Baltimore, Maryland (19th c.): 12; and Baltimore & Ohio Railroad 402, 407; cholera epidemic of 403; climate in 406; demographics of 400, 402; physicians of 406, 409–10; public health in 400; relations with Johns Hopkins Hospital 401

(*see also* Johns Hopkins Hospital, Baltimore); sick poor in 406; typhoid fever in 400, 402, 410; urban transportation in 401; Ward 19 399–400; Western Maryland Railway in 399

Bichat, Marie-François X.: and dissections at the Hôtel Dieu 310–12; empiricism of 309–12; new pathophysiology 312; organ pathology of 311–12; treatise on membranes 312. *See also* medicine, France; Hôtel Dieu, Paris

Billings, John S.: 404, 406–07; on hospitalism (*see* hospitalism); on medical educational (*see* education, medical; research, hospital); partiality for male attendants 1005; professorship in hygiene 406, 408

bloodletting (phlebotomy): 8, 19, 30, 36; and Aristides 35; and Brunonianism 271; in Byzantium 86; and cholera 441; and classical wound healing 55; and Cullen, William 247–49; and fevers 147; at the Hospital of St. John 138; and laboratory medicine 649; and leprosy 189; at Massachusetts General Hospital 347; in medieval monasteries 98, 103–04; at the Pantocrator Xenon 132; at Parisian hospitals 318; and plague victims 195, 211; by Sisters of Charity 318, 296; and tuberculosis 320–21. *See also* humoralism; therapeutics, medical

Boerhaave, Hermann: blistering schedule of 249; clinical observations of 271; and Edinburgh Medical School 239–40, 252–53 (*see also* Edinburgh Infirmary); and Haen, Anton de 271, 273–74; medical system of 240; as professor at University of Leyden 252–53; and Swieten, Gerard van 273

Boston, Massachusetts (19th c): demographics of 340–41; as financial center of New England 340; hospitals in 344–45, 348–49 (*see also* Massachusetts General Hospital, Boston); medicine in 360; rise of professional dentistry in 351; Society of Medical Improvement 357

Brown, John: 11; Brunonianism 256; classification of disease 270; critique of alcohol treatments 272 (*see also* medicine, Vienna); debates about opium 350; and Johann Duchau 270–73; and Frank, J. P.

(*see also* Frank, Johann P.); French criticism of 309; and Jackson, James, Sr. 347; his *Elementa Medicinae* 268; and Cullen, William 256, 268 (*see also* Cullen, William). *See also* Allgemeines Krankenhaus, Vienna; Scotland

Buenos Aires, Argentina (20th c.): hospital experiences of Guenter B. Risse vii–xii; medical school in x

Buffalo, New York (20th c.): consortium of community hospitals 550; economic problems in 515, 532; health care facilities in 519, 536; health in 517, 532–33, 536; Irish community in 514. *See also* Mercy Hospital, Buffalo, NY; Sisters of Mercy

Byzantine Empire: 73–87, 120–25; agricultural failures and famine in 74; Alexander of Tralles on spa-baths 121; Alexius Comnenus 117; Christianity as official religion 70–71; collapse of 70; demographic and economic decay in 70, 120–21; epidemics as crises of faith 83–85 (*see also* Joshua the Stylite); establishment of 70–71; hospitals in (*see xenodocheion*; *nosokomeion*); imperial capital 70–71; importance of local bishops in 79–81 (*see also* St. Gregory of Nazianzen; St. Gregory of Nyssa); infectious disease in 70; medicine in (*see* medicine, Byzantium); Moslem occupation of Syria and Palestine 121; municipal government in 70; Pantocrator Monastery and Xenon (*see* Pantocrator Xenon, Constantinople); political conditions in (*see* Constantinople); power of church in fifth century 71; profiteering of landowners 74; province of Cappadochia 84; reforms under Emperor Justinian 120; relations between Christians and Hellenized Jews 71; role of local town councils in 79; urban Christianity in (*see* St. Basil of Caesarea). *See also* Edessa, Anatolia

Cabanis, Pierre J. G.: hospital reformer 303, 307; medical "ideologue" 309–10. *See also* medicine, France

California, health care in: effects of Proposition 13 on 526; Kaiser Permanente 576;

Medi-Cal (Medicaid program of) 580, 626–27; public hospitals in 626; revolt of the patient in 644; State Assembly's health legislation 580; State Health Sciences Bond Issue 586. *See also* Moffitt Hospital, San Francisco; San Francisco General Hospital; University of California, San Francisco

caregivers: barber surgeons 153; caregiving as penance 152 (*see also* Sisters of Charity; Sisters of Mercy); caregiving as vocation 540; discipline of 152; inclusion in charges' prayers 152; monks as 101, 147, 152–53 (*see also* monasteries; Notker II); multidisciplinary teams of 682; pastoral activities 528, 549, 554; preference for male attendants 411; rationing of caregiving 154–55; role of lay brothers and sisters 152; sexual tensions among 152 ; Shanti Project volunteers 637–38, 652, 654–55, 663–64; threat of unionization by 555–56; widows as 150. *See also* Hospitallers; nursing; patient/physician relationship; physicians; women as caregivers

cathartics (purgatives): in "antiphlogistic" treatment 246; and Aristides 18; and Brunonianism 271; in Byzantine medicine 131–32; and cholera 441; for expulsion of poisons 19, 85; and French therapeutic skepticism 321; and leprosy 188–89; and plague 211. *See also* humoralism

Catholic Hospital Association (CHA): expanding role in the 1950s 522–23; ethics code of 523, 543, 545–46; Moulinier era 522–23; renewal and reform 543. *See also* hospitals, U.S., Catholic (20th c.)

Celsus: 54–55; on stomach disorders 54; on the *valetudinarium* 53; on wound healing 55. *See also* humoralism; medicine, Roman Empire; *valetudinarium*, civil

Cheyne, W. Watson: 386; disciple of Lister 385–86 (*see also* Lister, Joseph); at Edinburgh Infirmary 364–65, 381–85 (*see also* Edinburgh Infirmary (19th c.)). *See also* Mathewson, Margaret; surgery

cholera, Asiatic: administration of fluids in 442–45; "anticholerin" therapy for 441; in Baltimore ; as *cholera asphictica* 440;

cholera sicca 433; depleting treatments in 441; discovery of cholera vibrio (*see* Koch, Robert); employment of disinfectants in 442, 444; environmental theory of (*see* Pettenkoffer, Max von); Haffkine cholera preservative 422, 446; in Hamburg 423–27, 432–33, 435, 439–46; isolation of victims in 425; mortality from 445; pneumonia in 445; popular fears about 423; postmortem examinations in 440; stages of the disease 433, 444; stimulant treatment of 440, 444; symptoms of 422–23, 440

Christianity, early: Acts of Mercy (*see* St. Matthew); as basis for social solidarity 73–74; charity in 73–74, 80; concept of *hospitalitas* 5; healing in (*see* healing, early Christian); meaning of Christ's suffering 74; Origen's ascetic position 75; Pachomius' monastic tradition 75–76; St. Augustine's rules for monastic life 92, 152; salvation in 73–74; under Constantine 70–71; as urban phenomenon 73. *See also* Byzantine Empire

Clementia: admission to Rome's Lazaretto San Bartolomeo 209; diagnosis of bubonic plague 190, 195; under the care of plague doctors 212–13

Cologne (15th c.): 167; Melaten leper house (*see* Melaten leper house, Cologne); municipal council of 167; university and leper examination 169

Conant, Marcus: and Kaposi sarcoma (*see* Kaposi sarcoma); at University of California, San Francisco 631. *See also* medicine, U.S. (20th c.), AIDS

Constantinople: 11, 70–71; Justinian reforms in 120; Christodes Xenon 123–24; educated elite in 121; endowed *xenones* in 123; lay medicine in 119; philanthropy in 120; medical instruction in 121; as nucleus of imperial life 81; plague in 120; Pantocrator Monastery and Xenon (*see* Pantocrator Xenon, Constantinople); population of 120–21, 129; Samson Xenon 124, 139; trade in 121. *See also* Byzantine Empire; medicine, Byzantium

Corvisart, Jean N.: "meditations on death" 310; at the Hôpital de la Charité 313, and healing art 316, daily hospital rounds by 325; psychological aspects of illness 322; reintroduction of direct percussion 315; role of bodily constitution 320; Society of Medical Instruction 327. *See also* medicine, France

Crafts, Grace T.: hospital care as commodity 500; at Madison General Hospital 478, 480; rationing of resources 500–02; visits with patients 493–94. *See also* Madison General Hospital, Madison, Wis.

Cullen, William: 11; and bedside diagnoses 246; blistering schedule of 249; and bloodletting 247–49; and classification of fevers 243–45; debates about opium 350; at the Edinburgh Infirmary 235–36; French criticism of 309; and patient screening 236; personal appearance of 243; and postmortem examinations 310; and pulse-counting 243–44; and Royal College of Physicians, Edinburgh 236; system of medicine 245–46, 256; as university professor 235. *See also* Edinburgh Infirmary; medicine, Great Britain

Curschmann, Heinrich: gardens for healing 428, 430; and hospital construction 429–30; management style of 431–32; professional authority of 424; at St. Georg Hospital 427–28; and water filtration plant 431. *See also* Eppendorf General Hospital, Hamburg

Deaconess Sisters: and Florence Nightingale 369–70; influence on German nursing 437–38; Deaconess Training Institute, Kaiserswerth 437; role of volunteers 426–27. *See also* Eppendorf General Hospital, Hamburg

diagnosis, medical: anatomical clinical correlations (*see* medicine, France); bacteriological methods in cholera 424–25, 439 (*see also* laboratories); bone marrow studies 649; bronchoscopies in AIDS 649; diagnostic-related groups (DRGs) 580; differential among fevers 244–45; direct auscultation 316–17; direct percussion 243, 272, 315, 325; electrocardiography in 525–29, 535; functional bodily inventory 315; history-taking 314; imaging in 579, 677; indirect auscultation 316–317 (see also Laennec, René T.); indirect percussion 315; interpretation of symptoms 315; invention of the stethoscope 316–317; of leprosy 168–72, 175–76; linkage with prognosis 131; Lister's silver probe 365; medical certainty and status 315–16; at Moffitt Hospital, San Francisco 586, 610; pathological anatomy in 315; promise of bacteriology in 469; of skin diseases 118–19; truth telling and 492; of typhoid fever 414–15, 420; uroscopy in 102, 118; use of physical signs in Paris hospitals 292–293, 314–317; vital signs in head injuries 467; X-rays in 466, 470, 481–82

disease: AIDS (see Acquired Immunodeficiency Syndrome); cholera (see cholera, Asiatic); chronic conditions and aging 678; "consumption" 38; ecology of 4, 468; epidemic (see epidemics); ergotism 150; of heart (see heart disease); hepatitis B 622, 632; and immigration to America 468; influenza or English sweat 150; in joints (see joint disease); kidney failure (see end stage renal disease program); leprosy (see leprosy); linkage to industrialization and urbanization 468; malaria in Ancient Greece 26; Mediterranean region and disease pools 70; "phthisis' (tuberculosis) 318–19, 381–82; plague (see plague); scurvy 150; smallpox (see smallpox); stomach disorders 54; "synochus" fever 244–46; typhoid fever (see typhoid fever); and the urban Roman Empire 70; venereal syphilis 215

d'Uliva, Catharina: 90, 195, 212–13; admission to Rome's Lazaretto San Bartolomeo 209; diagnosis of bubonic plague 190, 195; under the care of plague doctors 212–13

Dumesnil, Jacques: 289–93, 317–25; admission to Paris' Necker Hospital 290; diagnosis of phthisis 319; under the care of Laennec, René T. 317–25

Duschau, Johann: 257–58, 268–73; admission to Vienna's Allgemeines Krankenhaus 268–70 (see also Allgemeines Krankenhaus, Vienna); diagnosis of fever and pneumonia 270; under the care of Frank, Johann. P. 270–73

Edessa, Anatolia, (5 c.): 11, 69–73, 86–87

Edinburgh, Scotland (18th–19th c.): 11, 236–43; air pollution in 235; and bills of mortality 234, 362; and Church of Scotland 231–32, 239–40; domestic servants in 232; and Drummond, George 240–41; and the Enlightenment 239–41; High Street in 241, 362; and Incorporation of Surgeons and Apothecaries 240; "Infirmary Sunday" in 234; New Town segregation 242; local presbytery of 234, 239; Royal College of Physicians 236, 240; Royal Infirmary of (see Edinburgh Infirmary (18th c.); Edinburgh Infirmary (19th c.)); and smallpox epidemics 234, 362; Royal Medical Society of 240; Town Council of 240; University of Edinburgh (see Edinburgh University)

Edinburgh Infirmary (18th c.): 231–36, 240–55; admission of patients 231–33; chores for patients 251; clinical lectures at 251–52 (see also Cullen, William); educational values at 236; establishment of 240–41; examination of female patients at 244; experimentation on patients 254–55; "feigned complaints" 249–50; female teaching ward 236; fundraising for 240–41; General Register of Patients 232, 234, 236; hospital life in 243–51; in-house infections 242–43; medical clerks at 236; and Monro, John 240; nursing at 247; post-mortem examinations at 255–56; ventilation at 242–43; subscribers to 240–41; surgery at 255–56; teaching ward 235–36, 251, 253–55; and treatment of the poor 232. See also Cullen, William

Edinburgh Infirmary (19th c): 361–66, 376–85; administration of chloroform at 363, 382, 384; admission of patients 365–66; affiliated convalescent home 385–86; amputation at 344, 365; bedside teaching 362–63; delays in surgery 381–82; High School building 362–63, 365; hospital dressers at 384–85; hospital life 379–85; at Lauriston Place 366; new surgical hospital 363; nursing 369–73; overcrowding in 362, 365, 381–82; post-operative experiences 383–84; reputation of 362; salubrity of

363, 366; shortage of beds at 385; shoulder surgery at (see Mathewson, Margaret); surgical staff at 372. See also Cheyne, W. Watson; Lister, Joseph

Edinburgh University (18th–19th c.): as alternative to Oxford and Cambridge 239; influence of University of Leyden on 240, 252–53; and Liston, Robert 363; matriculation statistics for 240; and Monro, John 240; reputation in British surgery 364; and Cullen, William 235; sponsorship of clinical lectures 252; and Syme, James 363, 365

education, medical: 576, 676; Boerhaave at Leyden 271; in Byzantium 77, 121; at cathedral schools 91, 108; at the Edinburgh Infirmary (18th c.) 251–56; in 18th century Vienna 273–77; at Eppendorf General Hospital 436; essay by Pinel 326; Jackson Sr. and Warren on 347; at Johns Hopkins Hospital 404, 408–11; Madison General internship 465, 481; in medieval monasteries 96–97; Mercy Hospital's residency program 515–16, 521; at Moffitt Hospital, University of California, San Francisco 597; in Padua 252; in Parisian hospitals 325–29; patients as teachers 292–93, 325–26; Pinel on 325–26; plans for Massachusetts General Hospital 347; reforms in post-Revolutionary France 302–03, 306; School of Salerno 108; Society of Medical Instruction in Paris 327; universities and hospitals 404, 408, 411, 576. See also academic medical centers, U.S.

end-stage renal disease (ESRD) program: and academic health centers 597; choices between dialysis and transplantation 590–91; dialysis treatments in 570, 572–73; eligibility for transplantation in 573; as entitlement program 609; and Samuel Kountz 594; Medicare coverage for 570, 572–73; statistics for 591

Enlightenment: 5, 8; in Austria 273; in Britain 236–43; in France 330; and pain 350; system- building in medicine 240, 245–46, 256

epidemics: AIDS (see Acquired Immunodeficiency Syndrome); in ancient Attica

26; in Byzantium 71, 73, 79, 85, 120; cholera (see cholera, Asiatic); Christians and 80; in Edessa 69–73, 86–87; erysipelas 341; hepatitis B 622, 632; in hospitals 341 (see also hospitalism); influenza 150, 477; linkage with famines 69–70, 83, 85–86, 122; and Mediterranean trade routes 39; plague (see plague); and the poor 150; smallpox 119, 234, 362; socio-political explanations of 434; in the Roman Empire 57; syphilis 215; typhoid fever (see typhoid fever). See also disease

Eppendorf General Hospital, Hamburg (19th c.): 12; administrative staff at 428, 431–32 (see also Rumpf, Theodor M.); building complex 428–31; cholera barracks in 432, 436, 439; clinical research and experimentation at 436, 440–443 (see also Hueppe, Ferdinand; Klebs, Edwin K.); cost-cutting measures at 424; disposal of bodies at 439–40; hospital life in 439–45; inauguration of 432; as isolation facility 425, 427–28; and Kast, Alfred 432, 436; lack of conveyances to 426, 429; length of stay at 432–33; location of 429; as medical institution 428–29; medical staff at 436; medical students at 426; nurses at 437, 447; open house at 432; patient discipline 437; planning and construction (see Curschmann, Heinrich); reporter's exposure to cholera at 422, 446; rotating admissions with St. George Hospital 425; Schede, Max 431; sterilization facilities at 447; systematic stool cultures at 424 (see also Fraenkel, Eugen); triage for cholera patients 432; ventilation at 429; volunteer nurses (see Deaconess Sisters); water filtration plant at 431, 447

F., Albert: 531–35, 546–53

finances, hospital: of the Allgemeines Krankenhaus, Vienna 264; in Ancien Régime France 293–94, 307; changes in the U.S. 681–83; of early Christian shelters 150–51, 155; of the Edinburgh Infirmary 240–44; Greek temple endowments 32–33, 37; of leper houses 182–83; Medicare and Medicaid; and

Nightingale nursing 905; patient payments in the U.S. 340–41, 349, 476–77, 484, 499–500, 502; in post-Revolutionary France 305–06; of U.S. hospitals 471–73, 478, 523, 625, 678

Fraenkel, Eugen: and cholera bacilli 425; at clinical laboratory of Eppendorf General Hospital, Hamburg 431. *See also* Eppendorf General Hospital, Hamburg

France (post-Revolutionary): Committee on Mendicity 301; Committee on Public Assistance 303–06; Committee on Salubrity 302–03; Consulate 307–08; Convention before Thermidor 304–05; Directory 306–07; expansion of medical corps in 304; home-based relief in 301–02; hospitals in (*see* hospitals, France (post-revolutionary); hospitals, Paris); Legislative Assembly in 303–04; National Constituent Assembly in 301–04; oath of loyalty to the Revolution 305; Paris (*see* Paris, France); physicians in (*see* medicine, France); repression of religion in 303–04; Thermidorean Convention 305–06

Frank, Johann P.: 265–78; and "antiphlogistic" therapeutics 270; and "asthenic" disease 270; and Brunonianism 268; and Capellini, Thomas 269–70; director of Allgemeines Krankenhaus 265; in Lombardy 265; and "medical police" 265–66; and pathological anatomy 277–78; patient selection and clinical instruction 269–70, 273; salubrity of hospitals 366–403; and Stifft, Joseph (*see* Stifft, Joseph); use of direct chest percussion 272

Galen: 17, 31; and Asclepius 30; healer-patient relationship 37; selecting a physician 17; rational therapeutics of 34; at the Asclepieion at Pergamon 33. *See also* Greece, Ancient; humoralism; medicine, Roman Empire

Germany: hospitals in (*see* hospitals, Germany); imperial epidemic legislation (*Reichsseuchengesetz*) 446–47; Imperial Health Ministry (*Reichsgesundheitsamt*) 435; *Krankenkassen* in 423; medicine in

(*see* medicine, Germany); *See also* Cologne; Hamburg, Germany

Gilman, Daniel C.: on mission of hospital 421–22; hospitals as hotels 408, and house staff 411; at Johns Hopkins Hospital 407–408; and Nurses Training School 411–12; on medical education 411

Giovanni, Cecilia di: admission to Rome's Lazaretto San Bartolomeo 209; diagnosis of bubonic plague 190, 195; under the care of plague doctors 212–13

Gottstine, Mary Ann: career at Mercy Hospital, Buffalo, NY 533–34, 547, 549, 551–53; on emotional factors in cardiac care 546–47, 549–51

Greece, Ancient: 27, 29; Aristotelian catharsis 30; attitudes toward health in 25; competition between gods 24–25 (*see also* Asclepius); disease and mortality in 25–26; divinity of nature in 27; healing craftsmen in (*see* medicine, Ancient Greece); health care in 27–28; incubation in temples 15–16, 27, 31 (*see also* Aristides, Aelius; Asclepius, cult of); malaria epidemic in Athens 26; rising individualism in 25; role of religion in daily life 24; social welfare (*philanthropia*) in 44–45; temple culture in 24–25 (*see also* Asclepius, temple of)

Haen, Anton de: *clinicum practicum* of 273–74; therapy of 271; as follower of Hippocrates 271; and autopsy 277; and Leyden's instructional model 274

Hamburg, Germany (19th c.): chaos in local hospitals 439 (*see also* Eppendorf General Hospital, Hamburg); cholera 422–23, 425–26, 434–35 (*see also* cholera, Asiatic; W., Erika); city cemetery at Ohlsdorf 426; hospital bed shortage 427; Imperial Health Ministry (*see also* Koch, Robert); chief medical officer 424–25, 434–35; local *Krankenkassen* 423, 427; municipal physicians in 423–24; population in 435; public health 435, 446–47; and religious nurses 437–38; tenements in 423; typhoid fever outbreaks in 435; water filtration plant in 431 healing: and the art of medicine 300, 311, 316, 635, 646, 661–62; (see also patient/physician relationship); and the art of nursing 646–51; based on love 647–48; as individual process 679–80; dying as healing experience 652–53; Eppendorf as place of 428; faith and emotion in 31; fundamental human experience 663; hospital space designed for 659, 681; hospitals as "healing machines" 300; importance of gardens for 428; laying-on-of-hands 330, 647; in modern hospitals 474–75, 680–81, 685; nature's power for 18–19, 342; personal narratives of 9–13; religious (see healing, early Christian; healing, pagan)

healing, early Christian: miracles in 122; Christ the Great physician 77, 79, 122; communal shelters in 74 (see also xenodocheion); cult of St. Cosmas and St. Damian 72, 79, 123; demonic possession and illness in 79; divine provision of remedies in 77; Edessa and 72; ideology of 74, 77–79; Gregory of Tour's on 96–97; and Matthew's Six Acts of Mercy (see St. Matthew); in monasteries 96, 105; medicine as charitable work 76–77 (see also St. Basil of Caesarea; St. Gregory of Nazianzen; St. Gregory of Nyssa); New Testament and use of medicines 78, 82; and relics 72, 78–79; sin theory of disease 78; tensions between Christian and lay healing 78, 96–97, 108; visitation to the sick 74; women in 80 (see also women as caregivers)

healing, pagan: Ancient Greek craftsmen (see medicine, Ancient Greece); cult of Isis and Sarapis 16; divinities for 57; in dreams 30–38; in Greek temples and Roman valetudinaria 57–58 (see also Asclepius, cult of); magic and 22; role of Apollo in 25

health care, U.S. (20th c.): for aging and chronic diseases 678; Committee on the Costs of Medical Care 503; consumerism in 471–72, 680–81; continuum of care 677; cultural changes in 678; definitions of health 4; education of patients in 677; emphasis on outcomes 678, 685; as en-titlement 7; epidemiological shifts and 678; escalating costs of 484–85; "focused settings" for 681; health insurance for 502–03; hospital industry in 681; hospitalization as system failure in 678; managerial revolution in 681–83; money taboo in 485, 499; non-profit organizations in 473

heart disease: 513–17, 531–35; arrhythmias in 549, 552; cardiac catheterization 548; danger of thrombophlebitis 525; extended rest treatment 526; golden age of cardiology 533; high incidence in the U.S. 517, 532; myocardial infarction 517, 525–26, 548–51; President Eisenhower's illness 531; symptoms of heart attack 517, 532; and use of electrocardiograph (EKG) 525, 529, 535

Hospital of St. John, Jerusalem: 138–53; admission to 141, 145; and Amalfi merchants 140; bequest by Baldwin I 140 to; building complex of 137; debt to Islamic hospitals 145; dedication to St. John the Baptist 140; description by John of Würzburg 137–38; destruction by earthquake 148; diet in 146–47; as early monastic shelter 137–40; fame in Western Europe 140–41; hospital life in 145–48 (see also Adolf of Cologne); increased endowment for 140; location 137; medicalization of 145; mission of 140–41; model for hospital organization 151–53; provision of physicians 145; reforms of Raymond du Puy 141; Regimen Sanitatis Salernitanum 147; religious ceremonies 146; Roger des Moulins 144; role of infirmarian 147–48; rule of Brother Gerard 140; St. John Order of the Hospital 141 (see also Hospitallers); the sick as Lords 141; spectrum of patients 141–42, 145; Theoderic von Würzburg 134–36, 138; therapeutic measures 147–48 (see also bloodletting)

hospitalism: 5, 366–68; at Allgemeines Krankenhaus 266–67, 269–70; and antiseptic surgery 373, 375; avoidance at the Eppendorf General Hospital 429; call for hospital reform 367; concerns of Johann P. Frank; decline of 386; erysipelas at the Massachusetts General Hospital 341; 18th century "hospital distempers" 366; "gateways to death" reputation 5; at the Hôtel Dieu in Paris 295, 297–98; John E. Erichsen on 367–68; linkage with overcrowding 368; need for ventilation 367; opinions of John S. Billings 368; postoperative surgical complications and 366; James Y. Simpson on 366–67

Hospitallers (Knights of St. John): and Augustinian rules 144–45; capture of Rhodes 148; creation through Papal bull 141; exemptions and privileges 142; Frankish origins 141; hospital network (see hospitals, Europe, (Middle Ages); impact of bubonic plague on 156; at Malta 156; military role of 143–44; model for the Order of the Holy Spirit 149; political and economic power of 141–42; preservation of the kingdom of Jerusalem 142; protection of pilgrims 142, 144; and Raymond du Puy 142–44; retreat to Acre and Cyprus 148; rules of feudalism and chivalry 141; struggles with the Papacy 156; types of membership 144

hospitals: administration (see administration, hospital); admission rituals 8; almshouses (see almshouses); architecture of (see architecture, hospital); basic aspects of institutional life 4–9; caregivers (see caregivers); Darwinian survival struggle 677; and demographics 677; documentation of activities 8; education and research in (see education, medical; research, hospital); evolution of 4, 675–79; finances (see finances, hospital); first International Hospital Congress 472; geographical location of 6; hygiene (see hospitalism; hygiene, hospital); individual personality 4; military and naval 218; new mergers and closings 3; organizational culture (see organization, hospital); patronage of (see patronage, hospital); political role of 4; as "pox houses" 214–15; range of activities in 7–8; religious role of (see religion);

reputation of 5; shifting boundaries 675–77; social control function (see isolation, hospital); utopian vision of 538; visiting hours in 8; welfare role of (see welfare)

hospitals, Byzantium: See xenodocheion

hospitals, Europe (Middle Ages): financial collapse of 154–56; Hôtel Dieu institutions 218; tensions between religious and lay healing 96–97, 108; network of 141–42, 149 (see also Hospitallers); uroscopy in 102 (see also Notker II). See also Hospital of St. John, Jerusalem; Pantocrator Xenon, Constantinople; St. Gall, monastic infirmary

hospitals, Europe, (early modern): administrative abuses in 218; and the Council of Trent 218; for beggars 218; Holy Spirit hospitals 218; Hôtel Dieu institutions 294–99, leper houses (see leper houses; Melaten leper house, Cologne); pesthouses (see lazarettos; lazarettos, Rome); Ospedale di San Bastiano in Florence 205; "pox houses" 214–15; visits from bishops 218; San Paolo Hospital, Florence 215; Santa Maria Nuova Hospital, Florence 154, 207, 214

hospitals, Europe (18th–19th c.): Austria's model institution (see Allgemeines Krankenhaus, Vienna); infirmaries in Britain (see hospitals, Great Britain (18th–19th c.)); in Germany (see hospitals, Germany); in France (see hospitals, France, (Ancien Régime); hospitals, France (post-Revolutionary))

hospitals, Europe (20th c.): 472–75; comparisons with Moffitt Hospital, San Francisco 610; full-time medical staffs 473–74; large wards 473;

hospitals, France (Ancien Régime): 293–99; and Academy of Sciences 295–96, 298; admission requirements 290–91; administration 294–95; donations and endowments 293–94; dual hospital system 294–95; financial corruption 293; funding sources for 294, 307; hôpitaux-générales or general hospitals 293; Hôtel Dieu institutions 294–95 (see also Hôtel Dieu, Paris); in Paris (see hospitals, Paris); religious caregivers 293; reputation 290; and welfare system 293–94, 330

hospitals, France, (post-Revolutionary): 300–08, 317–29; Anticatholicism in 304; appointment of physicians 308; bankruptcy of 305–06; clinical research in 327–28, 331; closure of establishments 305–06; dispensatory for 321; dominance of medical profession 309, 331 (*see also* medicine, France (18th–19th c.)); food and supplies 307; improvements in hygiene 308; installation of single beds 308; internship 327–28; jurisdiction over 306; lay personnel 308; as *maisons de santé* 304; medicalization of 303. 330; as museums of pathology 310; patient populations in 328, 330 (*see also* Hôtel Dieu, Paris); patient/physician relations at 309, 328–330; physical examinations in 330; postmortem examinations 310; private charity 308; reduction of overcrowding 300; resurgence of religious nursing orders 300, 330; seizure and sale of hospital properties 300, 305, 306 (*see also* hospitals, Paris); sources of medical knowledge 331 (*see also* medicine, France); status of 300; as symbols of moral corruption 304; as teaching institutions 306, 331; triage system in 307

hospitals, Germany, (19th c.): building boom 429; Moabit Hospital, Berlin 429; Robert Virchow Hospital, Berlin 429; St. Georg Hospital, Hamburg 424–429, 435–36. *See also* Eppendorf General Hospital, Hamburg

hospitals, Great Britain (18th–19th c.): admissions to 232–33; antiseptic surgery in (*see* Edinburgh Infirmary (19th c.)); dietary standards for 246; drug trials in 254 (*see also* Edinburgh Infirmary (18th c.); and Enlightenment values in 236–43; Glasgow Royal Infirmary 373; future role of 387; isolation wards in 386; "locked" venereal wards 234; in London 238; medicalization of 233; moral goals in 233–34; and the new nursing (*see* Edinburgh Infirmary (19th c.), nursing); religious roots of 237–38; turmoil in 385–86

hospitals, Islam (*bimaristan*): in Baghdad 305–06; in Damascus 305; Mansuri Hospital, Cairo 308; influence on Byzantine hospitals 311; institutional routines 310; medical control and staffing 308–10; modeled after Byzantine shelters 305 (*see also xenodocheion*); separate pharmacy 310–01; symbols of political and economic power 307–08; triage system in 309; use of wards 309

hospitals, Paris: crossinfection in 300 (*see also* hospitalism); dissections in 323–24; lack of moral rehabilitation 300; food shortages in 307; General Hospital (Bicêtre and Salpêtrière Hospices) 294, 296, 311; Hôpital de la Charité 311, 325; local Hôtel Dieu 294 (*see also* Hôtel Dieu, Paris); Hôpital Necker (*see* Necker Hospital, Paris); Hôpital St. Louis 289; population of 298; reduction in services 306–07; religious caregivers 294 (*see also* Sisters of Charity); surgical training in 325; under the Department of the Seine 306–07; use of patients for teaching 292–93

hospitals, U.S. (19th–20th c.): accountability of 475; administrative and social services of 471, 473; and American Hospital Association 475; and automobiles 491; buildings 473; board of trustees of 470; Catholic institutions (*see* hospitals, U.S., Catholic); closings and mergers of 677; death and dying in 468, 678–79; decentralized system 469; dietary department 483; dramatic image of 5; during the Depression 487; ethics of terminal care 678; finances of 471, 473, 523, 677; focus on intensive care 677; Hill-Burton Act 514, 577; holistic approaches in 677–78; as home substitutes 468, 472, 474; hotel-like atmosphere 474; ideology of self-sufficiency and competition 469; image 468, 499–500; institutions of first resort 467; insurance for 502–03; laboratory facilities in 473; as "Land that Never Sleeps" 680; maternity and pediatric services in 468, 471; and medical records 473–74; medical staffs in 470, 472–73; pastoral teams for 554, 683–84;

payments for services 476; as physicians' workshops 472, 504; popularity of private institutions 467, 472–73; redesign of patient care 681, 684–85; role of "hospitalist" 682; science ideology in 469, 472; shift to other facilities 677; as sources of civic pride 468; surgery in 469, 472; voluntary foundations 468. *See also* Johns Hopkins Hospital, Baltimore; Massachusetts General Hospital, Boston; Madison General Hospital, Madison, Wisconsin; Mercy Hospital, Buffalo, NY; Moffitt Hospital, San Francisco; San Francisco General Hospital, San Francisco

hospitals, U.S., Catholic (20th c.): as businesses 523; caregiving as vocation 540; as Church property 544; changes in nursing 524; charitable image 514–15; "conscience clause" 554; decline of 544; effects of Vatican II 540–42; encyclical of Pius XII 522; governance of 543; identity of 544, 533–54; influence of Medicare and Medicaid 536, 542; laypersons in 540–41; leadership of 542–43; links with the community 543; patients in 546. *See also* Mercy Hospital, Buffalo, NY

Hôtel Dieu, Paris: admissions to 299, 303–04; Augustinian nuns in 310; autopsies at 310, 312; chief surgeon Desault, Pierre J. 310; destruction by fire 295; eighteenth-century building complex 295; future role of 295–96; hygiene in 295, 298; medical and surgical services 154; medieval foundation for 294; number of beds 294; overcrowding 295; reconstruction plan for 295, 298–99; surgical training at 311, 325

Howard, John: at Edinburgh Infirmary 243; on European lazarettos 214; at the Hospice de Charité 297; salubrity of hospitals 366

Hueppe, Ferdinand: call for hospital reforms 447; critique of Rumpf's leadership 442; intestinal washings in cholera 442; volunteer at the Eppendorf General Hospital 427. *See also* medicine, Germany

humoralism: in Imperial Rome 53; basic notions of 18–20 (*see also* medicine, Ancient Greece); bodily excitement in 247; body as cooking vessel 19; bloodletting (*see* bloodletting); in Byzantine shelters 85–86; drainage of bad humors 342; holism of 20; individual constitution in 18; internal poisoning 19–20; nature's healing power 18–19, 342; miasma and contagion 197–98; in monastic practice 102 (*see also* therapeutics, medical); wound healing in 54

hygiene, hospital: at the Allgemeines Krankenhaus, Vienna 262–63, 266–67; danger of postoperative sepsis 366–678 (*see also* Edinburgh Infirmary (19th c.)); at Eppendorf General Hospital, Hamburg 429 (*see also* Curschmann, Heinrich); at the Edinburgh Infirmary 242–43 (*see also* Edinburgh Infirmary (18th c.)); as "gateways to death" 5; at Hôtel Dieu, Paris 295, 298; importance of single beds for 308; at Johns Hopkins Hospital, Baltimore 368, 405–06 (*see also* Billings, John S.); at Necker Hospital, Paris 296, 298; in pesthouses 207–08; Tenon, Jacques R. on 298, 366, 403 (*see also* Tenon, Jacques R.); whitewashing of walls 308. *See also* hospitalism

isolation, hospital: 8–9; of AIDS patients 637, 650; in British hospitals 386; at Eppendorf General Hospital 425, 427–28; for Hamburg's cholera patients 425; at Johns Hopkins Hospital 405–06; in pesthouses 202–04 (*see* lazarettos); of lepers (*see* leper houses); as social control in France 293; for venereal diseases 234

J., Warren: 619–23, 640–46, 649–58. *See also* patients, AIDS

Jackson, James, Sr.: on Brunonianism 347; chief of medicine 342; and conservative therapy 347; and foundation of Massachusetts General Hospital 345; pamphlet on education 347; retirement of 348; typhoid fever studies 347

Jerusalem: capture by Saladin 148; convent of St. Mary the Great 139; early hospice in 138; Easter pilgrimages to 135, 138; German Order of Hospital Knights 142–43; liberation by First Crusade 140; Holy Sepulcher in 134–35, 137, 139; description of 137 (*see also* Theoderic von Würzburg); death of Adolf of Cologne 135; Poor Knights of the Temple 144; Latin Kingdom and 140–42; population of 135; sponsorship of Jewish hospices in 138; Tower of David 137; Turkish invasion of 139–40; under Moslem rule 138–39. *See also* Hospital of St. John

Johns Hopkins Hospital, Baltimore (19th c.): 12, 402–08, 413–22; administration of 407–408, 412 (*see also* Gilman, Daniel C.); admissions to 401–02; appointment of faculty 406–07; architecture 403, 405–06; building complex 405–06; clinical chiefs 407 (*see also* Osler, William); construction process 404–07; design of (*see* Billings, John S.); hospital as hotel 408; hospital life in 413–20; hygiene in 405–06; image as House of God 422; inauguration of 408; isolation ward 405–06; Johns Hopkins on hospitals 402–03; and Johns Hopkins University 407, 411; location 401–02; management of patients 413–20 (*see also* typhoid fever); medical school 402, 406; nurses' training school 411–13 (*see also* nursing, U.S.; nursing staff and routines 407, 412; organization and personnel 406–08; patient demographics 402; relationships among staff members 413; reputation of 401; site for medical education and research (*see* education, medical; research, hospital); statue of Christ at 422; ventilation and heating 404, 406–07; and William H. Welch 406

joint disease: and amputation 343, 381; association with "scrofula" 342, 381; knee swelling 341–43; management of pain in 341, 343, 356; and pulmonary tuberculosis 342; shoulder abscess 365, 381; surgical mortality in 381; treatment with antiseptics 380–81; and "white" swellings 342

Jones, Diane: bonding with patients 649; "fish bowl medicine" 643 (*see also* health care, U.S.); night nurse at Ward 5 B 638; and nurses' "burnout" 654. *See also* nursing, U.S.; women, as caregivers

Joshua the Stylite: 11; famine and epidemic in Edessa 69–70, 72, 84, 86

Kaposi sarcoma ("gay cancer"): 627–30; opening of KS Clinic at UCSF 631; treatment with interferon 640. *See also* acquired immunodeficiency syndrome

Kelleher, Sister M. Annunciata: 554–57; and Mercy Hospital's CCU unit 533; and charitable Catholic traditions 542; and institutional modernization 537; religious identity of Mercy Hospital 545. *See also* Sisters of Mercy

Klebs, Edwin K.: at the Eppendorf General Hospital 427; treatments with "anticholerin" 441. *See also* cholera, Asiatic

Koch, Robert: at Eppendorf General Hospital 435; on cholera pathogenesis 434–35; conflict with Virchow, Rudolf 434; critique of Hamburg's leadership 435; discovery of the cholera vibrio 433 (*see also* cholera, Asiatic); need for preventive measures 433; opposition to his ideas 434, 446 (*see also* Pettenkoffer, Max von); public health legislation 446 (*see also* medicine, Germany); visit to Hamburg 435

laboratories: and bloodletting 649; and costly equipment 577; at Eppendorf General 424, 431, 439 (*see also* Fraenkel, Eugen); and Flexner Report 577; in modern hospitals 473; and other technical facilities 466 (*see also* technology, medical); and research at SFGH 626; role in diagnosis 410, 414, 677; scientific framing of disease 626; testing facilities for 589, 611 (*see also* academic medical centers, U.S.; use of biopsies 649, 661 (*see also* pathology); virology and AIDS 635, 642

Laennec, René T.: 12, 314–17; at Hôpital de la Charité 329; apprenticeship in Brittany 292; arrival in Paris 313; clinical-pathological correlations 312–13, 317; detection of "pectoriloquy" 319, 321, 323; diagnosis and management of "phthisis" (tuberculosis) 319–23 (*see also* Dumesnil, Jacques); and emotional status of patients 322; importance of pathological anatomy 313–14, 317; invention of the stethoscope 316–17; member of the Society of Good Works 292; resident physician 292, 316, 318 (*see also* Necker Hospital, Paris); textbook on chest diseases 317; use of the stethoscope 348. *See also* medicine, France

lazarettos (pesthouses): 17, 202–08; administration and organization 205–06; admission of plague suspects 202, 209; caregiving staff at 206–07; conditions in 207–08; contract physicians in 206–07; early institutions in Venice 202–05; as eighteenth-century quarantine stations 213–14; fear of removal to 195; Lazaretto de San Miniato, Florence 208; in leper houses or convents 190; location of 203; their makeshift character 190, 203–04; mortality in 210; in other Italian cities 203; permanent institution in Milan 203–05, 207; in Rome (*see* lazarettos, Rome); segregating function of 202–03; wave of European foundations 203, 205, 213–14

lazarettos, Rome (17th c.): 208–13; admission lists 209; anxiety and fear among inmates 210; clashes between religious and medical personnel 210; convent of San Eusebio 208; convent of Santa Maria de la Consolazione 208; disposal of the dead 209, 212–13; guarded by soldiers 209; isolation of plague suspects at 209; life in Lazzaretto San Bartolomeo 208–13; medical rounds 211; military escorts to 209; mortality rate at 210; number of inmates 209; nursing by Capuchin friars and lay volunteers 210; at other city hospitals 208; religious routines 210; suburban rehabilitation sites 208; transportation in wagons and litters 209; use of convicted criminals 209

leper houses: 179–90; admission rituals in

185; change in function 184; death and burial at 189–90; diet in 187–88; financial aspects of 182–83; Knights of St. Lazarus and "Lazar houses" 179–81; life in 184–90; medical management in 188–89; at Melaten 168 (*see* Melaten leper house, Cologne); municipal control of 183–84; number in the 13th century 181; nursing in 188; order and organization of 180–81, 187; origins of 179–80; selfmutilation for admission 189; separation of sexes 185

lepers: banishment from the community 172, 174–75; as Christ's "special poor" 174; Church's role in providing assistance to 177–78; denial and concealment by 170–71; diagnostic probe on 168, 172 (*see also* Thielen, Grette S.); function of parish panels 168; homelessness and unemployment 176–77; itinerant vagrants 180; judgments of moral corruption 172; needs for shelter and food (*see* leper houses); private seclusion 176; provision of special clothing 172; viewed as scapegoats 178–79

leprosy: 173–79, contradictory views on 174–75; bathing practices for 172; blood test for 170–71; in Byzantine Empire 173–74, 179; challenge to Christians 174; diagnostic signs of 168, 170–71 (*see also* lepers); "epidemic" of 177; humoral imbalance in 170; involvement of lay organizations in 177–78; meaning of *lepra* 173; medical examinations for 169–172 (*see also* Thielen, Grette S); medical opinions on 169, 171–172, 175–76; Old Testament references to 173; physical manifestations of 170; redemptive value of 174–75; role of Crusaders in 177; stages of social response to 176–78; types of disease 173–74

Lister, Joseph: 12, 373–78; admission of patients 365–66 (*see also* Edinburgh Infirmary (19th c.); his antiseptic system 373–77, 380, 387; and carbolic acid sprays and dressings 374–77, 380; appointment in Edinburgh 363–64, 373; new chair at King's College, London 364, 383–85; and Glasgow Royal Infirmary 373; critique of his antiseptic method 375, 377–78; early career of 363–64; employment of zinc chloride by 384; lectures on surgery 376; teaching cases of 380–81 (see also Mathewson, Margaret); use of silver probe 365; ward rounds of 377, 380, 383

Madison, Wisconsin: 12, 475–482; as natural hospital center 477; automobile accidents (see accidents, automobile); city-affiliated hospital (see Madison General Hospital Madison, Wisconsin); Dane County welfare payments 501; early 20th century development of 476–77; hospitals' occupancy rates in 464; influx of transients during the Depression 501; lack of road signs 488; Lorillard Co. tobacco warehouse in 463, 502; population in 1930 488; seat of state government 476; summer tourism in 490; University of Wisconsin Hospital in, 464. See also Wisconsin

Madison General Hospital, Madison, Wisconsin (20th c.): 12, 475–82; accidents and institutional mortality 464; accreditation 481; admission of injury cases 464 (see also trauma); bill collections 484, 500, 502; board of directors 475–76, 478, 481, 487; building additions 477, 479, 481; daily charges 483–84, 496; diagnostic department 466, 481, 500 (see also technology, medical); early history of 475–77; Emergency Room 463–64; financing of charity cases 478; and flu epidemic 477; hospital life in 492–99 (see also S., Paula); importance of paying patients 476–78, 482, 484, 499–500; internships at 465, 481; length of stay at 500; medical staff of 479 (see also Tormey, Thomas W.); municipal partnership 475–77; new admission rules 501–02; nursing at 480–81, 494–95; occupancy rates 464, 482, 500; operating deficits 502; patronage of Jackson, Reginald 477, 479; Social Services Department of 482, 484, 496–97, 501–02; training school for nurses 480 (see also Crafts, Grace T.)

Massachusetts General Hospital, Boston (19th c.): 12, 339, 344, 344–349; admission of patients 339, 347–49; affiliation with Harvard Medical College 346; amputation statistics 344; and Bigelow, Henry J. 343–44; board of trustees 340, 345, 348, 360; cases in the Boston Med. & Surgical Journal 347; chief of medicine (see Jackson, James Sr.); chief of surgery (see Warren, John C.); "deserving" charity patients 340, 348; epidemic of erysipelas 341; expansion of original building 343, 348; and Hayward, George 354–57; hospital life in 339–344, 352–57; influx of servants 340, 345; and the Massachusetts Legislature 345–46; Morton and ether or "letheon" (see anesthesia; Morton, William); nursing staff at 341, 343 (see also nursing, U.S.); origins 344–46; paying patients 340, 349; religious issues 347; reputation of 361; support from the Massachusetts Hospital Life Insurance Company 345; surgery under anesthesia 354–57 (see also Mohan, Alice); teaching and research 346–47; therapeutic conservatism at 342–44, 347

Mathewson, Margaret: 12, 361–66, 379–85; account of hospital experiences (see patients, narratives); admission to the Edinburgh Infirmary (19th c.) 365–66; diagnosis of tubercular joint disease 381–82 (see also joint disease); under the care of Joseph Lister 379–8

medicine, Ancient Greece: Hippocratic craftsmen or "Asclepiads" 18, 27–31, 34, 44; Hippocrates of Cos 27; issue of professional competence 17; rise of secular healing 29; role of the iatreia in 28, 44; theories of (see humoralism); therapeutics 31–32, 34–36. See also Aristides; Asclepius, cult of

medicine, Byzantium: Aetius of Amida's Sixteen Books on Medicine 121; basis in humoral theories 76–77, 132–34, (see also humoralism); education of physicians 77, 121; iatros 76–77; loss of social standing 122; Origen on physicians 77; physicians as Christians 77; physicians' income 122; professional fragmentation

124–25; prominence of medical profession 51, 76–77; Oribasius' medical encyclopedia 121; Paul of Aegina's *Epitome of Medicine* 121; secular healing and Christian care 122; surgery and cauterization 85–86. See also *xenodocheion*; Pantocrator Xenon, Constantinople

medicine, France (18th–19th c.): anatomical-clinical synthesis 312–13, 317, 331; creation of *écoles de santé* 306, 311; diagnosis and professional status 314–16; empirical approaches to knowledge 309; hospitals as professional workshops (*see* hospitals, Paris; Necker Hospital, Paris); importance of semeiotics 314; influence of Dupuytren, Guillaume 313; organ pathology 312 (*see also* Bichat, Marie-François X.); plan to reform medical education 302–03, 306; program of clinical instruction 325–29; quest for medical certainty 315; rejection of medical systems 309; role of "ideologues" 309, (*see also* Cabanis, Pierre J.G.; and Pinel, Philippe); Royal Society of Medicine 299; skepticism about causality 309; shortage of physicians 326; Society for Medical Instruction 327 (*see also* Corvisart, Jean N.); traditional cauterization and blistering 321; therapeutic skepticism 321; union of medicine and surgery 311–12

medicine, Germany, (19th c.): and Osler, William 433; Berlin conferences on epidemic disease 446; cradle of scientific medicine 433; ideology of 433–34, 436; limitations of scientific medicine 448; Munich Medical Society meeting 447; state support for 433–34; Union of German Medical Associations 436; University of Marburg 423; University of Munich 434; unregulated medical marketplace 436. See also Hueppe, Ferdinand; Klebs, Edwin K.; Koch, Robert; Pettenkoffer, Max von; Rumpf, Theodor M.

medicine, Great Britain, (18th–19th c.): Cullen's medical system (*see* Cullen, William); diffusion of Brunonianism to the Continent (*see* Brown, John); links to Leyden University (*see* Boerhaave, Hermann); Lister's antiseptic system (*see* Lister, Joseph); reputation of the Edinburgh Medical School 362 (*see also* Edinburgh University)

medicine, Roman Empire: *medici* in 17, 50–53, 56; pain treatment 55; practical orientation of 54; shelter for sick slaves and soldiers (*see valetudinarium*, civil and *valetudinarium*, military); stomach disorders, therapeutics in 54; surgery in 54–55; theory of health and disease (*see* humoralism); water cures 15, 20, 22, 54; wound management in 18, 52–55. See also Celsus; Galen

medicine, U.S. (19th–20th c.): academic (*see* academic medical centers, U.S.); devoted to AIDS (*see* medicine, U.S. (20th c.), AIDS); hospitals (*see* hospitals, U.S. (19th–20th c.)); physicians (see physicians, U.S.); *See also* Johns Hopkins Hospital, Baltimore; Massachusetts General Hospital, Boston; Madison General Hospital, Madison, Wisconsin; Mercy Hospital, Buffalo NY; Moffitt Hospital, San Francisco; San Francisco General Hospital, San Francisco

medicine, U.S. (20th c.), AIDS: amphotericin B therapy for 643–44, 649, 656 (*see also* San Francisco General Hospital Ward 5 B); art in 635, 661; brain biopsies and bronchoscopies 649; cost of care 661; critique of biomedicine 644; diagnostic efforts 622, 627–29, 640, 645, 649, 653, 658, 660, 663; limits of 659; physicians' fear of infection 632, 636, 643; San Francisco's model of care 13, 634, 658, 660–63; shift from hospitals 661; sulfa drugs in 643–44; treatment of 640, 649; use of pentamidine 643, 656. See also Abrams, Donald; Conant, Marcus; Volberding, Paul; Wofsy, Constance

medicine, Vienna: at the Allgemeines Krankenhaus (*see* Allgemeines Krankenhaus, Vienna; botanical research 275; clinical drug trials 275; reforms by Swieten, Gerard van 273; training at Bürgerspital 273–74; teaching at the Unierte Spital 274–75. See also Auenbrugger,

Leopold; Boerhaave, Hermann; Frank, Johann P.; Quarin, Joseph; Stoll, Maximilian; Stifft, Joseph

Melaten leper house, Cologne (15th c.): admission requirements 168–69, 172, 185; commission of prebendaries 169; destruction of buildings 185; and its tavern 184; life in 184–90; location outside city walls 181–82; municipal control over 183–84; papal protection for 182; patient census of 185; role of *Probemeister* in 168–69, 184–85

Melzer, Juliet S.: 596; opposition to the sale of organs 572; surgical operation on Faith T. 600; training in immunology 596; transplantation surgeon at UCSF 596

Mercy Hospital, Buffalo, NY (20th c.): 12, 513, 517–21, 535–40, 546–57; accreditation 518; adjacent nurses' home 518; affiliation with Georgetown University 521, 538–39 (*see also* O'Brien, John J.); Aid Society of 519; autopsy rate at 516; Cardiac Care Unit 533–34 (*see* Mercy Hospital Cardiac Care Unit); chief of medical staff 515–16; daily religious routines 528–30, 550; Electrocardiography Department 529; Emergency Room 513–14, 531–32, 534–35, 554–55; expansion of 520–21; food service at 537–38; fundraising campaign for 520; home-like atmosphere of 528; hospital life in 525–31, 546–53; house staff 527, 550–51; increase in admissions 535; Krupa, Francis, chaplain 528, 549, 554; McAuley Building 536–40, 554–55; Medicare and Medicaid at 535–36; mobile life-support unit 533, 555; nurses' shifts 524; pastoral program 554; reputation for cardiac care 515; residency in general medicine 515–16; staff privileges at 516; SUNY Buffalo affiliation 539; surgical practice 516; symbol of Catholic identity 519; Tissue Committee of 516; training school for nurses 519, 524; union activity at 555–56. *See also* Sisters of Mercy

Mercy Hospital, Cardiac Care Unit (CCU): 533–34; atmosphere in 546–47; configu-

ration and equipment 547; construction 533–34; early history 534; national antecedents 534; nursing staff 547–48; patient experiences of 534; transition to medical ward 551–52. *See also* Gottstine, Mary Ann.

Moffitt Hospital, San Francisco (20th c.):12, 576, 582–87; comparison with European hospitals 610; hospital life in 599–606; housing of research units 585; loss of patients from Medi-Cal 580–81; modernization of 586–87, 610; nursing model at 602; patients' impressions of wards in 582, 586; planning and opening of 584; transplantation surgery at (*see* UCSF Transplantation Service); as university hospital (*see* University of California, San Francisco)

Mohan, Alice: 339–44, 354–57, 360, 381

monasteries: 91–106; Benedictine rules 91–94; bloodletting in 98, 103–04, 131; breakdown of manorial system at 108; Cistercianism and its effects 107–08; Cluniac reforms 90; eclipse of intellectual leadership 108; economic power of 90–91, 93–94; hospitality and healing in 91, 94–97, 102–05; imperial control over 90–91; involvement with surrounding world 97, 108; location near streams 97; monasticism and hermitism 106–07; Monte Cassino 108–09; new form of social organization 92; overwhelmed by the needy 107; Pachomius's rules for 92, 96; preparation for death at 104; recovery of classical medical knowledge at 96; role of the *infirmarius* 100–01 (*see also* Notker II); St. Anthony's monastic ideals 91–92; St. Augustine's influence on 92; Second Lateran Council's effects on 108; sites of medical learning 5–96. *See also* St. Gall monastery

Morrison, Clifford: and dying 652–53; planning San Francisco General Ward 5B 637–39, 650; patient/nurse relationship 646; and reform of health care 662. *See also* San Francisco General Hospital Ward 5 B

Morton, William: attempt to patent ether anesthesia 358–59; dental practice of

357–58; experimentation with ether 352–53; use of "letheon" in amputation 354–55. *See also* Massachusetts General Hospital, Boston, (19th c.))

Necker Hospital, Paris (also Hôpital Necker and Hospice de Charité) (18th–19th c.): 290–93, 296–99; Academy of Sciences' Commission report on 296–97 (*see also* Tenon, Jacques R.); admission policies 290–93, 317; caregiving personnel 292; Committee on Mendicity reports on 301–02; costs of hospitalization at 292, 302; daily medical rounds 318; dietetics at 319; hospital routines 318; institutional mortality at 297; life in 317–23; "phthisis" (tuberculosis) at 318–19 (*see also* Dumesnil, Jacques); medical segregation of patients 291, 317–18; model institution 296–97; nursing at 322; postmortem dissection at 324; resident physician (*see also* Laennec, René T.); Sisters of Charity at 292, 296, 322 (*see also* Sisters of Charity); sponsorship of Necker, Suzanne C. 291, 296

New York State: Erie County's general practitioners 515; Erie County's incidence of heart attacks 532; malpractice crisis in 566; Mercy Health System of Western New York 566. *See also* Mercy Hospital, Buffalo, NY

Nightingale, Florence: 18, 366, 369–370; and Deaconess Institute, Kaiserswerth 369; and Edinburgh (see nursing, Edinburgh Infirmary); and Johns Hopkins Hospital 403, 411; and Sisters of Charity 369; and Training School in London 369–70

nosokomeion (nosocomium): 16; at Antioch 82–83; overlap of functions with Byzantine *xenodocheion* 82–83. *See also xenodocheion*

Notker II: care of Abbot Purchard I 99–101; court physician 100–01; function as *infirmarius* 91, 97; reputation as diagnostician 99–100; selection as abbot of St. Gall 105–06; as skilled uroscopist 102. *See also* St. Gall Monastery

nursing: and AIDS (*see* nursing, U.S. (20th

c.), AIDS); at the *Allgemeines Krankenhaus* in Vienna 263–64; Anglican Sisterhood of St. John's House 369; art of 495, 646–47 (*see also* caregivers); in early Christianity (*see* nursing, early Christian); at the Edinburgh Infirmary (*see* nursing, Edinburgh Infirmary); at the Eppendorf General Hospital 437–39, 447; home-like residences for 475; and issue of vocation 495; in medieval Byzantine Empire 129–30; and Florence Nightingale (*see* Nightingale, Florence); "paper nurses" 495; practical nursing in 20th century Europe 475; as "physician's hand" 495; Red Cross nurses 438; and relationships with patients 19; by religious personnel (*see* Deaconess Sisters, Sisters of Charity, Sisters of Mercy); at St. Thomas Hospital, London 369–70; staff at Massachusetts General Hospital 341, 343; in the United States (*see* nursing, U.S. (19th–20th c.))

nursing, early Christian: 71; opposition to secular medicine 78; power of faith 78; role of the *philoponoi* and *spoudaioi* 81; and religious conversion 80; and social welfare 71–73; supernatural cures 96–97; use of deacon system in 81; volunteers 83; *See also* healing, early Christian; medicine, Byzantium

nursing, Edinburgh Infirmary (19th c.): 369–73; Bell report on 369; and financial issues 372; influence of the Nightingales on 369–70, 373; Lister's relations with nurses 372; nurses' relationship with medical and surgical staffs 372–73; pre-Nightingale conditions 368–69; routines 379–80

nursing, U.S. (19th–20th c.): and AIDS (*see* nursing, U.S. (20th c.), AIDS); Bellevue Hospital Training School 411; cardiac care 547–48; clinical nurse specialist 548, 601; Catholic nurses 519, 523–24, 526, 529 (*see also* Sisters of Mercy); contemporary "reengineering" 681–82; expansion of training schools 411–12; Johns Hopkins Training School 411–13; at Massachusetts General Hospital 341–43; "mechanical" nurses 474; political power at SFGH 638; pre-World War I 474; "primary" care nurses 548; quest towards professional autonomy 538; role playing with physicians 601; team work in 638–39, 682; at UCSF's Moffitt Hospital 602

nursing, U.S. (20th c.), AIDS: and "burnout" 654; importance of empathy in 648; laying on of hands 647–48; "outing" of caregivers 647; patient advocacy and education 648–49; relationships with patients 649–50; religious motivations for 648; secular philosophy of 648; volunteers for Ward 5 B 638. See also Jones, Diane; Morrisson, Clifford

O'Brien, John J.: affiliation with Georgetown University 521; caring for patients (see O'H., Joseph); diagnosis of myocardial infarction 525– 27; interpretation of EKGs 529; director of medical education 521; and Mercy Hospital's cardiac care unit 534; and nuclear medicine 539; as spokesman for house staff 521, 526–27, 539; as staff internist 517

O'H., Joseph: 513–17, 525–31

organization, hospital: 6; Augustinian rules for 92, 152; at Benedictine infirmaries 92–94; Basil's Long Rules 77; charter for Hospital of St. John of Jerusalem 141; institutional routines 93, 127, 146–48; Hospitallers' model of 141, 144–45, 151–53; at Johns Hopkins Hospital 406–07; in lazarettos 205–06; at Madison General Hospital 501–02; order in leper houses 185–87; Pantocrator Xenon's typikon 120; regulations and statutes 92–94, 96, 145; rules and social control 234; separation of the sexes 155

Origen: justification for use of medicines 77; and lay physicians 78, 86; views of human body 74–75

Osler, William: appointment at Johns Hopkins Hospital 407; daily rounds of 409–10, 414; background of 408–09; on Hippocrates and the art of medicine 421; hospital routine of 409; and management of typhoid fever 415–20; and medical clinic model 409–10; selection of resident medical staff 409; on nurses and student nurses 412–13; textbook project 411; his therapeutic skepticism 415–16; typhoid fever metaphor 420; views on hospitals 421. See also Johns Hopkins Hospital, Baltimore

P., Nancy: 569–76, 599–607 See also UCSF Transplantation Service

pain: control in dentistry 350–51 (see also Morton, William); efforts at local suppression 350; linkage to nervous system 350; moral meaning of 350; and nitrous oxide 350, 352; in surgical operations 344, 352 (see also anesthesia); traditional views of 349–50; use of opiates in 341, 343, 350, 356

Pantocrator Xenon, Constantinople: 11, 128–30; administrative staff 129; admission of patients 130–31; ambulatory facility 129; charter or typikon of 120; description of 128; diet in 131; facilities for lepers 128; foundation by emperor John II Comnenus 120, 128; infirmary for sick monks 120, 128; inmate population 130; instruction of students 130; life in 130–34 (see also Prodromos, Theodoros); medical practices in 131; medical staff of 129–30; monastery complex 120, 128; nursing assistants 129–30; separate wards 128–29

Paris, France: Ancien Régime charity 293–94; demographics during the Restoration 290; hospitals in (see hospitals, Paris); parish of St. Sulpice and du Gros Caillou 290; population before the Revolution 293; social control and confinement in 293

pathology: and anatomical-clinical synthesis 312–13, 317, 331; and Bichat, Marie F. X. 312; and Frank, Johann P. 277–78; and Haen, Anton de 277; and Laennec, Rene T. 313–14, 316–17; museums of 310; and Welch, William H. 406

patient/physician relationship: attire 9–13; challenges to medical authority 643–45; communication and truthtelling 465, 497; emotions surrounding illness 9–11; Galen and 37; and education of patients

633, 643–44; medical paternalism 465; with nephrologists 603, 607 (see also Amend, William J.); new partnership 644, 680–81; patient passivity 465; replacement of traditional dyad 635; with transplant surgeons 603; voice of patients 9–10 (see also patients, narratives)

patients, AIDS: 639–46, 652–58; AIDS obituaries in the Bay Area Reporter 620; conflicting medical opinions and 644; death and dying of 622–23, 652–55; decision-making power of 644–45; drama about 623 (see also J., Warren); early optimism for a cure 639; education of 640, 643; erosion of self-esteem 645; experimentation with alternative medicines 645, 656; greater autonomy of 643–44; knowledge of diagnosis and treatment 643–44; lack of family support 646; new spirituality of 644; resentment and depression of 645; use of recreational drugs by 628–29

patients, cases (in chronological order): 11–13; Claudius Terentianus (2nd c. AD Alexandria) 38–41, 52–56; Aelius Aristides (2nd c. AD Pergamon) 15–20, 33–38; Purchard I (10th c. St. Gall) 87–91, 99–106; Theodoros Prodromos (12th c. Constantinople) 117–20, 130–34; Adolf of Cologne (12th c. Jerusalem) 134–38, 143–48; Grette S. Thielen (15th c. Cologne) 168–72, 184–90; Marina de Rossi, Catharina d'Uliva, Cecilia di Giovanni, and Clementina (17th c. Rome) 190, 195, 212–13; Janet Williamson (18th c. Edinburgh) 231–36, 243–51; Johann Duschau (18th c. Vienna) 257–58, 268–73; Jacques Dumesnil (19th c. Paris) 289–93, 317–25; Alice Mohan (19th c. Boston) 339–44, 354–57, 360; Margaret Mathewson 19th c. Edinburgh) 361–66, 379–85; John S. (19th c. Baltimore) 399–40, 413–20; Erika W. (19th c. Hamburg) 422–23, 439–45; Paula S. (20th c. Madison, Wisconsin) 463–67, 492–99, 504; Joseph O'H. (20th c. Buffalo, New York) 513–17, 525–31; Albert F. (20th c. Buffalo, New York) 531–35, 546–53; Faith T., Nancy P., and

Patty B. (20th c. San Francisco) 569–76, 599–607; Warren J. (20th c. San Francisco) 619–23, 640–46, 649–58

patients, narratives: 9–13; account of Joshua the Stylite 11, 69–70, 72, 84, 86; Aristides, Aelius 11, 15–20, 33–38; as ethnography 9; importance in cult of Asclepius 27; hospitalization as journey or pilgrimage 9; importance in historical discourse 9; interviews with B., Patty, P., Nancy, T., Faith 569–76, 599–607; letters of Terentianus, Claudius 11, 38–41, 52–56; model of Crichton, Michael 10; poems and letters of Prodromos, Theodoros 11, 117–20, 132–34; storytelling as healing 9; works of Frank, Arthur W. and Sacks, Oliver 10; written account of Mathewson, Margaret 361–66, 379–85

patronage, hospital: 6; and appointment of administrators 161; board of trustees in U.S. hospitals 340, 345, 475–76, 478, 487; in Byzantium 122–23; Church sponsorship 80–82, 150–51; city control of leper houses 183–84; importance of voluntarism 74; Joseph II's and the Allgemeines Krankenhaus, Vienna 261–62; jurisdictional disputes about 151; Knights of St. Lazarus 179; at Madison General Hospital 477, 479; municipal partnership in U.S. hospitals 475–77; Necker Hospital and Parisian aristocracy 291, 296; patients' prayers for benefactors 151; physicians as patrons 76–77; role of hospital orders (see Hospitallers); royal sponsorship 81, 149–50; subscribers to British infirmaries 237–39; support from European confraternities and municipalities 149–50; 13th century shift to lay patrons 149–51

Pettenkoffer, Max von: autoexperiment with cholera bacilli 446–47; and his environmentalist Bodentheorie 434, opponent of Robert Koch 434

physicians: at the Allgemeines Krankenhaus, Vienna 263, 267–68; in Ancient Greece 27–28; in Antonine Rome (see medicine, Roman Empire); charlatans among 17; drawn into hospital service 154; during plague epidemics 206–07; in France (*see* medicine, France); hazards of caregiving in Vienna 275; high honoraria in Byzantium 122; presence in Milan 154; lay *medici* 95; relationships with patients (*see* patient/physician relationship); shortage of in 13th century 153; surgeons' inferior status 153; in the U.S. (*see* physicians, U.S.)

physicians, U.S.: admission to hospital staffs 472; fear of "treadmill practice" 467; free care for the indigent 486; image and status of radiologists 466; income of 485–86; patronage of hospitals 472; polypharmacy in therapy 467; public relations during the Depression 486; specialization in the 1960s (*see* academic medical centers, U.S.); tensions between general practitioners and specialists 515–16

pilgrims: Adolph of Cologne 134–36; after the First Crusade 140–41; bathing in Jordan River 135; collection of Holy Land soil 139; Felix Farber 136; John of Würzburg 137–38; journeys of atonement 134–35; land route through Byzantium 139; landing at Acre 136; payment of tolls 139; protection by Templars and Hospitallers 136; role of Amalfian merchants 140; sea voyage 135–36; Theoderic von Würzburg 134–36

Pinel, Philippe: chief at the Salpêtrière 311; essay on clinical education 326; foe of polypharmacy 321; importance of diet 319; medical "ideologue" 309; nosology of 315; patients as teachers 325–26; psychological aspects of illness 328–29. *See also* medicine, France

plague: in Alexandria 80; in ancient Athens 21, 26; Antonine plague 70; *buboes* and other symptoms 194; celestial and terrestrial causes of 196; concepts of miasma and contagion in 197; Black Death in Europe 178, 191; domestic prevention of 195 (*see also* bloodletting; antidotes); flight from affected areas 192, 197; and humoralism 197–98, 211; of Justinian 191; in Marseilles 213; and the modern state 198–99; in Naples 190–91; periodic

visitations in Europe and Italian city-states 190–91, 201; religious views of 195–96; in Rome (*see* plague, Rome); in San Francisco 624, 630; treatment of 195, 211–12

plague, Rome (17th c.): convalescent care for 213; mortality among urban poor 191, 193; public health measures (*see* public health, Rome); reporting delays 191–92; status of "plague" doctors 206–07; terrorized population 194; transmission of 191; in Trastevere 190–95

Prodromos, Theodoros: 11, 117–20, 130–34; admission to hospital 119–20 (*see also* Pantocrator Xenon, Constantinople); chest complaints 132; at court 117; disfiguration of face 134; explanations of disease 131–32; friendship with Stephanos Skylitzes 117; and medical consultation 118; narrative of his illness 117–20, 132–34; note to Alexius Aristenos 118; possible case of smallpox 119; retirement 134; subjected to cauterizations 132–34; treatment of skin condition 132

public health: and AIDS 630–31, 640. 657; in Baltimore 400; deficiencies in Hamburg 435, 446–47; German imperial legislation on 446–47; plague measures in Italy and northern Europe 198–202; in San Francisco 622, 640, 657

public health, Rome (17th c.): 195–202; cancellation of religious ceremonies 196; cleansing procedures or *purga* 199; closure of city 199; concealment of cases 200–01; confinement in lazarettos 195 (*see also* lazarettos, Rome); disposal of clothing and bedding 206; fumigation of houses 193; Health Congregation activities 192–95; home visits by physicians 192, 194; inspection of city gates and closed houses 194; intelligence about plague 201; Papal aid 194; prompt burial of victims 198, 201; quarantine of Trastevere 193; segregation in homes 200–01; traffic of goods and persons 199; urban health boards 198–99, 201–02; violation of quarantine laws 194, 200

Purchard I: 87–91, 99–106; as abbot 90–91, 105–06; chapel construction of 105–06; and Hadwig, duchess of Swabia 87–88; injury of 101, 105; and Notker II 91; physical frailty of 89–90; riding accident of 88, 91

Quarin, Joseph: appointment of hospital staff 263–64; personal physician to Joseph II 262; plan for Vienna's almshouse 262; rationing of hospital supplies 264; resignation as hospital director 265;

religion: 73; Anglican theology 237; Calvinist beliefs 237–39; ceremonies during plague 196; Christian Byzantium 70–71, 73–79 (see also Christianity, early; healing, early Christian); Christ at Hopkins 422; Christian welfare 79–83; in daily Greek life 24; Egyptian healing cults in the Roman Empire 15–17 (see also healing, pagan); hospital as locus religiosus 106–07, 156; ministry in AIDS 655; partnership with science 422; pastoral care at Mercy Hospital 528, 549, 554; power of prayer and meditation 28–29, 528–29; religious services in U.S. Catholic hospitals 528–29, 531, 550; repression in post-Revolutionary France 303–04; in Roman health care 50, 56; role in ancient Greek life 24–25; specialized hospital chaplaincy 683–84; pestilence as punishment 195–96; prayers at the Asclepieion 28–29

research, hospital: on AIDS 633, 635, 640, 543; botanical 275; at Edinburgh Infirmary (18th c.) 254–55; drug trials in 18th century Vienna 271–73; experimental treatments at Eppendorf General Hospital 441–43; in French hospitals 327–28, 331; human experiments with ether anesthesia 357; at Moffitt Hospital 585; organ preservation studies 594–95, 598; patients as experimental subjects 578 (see also academic medical centers, U.S.,); at SFGH 626; systematic dissections at the Hôtel Dieu, Paris 310, 312

Roman Empire: agriculture in 42–47, 53; under Antoninus Pius 17–18; communi-
cations network of 43–44; distribution of grain in 45–46; Eastern provinces of 38–39; emperors as healing divinities 57; frontiers of 38–44; infectious diseases in 53; paterfamilias as caregivers 48; population of 42, 45–46; protection of commercial trade routes 39; religious pluralism of 57; role of religion in health care 50, 56; slavery in 46–48, 53; social welfare in 45–47; under Tiberius 43; under Trajan 38–41, 43–44; views of illness in 56–57. See also Aristides, Aelius; Roman Empire, army; Terentianus, Claudius

Roman Empire, army: 38, 41–44; burden of disease in 53; composition of 42, 52; capsarii in 50, 52; conditions in 42–43; defense of imperial borders 41–42; development under Augustus 41–42; diet in 54; Greek physicians in 51; health in 52–53; infectious disease in 39, 52–53; medical corps in 50–53; medical treatments in 42, 47–52; network of fortresses in 43–44; on northern frontier 40, 43–44; pay of 40, 42; physical fitness 52; professionalization of 39; provisioning of 43; public opinion of 39; reorganization under Trajan 40–41; Republican forces 41–42; social level of recruits 40. See also Terentianus, Claudius

Rome, Italy, (17th c.): capital of Catholicism 201; Caracalla Baths ruins 206; construction of St. Peter's basilica 192; gardens at Ripa 209; governance by congregations 192; island of San Bartolomeo 195; Jewish ghetto 193; Ospedale di Santo Spirito 149, 208, 218; Ospedale Santa Maria della Consolazione 192; outbreak of plague in (see plague, Rome); population 192; rule of Pope Alexander VII 192; San Salvatore della Corte tenement 190; suburban Trastevere 190–95; visits by pilgrims 192

Rossi, Marina de: 190, 195, 212–13; admission to Rome's Lazzaretto San Bartolomeo 209; diagnosis of bubonic plague 190, 195; under the care of plague doctors 212–13

Royal Infirmary of Edinburgh: see Edinburgh Infirmary (18th c.) and (19th c.)

Rumpf, Theodor M.: awarding health certificates 446; diagnosis of cholera 424; hospital director 423 (*see also* Eppendorf General Hospital, Hamburg); meeting with Robert Koch 435; opposition to new drugs 442, 444; supporter of bacteriology 424; and traditional therapy 448; use of saline infusions 443; work with volunteer physicians 427 (*see also* medicine, Germany)

S., John: 399–402, 413–20

S., Paula: 463–67, 492–99, 504

St. Augustine: rules for monastic life 92, 152; Christ as healer 79

St. Basil of Caesarea: appeals to the wealthy 76, 84; background of 76, 83; blueprints for an urban community 76; ecclesiastical and political leadership 76; foundation of the *Basileiados* shelter 84; and his brother St. Gregory of Nyssa (*see* St. Gregory of Nyssa); and his *Long Rules* 77; importance of cenobitic life 76; journey of life 87; medical knowledge of 83; social welfare 79; and St. Gregory of Nazianzen (*see* St. Gregory of Nazianzen); supporter of lay medicine 83

St. Benedict of Nursia: care of the sick 96; and daily routines 93; linkage to Johns Hopkins Hospital 422; original rule 92–94; responsibility of abbots 93

St. Cosmas and St. Damian: cult at monastic infirmaries 123; patron saints of medicine 79; shrines in Edessa 72

St. Gall, monastic infirmary: architectural plans for 98; bloodletting in 103–04; life in 99–106; need for herbarium 98; proximity to bloodletting house 98. *See also* Notker II

St. Gall, monastic shelter: architectural plans for 99; designation of *hospitale pauperum* 98–99

St. Gall monastery: Abbot Iso and lepers 100; appointment of abbots 90–91; architectural plan of 97–99; destination for pilgrims 89, 102; destruction of 89; and European monasteries 88 (*see also* monasteries); feudal politics 90; golden century of 89; *infirmarius* Notker I (*see* Notker II); institutional discipline 90;

and monastery of Reichenau 87–89; origins of 88–89; Otmar's foundation 100; Otto the Great 90–91; *portarius* Ekkehard 87; relics of St. Gallus 88, 102; reputation for medical learning 100; rule of abbot Purchard I (*see also* Purchard I); *scriptorium* of 88, 95–96; sponsorship of schools 89

St. Gregory of Nazianzen: and cauterization 86; critique of surgeons 86; description of Basil's shelter 84; friend of Basil of Caesarea 77; on medical practice 77

St. Gregory of Nyssa: brother of Basil of Caesarea 77; pagan shrines and epidemics 78–79; on prevalence of disease 78; support for secular medicine 78

St. Matthew: 5, 69, 74, 91, 109

Salvatierra, Oscar: 573, 593, 598; champion of veteran's health issues 598; director of the service 595; and 1984 National Organ Transplantation Act 599; partnership with nephrologists 595; political activist 598; president of the American Society of Transplant Surgeons 598; publications of 594–95; recruitment of surgeon Melzer, Juliet S. 596; use of donor-specific blood transfusions 596

San Francisco, California: bathhouses and sex clubs 621, 640, 645; *Bay Area Reporter* 620; bubonic plague and quarantine 624, 630; California Pacific Medical Center 679; Castro district in 621; gay community and organizations 621, 640; gay lifestyle and disease 629; gay sexual liberation and identity 621–22, 640–41; Haight-Ashbury Free Clinic 622, 640; Harvey Milk Club 640; hospice movement 662; incidence of sexually transmitted diseases 621–22; influx of gay population 621; public health officials 622, 640, 657; relations with UCSF 582–83 (*see also* University of California, San Francisco); and Toland Medical College 583; "Valley of the Kings" in 621. *See also* California, health care in

San Francisco General Hospital (SFGH): 12, 623–27, 633–39; affiliation with UCSF and Stanford 624–25; bubonic plague in 624; change in mission 625; charity patients 626; competition for patients with UCSF 634; decline in the 1950s 624; fear of AIDS patients 636–37; Infection Control Task Force and Merle Sande 632; inpatient Ward 5 B 622 (*see also* San Francisco General Hospital Ward 5 B); Medi-Cal patients in 626, 642–43; menace to the community 623–24; move to Potrero Hill 624; new Medical Center 625; 1915 hospital complex 624; origin of 623; out-patient ward 86 632–33 (*see also* San Francisco General Hospital Ward 86); political power of nurses 638; support from UCSF 626; threat of Medicare 625; and Toland Medical College 623; Trauma Center at 625. *See also* Abrams, Donald; Morrisson, Clifford; Volberding, Paul; Wofsy, Constance

San Francisco General Hospital, Ward 5 B: 12; call for volunteer nurses 628; caregiving teams 638–39; death and dying in 652–58; design and planning 637–39; donations to 650; early popularity 639; entertainment in 650–51; first Christmas at 651; focus on nursing 638; isolation techniques 650; length of stay 659; medical care from house staff 643; mortality statistics 642; presence of Shanti counselors 637–38, 652, 654–55, 663–64; opposition from gay community 637; religious conversion of dying patients 655; room arrangements 639; use of refrigeration blankets 650; visitors to 650–51

San Francisco General Hospital, Ward 86: clinical psychologists at 636; opportunistic infections 632; efforts at refurbishing 633; opening of 633; linkages to UCSF 635; Shanti Project volunteers 636; transfers from Moffitt Hospital 634–35

Scotland (18th c.): Church of Scotland 232, 239; and the Enlightenment 236–38; Edinburgh (*see* Edinburgh, Scotland); Glasgow Royal Infirmary 374; old Poor-Law 233; union with England 239. *See also* Edinburgh Infirmary (18th c.) and (19th c.)

Sisters of Charity: during the Ancien Régime 292, 296; in Baltimore 403; disbanded after the French Revolution 305; and

Florence Nightingale 369; at the Hôpital Necker, Paris 292, 322; oath of loyalty to the Revolution 305; 17th century origins 292; volunteers at Eppendorf General Hospital 426

Sisters of Mercy: apostolic mission 554, 556–57; authority of 516; collective decision-making 556; Collins, Sister M. Victorine 516; control of Mercy Hospital 524, 554; corporate development of 554, 556; early activities in Buffalo 518; effect of Vatican II on 541; establishment of convent and academy 518–19; first hospital on Tifft St. 519; Kelleher, Sister M. Annunciata (*see* Kelleher, Sister M. Annunciata); Kreuzer, Sister M. Sacred Heart 537; origins in Ireland 518; sponsorship of Trocair College 537; and staff education 557; teaching in South Buffalo 513–14; training in nursing 557; Walsh, Sr. Sheila M. 554, 556; Welch, Sr. Elizabeth 541

smallpox: in Byzantium and the Middle East 119; clinical manifestations 119; epidemics in Edinburgh 234, 362; humoral explanations of 131; treatment of 131–32

Starzl, Thomas E.: drug "cocktail" against organ rejection 588, first president of the American Society of Transplant Surgeons 590; importance of organ transplantation 569; role of patients 611

Stifft, Joseph: conflict with Frank, Johann P. 271; opposition to Brunonianism 268; Vienna's city physician 268

Stoll, Maximilian: at Allgemeines Krankenhaus, Vienna 275–76; chief at Trinity Hospital 263, 274–75; supporter of humoralism 271;

surgery: amputation in tuberculous joint disease 343, 381; and asepsis 385–87; body casts in fracture cases 492–93, 498; Byzantine surgeons 85–86; elective in imperial Rome 54–55; first amputation under ether anesthesia 354–57, 363; hospital hygiene and septic complications of 366–67; image of transplant surgeons 603; Lister's antiseptic system in 373–77, 387, 389; management of tubercular joint disease 363, 381; mortality from amputations 344; patients' fear of 381; patients' postoperative experiences 383–85; sterilization facilities for 447; surgical training in Paris 325; techniques of kidney transplantation 592–93, use of chloroform in 363, 382, 384; in wards of the Allgemeines Krankenhaus, Vienna 267; wound healing techniques in antiquity 52, 54–55

T., Faith: 569–76, 599–607

technology, medical: 11; bedside computer terminals 681; clinical laboratories and X rays 466, 470, 481–82; coronary arteriography 548; and depersonalization 470; echocardiography 548; electrocardiography 470, 525–26, 529, 533–35; hospital as house of high technology 677; imaging 579, 677; nuclear medicine 539; oscilloscopes and telemetry 534, 547–48; profit from 466, 471–72; refrigeration blankets in AIDS 650; updating of 471

Tenon, Jacques R.: chair of the Committee on Public Assistance 303; hospitals as a measure of civilization 289; hospitals as "healing machines" 300; salubrity of hospitals 298, 366; 1786 report on the Hospice de Charité 298; tour of British hospitals 298

Terentianus, Claudius: 38–41, 52–56; application to join the army 39–40; illness of 38–41, 54–56; as legionary 40; naval career of 38–40; spirituality of 56; Tiberianus, father of 39–40, 56; transfer to military camp 40; wounded in a riot 41

Theoderic von Würzburg: *Description of the Holy Places* 134–35; vision of the Last Judgment 364; walk through the Hospital of St. John of Jerusalem 138

therapeutics, medical: in AIDS; alcohol treatments in Vienna 272; "anticholerin" in cholera 441; antipyretic drugs 418; balneotherapy 47 (*see also* water treatments); bloodlettting (*see* bloodletting); cathartics or purgatives (*see* cathartics); cauterization in Byzantium 85–86, 132–34; cold water baths for typhoid fever 416–19; conservatism at Massachusetts General Hospital 342–44; creation of

blisters 249; cupping 18, 20, 54–55; emetics 248; hospital dispensatories for 267; imitation of natural healing 19–20; immunosuppression in transplantation 573–74, 588, 593; intestinal antisepsis in cholera 442, 444; issue of polypharmacy 321; in myocardial infarction 517, 525–27, 548–52; need for antidotes or *theriacs* 19; opiates for pain 341, 343; Osler's skepticism 415–16; *panaceas* 19; saline infusions for cholera 443–45; treatment of poisonings and wounds 18, 54–55

Thielen, Grette S.: 168–72, 184–90; Diedenhofen burgher 168; examination for leprosy at Metz 165; second probe in Cologne 168–72; management in leper house 185–90

Tormey, Thomas W.: application of a plaster jacket 498; attending surgeon at Madison General Hospital 465, 497; paternalism of 465; supervision of house staff 465–66; and spine fractures 492–97

transplantation, kidney: 587–94; advantage of living donors 574–75; and American Society of Transplant Surgeons 590; Belmont Report 590; cadaver transplants and Belzer, Folkert O. 589; combination therapy of Imuran and prednisone 593; complications of immunosuppression in 593–94; costs of 572–73; coverage by Medicare for 573; criteria for 570–71; employment of antilymphoblast globulin (ALG) 589, 593; experimental beginnings in Boston 587–88; "gift of life" issue 574–75; hospital experience as "rebirth" 604; immunosuppressant drugs 588; Kidney Transplant Dialysis Association 587; need for randomized clinical trials 590; pioneers in the field 594; at the University of California, Los Angeles 594; post-operative complications 606; preliminary tissue matching 592; requirements for transplantation units 589; surgical techniques in 592; at the University of Minnesota 590; use of cyclosporin 574, 593; *See also* UCSF Transplantation Service

transplantation of organs: 569, 606–11; central role of patients in 611; criteria for

570; Golden State Transplant Services 574; influx of foreign patients 596; insulation from economical issues 609; issue of "brain death" 571, 608; lack of planning 609–10; life-long immunosuppression 588, 591, 593; moral and ethical questions in 572–73; National Organ Transplantation Act 599, 607–08 (see also Salvatierra, Oscar); organ donations for profit 572; problems of procurement 571–72; as profitable "product line" 580; routine surgical procedure 609 (see also Starzl, Thomas E.); United Network for Organ Sharing (UNOS) 571, 607–08

trauma: administration of opiates in 466; application of plaster straps 467; complaints of backpain 464; check of vital signs 467, 493; dangers of concussion 493; drop in blood pressure 466; employment of tetanus antitoxin in 466; fracture of pelvis 466, 493; hip dislocation and leg fracture 101; management of spine fractures 493; prospects of long-term disability 498–99; rib fractures 466; scalp laceration 465–66; skull fracture 466; use of body casts in 493, 499; vertebral compression fracture 466, 492–93. See also accidents, automobile; S., Paula

typhoid fever: in Baltimore 400; in Buffalo 518; causative bacillus 402; cold water baths in 416–19; death in 420 (see also S., John); home care of 401; importance of nursing in 415; incidence among immigrants 401; intestinal hemorrhaging in 419; mortality statistics at Johns Hopkins Hospital 420–21; physical manifestations of 413–20; pathological findings in 420; pneumonia as complication 418–19; outbreaks in Hamburg 435; relapsing type 414–15; separation from typho-malarial fever 410; symptoms of 400–01

UCSF Transplantation Service: 569, 594–99; average patient stay 606; caregiving teams at 603; children, elderly and diabetics as surgical candidates 596; clinical challenges of diabetics 600; during Salvatierra's tenure 596–97 (see also Salvatierra, Oscar); early postoperative period 600–01; educational drawbacks for house staff 597; educational materials for patients 605; financial impact on UCSF's Hospitals and Clinics 595–97; first 1,000 kidney transplants 596; and immunologist Garovay, Marvin R. 596; inadequate facilities at Moffitt Hospital 582, 597; initial transplant by Najarian, John 594; leadership of Belzer, Folkert 594–95; organ procurement for 598; patient advocacy and education 602, 606; postoperative laboratory data 605; pre-and post- operative nursing 602; pre-transplant workups 574; reduced hospitalization 608; relations between surgeons and patients 603; role in the Department of Surgery 595–96; and staff psychiatrist Lauer, Roger M. 600, 604–05; 2,000 kidney transplants in 1983 598; world leader in kidney transplantation 569–97; work of in-patient coordinators Hopper, Susan and Devney, Peggy 599. See also Amend, William J., and Melzer, Juliet S.

University of California, San Francisco (UCSF): 576–87; affiliation with SFGH 583, 624–25; AIDS patients at 634; campus opposition to expansion 586; effects of Medi-Cal legislation on 580–81; financial support of SFGH 626; Hospitals and Clinics complex 576; kidney transplantations at (see UCSF Transplantation Service); Long Range Development Plan 586; move to Parnassus site 583; opening of KS Clinic 631; relations with the city 582–83; separate university branch 583; as Toland Medical College 582–83, 623; university hospital 583 (see also Moffitt Hospital, San Francisco) See also Abrams, Donald; academic medical centers, U.S.; Amend, William J.; Conant, Marcus; Melzer, Juliet S.; Salvatierra, Oscar; Volberding, Paul; Wofsy, Constance

valetudinarium, civil: in Columella, De Re Rustica 47; expansion of domestic responsibilities 48; medical practices in 53; Roman slaves as healers 46; slaves in 47–48; social welfare role of 47–48

valetudinarium, military: 41, 44–52; administration of 50; building complex 48–50; capacity of 49; care of soldiers 52–56; disease prevention in 52; dressers (*capsarii*) in 50; emergency care in 48; extant ruins of 48–50; at fortresses 43–44, 48, 53; heating of 50; as hospital forerunner 56–58; humoral medicine in 53–55; hygienic criteria for 48–50, 52; medical instruments in 49; nursing 50, 53; Persian peristyle plan for 49; precursors to 41–42, 48; as product of imperial policy 44, 48; religious shrines in 50; social control in 49; staff arrangements at 50–52; surgery in 49–50, 54–55; ventilation in 49; water cure at 54; wound treatment at 52, 54–55

Vienna, Austria (18th c.): 17; Bäckenhäusel lazaretto in 261; Bürgerspital in 261; center of the Habsburg Empire 257–58; decentralization of poor relief 259; demand for charitable services 261; hospital reform 260–61; population of 257; registered physicians and surgeons 273 (*see also* medicine, Vienna); reign of Francis II 258; university reform 273–74; venereal disease and tuberculosis in 258. *See also* Allgemeines Krankenhaus, Vienna; Austrian Empire

Volberding, Paul: background in oncology 635; and cases of Kaposi sarcoma 627 (*see also* Kaposi sarcoma); director of SFGH Division of AIDS Activities 631; fear of contagion 636; immersion into AIDS care 662; importance of social care 636; in-patient ward at SFGH 637, 643 (*see also* San Francisco General Hospital Ward 5 B); and KS Clinic 631; outpatient clinic at SFGH 631–32; patient education 633; patient transfer to SFGH 634; personal involvement with AIDS 634; research grant from NCI 635; teaching house staff 632; treatment of KS and lymphoma patients 641; trials with interferon 633, 640, 643; work in SFGH's Ward 86 633–35 (*see also* San Francisco General Hospital Ward 86). *See also* acquired immunodeficiency syndrome; medicine, U.S. (20th c.) AIDS

W., Erika: 422–23, 439–45

Warren, John C.: donation of religious books 347; first operation under surgical anesthesia 352–54; leg amputations by 344 (*see also* Mohan, Alice); pamphlet on education 347; professor of surgery at Harvard 341; purchase of surgical equipment 348; role in hospital foundation 345; removal of tumor 359; visits to the hospital 341 (*see also* Massachusetts General Hospital, Boston)

water treatments: in Antonine Rome 15, 20, 22, 35, 54; for cholera 443–45; diagnostic bathing for lepers 172; in Edessa 72; in monasteries 97, 104; as religious symbol 35–36; role at the Asclepieion 22–24, 28, 34–35; in Roman Imperial army 54; for typhoid fever 416–19. *See also* therapeutics, medical

welfare: altruism in Ancient Greece 44; in Ancient Egypt and Israel 44–45, 73–74; in Byzantium 81; care of strangers 94; Charlemagne's standardization of 95; decentralization in 18th-century Austria 259–61; "deserving" poor in 18th-century Edinburgh 233–34; in early Christianity 80; early poorhouses 94; hospitality to (Christ's) poor 106–07; in Imperial Rome 45–46; institutionalization of 109; involuntary pauperism 150; and new work ethic 217; Protestant reformation's views on 216–17; outdoor relief 218; *philanthropia* in Ancient Greece 44; and religious boundaries 216; restrictions in poor relief 216–17; role of urban laypersons in 109; Rome and the *pater familias* in 98–9; and "undeserving" poor 217

Williamson, Janet: 231–36; admission to Edinburgh Infirmary (18th c.) 236; diagnosis of fever 246; under the care of Cullen, William 243–51

Wisconsin: automobile accident compensation bill 501; Blue Cross medical insurance in 503; impact of Depression 501;

Medical Society of Milwaukee 486; need for drivers' licenses in 490; ratio of population to hospital beds in 467; state university 476

Wofsy, Constance: joining Ward 5 B 632 (see also San Francisco General Hospital Ward 5 B); expert in infectious diseases 636; work in Ward 86 633 (see also San Francisco General Hospital Ward 86)

women as caregivers: competition with surgical dressers 372 (see also nursing, Edinburgh Infirmary); domestic role in Ancient Greece 27–28; eroticism and physical attraction 413; ideology of German nursing 437–38; in Imperial Rome 41, 48; at Johns Hopkins Hospital 411–13; key role in early Christianity 80, 83 (see also nursing, early Christian); lack of job security in the U.S. 475; marginalized in the 13th century 152; menial chores for student nurses 495–96; Nightingale, Florence on 366; nurses as housekeepers 368–69 (see also Edinburgh Infirmary (18th c.)); nursing training as "voyage of service" 480 (see also nursing, U.S. (19th–20th c.)); plight of nightwatching 369; rivalry with physicians in post-revolutionary France 322; role of widows, 150; status of Nightingale's nurses 370–71; stereotype of "wild nurses" in 19th century

Germany 437; subservience to physicians 373, 495; views on Irish servants 339–41

xenodocheion (xenodochium or hospitalium): 79–83, 87, 99; administration of 123–24; admission rites 85; aristocratic guests in 99; association with springs 72; baths at 123; in Byzantium 122–25; caregivers at 124; at Cluny 99; death and dying in 86; early use of 71–72; ecclesiastical property of 122–23; example of Antioch 81–82; Fabiola and 94–95; foundations in the Latin West 94–95; funded by abbots 99; as guest room in imperial Rome 45; institutional regimen 85; license to practice in 124; linked to cathedral chapters 95; at monasteries and orphanages 82, 123; in Palestine 71–72, 82; post of nosokomos in 123–24; precursors to 72–73; private patrons for 122–23; protection and social control in 82; professional hierarchy in 124–25; role of ascetics in 83; roots in Jewish hostels 72; St. Basil's Basileiados model 84–85, 94; separation of the sexes 84; sponsorship in Edessa 71–72; status as locus religiosus 106; system of staff rotation in 124; and text Miracula Sancti Artemii 124; on Tiber Island 208; visits by physicians 124. See also Pantocrator Xenon, Constantinople

CPSIA information can be obtained
at www.ICGtesting.com
Printed in the USA
BVHW042145130319
542631BV00005B/10/P